The Child Protection Handbook

For Baillière Tindall:

Senior Commissioning Editor: Ninette Premdas
Project Development Manager: Karen Gilmour
Project Manager: Derek Robertson
Design Direction: George Ajayi

The Child Protection Handbook

Edited by

Kate Wilson BA(Oxon) DipSW DipCouns
Professor of Social Work,
University of Nottingham, Nottingham, UK

Adrian James BA MA PhD GDSA DASS
Professor of Applied Social Sciences,
University of Bradford, Bradford, UK

SECOND EDITION

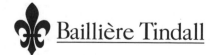 Baillière Tindall

EDINBURGH   LONDON   NEW YORK   PHILADELPHIA   ST LOUIS   SYDNEY   TORONTO 2002

BAILLIÈRE TINDALL
An imprint of Harcourt Publishers Limited

© Harcourt Publishers Limited 2002

❧ is a registered trademark of Harcourt Publishers Limited

The rights of Kate Wilson and Adrian James to be identified as editors of this work have
been asserted by them in accordance with the Copyright, Designs and Patents Act 1988

First published 2002

ISBN 07020 25844

British Library Cataloguing in Publication Data
A catalogue record for this book is available from the British Library

Library of Congress Cataloging in Publication Data
A catalog record for this book is available from the Library of Congress

The
publisher's
policy is to use
**paper manufactured
from sustainable forests**

Printed in China

Contents

Contributors   vii

Introduction to the second edition   1

Introduction to the first edition   3

Section 1 Understanding child abuse   7

1. Protecting children: a socio-historical analysis   11
   Nigel Parton

2. Patterns and outcomes   29
   Susan J Creighton

3. Child abuse: defining, understanding and intervening   50
   Kevin Browne

4. Characteristics of sexual abusers   71
   Stephen Frosh

5. Consequences and indicators of child abuse   89
   Helga Hanks and Peter Stratton

6. Gender and child abuse   114
   Brid Featherstone

7. Issues of ethnicity and culture   128
   Melanie Phillips

8. Disability and child abuse   147
   Margaret Kennedy

9. Abuse in institutional settings   172
   Ian Butler

Section 2 Managing the process of child protection   187

10. Child protection and the civil law   191
    Christina M Lyon

11. Making enquiries under Section 47 of the Children Act 1989   238
    Corrine Wattam

12. Assessment   253
    Margaret Adcock

13. Inter-professional cooperation and inter-agency coordination   272
    Brian Corby

14. Case conferences in child protection   288
    Margaret Bell

15. Protecting children: the role of the health visitor   305
    Sue Rouse

16. Enhancing the contribution of teachers to child protection   319
     Anne Peake

17. Court proceedings and court craft   342
     Mary Lane and Terry Walsh

18. The work of the guardian *ad litem*   355
     Ann Head

19. Child protection and the criminal justice system   369
     John Williams

     Section 3 Intervention and training issues in child protection   383

20. Partnership with parents   387
     Stephanie Petrie and Brian Corby

21. Individual work with children   403
     Margaret Compton

22. Non-directive play therapy with abused children and adolescents   423
     Virginia Ryan

23. Helping to prevent abuse: a cognitive-behavioural approach with families   442
     Katy Cigno

24. Working with abusing families   456
     Arnon Bentovim

25. Group work in child protection agencies   481
     Anne Bannister

26. Helping adult survivors of child sexual abuse   498
     Liz Hall and Siobhan Lloyd

27. Out-of-home care for the abused or neglected child: research,
     planning and practice   514
     June Thoburn

28. Child protection: the manager's perspective   538
     Paul Dyson

29. Safeguarding and promoting children's welfare: a question of competence? 552
     Pat Walton

30. Power and partnership: a case study in child protection*   571

* The author of this chapter has chosen to remain anonymous in order to protect the identity of the family described in the chapter.

Contributors

Margaret Adcock BA (Hons) MIFT

Margaret Adcock is a Social Work Consultant and has worked in Family Placement in the Local Authority as an Assistant Director at British Agencies for Fostering and Adoption and as a guardian *ad litem*. She now works in The Child Care Consultation Team in the Department of Psychological Medicine at Great Ormond Street Hospital, London.

Anne Bannister CQSW RDth AdDipPsych

Anne Bannister is a Child Protection Consultant and UKCP Registered Psychotherapist in private practice. Previously she set up and managed the Child Sexual Abuse Consultancy for NSPCC. She has taught on child protection and psychotherapy courses in many universities in the UK and abroad. She has published on child protection, child sexual abuse, psychodrama and dramatherapy, including *The Healing Drama* (1997) FAB and *From Hearing to Healing* (1998 reprint) Wiley. She is a Research Fellow at the Centre for Applied Child Studies, University of Huddersfield, and is currently engaged in doctoral research on treatment for sexually abused children. She is on the editorial board of *Research Matters*, published by Community Care and writes regularly on research in child protection.

Margaret Bell BA DipSocSci MPhil CQSW DPhil

Margaret Bell is a lecturer in Social Work at the University of York. Her teaching and research interests are largely in the field of child care and protection, with a particular focus on inter-agency issues, service user involvement and working in partnership. Recent funded research projects have included empirical studies of the involvement of families in and the experiences of children, of child protection investigations; the use of the Looking after Children materials in social work training and practice; the impact on children of witnessing domestic violence, and user perspectives on Family Group Conferences. Her practice experience includes work as a Guardian ad Litem, and wide experience of social work in the health field.

Arnon Bentovim MBBS FRCPsych FRCPCH BPAS DPM

Dr Arnon Bentovim is Director of The London Child and Family Consultation Service, and Honorary Consultant Child & Adolescent Psychiatrist to Great Ormond Street Children's Hospital and the Tavistock Clinic, and is Honorary Senior Lecturer at the Institute of Child Health, University College London. Since his appointment at Great Ormond Street Children's Hospital he has been concerned with the management of child abuse from the late 60's onwards. With colleagues he established assessment and treatment services for abused children and their families, on factors which lead to abusive behaviour in previously abused boys, family assessment approaches for children in need and their families, and has also published studies in various other aspects of child abuse including Induced Illness Syndrome – Muchausen by Proxy. He also consults to

SWAAY, a residential setting for the treatment of young people who have been abused, and are abusing others.

Kevin Browne BSc MSc PhD Med CBiol CPsychol
Kevin Browne has been researching family violence and child maltreatment for over 20 years and has published extensively on these subjects. He is an Executive Councillor of the International Society for the Prevention of Child Abuse and Neglect (ISPCAN) and is currently Consultant to the World Health Organisation (Europe) on Child Protection. As a Chartered Psychologist and a Chartered Biologist, he is currently employed by the School of Psychology at the University of Birmingham, as Professor of Forensic and Family Psychology. His most recent book is entitled *Preventing Family Violence*, is co-authored with Professor Martin Herbert and published by J Wiley (1997).

Ian Butler BA(Hons) MPhil CQSW
Ian Butler is a qualified social worker with considerable practice experience. He has worked in residential and field settings, mainly with children and their families, in the statutory, voluntary and independent sectors. He was an Assistant Director at the Rainer Foundation and is a Director of the Integrated Services Programme. He is an Honorary Member of the Council of the NSPCC. He also worked as a Parliamentary researcher before taking up a post as a lecturer in social work at Cardiff University. He was Director of Social Work Studies at Cardiff before moving to Keele University where he is now Professor of Social Work. His main research interests include children's accounts of their social worlds, the health care of looked after children and the practice of substitute family care. He is also interested in the development of social policy as it affects children and young people, especially young offenders.

Katy Cigno MA MA CQSW Accredited Practice Teacher
Katy Cigno is a Senior Lecturer in Social Work at the University of Hull and a Practice Teacher at Wakefield Housing and Social Care. She is a member of the British Association for Behavioural and Cognitive Psychotherapies and a former chair of the Cognitive Behavioural Social Work Group. Her main interests in teaching practice and research are children and families, learning disability in children and social care in Italy. She has published and lectured widely in these areas.

Brian Corby BA DipSA DipASS CQSW
Brian Corby is currently Reader in Applied Social Studies at the University of Liverpool. He has specialised in Child Protection Studies for many years and teaches on qualifying and post-qualifying courses. Recent publications include *Managing Child Sexual Abuse Cases* published by Jessica Kingsley in 1998. He has more recently been working on public enquiries into various forms of child abuse including abuse of children in residential care.

Susan J Creighton BSc MSc
Susan Creighton is a Senior Research Officer at the NSPCC, where she has been for over 20 years. Her main research has been on the epidemiology of child abuse

both from cases placed on Child Protection Registers and from more general national prevalence surveys. She has also researched and written on child deaths where abuse or neglect was implicated.

Margaret Crompton BA (English Lit) DipSocStud CertAppSocStud
Margaret Crompton is a self-employed writer/editor/lecturer. She has worked in a Bethnal Green settlement, for Leeds Children's/Social Service Departments, Lincolnshire SSD, as a guardian *ad litem*, and as a lecturer in Social Work at Bradford and Newcastle–upon–Tyne Universities. Her publications explore aspects of communicating with children/young people in a social work context. Preparing a training pack for CSQW on *Children, Spirituality, Religion and Social Work* (1996) led her to focus writing and teaching on developing understanding of spirituality and religion in relation to children/young people and social work and she has contributed to several conferences and training events. She also teaches adult education courses on, and writes about, English Literature.

Paul Dyson BA MSc CQSW
Paul Dyson is a Performance Manager in the East Riding of Yorkshire's Social Services. He has worked as a child care practitioner and manager for twenty five years. Additionally he has been a Senior Lecturer in Social Work.

Brid Featherstone BA CQSW DASS MA
Brid Featherstone is currently the NSPCC Reader in Applied Childhood Studies at the Centre for Applied Childhood Studies, University of Huddersfield. She has written widely on gender relations and child abuse. She is currently conducting research into fathers and child protection. She has worked as a practitioner and manager in the area of child abuse.

Stephen Frosh MA MPhil PhD
Stephen Frosh is Professor of Psychology at Birkbeck College, University of London, and (until October 2000) Consultant Clinical Psychologist and Vice Dean at the Tavistock Clinic, London. His books include *The Politics of Psychoanalysis* (Macmillan, 1999), *For and Against Psychoanalysis* (Routledge, 1994) and *Identify Crisis* (Macmillan, 1991). He is co-author, with Danya Glaser, of *Child Sexual Abuse* (BASW/Macmillan, 1993). He is also editor of the Macmillan series, *Basic Texts in Counselling and Psychotherapy*.

Liz Hall BA(Hons) PhD DipClinPsychol DipPsychotherapy
Liz Hall is a clinical psychologist and psychotherapist working in private practice in Lincoln. She qualified in 1974 having previously gained a PhD in the field of clinical psychology. She has worked with survivors in individual therapy for nearly twenty years in the voluntary sector, within the mental health services of the NHS and private practice. She is co-author with Siobhan Lloyd of *Surviving Child Sexual Abuse: a handbook for helping women challenge their past* published by Falmer Press in 1989 and revised in 1993. She is involved in training consultancy and supervision of other workers in the field of working with sexual abuse. She now contributes her knowledge gained through her work with adult

survivors to the care and placement of distressed families and their children within the care system through the provision of assessments for the legal and social services systems.

Helga Hanks BSc MSc DipPsych AFBPsS(Chartered) UKCT registered
Helga Hanks is a Consultant Clinical Psychologist and UKCP registered Psychotherapist and Family Therapist in the Department of Clinical & Health Psychology, St James's University Hospital, Leeds. She is also an Honorary Senior Lecturer in the Department of Psychology, Leeds University. She is one of the founder members of the Leeds Family Therapy and Research Centre (LFRTC) at Leeds University, which came into existence in 1979. She is the Centre's Clinical Director and one of the core staff who developed the MSc in Family Therapy in the Department of Psychology, Leeds University. Parallel to the involvement in family therapy she has worked in the area of child abuse and become well known working within a paediatric setting at St James's University Hospital. Her work in sexual abuse and failure-to-thrive is prominent. Together with a number of colleagues she was also involved in founding the Expert Witness Group (EWG) which developed guidelines for expert witnesses in child abuse cases. She has published and researched widely both in the area of family therapy and child abuse, and has been on radio and TV.

Ann Head MA Advanced Award in Social Work
Ann Head is a self-employed guardian *ad litem* in Oxfordshire, an appraiser of guardians *ad litem* in the South of England and an independent consultant. She has published some research on the placement of sexually abused children and has written on this subject and on the subject of sibling relationships. She has also written and lectured on the role of the guardian *ad litem* and on the subject of children's rights.

Ilan Barry Katz BA (Social Work) PhD
Ilan Katz is Head of Practice Development Unit NSPCC. He has worked as a social worker and manager mainly with children and disabled people. He heads a unit which is responsible for undertaking evaluative research, development and consultancy projects in the area of child protection and children's services. He has managed a number of research/development projects for the European Commission and for statutory and voluntary agencies in the UK. He has particular interests in children in the criminal justice system and in comparative research and has been involved with a number of research projects comparing children's services systems in the UK with those in other European countries.

Margaret Kennedy SEN.PSA(Oxon) CQSW AdvCert Child Abuse Studies
Margaret is an Independent Trainer and Consultant an all aspects of abuse of disabled children and adults. Her professional background is both nursing and social work. She is a renowned international and national speaker and writer in this area and works from a social model and feminist perspective. She represented disabled children on the BASPCAN National Executive for many years and is now on the Editorial Board of the new journal *The Journal of Adult Protection*. With colleagues she has formed PRODISCA, a training and

consultative consortium (www.prodisca.com). She is presently undertaking her MPhil/PhD on the subject 'Clergy Abuse of Adult Women'. Her work on Christianity and abuse has run parallel with her work on disability and abuse. She offers training and consultancy in this area also.

Mary Lane BA MSW LLB

Mary Lane graduated in Psychology in 1969 and qualified as a social worker in 1971. She specialised in child protection, adoption and fostering over 14 years and subsequently worked as a guardian *ad litem* for six years. During her social work career she has gained considerable experience in preparing cases for court with solicitors and barristers and in the witness box. In 1991 she began a new career in the legal profession and is currently a local authority solicitor, advising and representing Social Services in child protection and adoption litigation, and preparing social workers, and health and education professionals for giving evidence in court.

Siobhan Lloyd BA MSc DipCounselling BAC Accredited Counsellor CertSupervision

Siobhan Lloyd is Head of Counselling Services at the University of Aberdeen. She has also worked for more that twenty years in education, lecturing at different times in Social Work, Sociology and Women's Studies. She is a British Association Accredited Counsellor and she also has a small supervision practice.

Christina M Lyon LLB Solicitor of the Supreme Court

Christina Lyon is Queen Victoria Professor of Law and Director of the Centre for the Study of the Child, the Family and the Law at The University of Liverpool. She is also a fully qualified solicitor and sits in a part-time capacity as a Recorder in Her Majesty's Courts in Family and Crime. After working as a solicitor in private practice she became an academic lawyer and has since written extensively in the field of children, families and the law. She has recently completed research projects for the Calouste Gulbenkian (UK) Foundation, the Institute for Public Policy Research and UNICEF fund and has been consulted by a wide range of UK organisations with regard to the issues of human rights and children and legal issues effecting children and adults with learning disabilities and severely challenging behaviour. She is Chair of the National Youth Advocacy Service and a member of the Merseyside Guardian *ad litem* and Reporting Officers Committee and is regularly involved in the training of a wide range of professionals involving children and young people.

Nigel Parton BA CSQW MA

Nigel Parton is Professor of Child Care and Director of the Centre for Applied Childhood Studies at the University of Huddersfield. A social worker by training he has been writing and researching on child protection and child welfare for over twenty years and is the author of numerous books, articles and chapters on the topic. His most recent books are (as editor with Corrine Wattam) *Child Sexual Abuse: Responding to the Experience of Children* (John Wiley, 1999) and (with Patrick O'Byrne) *Constructive Social Work: Towards a New Practice* (Macmillan, 2000). He is also co-editor of the journal *Children and Society* published by John Wiley in association with the National Children's Bureau.

Anne Peake BEd MSc Mphil DipChProtection CPsychol
Anne Peake has worked as a Psychologist for Education and Social Services Departments in Liverpool, Harringey and Oxfordshire. She works with children and families and is particularly interested in consultation, family work and group work in Child Protection.

Stephanie Petrie MSocSci BA(Hons) DASS CQSW
Stephanie Petrie is currently a Lecturer in Social Work at the University of Liverpool. She held posts as a generic social worker and social services manager in local authorities and the voluntary sector form 1969 until 1995. She was a Honorary Fellow at the University of Hull for eleven years and in 1995 became a full-time academic initially at the University of Bradford and then the University of Lincolnshire and Humberside. She continues to undertake commissions as an independent social worker for legal and administrative proceedings.

Melanie Phillips BA (Hons) CQSW PgDipAppSocSci
Melanie Phillips is a black social worker of Asian origin. She has 20 years' experience in social services, initially as a social worker, working with children and families in London authorities, and subsequently providing training, supervision and consultancy on child care as well as undertaking research on child protection, practice teaching and on race equality. Melanie has written extensively in child protection and black families, and was recently a member of the Advisory Group which developed the *Framework for the Assessment of Children in Need and their Families* (DoH, 2000). She has also co-written a chapter in the *Practice Guide for the Assessment Framework on Assessing Black Families*.

Sue Rouse BSc RGN RHV PGDip HETC
Sue Rouse is a Lecturer in Health Visiting at the University of Hull. She has worked within the NHS as a Senior Nurse in Child Protection and as Director of Nursing and Clinical Services for a Community Trust. Within her current role, she is responsible for the educational preparation of Specialist Community Practitioners in Public Health Nursing (Health Visitors) as well as aspects of continuing professional education for qualified community practitioners.

Virginia Ryan BA*summa* PhD CPsychol BAPT CPT-P
Virginia Ryan is a child psychologist and play therapist who was trained in the United States and who has a longstanding clinical practice specialising in play therapy for children within statutory settings in the Hull area. As well as offering play therapy, Virginia is also an expert witness for the court and provides consultations, supervision and training to carers and/or other professionals. In addition to her clinical practice, Virginia is Senior Tutor and Supervisor on the University of York's post-qualifying MA/Diploma in Non-directive Play Therapy. She has written and presented extensively on the topic of non-directive play therapy.

Dr Peter Stratton BSc PhD DipPsychother FBPS UKCPFamily Therapist
Dr Peter Stratton is a developmental psychologist and UKCP accredited family therapist. He is a Senior Lecturer at Leeds University, and Director of Leeds

Family Therapy and Research Centre (LFTRC), a research clinic housed within the university psychology department. The clinic has an international reputation for its development of systematic approached to family treatment, founded in psychological theory. The clinic work provides a background, and generates data, for research into distressed human systems and techniques of consultation to such systems. His research currently uses a comprehensive qualitative methodology that he has developed to use casual attributions to investigate disturbed and abusive family relationships; blaming and responsibility in reconstituted families; family processes especially around food; and youth culture with specific reference to raves and associated drug usage. LFTRC houses four training courses in systemic family leading to a qualifying level MSc. These areas of expertise give him and internationally recognised authority on an exceptionally wide range of issues of family functioning.

June Thoburn BA MSW LittD
Professor Thoburn is a qualified social worker and currently is Dean of the School of Social Work and Psychosocial Studies at the University of East Anglia, Norwich. She has written widely on all aspects of child welfare, been a consultant to the Department of Health, and is often asked to provide expert evidence to the courts on complex child care cases. Her most recent completed research is on the permanent family placement of children of minority ethnic origin.

Pat Walton CQSW MA(Child Protection Studies) DipFamily Therapy
Pat Walton is a lecturer in the School of Social Work at Leicester University where she works on both the qualifying and post-qualifying programmes. Prior to joining the School in 1995, Pat had spent twenty-five years in local authority social work, initially in the field of adult mental illness. She qualified at the London University in 1985 as a family therapist and then specialised in child care / child protection social work. The focus of her MA research was the impact on mothers of child sexual abuse. Following the publication of the study, Pat continued to work with her research participants in establishing a support network for mothers. Having written and taught programmes accredited within the CCESTW post-qualifying framework since 1995, Pat has recently contributed to a successful tender to develop one of the new PQ Child Care Award programmes.

Corrine Wattam BA CSQW DASS PhD
Corrine Wattam is currently Professor of Child Care at the University of Central Lancashire, having previously been NSPCC Reader at the University of Huddersfield and co-ordinator of CAPCAE (Concerned Action for the Prevention of Child Abuse in Europe). She has researched and published widely in the field of child protection and has a particular interest in risk assessment, prevention and the perspective of those who have direct experience of child maltreatment. Professor Wattam has been involved in research projects for the European Commission and the WHO on child abuse prevention. She continues to research in this area and recent projects include studies on family support and

social inclusion, participation in a national prevalence study on child abuse and a study on child death.

Terry Walsh

Terry Walsh has over thirty years experience in the law dealing with all aspects of litigation. He holds a part-time judicial appointment in both the criminal, family and civil fields of court work as a Recorder. He is authorised to exercise rights of audience in the Higher Courts by the Council of the Law Society for all cases (criminal and civil). He is an original member of what is now the Law Society's Children Panel and a member of the Solicitors Family Law Association. When he is not advising clients or appearing in court on child care, crime, civil or matrimonial disputes, he lectures fellow professionals from time to time on aspects of child law or court work generally. He is co-author of *Child Care and the Courts*. He is a recognised adoption expert and is legal adviser to an independent adoption agency. He is former president of the Bradford Law Society.

John Williams LLB(Wales) LLB(Cantas) Barrister

John Williams is a Professor of Law and Head of the Law Department at the University of Wales, Aberystwyth. He writes on areas relating to social work and the law with special reference to children and vulnerable adults. His most recent research involves examining the working of appropriate adult schemes. In addition to these areas of research, he has an active interest in information technology and the law. As a training consultant with the British Association for Services for the Elderly, he regularly provides training for social workers, health care professionals and the voluntary sector in Wales and England. Between 1993–99 he was a member of the Human Fertilisation and Embryology Authority and chaired the Information Committee. He is an active member of the CAB.

Note

The author of Chapter 30 was employed in a local authority social services department in the North of England when the work described in that chapter was carried out. The name of the author has been withheld to protect the identity of the family who are described in the chapter.

INTRODUCTION TO THE SECOND EDITION

Just as we opened the introduction to the first edition with a quotation from the press that reflected concerns at that time, so it is salutary to note that we are able to do so again for this revised edition. The headline 'Cruelty and neglect kill 1000 children in decade' introduces an article that appeared in the *Independent* (Friday, 4 February 2000). This describes what are seen as the continued failures of the child protection system in the wake of the sentencing of Gary Davis to life imprisonment for the murder of his 4-year-old stepson, whose mother was also sentenced to 2.5 years on two charges of cruelty.

The first edition of the handbook was planned and written soon after the implementation of the Children Act 1989, which together with other key documents (for example, *Working Together*, HMSO, 1991; *Memorandum of Good Practice*, HMSO, 1992) brought about unprecedented changes in policy and practice in the care and protection of children in the UK. The success and popularity of the *Handbook* demonstrates that it met a need for an authoritative, informative and accessible book which addressed key areas of child protection practice.

The period since the publication of the first edition has been one of change and development, as well as of consolidation. The publication of *Messages from Research* (HMSO, 1995) signalled an attempt to shift the focus of practice by ensuring that greater numbers of children would be considered within the framework of children in need provided by the Children Act 1989, rather than through child protection procedures. The revisions of two key policy documents (*Working Together to Safeguard Children* and the *Framework for Assessment* which replaces the 'Orange' book) attempt to incorporate the additional lessons that have been learned from those cases of neglect and abuse that have occurred since the 1988 Cleveland Inquiry. For *The Child Protection Handbook* to continue to meet the needs of its readers, therefore, it was essential that it should be revised, both to incorporate as much of this new guidance as possible, and also to describe developments which have taken place in other areas of practice.

It is also clear that the debate about and practice in relation to child protection has moved on and that, perhaps most importantly of all, there has been a significant shift in the political context of policy and practice following the election of a New Labour government in 1997. Although not intended as a direct contribution to the child protection debate, this change is reflected most clearly in the publication by the Home Office in 1998 of the Green Paper on the family, *Supporting Families: A Consultation Document* (The Stationery Office, 1998). This marked the first step in the first-ever attempt by *any* government to craft the beginnings of a family policy. However, it also reflected the push from New Labour to develop not only 'joined up thinking' in terms of policy but, closely related to this, 'joined up practice', whether this is viewed in terms of relationships between government departments or the coordination of the wide range of agencies responsible for delivering services to local communities.

This new approach has led to increasing stress being placed on evidence-based practice but also on holding public services to account, not only to the Treasury but also to service-users, and is reflected in the continuing concern about effectiveness in the use of public money. Another recent article in the press reflects this shift of emphasis towards concerns about effective performance:

The Government has identified 17 failing social services departments ... The departments were assessed against 35 performance indicators ... The report showed that on average, one in 10 children on the child protection register did not have their case reviewed when it should have been. Eight authorities assessed less than two-thirds of cases, and 10 authorities were not able to provide information. Children's charities said yesterday that it was unacceptable that only 33 of the 150 authorities reviewed all child protection cases.

(*Independent*, Wednesday, 24 November 1999)

In addition, however, there have been other important shifts in the debate about child protection which, although not unrelated to this change of political emphasis, must be recognised and addressed separately. This is arguably most evident in the way in which the phenomenon of child abuse has begun to be reconstructed, with a shift away from the medico-social model so in evidence in early child abuse inquiries towards a socio-legal model, in which emphasis has increasingly been placed on investigating, assessing and weighing 'forensic evidence' in the context of allegations of child abuse.

Such changes made it necessary for us to reconsider the coverage of the second edition. As a result of this, some chapters have been dropped whilst some significant new chapters have been included. The process of the reconstruction of child abuse is clearly identified in one of the most significant new chapters, that by Nigel Parton, in which he reviews the changing dimensions of this debate and identifies the most recent shift towards *supporting* the majority of families who come in to the child protection system and on meeting children's needs, whilst preserving major child protection interventions for the most high-risk families. Another phenomenon which has attracted increasing concern and publicity since the publication of the first edition has been that of so-called 'institutional abuse', and we are pleased to be able to include a chapter by Ian Butler on this important issue.

In the context of such changes, three other areas have become of increasing importance and are reflected in the coverage of this new edition. Firstly, and quite apart from its increasing significance in the context of supporting families, there has been a growing concern and debate about the gendered nature of child abuse itself but also of the responses of agencies and practitioners. Secondly, and particularly as a consequence of the shift of emphases to which we have referred above, the role of senior managers in social services departments has become increasingly critical in terms of providing the effective and coordinated responses sought by all professionals concerned with child protection. And thirdly, reflecting in part the thinking that is evident in the government's proposals outlined in *Supporting Families*, is the importance of health visitors as front-line family workers who can play such a critical role in the identification and prevention of child abuse. We therefore welcome the introduction of three other completely new chapters – on gender by Brid Featherstone, on the managerial perspective by Paul Dyson, and on the role of the health visitor by Sue Rouse.

All of the chapters that have been retained from the first edition have been revised to varying degrees, depending upon the focus of each chapter and the extent to which the changes outlined above have had an impact on the issues under consideration. In the case of some chapters, the original authors were unable for various reasons to make the necessary revisions and in such cases we have sought the assistance of alternative authors in order to retain and revise these important chapters. Throughout, however, we have sought not only to maintain the very highest standards of contribution but to retain the qualities essential to the success of a handbook such as this – that it should be up-to-date and informative; that it should be comprehensive and provide all professionals concerned with child protection with an accessible source of authoritative guidance, combined with advice on further reading; and that it should be readable.

As we acknowledged in the Introduction to the first edition

In all probability, few will have either the time or the inclination to read this book from cover to cover and it was not our expectation that it should be used in this way. Rather, we envisaged a book which would find a place on the reading lists for courses for every profession involved in working with child abuse and providing child-protection services. We also envisaged a book which would find a place as a source of reference on the bookshelves or desks of busy practitioners in whatever setting they practice or to whatever profession they belong.

We hope that we have been able to achieve these aims in this new edition and, as editors, we are grateful to all of those who have contributed to this project and to the publishers for giving us the opportunity to bring the original book up to date.

Kate Wilson
Adrian L. James

INTRODUCTION TO THE FIRST EDITION

At the time of writing the introduction to this *Handbook*, child abuse and the failure of child protection agencies and procedures to ensure that children are protected against abuse are in the papers – once again. 'Social work muddle led to girl's death', read the headlines. 'Child protection arrangements which should have saved a 3-year-old girl from prolonged abuse and eventual murder collapsed in an unco-ordinated muddle, according to a report on Nottinghamshire social services', continues the story (*The Guardian*, 8.2.94).

The seemingly frequent, repeated occurrences of such failures, so long after the sad death of Maria Colwell first brought child abuse to the attention of the British press and public, provides both the context and the rationale for this *Handbook*. It is a phenomenon which stirs deep-seated emotion in all of us, not least because of our apparent failure to 'get it right'. This seems all the more remarkable in view of the by now considerable body of knowledge which welfare professionals of various kinds have about the nature, causes and distribution of child abuse. To this must also be added the substantial body of guidance, gleaned from hard-won experiences in the many cases of child abuse which have come to our attention over the past two decades, about the procedures which ought to be established and followed by agencies involved in the care and protection of children.

Such failures, which all too often result in tragic consequences of the type mentioned above, inevitably attract a great deal of attention and criticism for those most centrally involved – in most cases social workers – and this is often justified. What we do not and cannot know about, however, are the many cases in which this knowledge and these guidelines have been used to good effect and, as a result, have avoided many potential tragedies. Such is the nature of the work of caring professionals, of the news media and of the public conscience.

This realisation also gives us some important clues, however, about the limits of our capabilities for dealing with such issues and about how further progress can be made. It is becoming clear that no matter how much knowledge we accumulate and how many lessons we learn from our previous experience, the nature of human problems and human responses to them is such that tragedies will continue to occur. Unless we are able to accept as a society previously unconsidered levels of intervention in the lives of many families in the name of prevention and to provide the vast resources which would be necessary for such a 'service', child abuse will continue to occur, and occasionally children will die as a consequence. Indeed, even if such levels of intervention were conscionable and could be resourced, it is difficult seriously to entertain the prospect that we should ever be able to eradicate child abuse entirely. If this is, indeed, the case the way forward must lie in another direction.

A major problem for those whose contact with children is such that they can be deemed to be the 'front-line' workers in the field of child protection – social workers, health visitors, teachers, doctors or members of related professions – is that, by and large, they are very busy. Indeed, they are so busy that they have little or no time to keep fully abreast of the latest research, the latest thinking and the latest guidance relating to child abuse and protection. There are therefore often gaps in their knowledge, or it is out of date and consists of what (in some cases all-too-little) training they received whilst working for their professional qualifications, which may have been some years ago.

Furthermore, different professions have different responsibilities and priorities, and therefore place a different emphasis on child protection, not only in pre-qualifying training but also in post-qualifying training and day-to-day practice. Those such as social workers specialising in child protection and guardians *ad litem* might therefore reasonably be expected to be better informed than teachers, even though the latter may have substantially more face-to-face contact with much larger numbers of children. All, however, are hard-pressed public servants, most of whom work in an organisational context in which the principal means of achieving the objective of providing value for public money in service delivery is frequently that of reducing unit costs.

In such circumstances, training is often one of the first areas of activity to be cut back. Such a context is not conducive to keeping abreast of theoretical and practical developments in child abuse and protection, important though this is universally recognised to be. This same imperative, and the difficulty of complying with it, can also serve to increase the anxiety levels of those in the 'front line', where the pressures, uncertainties and responsibilities of practice are already a heavy burden. The fact that agencies may be less able to resource the necessary training does not necessarily remove from practitioners the feeling of personal and professional responsibility for keeping abreast of such developments, however. Their problem is how best to accomplish this.

An additional difficulty mirrors one of the continuing problems of practice – that of how to communicate effectively about theoretical, research and practice knowledge across professional and disciplinary boundaries. This has been a central issue in many child abuse inquiries and is one which is embedded in the way in which training is traditionally organised (for individual groups of professionals, often entirely in isolation from other professionals working, at least in part, in the same or overlapping areas) and knowledge is most often disseminated (through profession-specific rather than multi-disciplinary channels). Thus, for example, the medical discourse about child abuse and the social work discourse have proceeded with a much higher level of separation that is desirable, communicating largely through their own professional journals and their own professionally orientated conference networks. Neither has made consistent or effective attempts to break out of their respective frameworks to engage with each other, let alone with other professionals, such as teachers. There is therefore also a problem about how best to accomplish this.

This is the rationale for this *Handbook*. In producing it, our three main objectives were:

- to produce a reader and a sourcebook which brings together a series of reviews, by nationally and internationally recognised experts in various fields related to the emotional, physical and sexual abuse of children, providing succinct accounts of issues of both policy and practice, as well as an up-to-date review of research and other relevant literature;
- to produce a reader which, by virtue of its coverage and presentation, makes key information about child abuse accessible, comprehensible and helpful to a wide range of professionals, at both qualifying and post-qualifying levels, who have an interest in and need to know about child abuse; and
- to produce a reader which is coherent enough to be read as a whole but in which the contributions are of sufficient substance and relevance to be read or referred to independently.

These are, perhaps, ambitious objectives and it is inevitable that in covering such a wide range of issues there will be some variations. These are reflected not only in different writing styles, but in the balance between theoretical and practical issues, between a macro analysis of concepts and theories and a micro analysis of skills and behaviours. Such variations are not a weakness but a strength, an inevitable consequence of producing such a book. They reflect the complex nature of child abuse itself, the debate surrounding it and the many different levels of knowledge and skills which are integral to an understanding of child abuse and to high standards of professional practice in providing services for the protection of children.

Having said this, it is also inevitable that the individual chapters reflect both current concerns and preoccupations, and also the level of knowledge available about certain aspects of child maltreatment. One result of this is that in a number of chapters, issues concerning child sexual abuse are addressed virtually to the exclusion of other forms of abuse. Sometimes this reflects the way in which a service has grown from the identification of a particular need. Services for adult victims of sexual abuse, for example (discussed in the chapter by Liz Hall and Siobhan Lloyd, Section III), were substantially developed as a result of the early help given to women through women's support networks, and little work has been done with victims of physical or emotional abuse who on the whole have not come together as an identifiable group. In other areas such as family therapy, practice with families involving incestuous abuse arose out of earlier work with physical abuse, and the emphasis on the former in Tilman Furniss and Liza Bingley Miller's chapter (Section III) reflects a current concern to develop practice with what are seen to be problems of particular complexity.

The amount and quality of the research cited in different chapters also reflects wider policy issues. The range of the research cited in the chapters on the early stages of the protective process (for example, the chapters on investigation and case conferences in Section II) contrasts with the paucity of research material which can be drawn on to support the discussion on children with disabilities who have been abused. June Thoburn's discussion of research findings concerning out-of-home care for children highlights the absence of any similar detailed work on therapeutic services for children, a point we explore further in the introductory chapter to Section III. This imbalance reflects large differences in resources allocated to different aspects of the protective process. To some extent, any book that tries to provide a 'state of the art' picture of child protection will reflect this imbalance, although it will also try, as we do here and other writers do throughout, to highlight deficiencies in the current state of knowledge and practice. Christine Hallett returns to this theme in the final chapter.

As far as possible, however, given the diverse nature of the topics covered, each chapter provides: an introduction to the general issues to be addressed; a review of recent literature and research; an analysis of policy issues where this is appropriate; discussion of the implications for practice of the issues raised; a summary of the key issues followed by a conclusion; a bibliography and, finally, recommendations for further reading which have been annotated to give guidance to those wishing to pursue particular issues further. We have sought throughout to ensure that the emphasis is on communicating as clearly and simply as possible, avoiding jargon wherever possible.

In order to facilitate further ease of use, we have organised the book in sections which bring together contributions dealing with broadly comparable issues. Section I is concerned with our understanding of child abuse, not only in terms of what we 'know' about it – what 'it is', how often it 'occurs', who 'does' it and what 'causes' it – but also the social processes which define our knowledge and understanding of these key areas of 'knowledge' about child abuse.

Section II contains those chapters which contribute primarily to the analysis of the frameworks (such as that provided by the law), structures (such as case conferences and courts of law) and processes (such as assessment, monitoring and inter-professional co-operation) which have been developed for and are integral to the process of managing the process of child protection.

Section III includes chapters which focus on both the context and the main methods which can be employed when working with families where abuse has occurred, and with those adults and children who have experienced abuse. The final section addresses training issues, both at the level of general trends and specific issues in terms of content, and concludes with an overview and summary of the main issues to have emerged from all the contributions.

In all probability, few will have either the time or the inclination to read this book from cover to cover, and it was not our expectation that it should be used in this way. Rather, we envisaged a book which would find a place on the reading lists for courses for every profession involved in working with child abuse and providing child protection services. We also envisaged a book which would be a useful source of reference on the bookshelves or desks of busy practitioners in different professions everywhere.

We are grateful to a number of colleagues and friends for their advice and encouragement during the development of this book; to the anonymous assessors for their comments; and to Hilary Woodward for her particular help.

Kate Wilson
Adrian L. James

UNDERSTANDING CHILD ABUSE

An understanding of child abuse, and how it is defined and interpreted in its historical and cultural context, is of central importance to all of those who are concerned with child abuse and child protection, be they researchers, lawyers, social workers, health visitors, teachers or police officers. Without greater clarity about how we define child abuse, we cannot begin to ask questions about incidence and distribution (How frequently does it occur? Where does it occur most, either geographically or demographically?). Nor can we ask questions about who is responsible for abuse or what are its causes. And until we can provide some answers to these questions, we cannot even begin to answer the crucial question 'What remedies might there be?'

The analysis of other important issues depends on the answer to this pivotal question of what we understand by child abuse. Thus, until we can define child abuse, we cannot begin to determine or understand what is *not* child abuse, a matter which is clearly of equal importance; we cannot understand *why* some closely related behaviours are defined as abusive and others are not; we cannot identify what social and political dynamics underpin the process by which such 'knowledge' is defined; and we cannot address the question of why such definitions are historically specific – why, for example, what was reasonable physical chastisement of a child 100 years ago would today, in all probability, be considered abuse.

Section 1 addresses these and related issues. In the first chapter, which is new to this second edition, Nigel Parton offers a valuable historical overview of the development of the debate about child abuse. In particular, he draws attention to the progressive shift of emphasis away from the medical model, which dominated the debate surrounding the 'discovery' of child abuse in the 1960s, towards the socio-legal model that has become so important in recent years. The emphasis this places on legal expertise and the importance of forensic investigation and the assessment of evidence in the context of legal proceedings has done much to reshape practice. Importantly, in terms of the other chapters in this second edition, he charts the emergence of the recent emphasis on the identification of 'high-risk' cases and the much broader focus on the provision of support for the much larger number of families that become involved in the child protection system but in relation to whom there are fewer concerns.

In the following chapter, Susan Creighton goes on to address the question of the incidence of child abuse, to discuss some of the research issues that need to be addressed when studying child abuse, and to clarify the factors that practitioners need to bear in mind when making use of data about the incidence and prevalence of child abuse to inform their work. Such issues are of particular importance in enabling those working with children to have an informed awareness of the probability of there being abused children amongst those with whom they come into contact, some of the likely characteristics of those children, and the likely levels of incidence of such cases. In concluding, she draws attention to the impact of increased reporting of child abuse in recent years combined with cutbacks in local authority resources. This, she argues, has led to priority being given to child protection at the expense of child care, thus echoing the distinction drawn in the previous chapter. Since this is similar to her conclusion at the end of her original chapter in the first edition, it suggests that in her view attempts to shift the focus from child protection to child care have had so far little impact.

In Chapter 3, Kevin Browne delineates some of the issues and problems inherent in defining child abuse and considers some of the different theories of causation which have emerged. He considers different intervention strategies, in particular those which operate at the third level of treatment, i.e. after violence to the child has occurred, and concludes by stressing that those involved in the treatment of abusing families should be concerned not just with inhibiting violence towards the children, but also with developing a secure relationship between parent and child.

Some of these issues are developed further by Stephen Frosh who, in Chapter 4, discusses the characteristics of child abusers and, in particular, those who abuse sexually. In doing so, he distinguishes between child sexual abuse and sexual offending more generally by considering the relationship between non-sexual and sexual abuse and the extent to which the latter is concerned with sexual gratification as distinct from the use of power. He also usefully considers the reliability and limitations of the empirical evidence which is currently available and the implications of this for the choice of treatment method.

In Chapter 5, Helga Hanks and Peter Stratton go on to consider the effects of abuse on children, distinguishing between the effects of physical, emotional and sexual abuse, and the effects of neglect. Throughout this discussion, they develop an interactive model. In this, they consider children as active and self-conscious actors rather than passive recipients of abuse, exploring how they react to and attempt to moderate the consequences of the abuse, and the role that the personality and characteristics of the abuser can play in shaping the child's adaptations. The chapter outlines both the direct physical and behavioural consequences of abuse, the psychological consequences and secondary consequences on other aspects of a child's life. They conclude by considering the longer-term consequences of abuse in terms of later childhood, adolescence, adulthood and the victim as parent, exploring in the process the possibility of a cycle of abuse.

The following chapter, by Brid Featherstone, is a new chapter in this edition of the *Handbook*. The contribution of feminist writers to a wide range of discourses has been of enormous significance and the analysis of issues of gender has become increasingly more sophisticated since the early days of the emergence of the women's movement. Given the growing awareness of the impact of gender in terms of family functioning and interpersonal relationships, the discussion in this chapter of the significance of gender in the structuring and conduct of family relationships and, in particular, on the significance of the changing nature of masculinity, provides an important introduction to the significance of gender to our understanding of and practice in relation to child abuse.

The study of relatively new areas of interest rarely, and perhaps inevitably, proceeds in a uniform way. As a consequence of more immediate and mainstream concerns that follow the 'discovery' of a phenomenon like child abuse, such as the need to delineate its prevalence and understand its causes, minority issues such as those relating to ethnicity and culture or to disability, tend initially to be marginalised. Chapters 7 and 8 draw attention to this process of marginalisation and seek to rectify it. Melanie Philips highlights the persistent failure of policy-makers and practitioners to address the needs of black families and calls for a thorough rethinking of practice. She questions the relevance of the theoretical models commonly used in child protection and asks whether they are universally applicable or whether they simply reinforce stereotypical views of black families. The solution, she argues, lies in developing an approach to working with families from black cultures in a way which challenges racist myths and assumptions through much more open discussion with the families themselves.

In Chapter 8, Margaret Kennedy also explores the myths that relate to abuse and the disabled child and points to the almost complete lack of research in the UK into the prevalence or incidence of abuse of disabled children. In the process, she contributes to the debate outlined in previous chapters about definitions of abuse, identifying some forms of abuse unique to children with disabilities. She suggests that an integrated ecological model of abuse moves away from the dependency-stress model, and provides a structural framework for understanding the abuse of disabled people. She also identifies the greater resistance of adults to disclosures of abuse by children with disabilities and some of the problems of identifying abuse using behavioural indicators and of communication, both in the context of identification and any subsequent therapy. Echoing Melanie Phillips, she questions the suitability of current child protection services for coping with the needs of children with disabilities and calls for the development of a new and more sensitive approach which challenges stereotypes and which acknowledges the unique needs of disabled children. Finally she considers the implications for disabled people of recent policy developments under the *Quality Protects* initiative (Department of Health, 1998) and the new assessment framework (Department of Health, 2000).

Chapter 9, by Ian Butler, is another new addition to the second edition of the *Handbook*, one which also reflects recent developments and concerns. Institutional abuse is a facet of child abuse that has only recently been 'discovered' and made public in the context of a number of high profile scandals. In addition to considering the implications of these, however, this chapter also considers the importance of institutional abuse and the abusive potential of institutional practices in the care of children living away from home, as well as abuse within institutions. More telling, perhaps, is the recognition that the way in which we construct and understand childhood is deeply embedded in practices that lead all too often to the marginalisation of children and a failure to involve them actively in the processes and practices of child care.

Protecting children: a socio-historical analysis

Nigel Parton

**INTRODUC-
TION**

Over the last 30 years in the UK the issue of child abuse and what to do about it has been the subject of considerable political and media interest (Franklin & Parton 1991, Aldridge 1994) and has thrust the activities of social workers and other professionals into the public eye. As a consequence, the role, priorities and focus of policy and practice have shifted in important ways. While it is generally agreed that child abuse is a problem we should do something about, there has been intense argument about what the nature of the problem is, what we should do and how we should do it. Not only have we witnessed significant changes in the area of child protection but these developments have had important, sometimes unintended, consequences for child welfare policy and practice more generally. As a result, we are now living through a major period of debate and change concerning how child protection can be refocused, particularly in terms of its relationship with more wide-ranging preventative measures for the support of the family and the provision of services for children in need (Parton 1997).

My central argument is that there has been an important shift in the relationships and hierarchies of authority between different agencies and professionals in key areas of decision-making. While at the time of its modern (re)emergence in the 1960s, child abuse was constituted as essentially a medico-social problem, where the expertise of doctors was seen as focal, increasingly it has been constituted as a socio-legal problem, where legal expertise takes pre-eminence. Whereas previously the concern was with diagnosing, curing and preventing the 'disease' or syndrome, increasingly the emphasis has become investigating, assessing and weighing 'forensic evidence'. While social workers and social service departments have been seen as the lead and key agency throughout this period, the focus and priorities of both their work and that of other charitable and statutory agencies in the child welfare field, have been reconfigured as a result. However, at the time of writing we are witnessing a serious attempt to 'refocus' child protection policy and practice, in order to achieve a much greater emphasis on family support and meeting children's needs.

The purpose of this chapter is to outline and analyse the crucial factors that have influenced and circumscribed the policies and practices we now call child protection and how these differ from what went before. More particularly, I will identify the central tensions that have been embedded in policies and practices, as well as the outcomes now showing themselves and to which policy-makers are attempting to respond and for which there are significant future implications. *The question which has to be addressed and which has been a central issue for the liberal state since the mid-nineteenth century is how can we devise a legal basis for the power to intervene in the private family to protect children which does not convert a sizeable proportion of families into clients of the State?* Such a problem is posed by the contradictory demands of, on the one hand, ensuring that the family is experienced by its members as autonomous and the primary sphere for rearing children, while on the other recognising there is a need for intervention in some families where they are seen as failing in this primary task and in a context where such laws are supposed to act as the general norms applicable to all (Parton 1991). What will become evident is that current arrangements are seen as getting this balance badly wrong, even according to the essential principles and criteria set out in the Children Act 1989 and the various official guidelines that go with it. This is a significant issue for liberalism more generally, which is based on a vision of society where government is based on the exercise of freedom and where the relationship between liberty and discipline, freedom and rule, while interdependent, should be subject to continual re-negotiation and fine balancing (Parton 1998).

Discovery of child abuse and its subsequent disappearance

For a phenomenon to take on the guise of a social problem requiring some form of state intervention it first has to be defined and constituted as such. While, as I shall argue below, the last 40 years have been key, it is clearly wrong to assume that child abuse and hence child protection practices are of such recent origin. The late nineteenth and early twentieth century is in many respects the period that provided the foundations and many of the central elements for what has more recently developed. What Linda Gordon (1989) calls the era of 'nineteenth century child-saving' (p. 20) lasted until World War I, when child abuse effectively disappeared as a subject of social concern until it was 'rediscovered' by American paediatricians as the 'battered baby syndrome' nearly half a century later.

Gordon (1989) and Parker (1995) argue that child welfare only becomes an issue when women's voices are being heard strongly and, in the latter half of the nineteenth century, middle-class women used their increased leisure time to engage in charitable work. Thus the welfare of children as well as the fear of delinquency became a focus. The latter, however, remained a major preoccupation (Hendrick 1994). The huge growth in voluntary organisations followed the riots, famines and hard winters of the 1850s and 1860s, which overwhelmed the Poor Law's always limited capacity to provide relief. Stedman Jones (1971) argues that 'in all known traditional societies the gift has played a central status-maintaining function' (p. 251): to give is to assert superiority, to receive without repayment is to accept an obligation to behave 'properly'. To regulate all this charitable work the Charity Organisation Society was set up in 1869, its agents conscientiously investigating the home circumstances of the needy to ensure they were morally deserving.

From such encounters grew a widespread concern (among the middle classes) about child cruelty and neglect (among the poor) and the first Society for the Prevention of Cruelty to Children was established in 1883, modelled on the SPCCs being established in America. The National Society for the Prevention of Cruelty to Children (NSPCC) was formed in 1889 and was hugely successful in organising the public and political campaign which produced the first legislation specifically to outlaw child cruelty and give public agencies powers to protect and remove children (Parton 1985).

The activities of the NSPCC were of great significance in this period. Ferguson (1990) has analysed cases drawn from case files of the period and has shown how the new discourse of child protection was being constructed. NSPCC inspectors worked ostentatiously in the homes of poor communities describing, classifying and assigning deviancy. Here were 'social actors actively constructing the foundations of modern forms of knowledge, of therapeutic and cultural practice: in short, a professional culture that would take child protection into the twentieth century' (Ferguson 1990, p. 135). Indeed, many of the dilemmas of modern practice were here (Ferguson 1996, 1997) as inspectors advocated for clients, pondered the advisability of rehabilitating children and sought to reform and change abusing parents.

And yet, after 1918, much of this activity disappeared from view. Parker (1995) suggests a number of reasons for this: the decline of the women's movement following the granting of universal suffrage, for example, and changes in the NSPCC, to whom the Government was happy to leave the responsibility for child cruelty and which became more bureaucratic and less campaigning. Ferguson (1996, 1997) has argued that the general approach of the NSPCC to publicising child deaths shifted considerably during this period. In the nineteenth and early twentieth centuries the NSPCC was not afraid to discuss publicly the deaths of children about whom they had direct knowledge and with whom they were working. The child death statistics were always included in its annual report. It seems that, paradoxically, the existence of child death was viewed as a sign that child protection was working well. It was highly publicised because it meant that increasing numbers of vulnerable children were being reached by its workers and hence they were fulfilling a valuable role. By the 1920s, Ferguson argues, this approach had been transformed so that death in child protection cases ceased to be made public, not because the problem was solved but because knowledge about it was, in effect, repressed by the NSPCC and others. Disclosure of deaths 'threatened the authority, optimism and trustworthiness of the expert system' (Ferguson 1997, p. 223).

The 1948 Children Act was shaped, in part, by an inquiry into the much publicised death of a child in foster care in 1945 but intrafamilial abuse was hardly on the agenda. Instead, the creation of local authority Children's Departments and the abolition of the last remains of the hated Poor Law seemed to usher in a new, enlightened age in which families would be helped to stay together after the terrible experiences of war and evacuation. Neglect was seen as the main problem and families would be supported by preventive work from the newly professionalised social workers. As in the past, fears about child mistreatment centred on the link between neglect and delinquency and the threat to public order this would entail (Parton 1999). The earlier concerns about child abuse, as an issue in its own right, had all but been erased from public policy and professional practice.

The (re)emergence of child abuse as a socio-medical reality in the context of welfare reformism

The establishment of the local authority child care service in the post-war period can be seen as a particular instance of the growth and rationalisation of social interventions associated with the establishment of the welfare state at that time (Rose & Miller 1992). The key innovations of welfarism lay in the attempts to link the fiscal, calculative and bureaucratic capacities of the state in order to encourage national growth and well-being. This was to be achieved via the promotion of *social* responsibility and the mutuality of *social* risk, and was premised on notions of *social* solidarity (Donzelot 1988).

A number of assumptions characterised welfarism: the institutional framework of universal social services was seen as the best way of maximising welfare in modern society, whilst the nation state worked for the whole society and was the best way of progressing this. The social services were instituted for benevolent purposes, meeting social needs, compensating socially caused 'diswelfares' and promoting social justice. Their underlying functions were ameliorative, integrative and redistributive. Social progress would continue to be achieved through the agency of the state and professional intervention, so that increased public expenditure, the cumulative extension of statutory welfare provision and the proliferation of government regulations backed by expert administration represented the main guarantee of equity, fairness and efficiency. At the same time, social scientific knowledge was given a pre-eminence in ordering the rationality of the emerging professions, who were seen as having a major contribution to developing individual and social welfare, thereby operationalising increasingly sophisticated mechanisms of social regulation.

Children's Departments attempted to establish, for the first time, a professional State-sponsored child welfare service that saw the family as an object of positive social policy (Packman 1981). Heywood (1978) has argued that legislation was passed in 'a fresh and hopeful atmosphere' and that by the 1948 Act 'the old paternalistic pattern of the poor law was brought to an end, and services which the individual could claim as a right were substituted' (pp. 148–149). The aim was not to punish bad parents but to act in the interests of children. As the emphasis was on the strength and formative power of the natural family, this meant trying to maintain children in the family (Holman 1996). It heralded an era where families were encouraged and helped to care for their own children, in their own homes, and underlined the importance of both the home and the child's own parents to his or her development. Where children could not live or remain at home, the priority was on placing them with foster parents rather than the large and often impersonal institution as previously. Increasingly, the emphasis was on developing preventative services thereby stopping children coming into local authority care in the first place. This emphasis was given legislative expression by the 1963 Children and Young Persons Act.

The practice of local authority social work with children and families during the post-war period up until the early 1970s was thus imbued with a considerable optimism, for it was believed that measured and significant improvements could be made in the lives of individuals and families via judicious professional interventions. Social work operated quietly and confidently, and in a relatively uncontested way, which reflected a supportive social mandate. It was allowed wide professional discretion. It also harmonised with a central plank of the post-war reconstruction – that a positive and supportive approach to the family was required so that the State and the family could work in partnership to ensure that children were provided with the appropriate conditions in which to develop.

The high point of this optimistic growth, and the institutionalisation of social work in the context of welfarism, came with the establishment of the larger and more wide-ranging local authority social service departments in 1971. It reflected the belief of the Seebohm Report (1968) that social problems could be overcome via State intervention, by professional experts with social scientific knowledge and skills in the use of relationships, and envisaged a progressive, universal service available to all and with wide community support. Interventions in the family were not conceived of as a potential source of antagonism between social workers and individual family members, whether parent(s) or child(ren). Indeed, the latter were not seen as having interests or rights distinct from the unitary family itself. When a family required modification, this would be via social casework, help and advice and if an individual did come into State care, this was assumed to be in their best interests. The law was not conceptualised as in any significant way constituting the nature of social work, or significantly informing the skills required of social workers and the types of relationships deemed appropriate for work with clients. When more coercive aspects were drawn upon, these were primarily seen as a tool for fulfilling the more significant therapeutic goals. It was in this context that child abuse was (re)discovered in the 1960s and 1970s.

There are two important issues to note about the modern (re)discovery of child abuse. First, it was discovered in the USA and then quickly imported into the UK, particularly via the NSPCC and a number of other social work and health professionals (see Parton 1985 for a detailed analysis of this process). As a consequence, policy and practice in the UK, and most other English-speaking Western societies, were heavily influenced by developments and changes in knowledge, policy and practice in the USA. It is only in very recent years that policy-makers, practitioners and researchers in the UK have looked to mainland Europe for different ways of thinking and different models of practice (see, for example, Cooper *et al.* 1995, Harder & Pringle 1997, Hetherington *et al.* 1997, Pringle 1998).

Second, and perhaps most significantly, the initial (re)discovery took the form of the 'battered baby syndrome' following the publication of the highly influential paper by Henry Kempe and his colleagues (Kempe *et al.* 1962) from Denver, Colorado. Unlike developments in the nineteenth century it was professionals, particularly medical professionals, rather than victims, survivors, community groups and the women's movement who not only brought the issue back to public attention but, in the process, conceptualised it in certain ways. It was defined as a 'syndrome' or 'disease' and hence something in which professionals, particularly doctors, were seen as experts.

It is quite clear that the term 'battered baby syndrome' was specifically chosen, as opposed to 'physical abuse', in order to appeal to as wide an audience as possible, including conservative paediatricians. Kempe wanted no hint of legal, social or deviancy problems – the problem was *medicalised*, so that medical experts and medical technology (for example the use of the X-ray to identify old and otherwise hidden injuries) was seen as key.

The original article (Kempe *et al.* 1962) claimed that the syndrome characterised a clinical condition in young children, usually under the age of 3, who had received serious physical abuse, usually from a parent, and that it was a significant cause of childhood disability and death. It argued that the syndrome was often misdiagnosed and that it should be considered in any child showing evidence of possible trauma or neglect, or where there was a marked discrepancy between the clinical findings and the story presented by parents. The use of X-rays to aid diagnosis was stressed, and it was argued that the prime concern of the physician was to make the correct diagnosis and to make certain that a similar event did not occur again. The authors recommended that doctors should report all incidents to law enforcement or child protection agencies. It was also said that the problem was not simply concerned with poverty and that the characteristics of the parents were that: 'they are immature, impulsive, self-centred, hypersensitive and quick to react with poorly controlled aggression' (Kempe *et al.* 1962, p. 19). Such an approach was to have an enormous influence on the way child abuse was thought about for many years to come.

While the 'battered baby syndrome' proved the dominant underlying metaphor, it is also clear that the category of child abuse was quickly subject to various 'mouldings' (Hacking 1988, 1991, 1992) and 'diagnostic inflation' (Dingwall 1989, p. 29). By the 1980s it included emotional abuse, neglect, sexual abuse, children at risk, as well as physical abuse, and it was no longer focused only on children but could include young people up to adulthood, i.e. 18 years old.

However, it was the public inquiry into the death of Maria Colwell which was to catapult the issue of child abuse and the practices of health and welfare professionals, particularly social workers, into the centre of public, political and media attention. This hastened the introduction of a range of new policies, practices and procedures, thereby placing the issue at the top of professional agendas (Secretary of State for Social Services 1974; see Parton 1985 for a detailed analysis of the nature and impact of the Maria Colwell case).

The system of child abuse management was effectively inaugurated with the issue of a Department of Health and Social Security circular (DHSS 1976*b*) in the wake of the death of Maria Colwell. The roles of paediatricians, general practitioners (GPs), health visitors and social workers were seen as vital, and the social services department, as the statutory child care agency, was central. The police at this stage were not seen as crucial and it was not until a further circular in 1976 (DHSS 1976*b*) that it was recommended that a senior police officer should be included on all area review committees and case conferences.

The collapse of the welfare consensus in child care

The optimism and confidence evident in social work and the welfarist child welfare system more generally was increasingly subject to a number of critiques from the mid-1970s onwards and these increased further during the 1980s. Some of the anxieties emanated from within social work itself and concerned the apparent poor, and even deteriorating, quality of child care practice in the newly created social service departments (Parker 1980). More widely, however, a whole variety of different concerns were developing which became increasingly important in influencing the parameters of the debate. While the criticisms represented somewhat different, though overlapping, constituencies, their net effect was to undermine the optimistic welfare consensus in child welfare, and also to undermine the 'medicalised' conceptualisation of child abuse that was dominant from the moment of its (re)discovery.

From the 1960s onwards, with the growth of the women's movement and the recognition of violence in the family, it was recognised that not only might the family not be the haven it was assumed to be but that women and children were suffering a range of abuses at the hands of men. Much early campaigning was directed to improving the position of women and it was only from the mid-1970s, with the growing concerns about sexual abuse, that energy was directed to the position of the children (Parton 1990). Such critiques helped to disaggregate the interests of individual family members and supported the sometimes contradictory development during the period of the Children's Rights movement (Freeman 1983, Franklin 1986, 1995).

Secondly, the growth from the late 1960s was of a more obviously civil liberties critique. This concentrated upon the apparent extent and nature of intervention in people's lives that was allowed, unchallenged, in the name of welfare (Morris *et al.* 1980, Taylor *et al.* 1980, Geach & Szwed 1983). Increasingly, liberal due process lawyers drew attention to the way the administration of justice was unfairly and unjustly applied in various areas of child care and to the need for a greater emphasis on individual rights. During the mid 1980s, the parents' lobby gained its most coherent voice with the establishment of Parents Against INjustice (PAIN). This organisation was to prove influential in ensuring that the rights of parents and of children to be left at home, free of State intervention and removal, were placed on the political and professional agendas. As a result, State intervention, via the practices of health and welfare professionals as well as parental violence, were identified as being actively and potentially abusive.

However, it was child abuse inquiries that provided the key catalyst for venting major criticisms of policy and practice in child welfare and the competencies of social workers. While these were evident from 1973 onwards following the death of Maria Colwell (Secretary of State for Social Services 1974, Parton 1985), they gained a new level of intensity during the mid-1980s through the inquiries into the deaths of Jasmine Beckford (London Borough of Brent 1985), Tyra Henry (London Borough of Lambeth 1987) and Kimberley Carlile (London Borough of Greenwich 1987). It was public inquiries which provided the vehicles for political and professional debate about what to do about child abuse in a very public way and in the full glare of the media (Franklin & Parton 1991, Aldridge 1994). Not only did they provide detailed accounts of what had gone wrong in the particular cases, they commented critically on the current state of policy and practice more generally and made recommendations as to what should be done (DHSS 1982, DOH 1991) (see Corby, Chapter 13, in this volume).

Up until the mid-1980s, the 30-plus inquiries had all been concerned with the deaths of children at the hands of their parents or caretakers. All the children had died as a result of physical abuse or neglect and had often suffered emotional neglect and failure to thrive. The child care professionals, particularly social workers, were perceived as having failed to protect the children with horrendous consequences. The deaths were viewed as particular instances of the current state of policy, practice, knowledge and skills and the way systems operated and inter-related (Hallett & Birchall 1992). Crucially, professionals, particularly social workers, were seen as too naïve and sentimental, with parents failing to concentrate on the interests of the children and to use the statutory authority vested in them. The emphasis in inquiry recommendations was on encouraging social workers to use their legal mandate to intervene in families to protect children, to rationalise the multidisciplinary frameworks, and to improve practitioners' knowledge of the signs and symptoms of child abuse so that it could be spotted in day-to-day practice.

However, the Cleveland inquiry (Secretary of State for Social Services 1988) provided a rather different set of concerns and circumstances, and a different set of interpretations of what was wrong and how we should respond. The Cleveland affair broke in early summer 1987 and was focused on the activities of two paediatricians and social workers in a hospital in Middlesbrough, a declining chemical and industrial town in the North East of England. During a period of a few weeks over a hundred children were removed from their families to an emergency Place of Safety (the hospital) on the basis of what was seen by the media and two local Members of Parliament as questionable diagnoses of child sexual abuse. As a result, a number of techniques for diagnosing and identifying sexual abuse developed by paediatricians and child psychiatrists (particularly the anal dilation test, the use of anatomically correct dolls and 'disclosure' work) were subjected to close scrutiny. Not only was it the first scandal and public inquiry into possible over-reaction, it was also the first on sexual abuse and the first where medical science, as well as social work, was put under scrutiny (see Parton 1991 for a more detailed analysis). Unlike most developments up until this point, which had carried the imprint of thinking in the USA, developments in Cleveland were a very British affair and had a history and impact, both in this country and abroad, of their own (see Hacking 1991, 1992).

This time it seemed professionals, including paediatricians as well as social workers, had failed to recognise the rights of parents and had intervened prematurely in families where there were concerns about sexual abuse. While the reasons for the crisis were again seen as residing primarily in inter-agency and inter-professional misunderstandings, in poor coordination and communication, and in the legal context and content of child abuse work, the emphasis was rather different. Now, not only did the law itself need to be changed but there was a need to recognise that professionals should be much more careful and accountable in identifying the 'evidence', legally framed, for what constituted sexual abuse and child abuse more generally. It was not only a question of getting the right balance between family autonomy and State intervention but also getting the right balance between the power, discretion and responsibilities of the various judicial, social and medical experts and agencies. In this respect, the judiciary was seen to be central to future decision-making.

There were some other issues associated with Cleveland, however, which meant its impact and significance made it of a different order to the public inquiries which had gone before. Cleveland was about sexual abuse, and the issue of sexual abuse touches a range of sensitivities which were rarely evident in earlier concerns about physical abuse and neglect: it reaches into the most intimate, hidden and private elements of family life and adult–child relations; it represents a major set of debates around patriarchy and male power and thereby opens up a range of political arguments around gender never evident in the official discourse previously; and, for the first time, the issue threatened middle-class and professional households. No longer could child abuse be seen as only associated with the marginalised and the disreputable sections of society. It seemed to permeate 'normal' families.

Thus while quite different in their social location and their focus of concern, we can see a growing set of constituencies developing from the mid-1970s which criticised the post-war welfarist consensus in relation to child welfare and the medico-scientific dominance in relation to child abuse. These were most forcefully articulated in and through child abuse inquiries. What emerged were arguments for an approach where there was a greater reliance on individual rights firmly located in a reformed statutory framework, and where there was a greater emphasis on legalism. Within this emphasis, the rule of law as ultimately judged by the court, took priority over those considerations which may be deemed, by the professional 'experts', as optimally therapeutic or 'in the best interests of the child'. By the late 1980s/early 1990s therefore we can see a distinct shift in the dominant discourse concerning child abuse, away from the 'socio-medical' to the 'socio-legal', which had a series of implications for the way policy and practice was framed and operated.

Such development need to be located in the context of the more wide-ranging changes that were taking place in the political environment. During the 1970s an increasing disillusion was evident about the ability of the social democratic State both to manage the economy effectively and to overcome a range of social problems through the use of wide-ranging State welfare programmes. The growth of what has been termed the New Right (Levitas 1986) proved particularly significant in shifting the nature of political discourse in the 1980s. For the New Right, the problems in the economic and social spheres were closely interrelated. They were seen to emanate from the establishment and increasing pervasiveness of the social democratic welfare State. The prime focus for change was to be the nature, priorities and boundaries of the State itself. The strategy consisted of a coherent fusion of the economic and the social. It had its roots in an individualised conception of social relations whereby the market is the key institution for the economic sphere, while the family is the key institution for the social sphere. The family is seen as an essentially private domain from which the State should be excluded but which should also be encouraged to take on its natural caring responsibilities for its members, particularly children. The role of the State should thus be reduced to: (a) ensuring that the family fulfils these responsibilities and (b) ensuring that no one suffers at the hands of the violent and strong.

Freedom, while central, is constructed in negative terms – as freedom from unnecessary interferences. Clearly, however, a fine balance has to be struck between protecting the innocent and weak, and protection from unwarrantable interference – particularly from the State. In such circumstances, the law becomes crucial in defining and operationalising both 'natural' rights and 'natural' responsibilities. Not only must it provide the framework to underwrite contracts between individuals and between individuals and the State, it also aims to make the rationale for intervention by State officials into the natural spheres of the market and the family more explicit and their actions more accountable.

Recent legislative changes and practice guidances

It is in this context that we need to understand the Children Act 1989. In many respects the Act was not consistent with other pieces of social legislation that were being introduced at the time. Many of its key principles seemed to be much more in line with the premises of social democratic welfarism than with those of the New Right. The Act took much of its inspiration from the Short Report (Social Services Committee 1984), and the Review of Child Care Law (DHSS 1985*a*). Consequently the central principles of the Act encouraged an approach to child welfare based on negotiation with families, and involving parents and children in agreed plans. The accompanying guidance and regulations encouraged professionals to work in partnership with parents and young people (see Petrie and Corby, Chapter 20, in this volume). Similarly the Act strongly encouraged the role of the State in supporting families with children in need through preventative work, thus keeping the use of care proceedings and emergency interventions to a minimum.

However, the Act was centrally concerned with trying to construct a new set of balances, related to the respective roles of various State agents and the family in the upbringing of children. While it would be inappropriate to see the legislation as a direct consequence of Cleveland and other child abuse inquiries, it was child protection that in effect was its central concern (Parton 1991). Notions of individual rights and legalism framed the legislation in ways not evident previously. The other key element to emerge was in terms of the *criteria* to be used for making decisions. The assessment of *high risk* has become central (Parton & Parton 1989*a*, 1989*b*, Parton 1991, 1998, Parton *et al.* 1997). In the Children Act, *high risk* is framed in terms of 'significant harm'. The criterion for State intervention under the Children Act is 'that the child concerned is suffering, or is likely to suffer significant harm' (section 31(92)(a)). For the first time the criterion for State intervention includes a prediction of what may or is likely to occur in the *future* (see Lyon, Chapter 10, in this volume).

Since the mid-1980s, the idea of dangerousness or the identification of 'high risk' has become a major topic in discussions of reforming systems of State social regulation more generally (Bottoms 1977). Indeed, assessments of actual or potential 'high risk' have become *the* central concern and activity. However, in a context where the knowledge and research for assessing and identifying 'high risk' are themselves contested, and where the consequences of getting that decision wrong are considerable, it is not surprising that it is not seen as appropriate to leave the decision to the health and welfare experts alone. The decisions and the accountability for making them need ultimately to be lodged with the court and be based on *forensic evidence*. So, while assessments of high risk are central, they are framed in terms of making judgements about what constitutes actual or likely 'significant harm'. The implication is that the legal gaze, and the identification and weighing of forensic evidence, should cast a shadow throughout child abuse work and child welfare more generally, but should be subjected to a variety of checks and balances set in place via the need to work in partnership with children and families, and 'working together' with a range of agencies and professionals.

Law-and-order agencies thus moved centre stage in a way that was not evident previously. For example, the key investigating statutory agencies were identified as the police and social services departments for cases that 'involve both child care and law enforcement issues' (Home Office *et al.* 1991, para. 5.14.4). Social workers were still central, not as social caseworkers or counsellors but as key workers, coordinating and taking central responsibility for assessing *risk* and monitoring and evaluating progress. This was to take place in a context where formalised procedures inform the work, thereby potentially making policy and practice more explicit and accountable.

This was reinforced by the practices and procedures set in place following the Criminal Justice Act 1991, and the *Memorandum of Good Practice on Video Recording Interviews with Child Witnesses for Criminal Proceedings* (Home Office 1992). The mechanisms for gathering forensic evidence for the purpose of the criminal prosecution of offenders and the civil protection of the child were effectively combined (Wattam 1992; and Wattam, Chapter 11, in this volume). The *Memorandum of Good Practice* attempted to harmonise 'the interests of justice and the interests of the child' (Home Office 1992, foreword), for it had long been recognised that the criminal courts were not an appropriate vehicle for receiving the evidence of children who were usually the key witness in prosecution cases against adults, particularly in child sexual abuse cases. Not only were the children not believed but the processes of giving evidence, examination and cross-examination could themselves be seen as abusive of children. In 1988 the Government decided to allow child witnesses to give evidence from outside the courtroom via a special television link and to ease the rules about child witnesses (see Williams, Chapter 19, in this volume). This innovation was extended in the Criminal Justice Act 1991. For the first time, video recordings of earlier interviews with police and social workers could be played to the court as part of the trial. The *Memorandum of Good Practice* produces guidance about how this can be done which, while attempting to be sensitive to the child, crucially ensures that the video constitutes forensic evidence that will stand up in a criminal court. The introduction of the Criminal Justice Act provisions together with the *Memorandum of Good Practice* not only underlined the role of the police in child protection, it had the effect of raising the threshold for identifying what constitutes a child protection case.

By the mid-1990s we can thus characterise the nature of child protection work in the UK in terms of the need to identify 'high risk', in a context where notions of working together were set out in increasingly complex yet specific procedural guidelines, and where the work was framed by a narrow emphasis on legalism and the need for forensic evidence.

The 'refocusing' of children's services

For all the changes introduced in the early 1990s, major problems have continued. The number and range of public inquiries have not subsided and child abuse tragedies of both under- and over-prevention continually feature in the media and now include numerous inquiries into abuse in children's homes (see, for example, the Welsh Office 1996; and Butler, Chapter 9, in this volume). A major debate has now opened up about the future direction of policy and practice. The central issue is how policies and practices in child protection integrate with, and are supported by, policies and practices concerned with family support for children in need. Increasingly it seems there is a major tension between the two and that this is posing major problems for politicians, policy-makers, managers, practitioners and users of child welfare services. What we are currently witnessing is a major debate about whether and how policy and practice can be reframed, so that it is consistent with the original intentions and principles of the Children Act 1989 in terms of prioritising family support for children in need.

Two key catalysts for these debates were the publication of the Audit Commission (1994) report *Seen But Not Heard: Coordinating Community Child Health and Social Services for Children in Need* and the launch by the Department of Health (1995) of *Child Protection: Messages from Research*. The Audit Commission Report suggested that the aspirations and central aims of the Children Act were not being achieved and it made a number of recommendations to try to move policies and practices forward. It argued that children were not receiving the help they needed because local authority and community child health services were poorly planed and coordinated, resulting in much of the £2 billion being wasted on families who do not need support. Central to the Report's recommendations was that local authorities and the health service should produce strategic children's services plans to target resources more effectively. The focus of these should be on identifying and assessing need, then producing flexible and non-stigmatising services, with a particular emphasis on the role of care managers who would coordinate provision. More emphasis should be placed on prevention and less on reactive interventions and reliance on expensive residential services. The problems in developing the family support aspirations of the Children Act were also identified in a number of other studies (Aldgate *et al.* 1992, 1994, Giller 1993, Colton *et al.* 1995, Social Services Inspectorate 1995) and explicitly referred to in the Children Act Report 1993 (DOH 1994).

The central themes and recommendations in the Audit Commission Report reflected, and were in part informed by, the findings and conclusions of a number of a major Department of Health funded research projects (Birchall & Hallett 1995, Cleaver & Freeman 1995, Farmer & Owen 1995, Ghate & Spencer 1995, Gibbons *et al.* 1995a, 1995b, Hallett 1995, Thoburn *et al.* 1995) and there is no doubt that the launch of the research overview document *Child Protection: Messages from Research* (DOH 1995) on 21 June 1995 proved something of a watershed in thinking about child welfare policy and practice.

The decision to fund the research programme in the 1980s was a direct consequence of the fall-out from the Cleveland inquiry (Secretary of State for Social Services 1988) and the apparent paucity of knowledge in the area of child abuse, and the manifest confusions in the reactions of the investigative agencies. The programme of research aimed to explore different aspects of child abuse which would, in combination, help to provide a more comprehensive assessment of current practices. The primary focus was the processes and outcomes of child protection interventions.

Messages from Research argued that any '*incident* has to be seen in *context* before the extent of its harm can be assessed and appropriate interventions agreed' (DOH 1995, p. 53, original italics), and that the studies demonstrate that 'with the exception of a few severe assaults and some sexual maltreatment' (p. 53) long-term difficulties for children seldom follow from a single abusive event or incident – rather they are more likely to be a consequence of living in an unfavourable environment, particularly one that is *low in warmth and high in criticism*. Only in a small proportion of cases in the research was abuse seen as extreme enough to warrant more immediate and formal child protection interventions to protect the child. It suggests that if we put to one side the severe cases (p. 19), 'the most deleterious situations in terms of longer-term outcomes for children are those of *emotional neglect* (p. 20), where the primary concern is the *parenting style* which fails to compensate for the inevitable deficiencies that become manifest in the course of the 20 years or so it takes to bring up a child'. Unfortunately, the research suggested that these are just the situations where the current operation of the child protection system seemed to be least successful. What was demonstrated was that there was little evidence that children referred to social service departments were suffering harm unnecessarily at the hands of their parents, as implied by most child abuse inquiries, and practice was thus *successful* according to a narrow definition of child protection. This was, however, at a cost. Many children and parents felt alienated and angry, and there was an over-emphasis on forensic concerns, with far too much time spent on investigations and a failure to develop longer-term coordinated treatment, counselling and preventative strategies (Cleaver & Freeman 1995, Farmer & Owen 1995).

Perhaps most crucially, valuable time and resources were seen as being wasted, particularly on investigations, with little apparent benefit. This was also a major conclusion in the *Audit Commission Report*. In both, the key research was the study carried out by Gibbons *et al.* (1995*a*) on the operation of the child protection system. This research, based in eight local authorities, over a 16-week period in 1992, identified all children referred for a new child protection investigation (1888 cases) and tracked their progress through the child protection system for up to 26 weeks via social work records and the minutes of case conferences. What was seen as particularly significant was the way a series of filters operated. At the first, 25% were filtered out by social work staff at the duty stage, without any direct contact with the child or family. At the second, the investigation itself, another 50% were filtered out and never reached the initial case conference. Just 15% were placed on the child protection register. Thus six out of every seven children who entered the child protection system at referral were filtered out without being placed on the register. In a high proportion (44% of those actually investigated) the investigation led to no further action at all. There was no intervention to protect the child nor were any services provided. In only 4% of all the cases referred were children removed from home under a statutory order at any time during the study. These findings were reflected in many of the other studies.

In the light of the evidence, *Messages from Research* made a number of suggestions about how 'children's safety' could be improved. It emphasised: the importance of sensitive and informed professional–client relationships, where honesty and reliability are valued; the need for an appropriate balance of power between participants where serious attempts are made at partnership; a wide perspective on child protection which is not simply concerned with investigating forensic evidence but also with notions of welfare, prevention and treatment; that priority should be afforded to effective supervision and the training of social workers; and that generally the most effective protection from abuse is brought about by generally enhancing children's quality of life. More specifically in terms of current policy, it called for a refocusing of child protection work which prioritises the provisions of Section 17 and Part 3 of the Children Act 1989 for helping and supporting families with 'children in need', thereby keeping notions of policing, surveillance and coercive interventions to a minimum. It similarly suggests that Section 47 should be read essentially as the power to enquire in the first instance rather than simply being required to undertake the forensically determined investigation. These issues have proved central to the recent redrafting of government guidance in terms of *Working Together to Safeguard Children: New Government Proposals for Inter-agency Cooperation* (DOH 1999) and the introduction of the *Framework for the Assessment of Children in Need and their Families* (DOH 2000).

New Labour, family support and safeguarding of children

In many respects it seems that the election of the New Labour Government in May 1997 has taken these issues and concerns forward in ways not evident previously. A number of statements from both the Home Office and the Treasury, as well as the Department of Health, suggest that Ministers are keen to broaden the 'refocusing' initiative, beyond simply family support and child protection, to embrace a much wider concern with parenting, early intervention, supporting the family and regenerating the community more generally. This is to be a key responsibility for local authorities, rather than just social service departments, and repositions the role of voluntary agencies, health trusts and education authorities, which are seen as developing accessible, non-stigmatising preventive services, and where early years services and health visitors will play a key role. New Labour came into power with a quite distinctive political agenda which not only reframes how support for families is considered but has fundamental implications for the future of welfare policy more generally (Jordan 1998).

New Labour has developed a number of policies directly concerned with services for children which directly inform and support the core of its welfare reforms (Jordan 1998). It has become apparent that the government's political agenda over the next few years includes: early intervention; community support; multi-agency working; and a focus on families. As Paul Boateng (1999) wrote while Parliamentary Under-Secretary of State for Health:

This government is committed to ensuring that we support families, especially in their parenting role, so as to give children the best start of life. We are committed to supporting families when they seek help, and before they reach crisis point, and to making the best use of scarce public resources. It is because of that that we see the importance of early intervention. The evidence is that early intervention works. (p. 14)

Perhaps the clearest example of these developments is the introduction of the Sure Start programme. This is based on the assumption that even when chains of causation cannot be incontrovertibly established, successful efforts to reduce known risk factors and increase protection factors across a broad population can achieve a desirable preventive effect (Utting 1998). During the discussions that paved the way for Sure Start, Tessa Jowell, the Minister for Public Health, provided something of a mission statement for the New Labour government's reshaping of children's services:

We want services to be flexible and responsive to the needs of each child so everyone can get the best possible start to life. If Government departments work together, not only can we give best value to the children but we can also get value for money by cutting the costs of crime and unemployment which can so easily follow if children do not get help at an early age.

(HM Treasury News Release, 21 January 1998)

As this illustrates, the reform of children's services is primarily informed by concerns related to the prevention and reduction of crime and unemployment, not child abuse. This is not to say that the former are not relevant to the latter but that concerns around what to do about child protection are not as dominant as previously, and where they are, this is particularly in terms of ensuring there is a major overhaul of children's residential services in the light of a series of scandals throughout the 1990s. It is as if the debates prompted by *Messages from Research* (DOH 1995) have been overtaken by other more wide-ranging policies and priorities being introduced by New Labour concerned with supporting the family, parenting and early intervention.

At the same time, however, the 1990s has seen an increased moral and punitive backlash against child abusers, particularly child sex abusers and paedophiles, as evidenced by the massive media coverage at the outrage of the community related to the release of the convicted sex offenders Robert Oliver and Sydney Cooke in 1998. There were also important changes introduced in the 1997 Sex Offenders Act and the 1998 Crime and Disorder Act, including the introduction of a register for sex offenders and a Sex Offender Order. The 1990s have thus witnessed an increasing ambivalence about what to do, for while policy has increasingly stressed the importance of softer, more supportive preventive services for parents and carers, there is also evidence of an increasing punitive element towards abusers themselves, which emphasises exclusion and incarceration rather than inclusion and community support.

Conclusion

As I have tried to illustrate throughout this chapter, the tensions and contradictions that lie at the core of child protection policy and practice, while they will take slightly different forms at different times and in different places, are inherent issues for the liberal State and in many respects have been heightened over the last 30 years in the light of the developments I have analysed. There are a number of key themes. Firstly, the nature of the problem of child abuse has been officially broadened well beyond its original conception of the 'battered baby syndrome' (Dingwall 1989) and now includes neglect, physical abuse, emotional abuse and, most recently, organised abuse (Home Office *et al.* 1991). The definitions are essentially broad and all inclusive, and while we do not have a mandatory reporting system, such as that in the USA, health and welfare professionals may be found morally and organisationally culpable if they do not report their concerns to an appropriate investigating agency, essentially social services departments.

Secondly, and directly related to this, public, professional and political awareness has grown considerably. This was reflected in the 1980s by the tremendous increase in the number of cases on child protection registers. Perhaps of greater significance, however, is the dramatic increase in referrals requiring investigation, now estimated at running at about 160 000 (DOH 1995). It is literally the case that individuals – children, adults and professionals – now have a discourse for describing, understanding and communicating their experiences in a way that did not previously exist.

Thirdly, this broadening definition, and the growth in awareness and referrals has taken place in a context where social workers and others now have a clear responsibility not only to ensure that children do not suffer in the family but also that parental responsibility and family autonomy are not undermined. The discourse of child protection subsumes within it not only the protection of child from significant harm but also the protection of the parents and family privacy from unwarrantable State interventions. The notion of 'safeguarding children', which has recently appeared in Government guidance, is the most recent term introduced to try and reframe and address this central issue.

Fourthly, these developments have taken place in a changing economic and social environment which has had a direct impact on social services departments and social work practice with children and families. The amount of need and potential clients has grown as increasing sections of the population have become marginalised and excluded from the mainstream of the economy and as the incidence of poverty, deprivation and insecurity have increased (Utting 1997). However, not only have other State health and welfare services had insufficient resources for the demands made of them but social services departments have been subject to continual resource constraint and cutback, even when we take into account the extra resources made available by the New Labour Government.

This increased actual and potential demand in the context of reduced resources means that social services departments are finding it almost impossible to develop the more wide-ranging preventative family support strategies included in the Children Act 1989. Priorities and choices have to be made, not just between the more traditional child welfare responsibilities and responding to child abuse, but also choices and priorities in relation to child abuse itself. It is in this respect that the investigation of 'high risk' has taken on a particular significance and gets to the heart of what it is to do child protection work. The focus becomes differentiating the 'high risk' from the rest, so that children can be protected, parental rights and responsibilities can be respected, and scarce resources directed to where they will, in theory, be most effective. Resources and skills are focused on investigating, assessing and sifting out 'high risk', particularly when 'high risk' cannot be clearly demarcated. Where there is insufficient knowledge to demonstrate that the family or situation is safe, systems monitoring, observation and surveillance take on a major significance (Parton 1998).

The child protection system has been set up essentially to identify actual or significant harm and this has been dominating the provision and priorities of child welfare services more generally since the early 1970s. Increasingly, however, the priorities have been framed according to legalistic criteria where the identification of forensic evidence is central, even when the case is not strictly provable. Where cases cannot be so constructed, or where the weight of evidence is not sufficient, the case is quickly filtered out of the system. What the current system does is provide mechanisms and rationales, however administratively and professionally time-consuming these might be for controlling demand and thereby prioritising work. Unfortunately, the way the current system operates is not only contrary to the Children Act, it leaves children and families vulnerable and exposed. It is too early to say how far the recent changes introduced under New Labour may change this situation.

Annotated further reading

Parker R 1995 A brief history of child protection. In: Farmer E, Owen M (eds) Child Protection Practice: Private Risks and Public Remedies. HMSO, London
As the title suggests this provides a brief and very accessible introduction to the historical contexts and influences upon child protection policy and practice in the nineteenth and twentieth centuries.
Parton N 1985 The politics of child abuse. Macmillan, London
The primary concern in this quite detailed analysis is why child abuse emerged as such a significant social problem in Britain in the late 1960s and 1970s and the way this impacted on child welfare practice more generally.
Parton N 1991 Governing the family: child care, child protection and the State. Macmillan, London
This takes on further the story in the earlier book and pays particular attention to the social influences behind the Children Act 1989, particularly the impact of the 'Cleveland affair'.
Ferguson H 1997 Protecting children in time. Child and Family Social Work 14: 205–218
This is particularly interesting in the light it throws on early policy and practice at the turn of the twentieth century and the earlier years of the twentieth century, and the similarities and differences with more recent developments.
Hendrick H 1994 Child welfare: England 1872–1989. Routledge, London
While not exclusively concerned with child protection, this book provides a comprehensive analysis and resource for anyone wishing to explore the historical contexts of childhood and child welfare policy and practice more generally.

References

Aldgate J, Tunstill J, McBeath G 1992 National monitoring of the Children Act: Part III Section 7 – the first year. Oxford University/NCVCCO, Oxford
Aldgate J, McBeath G, Ozolins R, Tunstill J 1994 Implementing Section 17 of the Children Act – the first 18 months. Leicester University School of Social Work, Leicester
Aldridge M 1994 Making social work news. Routledge, London
Audit Commission 1994 Seen but not heard: coordinating child health and social services for children in need. HMSO, London
Barclay P 1995 Joseph Rowntree Foundation: inquiry into income and wealth, Vol. 1. Joseph Rowntree Foundation, York
Birchall E, Hallett C 1995 Working together in child protection. HMSO, London
Boateng P 1999 The Government's role in early intervention. In: Bayley R (ed) Transforming children's lives: the importance of early intervention. Family Policy Studies Centre, London
Bottoms A E 1977 Reflections on the Renaissance of dangerousness. Howard Journal of Penology and Crime Prevention 16 (2): 70–96
Cleaver H, Freeman P 1995 Parental perspectives in cases of suspected child abuse. HMSO, London
Colton M, Drury C, Williams M 1995 Children in need: family support under the Children Act 1989. Avebury, Aldershot
Cooper A, Hetherington R, Bairstow K, *et al.* 1995 Positive child protection: a view from abroad. Russell House, Lyme Regis
Department of Health (DOH) 1991 Child abuse: a study of inquiry reports 1980–1989. HMSO, London
Department of Health (DOH) 1994 Children Act Report 1993. HMSO, London
Department of Health (DOH) 1995 Child protection: messages from research. HMSO, London
Department of Health (DOH) 1999 Working together to safeguard children: new Government proposals for inter-agency cooperation. Consultation Paper. The Stationery Office, London
Department of Health (DOH) 2000 Framework for the assessment of children in need and their families. The Stationery Office, London
Department of Health and Social Security (DHSS) 1976a Non-accidental injury to children. Local Authority Social Services Letter (74), (13)
Department of Health and Social Services (DHSS) 1976b Non-accidental injury to children: the police and case conferences. Local Authority Social Services Letter (76), (26)
Department of Health and Social Security (DHSS) 1982 Child abuse: a study of inquiry reports 1973–1981. HMSO, London
Department of Health and Social Security (DHSS) 1985a Review of child care law: report to Ministers of an interdepartmental working party. HMSO, London
Department of Health and Social Security (DHSS) 1985b Social work decisions in child care: recent research findings and their implications. HMSO, London
Dingwall R 1989 Some problems about predicting child abuse and neglect. In: Stevenson O (ed) Child abuse: public policy and professional practice. Harvester-Wheatsheaf, Hemel Hempstead
Donzelot J 1988 The promotion of the social. Economy and Society 17 (3): 395–427

Farmer E, Owen M 1995 Child protection practice: private risks and public remedies. HMSO, London

Ferguson H 1990 Rethinking child protection practices: a case for history. In: The Violence Against Children Study Group, 'Taking Child Abuse Seriously'. Unwin Hyman, London

Ferguson H 1996 The protection of children in time. Child and Family Social Work 1 (4): 205–218

Ferguson H 1997 Protecting children in new times: child protection and the risk society. Child and Family Social Work 2 (4): 221–234

Franklin B (ed) 1986 The rights of children. Basil Blackwell, London

Franklin B (ed) 1995 A comparative handbook of children's rights. Routledge, London

Franklin B, Parton N (eds) 1991 Social work, the media and public relations. Routledge, London

Freeman M D A 1983 The rights and wrongs of children. Francis Pinter, London

Geach H, Szwed E (eds) 1983 Providing civil justice for children. Arnold, London

Ghate D, Spencer L 1995 The prevalence of child sexual abuse in Britain. HMSO, London

Gibbons J, Conroy S, Bell C 1995*a* Development after physical abuse in early childhood: a follow-up study of children on protection registers. HMSO, London

Gibbons J, Gallagher B, Bell C, Gordon D 1995*b* Development after physical abuse in early childhood: a follow-up of children on protection registers. HMSO, London

Giller H 1993 Children in need: definition, management and monitoring: a report for the Department of Health. Social Information Systems, Manchester

Gordon L 1989 Heroes of their own lives: the politics and history of family violence. Virago, London

Hacking I 1988 The sociology of knowledge about child abuse. Nous 2: 53–63

Hacking I 1991 The making and moulding of child abuse. Critical Inquiry 17 (Winter): 253–288

Hacking I 1992 World-making by kind-making: child abuse for example. In: Douglas M, Hull D (eds) How classification works: Nelson Goodman among the social sciences. Edinburgh University Press, Edinburgh

Hallett C 1995 Inter-agency coordination in child protection. HMSO, London

Hallett C, Birchall E 1992 Coordination and child protection: a review of the literature. HMSO, London

Harder M, Pringle K (eds) 1997 Protecting children in Europe: towards a new millennium. Aarlborg University Press, Aarlborg

Hendrick H 1994 Child welfare: England 1872–1989. Routledge, London

Hetherington R, Cooper A, Smith P, Wilford G 1997 Protecting children: messages from Europe. Russell House, Lyme Regis

Heywood J S 1978 Children in care: the development of the service for the deprived child, 3rd edn. Routledge and Kegan Paul, London

Hills J 1995 Joseph Rowntree Foundation: inquiry into income and wealth, Vol. 2. Joseph Rowntree Foundation, York

Holman R 1996 Fifty years ago: the Curtis and Clyde Reports. Children and Society 19 (3): 197–209

Home Office in conjunction with the Department of Health 1992 Memorandum of good practice on video recording interviews with child witnesses for criminal proceedings. HMSO, London

Home Office, Department of Health, Department of Education and Science, Welsh Office 1991 Working together under the Children Act 1989: a guide to arrangements for inter-agency cooperation for the protection of children from abuse. HMSO, London

Households below average income 1979–1990/91. 1993 HMSO, London

Jordan B 1998 The new politics of welfare. Sage, London

Kempe C H, Silverman F N, Steel B F, *et al.* 1962 The battered child syndrome. Journal of the American Medical Association 181: 17–24

Levitas R (ed) 1986 The ideology of the New Right. Oxford Polity Press, Oxford

Lindsey D 1994 The welfare of children. Oxford University Press, Oxford

London Borough of Brent 1985 A child in trust: report of the Panel of Inquiry investigating the circumstances surrounding the death of Jasmine Beckford. London Borough of Brent, London

London Borough of Greenwich 1987 A child in mind: protection of children in a responsible society, report of the Commission of Inquiry into the circumstances surrounding the death of Kimberley Carlile. London Borough of Greenwich, London

London Borough of Lambeth 1987 Whose child? The report of the Panel appointed to inquire into the death of Tyra Henry. London Borough of Lambeth, London

Morris A, Giller H, Szwed E, Geach H 1980 Justice for children. Macmillan, London

Packman J 1981 The child's generation, 2nd edn. Basil Blackwell/Martin Robertson, Oxford

Parker R (ed) 1980 Caring for separated children: plans, procedures and priorities. A report by a Working Party established by the National Children's Bureau. Macmillan, London

Parker R 1995 A brief history of child protection. In: Farmer E, Owen M (ed) Child protection practice: private risks and public remedies. HMSO, London

Parton N 1979 The natural history of child abuse: a study in social problem definition. British Journal of Social Work 9 (4): 431–451

Parton N 1985 The politics of child abuse. Macmillan, London

Parton N 1990 Taking child abuse seriously. In: The Violence Against the Children Study Group (ed) Taking child abuse seriously: contemporary issues in child protection theory and practice. Unwin Hyman, London

Parton N 1991 Governing the family: child care, child protection and the State. Macmillan, London

Parton N 1996 Child protection, family support and social work: a critical appraisal of the Department of Health research studies in child protection. Child and Family Social Work 1 (1): 3–11

Parton N (ed) 1997 Child protection and family support: tensions, contradictions and possibilities. Routledge, London

Parton N 1998 Risk, advanced liberalism and child welfare: the need to rediscover uncertainty and ambiguity. British Journal of Social Work 28 (1): 5–27

Parton N 1999 Ideology, politics and policy. In Stevenson O (ed) Child welfare in the UK, 1948–1998. Blackwell Science, Oxford

Parton C, Parton N 1989*a* Child protection: the law and dangerousness. In: Stevenson O (ed) Child abuse: public policy and professional practice. Harvester Wheatsheaf, Hemel Hempsted

Parton C, Parton N 1989*b* Women, the family and child protection. Critical Social Policy 24: 38–49

Parton N, Thorpe D, Wattam C 1997 Child protection: risk and the moral order. Macmillan, London

Pringle K 1998 Children and social welfare in Europe. Open University Press, Buckingham

Rose N, Miller P 1992 Political power beyond the State: problematics of Government. British Journal of Sociology 43 (25): 173–205

Secretary of State for Social Services 1974 Report of the inquiry into the care and supervision provided in relation to Maria Colwell. HMSO, London

Secretary of State for Social Services 1988 Report of the inquiry into child abuse in Cleveland. Cmnd 412. HMSO, London

Seebohm Report 1968 Report of the Committee on Local Authority and Allied Personal Social Services. Cmnd 3703. HMSO, London

Social Services Committee 1984 (HC 360) Children in care. HMSO, London

Social Services Inspectorate 1995 An analysis of a sample of English services plans. HMSO, London

Stedman Jones C 1971 Outcast London. Penguin, Harmondsworth

Taylor L, Lacey R, Bracken D 1980 In whose best interests? Cobden Trust/Mind, London

Thoburn J, Lewis A, Shemmings D 1995 Paternalism or partnership? Family involvement in the child protection process. HMSO, London

Unsworth C 1987 The politics of mental health legislation. Oxford University Press, Oxford

Utting D (ed) 1998 Children's services: now and in the future. National Children's Bureau, London

Utting W 1997 Children in the public care: a review of residential care. The Stationery Office, London

Wattam C 1992 Making a case in child protection. NSPCC/Longman, London

Welsh Office 1996 Report of the examination team on child care procedures and practices in North Wales. HMSO, London

2

Patterns and outcomes

Susan J. Creighton

INTRODUCTION

How many children in the UK have been abused? What are the chances of a baby born this year being abused by the time she or he is 18 years old? In the average classroom how many children are recovering, or not, from past abuse and how many are still suffering, or not, from continuing abuse? Is abuse sexual abuse, or does it include other forms of abuse as well? Are particular children more, or less, at risk of abuse?

Professionals working with children need to know the answers to these and other similar questions. They need to know so they can respond sensitively to individual children potentially in need, and confidently institute their local child protection procedures for those children they identify as in need of protection.

Estimates of abuse range from 'one in two girls and one in four boys will experience some form of sexual abuse before their 18th birthday' (Kelly *et al.* 1991) to 5100 children registered in the sexual abuse category in England during the year 1 April 1999 to 31 March 2000 a rate of 0.40 per 1000 population under the age of 18 years in 1999–2000 (DOH 2000). The discrepancy between these two estimates creates confusion in the minds of the general public and professionals alike. This chapter attempts to outline the reasons behind such a discrepancy. It aims to clarify the factors that practitioners need to consider when using incidence or prevalence figures for abuse and how these impinge on their work with children.

Review of frequency literature

Estimates of the frequency of child abuse are usually derived from either incidence or prevalence studies. Incidence refers to the number of new cases occurring in a defined population over a specified period of time – usually a year. Prevalence refers to the proportion of a defined population affected by child abuse during a specified time period – usually childhood.

There are five levels of professional recognition or public awareness of child abuse and neglect:

Level 1

Those children who are reported to protective agencies such as social services, the police or the National Society for the Prevention of Cruelty to Children (NSPCC) as having been abused or neglected, regardless of whether they are subsequently registered or not.

Level 2

Those children who are 'officially known' to a variety of investigatory agencies, such as social services, health services and the police for reasons other than abuse or neglect. These could include matrimonial disputes, delinquency, 'children in need of control', truancy, nutritional and hygiene problems. These children are not regarded by the community as abused or neglected in the same sense as Level 1 children are, and they are unlikely to receive assistance which specifically targets abuse and neglect.

Level 3

Abused and neglected children who are known, and of concern, to other professionals such as schools, hospitals, GPs, day care facilities and mental health agencies but are not reported as abused or neglected. These children may be thought of as 'children in need' (Children Act 1989) but not as children in need of protection. Alternatively, some professions may feel that they are better able to help these children and their families outside the child protection system, or they may not trust the child protection system to handle the problem effectively, or they may not wish to become involved in the investigative process (NB see 'Implications for practice' below for a discussion of mandatory reporting).

Level 4

Abused and neglected children recognised as such by neighbours, relatives or by one or both of the involved parties – the perpetrator and the child. None of these individuals, however, have reported it to a professional agency.

Level 5

Children who have not been recognised as abused or neglected by anyone. These are cases where the individuals involved do not regard their behaviours or experiences as child maltreatment and/or where the situations have not yet come to the attention of outside observers who would recognise them as such.

It is helpful to bear these five levels of awareness and/or discovery in mind when looking at the cases which are most likely to be included in incidence and prevalence studies.

Incidence studies are mainly concerned with reported and recorded cases of abuse to children – Level 1 children. Many cases of child abuse do not come to the notice of potential reporting authorities. Prevalence studies attempt to find out these hidden cases by asking a sample of adults if they were abused during their childhood, regardless of whether or not that abuse came to light and was reported.

In the UK, the best known incidence studies of child abuse are drawn from children placed on child protection (previously child abuse) registers (Creighton 1992, DOH 2000). The best known prevalence studies are the MORI (Baker & Duncan 1985) and Childwatch (BBC 1987) surveys of child sexual abuse. The Childwatch survey included questions on child abuse other than sexual abuse, but it concentrated on the sexual abuse cases when presenting its findings. This is interesting in view of the fact that more people reported having been emotionally or physically abused as children than sexually abused. More children are also registered annually as having been physically abused than as having been sexually abused (DOH 2000). Yet, apart from the Childwatch survey, all the child abuse prevalence studies conducted in the UK, and the majority in the USA, have been on sexual abuse. This may be because of the different age distributions of the different types of abuse. The youngest age group, the 0–1-year-olds, are more vulnerable to physical abuse and neglect (Creighton 1992), whereas the average age of the children registered for sexual abuse was 9 years 7 months. Adults' recall of childhood experiences is very limited for the first 3–4 years of their lives, so if the physical abuse or neglect ceased before they were 4, they may well have no memory of it. The preponderance of child sexual abuse prevalence studies in the literature and the media has led to a sizeable proportion of the general public equating child abuse with child sexual abuse. Children have been murdered (e.g. in 1991 Claire McIntyre, Karin Griffin, Angela Flaherty and Sarah Furness were all killed) following sexual abuse, but usually by strangers or acquaintances, not family members. Many more children die following physical abuse or neglect (Home Office 2000), mostly at the hands of their immediate caretakers. Abuse within the family has, up to now, been the major concern of professionals working in child protection.

Incidence studies

In 1998, two people were found guilty of or were cautioned for the offence of 'infanticide', 674 for 'cruelty to or neglect of children' and 14 for 'abandoning a child aged under 2 years'. A further 78 were found guilty of or were cautioned for the offence of 'unlawful sexual intercourse with a girl under 13 years', 511 for 'unlawful sexual intercourse with a girl under 16', 72 for 'incest' and 264 for 'gross indecency with a child' (Home Office 2000). Criminal statistics represent the most extreme end of the child abuse recognition continuum, where it is not sufficient for children to be recognised and reported as abused. The perpetrators of abuse also have to be recognised and reported, and sufficient evidence gathered to mount a successful prosecution.

The next level of public recognition are those cases which are officially recorded as child abuse. In the UK, these are the children who are placed on child protection registers. In the Netherlands they are those verified by the 'confidential doctor' system, and in the USA they are those substantiated by the Child Protection Services in each State under the Child Abuse and Neglect Prevention and Treatment Act (1974). Not all children who are reported as abused or neglected will be officially recorded as such. In England and Wales, various studies (Association of Directors of Social Services (ADSS) 1987, Giller *et al.* 1992, Gibbons *et al.* 1995) have shown that for every ten children referred for child protection only two will be registered. The remaining eight will be filtered out during the course of investigation and case conferencing. In the USA, approximately 32% of reports of maltreatment are substantiated (Daro 1996). In the Netherlands, every report to the confidential doctors is verified by the Office (Pieterse & Van Urk 1989). Many reports are incomplete, too short or sometimes unreliable, and further enquiry is necessary. Only the verified cases are accepted.

Table 2.1 shows the officially recorded cases of child maltreatment in various countries.

The wide variations in rates per 1000 children and the breakdown in cases reflect a number of factors. These include the length of time the reporting system has been operating, the general level of public awareness and willingness to report, and the criteria for recording, in addition to the underlying levels of abuse and neglect in the country. Mandatory reporting was established in the USA in 1974 with the passage of the Child Abuse Prevention and Treatment Act. Non-mandatory guidance on the management of cases of non-accidental injury to children, including the establishment of registers, was issued by the Department of Health in late 1974 (Department of Health and Social Security (DHSS) 1974). Similar guidance was offered in Wales. Four 'confidential doctors' were introduced in the Netherlands as an experiment on 1 January 1972 for 2 years. After this, a governmental institute for the prevention of child abuse and neglect was established. Official reporting appears to have started at similar times in the Netherlands, the USA and the UK. The resources made available and the public and professional awareness campaigns in the different countries varied enormously.

Officially recorded cases of child abuse and neglect are at Level 1 of the professional recognition continuum. There have been two incidence studies which

Table 2.1
Official records of child maltreatment

Country	Year	Number of cases	Rate per 1000	Breakdown of cases (%)		Source
Australia	1 July 1995–30 June 1996	29 833	5.8	Emotional Neglect Physical Sexual	31 25 28 16	Broadbent & Bentley (1997)
Canada (Ontario)	March–June 1993	12 309	5.6	Emotional Neglect Physical Sexual	8 36 34 28	Trocme et al. (1994)
England	1 April 1999–31 March 2000	29300	2.6	Emotional Neglect Physical Sexual	17 44 32 17	Department of Health (2000)
Scotland	1 April 1997–31 March 1998	1919	1.7	Emotional Neglect Physical Sexual	9 27 43 20	Scottish (1999) Executive
USA	1995	996 000	15.0	Emotional Neglect Physical Sexual Other	3 54 25 11 6	Daro (1996)
Wales	1 April 1998–31 March 1999	2516	3.7	Emotional Neglect Physical Sexual	18 39 37 17	Welsh Office (1999)

attempted to ascertain cases from all professionals, i.e. Levels 1 through 3, one in the USA and one in Northern Ireland. The US Department of Health and Human Services commissioned research into the national incidence of child abuse and neglect in 1980, 1986 and 1993. The 1993 survey (US Department of Health and Human Services 1996) looked at all the cases reported to the Child Protective Services staff, as well as cases reported by a variety of professionals in other agencies who served as 'sentinels'. They were asked to be on the lookout during the study period for cases meeting the study's definitions of child maltreatment. These definitions were designed to be clear, objective and to involve demonstrable harm to the child. The research found that, in 1993, just under 1 553 800 children, a rate of 23.1 per 1000 nationwide, experienced abuse or neglect as defined by the study. Only 9% of these children were cases investigated by the Child Protective Services. Non-investigatory agencies (which included schools, hospitals, social services and mental health agencies) recognised seven times the number of child victims than did investigatory agencies (police/probation service/courts and public health agencies). The most frequent type of abuse was physical, followed by sexual and then emotional abuse. The relative incidence rates for these were 5.7 for physical, 3.2 for sexual and 3.0 for emotional abuse per 1000 children. The overall incidence rate for abuse was 11.1 per 1000 children. Educational neglect (i.e. permitted chronic truancy or inattention to special educational needs by parents) was by far the most frequent form of neglect, with an incidence rate of 5.9 per 1000 children. This was followed by physical neglect, at a rate of 5.0, and then emotional neglect with an incidence rate of 3.2 per 1000 children. The overall incidence rate for neglect was 13.1 per 1000 children. These were calculated using the stringent criterion that the child had to have already experienced demonstrable harm as a result of maltreatment in order to be included. The incidence of both abuse and neglect had more than doubled since the 1980 survey.

The other study was conducted in Northern Ireland by the Research Team from the Departments of Child Psychiatry, Royal Belfast Hospital for Sick Children, and Epidemiology and Public Health at Queen's University, Belfast (1990). This was a research study of the annual incidence of child sexual abuse in Northern Ireland during a 1-year period, 1 January 1987–31 December 1987. It was a multi-source notification study whereby all professional staff from all agencies concerned with children completed a specially designed notification form when they came across a case of sexual abuse which fulfilled the study definition. These staff were interviewed later by one of the researchers and the information recorded on a standard questionnaire. In the year prior to data collection, 1986, the researchers contacted all the possible agencies likely to come across cases of child sexual abuse, explained the study to them and gained their cooperation. Information was sought for cases which were:

1. Suspected – when the reporter has been given any reason at all to believe that an incident of child sexual abuse may have occurred.
2. Alleged – where someone communicates to the reporter that an incident of sexual abuse has occurred.
3. Established – where the reporter and others are satisfied that an incident of child sexual abuse has occurred.

The incidence rate for established cases of child sexual abuse in Northern Ireland discovered by the study was 1.2 per 1000 children under 17 years. This contrasts with the sexual abuse registration rate over a similar period in England of 0.36 (DOH 1989). It may be that the underlying rate of child sexual abuse is higher in Northern Ireland than in England, but it seems more likely that the methods employed in this study pick up cases that would not normally be reported.

Incidence studies which attempted to ascertain cases at Level 4, where no professional agency is involved, are those conducted in 1975, 1985 and 1995 by the Family Violence Research Program at the University of New Hampshire (Straus 1979, Straus & Gelles 1986, Straus *et al.* 1998). The 1975 and 1985 studies were of a nationally representative selection of American families with at least one child aged between 3 and 17 years living at home. One of the parents was interviewed and the studies attempted to determine whether physical abuse had occurred and at what levels of severity. Abusive violence was ascertained when the parent acknowledged that they, or their spouse, had 'punched, kicked, bitten, hit with an object, beaten up or used a knife or gun' on their child in the last year. The 1986 study obtained a rate of one in every ten American children aged between 3 and 17 years subjected to severe physical violence each year. Compared to the rate of officially reported cases of physical abuse (Schene 1987), 'only one child in seven who is physically injured is reported'. Both these studies only included children aged between 3 and 17 years, whereas the youngest age groups, the 0–1-year-olds and the 2–3-year-olds, are the most vulnerable to physical abuse (DOH 2000). Hence, the rates the authors obtained for the older age groups are likely to be underestimates of the incidence of physical abuse to all children in America. The 1995 study (Straus *et al.* 1998) included a nationally representative sample of US children under the age of 18 and a revised measure. They found a rate of severe physical assault against children of 49 per 1000, over eight times greater than that uncovered in the Third National Incidence Study (US Department of Health and Human Services 1996).

Prevalence studies

Prevalence studies of child abuse have been almost entirely confined to child sexual abuse. Table 2.2 summarises the main prevalence studies of child sexual abuse conducted outside the UK. The percentage of adults and adolescents affected varies from 6.8–54% of women and girls and 3–25% of men and boys.

The earliest prevalence studies (e.g. Finkelhor 1979) were usually conducted on samples of college students on social science courses. Social science students have the advantage of providing a captive sample but are probably not representative of the population as a whole. The studies included in this table concentrate on samples drawn from the entire population. The wide variations among them probably reflect the differences in the methods used rather than significant geographical variation. These include items such as definitions used, how the sample was chosen and approached, the methods used to get the information from the respondents and how many refused to participate. The methodological issues involved in these studies will be discussed later in this chapter but brief details are included in Table 2.2. The factor with the greatest effect on the prevalence figures is whether or not the definition of child sexual abuse used includes non-contact experiences such as exposure, in addition to contact experiences. Table 2.2 shows whether or not the definition included contact and non-contact experiences in the prevalence figures.

In the UK prior to 1995, there had been only two prevalence studies which had attempted to use a nationally representative sample; the MORI poll reported by Baker & Duncan (1985) and the BBC Childwatch Survey (1987), the full results of which were never published. The MORI poll examined the prevalence of child sexual abuse, whilst the BBC Childwatch Survey (1987) asked about all forms of child abuse but only released the sexual abuse data. Table 2.3 summarises the main prevalence studies conducted in the UK with brief details of the methods employed. The 90% prevalence produced by the 1986 BBC Childwatch Survey is what you might expect from a self-selected sample. If you produce a high-profile TV programme on a particular social problem and then invite viewers who have experienced this problem to write in and complete a questionnaire on it, you might expect a 100% prevalence of the problem among the returned questionnaires. This survey really highlights the relevance of the methods employed in these studies.

Methodological factors

The factors that need to be taken into account when planning or assessing studies of the frequency of childhood maltreatment include:

- Definitions
- Method of sampling
- Case ascertainment
- Measurement tools
- Bias
- Generalisability
- Comparability.

Definitions

The definition of childhood sexual abuse used in the MORI survey (Baker & Duncan 1985) was:

Table 2.2
Prevalence studies of child sexual abuse outside the UK

Country	Authors	Sample	Method	Response rate (%)		Prevalence
USA	Russell (1983)	930 women 18+, random sample, San Francisco	Face-to-face interviews	50	< 18	38% involving contact 54% including non-contact
					< 14	28% involving contact 48% including non-contact
Canada	Badgley et al. (1984)	Representative population study 18+, over 2000 men and women	Hand-delivered questionnaires	94		42% women including 25% men } non-contact 10% girls involving contact
USA	Siegal et al. (1987)	Two-stage probability sample of 3132 adults (male and female), Los Angeles	Mental health survey; face-to-face interviews	68	< 14	6.8% women } 3.8% men } involving contact
USA	Finkelhor et al. (1990)	Sample of 2626 adults (male and female)	Telephone interviews	76		27% women 16% men} largely involving contact
New Zealand	Anderson et al. (1993)	Random sample of female electorate Dunedin (n = 1920)	Health survey postal questionnaire followed by face-to-face interviews	73 (< 65 years)	< 16 < 12	25% involving contact 32% including non-contact 16% involving contact 20% including non-contact
Finland	Sariola & Uutela (1994)	Random sample of 15- to 16-year-olds in schools (n = 7349)	Self-administered questionnaire done in school nurse's room or in class room	96		8% girls 3% boys
Switzerland	Halperin et al. (1996)	Representative sample of adolescent population aged 13–17 years in schools in Geneva (n = 1116)	Self-administered questionnaire following information session	93.5		20.4% girls 3.3% boys } involving contact 33.8% girls 10.9% boys } including non-contact
Canada	McMillan et al. (1997)	General population survey of residents aged 15+ Ontario (n = 9953)	Health survey; self-administered questionnaire as part of interview	66		12.8% women 4.3% men } including non-contact 11.1% women 3.9% men } severe sexual abuse*

* included 'threatened to have sex with'.

Table 2.3
Prevalence studies of child sexual abuse in the UK

Authors	Sample	Method	Response rate (%)	Prevalence
Nash & West (1985)	223 female GP patients aged 20–39 years	Questionnaire and face-to-face interviews	53	42% including non-contact 22% involving contact
BBC Childwatch (1986)	Almost 3000 self-selected viewers, male and female	Viewers wrote in for and completed questionnaires	75	90%
Baker & Duncan (1985)	Nationally representative sample of adults aged 15+ in Great Britain, 2019 men and women	Face-to-face interviews in homes	87	12% female } including 8% male } non-contact
BBC Childwatch national interview survey (1987)	Probability sample of 2041 adults aged 16 + in UK	Interviews (full results not published)	Not known	3% of sample} involving contact
Kelly et al. (1991)	1244 polytechnic students aged 16–25 years	Questionnaires in class	97	59% women} including 27% men } non-contact 27% women} involving 11% men } contact
Creighton & Russell (1995)	Nationally representative quota sample of adults aged 18–45 in Britain (n = 1032)	Face-to-face interviews in homes including self-completion questionnaire for sensitive topics	96	24% female} including 9% male } non-contact 17% female} involving 6% male } contact
NSPCC (2000)	National random sample of adults aged 18–24 in UK (n = 2869)	Face-to-face computer assisted interviews in homes including self-completion for sensitive topics	65	20% female} including 10% male } non-contact 15% female} involving 6% male } contact

A child (anyone under 16 years) is sexually abused when another person, who is sexually mature, involves the child in any activity which the other person expects to lead to their sexual arousal. This might involve intercourse, touching, exposure of the sexual organs, showing pornographic material or talking about sexual things in an erotic way.

Ten per cent of their respondents (12% female, 8% male) reported that this had occurred to them. The definition employed by Siegal *et al.* (1987) in their mental health survey took the form of the question:

In your lifetime, has anyone ever tried to pressure or force you to have sexual contact? By sexual contact I mean their touching your sexual parts, or sexual intercourse?

Respondents who answered affirmatively were asked if they had ever been forced or pressured for sexual contact before the age of 16 years (childhood sexual assault). These specific questions, which focus on the nature of the behaviour – contact and pressured – plus the age when it happened (under 16 years), led to a prevalence figure of 5.3% (6.8% women, 3.8% men). This is one of the lowest figures for the studies but is very similar to that for the 'contact' cases in the Baker & Duncan study (derived from their Table 3, page 461). Kelly *et al.* (1991) provide a detailed breakdown of the influence of definitions on prevalence findings in their study (see their Appendix C, page 20). As the definitions get more 'serious' (in the sense of more intrusive and unwanted contact), so the numbers affected drop from 59% for the widest definition to 5% for the most serious.

Method of sampling

The four most commonly used methods in maltreatment studies have been: volunteer (e.g. BBC 1986), quota (e.g. Baker & Duncan 1985, BBC 1987), random (e.g. Russell 1983) and national random (e.g. Badgley *et al.* 1984). Volunteer samples are obviously going to be biased towards those with something to report. Quota samples – in which people or households are approached until the required quota of subjects is obtained – run the same risk: that those choosing to participate will not be typical of the general population. Random samples, where each person in a population has an equal probability of being included in the sample, are preferred. Ideally, it should be a national random sample. A random sample in only one area might give the prevalence for that area but not be suitable for generalisation to other areas.

Case ascertainment

Even if a random sample of the population has been approached, the actual cases ascertained can be biased due to factors relating to: the subject, the interviewer and the measurement tool (the questionnaire). In such an emotive area as child maltreatment, subjects can either fail to recognise themselves as abused (Berger *et al.* 1988) or repress memories of parental abuse and fail either to recall or report them. The gender, age and ethnicity of the interviewer in relation to the subject have all been shown to affect the likelihood and accuracy of the responses. Both men and women prefer to be interviewed about sexual topics by a woman, even adolescent males who have been abused by a woman (Kaplan *et al.* 1991).

The way the survey questionnaire is introduced can affect the likelihood of getting any answers. A survey presented as one on child sexual abuse is more likely to encounter a refusal than one on general health or attitudes.

Measurement tools

The wording of the questions or their position in the questionnaire (or interview) can have an impact on subject response. Questions need to be clear, simple and unambiguous. Sensitive questions which at the beginning of an interview may inhibit responses may, if placed at the end, be answered. Respondents are more likely to be engaged in the survey by a personalised approach but they may be embarrassed to answer personal questions. Surveys such as Badgley *et al.*'s (1984) study, which employed a personal approach coupled with a self-completed questionnaire, were very successful. The use of computers in surveys has also helped respondents to feel freer to divulge sensitive information (Turner *et al.* 1998). Computer-assisted personal interviewing (CAPI), where the interviewer uses a pre-programmed computer rather than a paper questionnaire, is now widely used in social surveys. Computer-assisted self-interviewing (CASI) is the computerised version of the self-completion questionnaire. The interviewer hands the computer over to the respondent for the more sensitive questions, and also demonstrates the complete confidentiality of their answers. The programme is set up to prevent the interviewers having any access to the CASI answers.

It is very important to get a high response rate to the survey. Those people who refuse to answer questions are unlikely to be like those who agree, particularly in relation to child maltreatment. If only half the people you approach agree to answer the questions, then a high rate among them is misleading. The other half who refused may have done so because they were not affected. This effectively halves the prevalence estimate reported. A low response rate has the effect of turning a random sample into more of a volunteer sample. Although there is no simple acceptable response rate, rates lower than 80% are considered undesirable (Markowe 1991).

Missing data pose a similar problem. If a particular question is not answered by the majority of the respondents, the answers gained cannot be considered representative of the sample as a whole. It is important to pre-test and pilot the questionnaire or survey instrument to avoid including questions that will not be answered.

Bias

Bias is any trend in the collection, analysis, interpretation, publication or review of data that can lead to conclusions that are systematically different from the truth. Bias can be introduced in the ascertainment of cases, the design of a survey and the sample method employed. In child abuse reporting, it has been shown that the children of the middle and upper classes are less likely to come to the attention of the child protection agencies than those of the poor and disadvantaged. The perceived social status of the parents also affects the level of suspicion of experienced professionals about the possible non-accidental nature of an injury (O'Toole *et al.* 1983). Higher social class parents were less likely to be judged as abusive than lower class parents. Nurses and more experienced professionals were not affected by this social class bias. There are also likely to be reporting and substantiation biases in cases involving ethnic minorities, disabled children or children in out-of-home care. Hong & Hong (1991), using a sample of Californian students, found that the Chinese were more tolerant of parental conduct than the Hispanics and Whites, and were less likely to ask for investigation by protective agencies in potential cases of child abuse and neglect. Nunno (1992) reported a survey of complaints of maltreatment of children in out-of-home care in the USA in 1989. Only 27% of these complaints were substantiated by child protection workers compared to 53% for familial maltreatment reports.

In addition to the characteristics of the child, the characteristics of the reporter – professional or other – has an effect on the process. In the USA, cases of child abuse reported by non-mandated sources, e.g. neighbours and schools, are less likely to be substantiated than cases reported by mandated sources, e.g. child protection services (Eckenrode *et al.* 1988). Similarly, in the UK, Stevenson (1989) has described the relative status and perceived powers of the different agencies involved in child protection. These are all factors which can lead to bias in the recognition, reporting and registering of cases of child abuse.

Generalisability

If a prevalence or incidence study is thought to be methodologically sound, the next step is to assess how far it can be generalised. Are students in further education colleges, as in Kelly *et al.*'s (1991) sample, or students on social science courses (Finkelhor 1979) representative of all students? Are students representative of all young adults? Follow-up studies of abused children (Zimrin 1986, Finkelhor 1988, Wind & Silvern 1992, Kendall-Tackett *et al.* 1993) would seem to indicate that the loss of self-esteem, the development of behavioural problems and the inability to concentrate often found in abused children would make them less likely to go into further education than other young adults. Although the problem of generalisability is not easily satisfied it should always be considered.

Comparability

Can we compare child abuse or maltreatment in the USA or Canada with that in the UK – or that reported in London with that in Newcastle? Can the results of one study be directly compared with that of another? These are likely to be subjective judgements to some extent, but comparison of the methodological factors discussed in this section should help to provide a more objective basis for such a judgement.

Time trends

One of the most interesting areas of comparability in child maltreatment is between different times. Has child maltreatment increased or decreased over the years, or have individual types of abuse changed? Do increases or decreases in reported rates reflect actual changes in maltreatment levels or changes in professional and public awareness and willingness to report? There have been a number of studies that have looked at changes in officially reported cases and in the incidence and prevalence rates of child maltreatment over time. The next section deals with trends in reported cases in the Netherlands (Pieterse & Van Urk 1989), the USA (Daro & Mitchel 1990, McCurdy & Daro 1993) and the UK (Creighton 1992) over a similar time period.

Reported cases

In the Netherlands, Pieterse & Van Urk (1989) compared the data on reports received by the 'confidential doctor' system in its first official year, 1974, with that of 1983. They found a threefold increase in the number of verified cases over the 10 years, for both boys and girls. The incidence (number of cases per 1000 children) increased fourfold from 0.19 per 1000 children in 1974 to 0.71 in 1983. The types of abuse reported and verified had changed, from a preponderance of physical abuse cases in 1974 (64% of cases) to a preponderance of emotional abuse/neglect in 1983 (50% of cases). There were only seven cases of sexual abuse reported in 1973 compared to 189 (7% of all cases) in 1983. The increases in all types of abuse were mostly in the older age group, the 12–17-year-olds, for both boys and girls. There was an increase in the detection of child fatalities but a decrease in the severity of physical abuse. No change was found in the identity of the suspected perpetrators – primarily fathers and/or mothers – or in the social conditions of the families. There was a decrease in the percentage of married parents and a corresponding increase in single mothers. There was an encouraging increase in the numbers of victims residing at home rather than in children's homes which the authors attributed to the improvement in aftercare for these children.

In the USA, the rate of children reported for child abuse and neglect between 1985 and 1992 increased 50% from 30 per 1000 children in 1985 to 45 per 1000 in 1992 (McCurdy & Daro 1993). Between 1980 and 1985, there had been an average 11.4% annual increase in reports (Daro & Mitchel 1990). The rapid increase in reported cases between 1985 and 1992 was attributed to the increased economic stress caused by the recession, an increase in substance abuse and increased public awareness leading to greater reporting.

The different types of abuse reported in the USA did not show the changes that the Netherlands data did. In the USA, cases of neglect were most likely to be reported (45% in 1992), followed by physical abuse (27%), sexual abuse (17%), emotional maltreatment (7%) and other (8%). As in the Netherlands between 1974 and 1983, the rate of confirmed child maltreatment fatalities in the USA had risen steadily between 1985 and 1992 from 1.3 per 100 000 children in 1985 to 1.94 per 100 000 in 1992. As McCurdy & Daro (1993) report: 'This means that more than three children die each day in the US as a result of maltreatment' (p. 13).

By contrast, in the UK one to two children are killed each week (Home Office 2000). As with deaths, the reporting or registration rates for child maltreatment are much lower in the UK than in the USA, although they have also shown increases over the years. The registration rate trebled over 7 years from 1.16 per 1000 children in 1984 to 3.40 per 1000 children in 1990 (Creighton 1992). This was largely due to the change from Child Abuse Registers to Child Protection Registers in 1988 following the DHSS guidance *Working Together* (DHSS 1988). This led to a massive increase in registrations in the 'grave concern' category, i.e. children who had not been abused but were thought to be at significant risk of abuse. In the UK, registers were initially 'Non-Accidental Injury Registers' between 1975, when most were established, and 1980 when they became Child Abuse Registers. Cases of physical abuse are the only type of abuse to have been reported since 1975. Between 1976 and 1979, the registration rate for cases of physical abuse remained steady but increased gradually from 1979 to 1984. There was a marked increase between 1984 and 1985, and between 1985 and 1990 the rate fluctuated from year to year. The physical abuse rate ranged from 0.44 in 1976 to 1.02 per 1000 children under 15 years in 1989 (Creighton 1992).

Among the abused children placed on UK registers between 1980 and 1990, cases of physical abuse predominated, followed by sexual abuse, neglect and emotional abuse. Given the historical evolvement of registers from non-accidental injury, through child abuse to child protection registers it is not surprising that registrations for physical abuse predominated until fairly recently. Before 1994 they were followed by cases of sexual abuse, neglect and emotional abuse. The rate of registrations for sexual abuse increased most between 1985 and 1986, reaching a peak of 0.65 per 1000 children under 17 years in 1987 (Creighton & Noyes 1989), after which it declined. The sudden increase in reported cases of sexual abuse in Cleveland (Butler-Sloss 1988) was in 1987. Whether the decline in registered cases of sexual abuse following 1987 was due to fewer cases being recognised, or greater caution in reporting and registering them, could not be determined. The register data (Creighton 1992) showed evidence of increased caution in cases of sexual abuse with regard to assessing severity and the suspected perpetrator. It failed to show any evidence of workers assigning cases they would have registered as sexual abuse in the past to the grave concern category instead. There was also a slight increase between 1988 and 1989 before declining again in 1990. It is unfortunate that the changes in registration criteria introduced by the new guidance *Working Together under the Children Act, 1989* (Home Office *et al.* 1991) mean that the registrations for sexual abuse from 1991 are not comparable with those from 1988 to 1990. The 1991 guidance excluded the grave concern category as a separate reason for registration. Children who were thought likely to be physically, sexually or emotionally abused or neglected were to be registered in the appropriate category. This means that the registrations for sexual abuse from 1991 will include both children who have been sexually abused and children thought likely to be sexually abused. It will not be possible to see if the decline in registrations for actual child sexual abuse between 1987 and 1990 has continued or reversed. In recent years registrations for neglect, and to a lesser extent, emotional abuse, have increased so that by 31 March 2000 there were more neglect than physical injury registrations, a profile of reported abuse more similar to that of the USA.

As in the Netherlands, there was a decline in the rate of serious and fatal injuries in the early years (1975–1976) of the registers (Creighton 1992). From 1976 to 1984 the rate remained fairly stable but there was a marked increase between 1984 and 1985. From 1985 to 1990, the rate of serious and fatal injuries fluctuated but at a higher rate than that between 1976 and 1984 (Creighton 1992). The DOH does not collect information on the severity of the injuries inflicted on children registered in the physical injury category so there are no comparative data for the last decade.

As registers became established, more older children were placed on them, particularly for sexual abuse but also for physical injury. The Netherlands data showed an increase in older children being reported to the confidential doctors between 1974 and 1983. In the UK, the average age of the children registered for physical abuse increased from 3 years 8 months in 1975 to 7 years 1 month in 1990 (Creighton 1992). Boys have been consistently over-represented amongst the children registered for physical abuse, whilst the overwhelming majority of children registered for sexual abuse have been girls. More boys than girls have been registered for neglect.

The family situation of the children registered in the UK changed over the years from 1975 to 1990, with fewer children living with both their natural parents and more living with their natural mother alone and with their natural mother and a father substitute. The Netherlands data showed a similar decrease over the years in children living with both their natural parents and an increase in mothers alone, but they do not include information on father substitutes. In the UK generally, there were major demographic changes over the period of the NSPCC register research (Central Statistical Office (CSO) 1993), with increases in divorces and the numbers of single mothers. In spite of these changes, and some of the more lurid headlines in the tabloid press, the majority of UK children continue to live with both their natural parents. This was not the case for the children placed on Child Protection Registers in England. By 1990, just over a third of the registered children were living with both their natural parents (Creighton 1992). The registered children were eight times more likely to be living with a father substitute than children nationally from similar social classes.

The three studies on the officially reported cases of child maltreatment in the three countries, the Netherlands, the USA and the UK, show some differences but more similarities. Over the different time periods covered by each they all show increases in the numbers of children officially reported as having been maltreated.

Incidence and prevalence changes

There have been two major studies looking at incidence rates of child maltreatment at different times, both conducted in the USA. The first, the three National Incidence Studies (NIS-1, NIS-2 and NIS-3) (US Department of Health and Human Services 1988, 1996, Sedlak 1990) were conducted in 1980, 1986 and 1993. They collected all cases of child maltreatment recognised and reported to the study by 'community professionals' in a national probability sample of 29 counties throughout the USA where the child had experienced demonstrable harm as a result of the maltreatment. The data included all the cases reported to the Child Protection Services (CPS) staff during the study period, plus cases coming to the notice of other non-CPS agencies (such as hospitals and schools, etc.) who were acting as 'sentinels' on the lookout for such cases during the study. The data coming to light here would cover Levels 1 through 3 of public awareness outlined at the beginning of this chapter. The second study, from the Family Violence Research Program (Straus 1979, Gelles & Straus 1987), attempted to assess the physical abuse conducted at public awareness Level 4 by asking a nationally representative sample of parents with a child aged 3 through 17 years at home about their behaviour towards a randomly selected child in the last year. They conducted national surveys in 1975 and 1985. The two sets of studies produced very different findings.

The first two National Incidence Studies (NIS-1 and NIS-2) found a significant increase (51%) in the incidence of maltreatment cases coming to the attention of their survey respondents in 1986 compared to 1980. This was largely due to cases of abuse (53% increase), as no form of neglect showed reliable changes in incidence rate since the earlier study. Emotional abuse also showed no change in incidence rate in 1986 compared to 1980. The significant rises in incidence rates were in cases of sexual abuse, where the rate tripled between 1980 and 1986, and physical abuse where it increased by 39%.

By contrast, the two national surveys conducted by the Family Violence Research Program in 1975 and 1985 showed a 47% decrease in the rate of child physical abuse between 1975 and 1985. The disparity between these two sets of findings for the physical abuse of children can be explained if we look at the definitions employed and the actual rates in the two studies.

The National Incidence Studies used a definition of physical abuse which specified that the child must be live-born and under 18 years of age at the time of the abuse, the abusive behaviour must have been non-accidental and avoidable, the perpetrator had to be either a parent or adult caretaker (over 18) and the child must have suffered demonstrable harm. The incidence rates they discovered were 3.1 per 1000 children in the population in 1980 and 4.3 per 1000 in 1986. By 1993 this had increased to 5.7 per 1000 children.

The Family Violence Research Program surveys used a definition of physical child abuse which included acts of behaviour by a parent to a child between the ages of 3 and 17 years which had a relatively high probability of causing an injury. These included: kicking, biting, punching, hitting with an object, beating up and threatening or using a knife or gun on the child. The incidence rates they found for these types of behaviour were 140 per 1000 children in 1975 and 107 per 1000 in 1985. Although this 1985 figure represents a considerable decrease compared with the 1975 figure, it is still nearly 25 times greater than the 1986 incidence figure found in the National Incidence Study.

The severe violence inflicted on children uncovered by the Family Violence Research Program surveys may not have caused any noticeable injuries or demonstrable harm. Very few of the children so affected would have been reported, or recognised, as abused to either child protection or other agencies. Schene (1987) estimated, on the basis of the 1985 national survey incidence rate and the official reported rate for that year, that only one physically abused child in seven was reported.

Changes in childhood sexual abuse prevalence rates over the years have been assessed by comparing a number of studies conducted in the 1970s and 1980s with that of Kinsey and his co-workers in the 1940s (Kinsey *et al.* 1953). Feldman *et al.* (1991) reviewed the Kinsey report and 19 prevalence studies reported since 1979 using predetermined criteria for quality of information, commonality of definitions of childhood sexual abuse and research design. They found that the more recent studies, with the strongest methodology and where definitions of childhood sexual abuse were similar, reported prevalence figures similar to those of Kinsey in the 1940s, in spite of differences in study designs and populations surveyed. Using a definition close to Kinsey's, i.e. girls younger than 14 years of age having sexual contact with an adult male at least 5 years older, and the studies with the best research design gave three studies, including Kinsey's. The other two were reported in 1984 (Badgley *et al.*) and 1987 (Siegal *et al.*), and all three produced prevalence figures of between 10 and 12% for girls younger than 14 years of age. Feldman *et al.* (1991) concluded that the increased number of reports of child sexual abuse was not due to a true increase in prevalence but to changes in legislation and public awareness. They stressed that this should not deter child protection professionals from continuing to provide treatment and preventative services to sexually abused children.

Implications for practice

There are a number of implications for practitioners to be drawn from the review of the literature in the previous section. The most important of these is probably the fact that, in spite of the varying estimates produced by the different studies, there can be no doubt that there is a large base group of children who have been, or are being, maltreated. What is also clear is that only a fraction of them are being reported to child protection practitioners. Before feeling overwhelmed by the size of the problem confronting them, practitioners should also bear in mind that the majority of children are not abused or maltreated. The importance of incidence and prevalence studies on child maltreatment is in giving practitioners a sense of the base underlying rate of the problem and the characteristics of that population. It is against that background of knowledge that they can look at the individual cases referred to them and assess the likelihood that they are cases of maltreatment.

The finding that, even with vastly increased reporting rates, only one American child in seven who was physically injured was reported (Schene 1987, commenting on the Gelles & Straus survey) has implications for intervention. Are practitioners concerned only about the cases which come to light or the abusive behaviour *per se*? Gelles & Straus (1987) quote Erikson's theory that 'the number of acts of deviance that come to community attention is a function of the size and complexity of the community's social control apparatus – in this case, the child protection system'. There is increasing concern (Dingwall 1989, Parton & Parton 1989) that social control is taking over from social support in the child welfare services. Child protection is taking increasing priority over child care. As more and more resources are put into increasing the size and complexity of the child protection system, and hence identifying more 'cases', there seem to be fewer resources available for the treatment and monitoring of these identified cases. There is a worrying dearth of research and evaluation studies into the effectiveness of the various forms of intervention in child abuse and neglect cases both in the UK and the USA. As Starr (1990) argues, 'Without such studies we cannot determine the effectiveness of treatment and prevention efforts that, while well intended, may have no effects on the participating parents and children, or, worse still, may have unintended negative consequences.'

Child protection practitioners are compelled to intervene in identified cases of child abuse and neglect for largely negative reasons. These include the social control system within which they work, the fear that if they do not intervene the child will die or be seriously damaged, and the longer-term adverse effects on the abused child deprived of treatment.

These are powerful motivators for action, though contrary to the general ethos of help and support that brought many practitioners into the child welfare services. The available evidence from the prevalence, incidence and other studies is not encouraging. It implies that the more the child protection system is expanded, the more cases of child abuse and neglect will come to official recognition. Intervention, tragically (e.g. Jasmine Beckford, Tyra Henry), does not always save a child's life. The findings on the long-term effects of child abuse and neglect are equivocal. Prevalence studies on general populations reveal large numbers of adults, abused as children, who appear not to have suffered long-term adverse consequences. Similarly, follow-up studies of abused children (Toro 1982, Finkelhor 1988, Kendall-Tackett *et al.* 1993) have found that about a third of the victims show no symptoms of abuse in the short-term, and larger numbers none in the longer term. Socio-economic status and related factors may be more important than abuse in determining the course of child development. More research needs to be conducted into those factors which protect individual children, and which are the cases of abused and neglected children and their families where practitioners can most usefully intervene. Practitioners should also be lobbying for a radical re-appraisal of the child protection system, to assess whether it provides the most effective use of human and financial resources, e.g. the programme of research funded by the DOH and summarised in their publication *Child Protection: Messages from Research* (DOH 1995). Gelles & Straus (1987), speculating about the reasons behind the decrease in incidence rates over the 10 years 1975–1985, suggest that changes in attitudes and cultural norms regarding the social acceptability of family violence may have led to changes in overt behaviour. Public education campaigns play a vital role in attempting to change such attitudes.

The wide differences between the reported rates and types of abuse in the different countries also have implications for practitioners. Is the USA intrinsically more abusive to its children than such European countries as the UK and the Netherlands, as the relative reporting rates would suggest? Or does mandatory reporting, a massive public education programme and nationally available treatment programmes lead to a narrowing of the gap between actual and reported incidence? There have been no incidence studies similar to those of Gelles and Straus conducted in the UK which could throw light on underlying incidence rates here. Pieterse & Van Urk (1989) advocated mandatory reporting in the Netherlands in an attempt to reduce the discrepancy between the two countries' reported rates. Would mandatory reporting in the UK lead to more reports than the present non-mandatory inter-agency collaboration? Although UK professionals are not statutorily required to report cases of child abuse, most of them have some reporting duty written into their codes of ethics. Not to report a case would be an exception in the UK. In the USA, with mandatory reporting, the National Committee for Prevention of Child Abuse found a 40% substantiation rate for reports in 1992 (McCurdy & Daro 1993). In the UK, with a non-statutory system of referring, only 15% of child protection referrals in eight local authority social services departments in 1991 were subsequently registered (Gibbons *et al*. 1995). A non-statutory system does not seem to lead to a decrease in initial referrals in relation to final registration.

The UK differed from the USA in the 1980s and early 1990s in registering so few cases of neglect, and from the Netherlands in the small number of cases of emotional abuse registered. The fact that Child Protection Registers were initially Non-Accidental Injury Registers until 1980 may have led to a professional bias towards physical abuse in the UK at the expense of other forms of abuse. Gibbons *et al*. (1995) found that only 7% of the cases initially referred for neglect reached the register and most were screened out of the system at an early stage, usually without the offer of other services. Very few cases of emotional abuse were referred initially. The child protection system in the UK is a very reactive one, designed to rescue children in immediate danger and, as such, unsuited to the more insidious effects of neglect or emotional abuse. Neglected and emotionally abused children may not be in immediate need of protection but they are nevertheless 'in need'. Practitioners should be aware of, and be responsive to, those needs. The recent increases in registrations for both neglect and emotional abuse (DOH 2000) could be indicative of such responsiveness.

Finally, practitioners need to be aware of the methodological factors underlying the various published studies of child abuse and neglect incidence and prevalence. In child protection, practitioners walk a tightrope between either too much (e.g. Cleveland) or too little (e.g. Kimberley Carlile) intervention in the public's mind. In choosing either to intervene or not to intervene in a particular case, they need to be able to speak authoritatively about the population base they are drawing from. How rare is this particular type and severity of abuse in the general population? Does this case share any of the characteristics of cases identified in the most rigorous studies? Might various biases be operating in the reporting or ascertainment of this case? The more aware practitioners are of these factors, the more likely they are to make a convincing case for either intervention or non-intervention.

Summary

This chapter has looked at the five levels of public and professional awareness of child abuse and neglect on which any estimate of the frequency of the problem will be based. The UK is at the first levels of official reporting of cases of child abuse and neglect in its incidence figures.

The incidence and prevalence studies reviewed have shown wide variations, between and within countries, in the rates of child maltreatment reported and the different types of child abuse. A large part of these differences may be due to the methods employed in the studies, in particular the definitions used and possible sources of bias. A broad definition of abuse, say sexual abuse not involving contact, will ascertain many more cases than one involving only contact or penetrative acts. With any socially deviant act, particularly one that attracts the moral opprobrium that child abuse and neglect does, the possible sources of bias increase. Social class, ethnicity, perceived status, experience and the characteristics of the children themselves are all factors that can lead to bias in the recognition, reporting and registering, or substantiation, of cases of child abuse and neglect.

The methodological factors of generalisability and comparability of prevalence and incidence studies are particularly important for practitioners. It is against these that they have to weigh up their own individual referrals and decide whether, or to what extent, they should intervene.

Examination of the changes in incidence and prevalence rates of child maltreatment over time have shown increases in reported cases, decreases in the incidence of physical abuse and no change in the prevalence of child sexual abuse. Possible reasons for the discrepancies between these findings are discussed. The role of public education and a change in public attitudes towards violence within families, and their effect in reducing the incidence of physical abuse of children, is stressed.

The gap between actual and reported cases has important implications for practitioners, as has the somewhat negative controlling ethos of current child protection practices. Practitioners can feel helpless in the face of an ever increasing number of child maltreatment referrals and the possible consequences of not intervening. Incidence and prevalence studies provide a picture of the underlying base rate of maltreatment and the characteristics of the abused population. Research is needed into identifying those children and families where intervention is vital and those which can be diverted into less controlling and more supportive systems.

Conclusions

In the UK, the television companies – the BBC's Childwatch and Channel 4's MORI poll – were the agencies first concerned with finding out the underlying frequency of child abuse. They were the first studies to attempt to discover how many children nationally had been abused (the prevalence rate). The prevalence they were concerned with was that of child sexual abuse. Other prevalence studies, also of child sexual abuse, have been on nationally unrepresentative samples such as GP patients or college students. Incidence studies in the UK have been drawn entirely from cases of child abuse and neglect reported each year. The evidence from studies in the USA and Canada indicates that actual rates of abuse are much higher. Research should be conducted in the UK to ascertain what is the gap between actual and reported cases of abuse. The NSPCC has commissioned two national prevalence studies of abuse. The first (Creighton & Russell 1995) looked at childhood physical and sexual abuse, and the second (NSPCC 2000) at all four types of abuse: physical, sexual, emotional and neglect. An incidence study of physically abusive parental behaviour, similar to that of the Family Violence Research Program in the USA, should also be conducted in the UK.

The increases in reported incidence rates over the years, accompanied in recent years by the recession and cutbacks in local authority resources, have led to child protection taking increasing priority over child care. It is to be hoped that the Children Act 1989, with its emphasis on providing services for all children in need, will help to reverse this trend. Neglected and emotionally abused children, who are as equally needly as physically and sexually abused children, tend to get disproportionately filtered out of the child protection system in the UK but with no compensating services. A revised system, focusing on children in need and not just on those in need of immediate protection, is more likely to tackle the adverse effects of child abuse and neglect.

Annotated further reading

Creighton S J 1992 Child abuse trends in England and Wales 1988–1990 and an overview from 1973–1990. NSPCC, London
Provides an overview of the trends in registered cases of child abuse and neglect in the UK over 18 years. It also examines the characteristics of the different types of abuse, the children, their parents, suspected perpetrators and families in addition to the management of the cases.
Creighton S J, Russell N 1995 Voices from childhood. A survey of childhood experiences and attitudes to child rearing among adults in the United Kingdom. NSPCC, London
Provides data on a nationally representative sample of adults' childhood experiences including physical and sexual abuse and attitudes to acceptable and unacceptable parental disciplinary methods.
Department of Health (DOH) 1995 Child protection: messages from research. HMSO, London
Provides an overview of research on the child protection system in England including summaries of the individual projects.
Finkelhor D 1994 The international epidemiology of child sexual abuse. Child Abuse and Neglect 18 (5): 409–417
Provides an overview of child sexual abuse surveys in 21 countries.
Kelly L, Regan L, Burton S 1991 An exploratory study of the prevalence of sexual abuse in a sample of 16–21-year-olds. PNL: Child Abuse Studies Unit, London
Provides an extremely useful breakdown of prevalence rates by different definitions of sexual abuse.
Markowe H 1988 The frequency of child sexual abuse in the UK. Health Trends 20 (1): 2–6.
Provides a concise survey of UK sexual abuse frequency studies and detailed consideration of their methodological weaknesses.
Pilkington B, Kremer J 1995 A review of the epidemiological research on child sexual abuse: community and college student samples. Child Abuse Review 4 (2): 84–98
Provides a summary of prevalence studies on child sexual abuse in community samples from the 1920s to 1990.
Research Team 1990 Child sexual abuse in Northern Ireland. Greystoke Books, Antrim
Provides a detailed report on the methodology of mounting a national incidence study and details of the cases ascertained.

References

Anderson J, Martin J, Mullen P, Romans S, Herbison P 1993 Prevalence of childhood sexual abuse experiences in a community sample of women. Journal of the American Academy of Child and Adolescent Psychiatry 32 (5): 911–919
Association of Directors of Social Services (ADSS) 1987 Child abuse: incidence of registrations for child abuse between 1985 and 1986 (Press Release). Berkshire Social Services Department
Badgley R F, Allard H A, McCormick N, *et al.* 1984 Sexual offences against children, Vol. 1. Report of the Committee on Sexual Offences Against Children and Youths. Minister of Supply and Services, Ottawa, Canada
Baker A W, Duncan S P 1985 Child sexual abuse: a study of prevalence in Great Britain. Child Abuse and Neglect 9: 453–467
BBC 1986 Childwatch – overview of results from 2530 self-completion questionnaires. BBC Broadcasting Research (unpublished)
BBC 1987 Childwatch – national survey on child abuse. BBC Press Briefing, 9 July
Berger A M, Knutsen J F, Mehm J G, Perkins K A 1988 The self-report of punitive childhood experiences of young adults and adolescents. Child Abuse and Neglect 12 (2): 251–262

Broadbent A, Bentley R 1997 Child abuse and neglect Australia 1995–1996. Canberra: Australian Institute of Health and Welfare, cat no. CWS 1 (Child Welfare Series no. 17)

Butler-Sloss L J E 1988 The report of the inquiry into child abuse in Cleveland 1987. HMSO, London

Central Statistical Office 1993 Social Trends 23, 1993 Edn. HMSO, London

Creighton S J 1992 Child abuse trends in England and Wales 1988–1990 and an overview from 1973–1990. NSPCC, London

Creighton S J, Noyes P 1989 Child abuse trends in England and Wales 1983–1987. NSPCC, London

Creighton S J, Russell N 1995 Voices from childhood. A survey of childhood experiences and attitudes to child rearing among adults in the United Kingdom. NSPCC, London

Daro D 1996 Current trends in child abuse reporting and fatalities: NCPA's 1995 annual fifty-state survey. APSAC Advisor 9 (2): 21–24

Daro D, Mitchel L 1990 Current trends in child abuse reporting and fatalities: the results of the 1989 annual fifty-state survey. Working Paper No. 808. National Center on Child Abuse Prevention Research, Chicago

Department of Health (DOH) 1989 Survey of children and young persons on Child Protection Registers. Year Ending 31 March 1988 – England. Government Statistical Service, London

Department of Health (DOH) 1995 Child protection: messages from research. HMSO, London

Department of Health (DOH) 2000 Children and young people on Child Protection Registers. Year ending 31 March 2000 – England. Personal Social Services Local Authority Statistics. National Statistics, London

Department of Health and Social Security (DHSS) 1974 Non-accidental injury to children. Local Authority Social Services Letter (74), (13)

Department of Health and Social Security, Welsh Office 1988 Working together: a guide to arrangements for inter-agency cooperation for the protection of children from abuse. HMSO, London

Dingwall R 1989 Some problems about predicting child abuse and neglect. In: Stevenson O (ed) Child abuse: professional practice and public policy. Harvester Wheatsheaf, Herts, ch 2

Eckenrode J, Munsch J, Powers J, Doris J 1988 The nature and substantiation of official sexual abuse reports. Child Abuse and Neglect 12 (3): 311–319

Feldman W, Feldman E, Goodman J T, *et al.* 1991 Is childhood sexual abuse really increasing in prevalence? An analysis of the evidence. Pediatrics 88 (1): 29–33

Finkelhor D 1979 Sexually victimized children. Free Press, New York

Finkelhor D 1988 Initial and long-term effects of child sexual abuse. Paper at SRIP Conference, Leeds

Finkelhor D, Hotaling G, Lewis I A, Smith C 1990 Sexual abuse in a national survey of adult men and women: prevalence, characteristics and risk factors. Child Abuse and Neglect 14 (1): 19–28

Gelles R J, Straus M A 1987 Is violence toward children increasing? A comparison of 1975 and 1985 national survey rates. Journal of Interpersonal Violence 2: 212–222

Gibbons J, Conroy S, Bell C 1995 Operating the child protection system. HMSO, London

Giller H, Gormley C, Williams P 1992 The effectiveness of child protection procedures. An evaluation of child protection procedures in four ACPC areas. Social Information Systems Ltd

Halperin D S, Bouvier P, Jaffe P D, *et al.* 1996 Prevalence of child sexual abuse among adolescents in Geneva: results of a cross-sectional survey. British Medical Journal 312: 1326–1329

Home Office 2000 Criminal statistics: England and Wales 1998. Cmnd 4649 The Stationery Office, London

Home Office, Department of Health, Department of Education and Science, Welsh Office 1991 Working together under the Children Act 1989: a guide to arrangements for inter-agency cooperation for the protection of children from abuse. HMSO, London

Hong G K, Hong L K 1991 Comparative perspectives on child abuse and neglect: Chinese vs. Hispanics and Whites. Child Welfare 70 (4): 463–475

Kaplan M J, Becker J V, Tenke C E 1991 Influence of abuse history on male adolescent self-reported comfort with interviewer gender. Journal of Interpersonal Violence 6 (1): 3–11

Kelly L, Regan L, Burton S 1991 An exploratory study of the prevalence of sexual abuse in a sample of 16–21-year-olds. PNL: Child Abuse Studies Unit, London

Kendall-Tackett K A, Williams L M, Finkelhor D 1993 Impact of sexual abuse on children: a review and synthesis of recent empirical studies. Psychological Bulletin 113 (1): 164–180

Kinsey A C, Pomeroy W B, Martin C E, Gebhard P H 1953 Sexual behaviour in the human female. W B Saunders, Philadelphia, Pennsylvania

McCurdy K, Daro D 1993 Current trends in child abuse reporting and fatalities: the results of the 1992 annual fifty-state survey. National Center on Child Abuse Research, Working Paper No. 808. NCPCA, Chicago

Markowe H L J 1988 The frequency of child sexual abuse in the UK. Health Trends 20 (1): 2–6. HMSO, London

Markowe H L J 1991 Epidemiological assessment of studies of child abuse. Paper given at BASPCAN conference 'Turning Research into Practice', Leicester

McMillan H L, Fleming J E, Trocme N, *et al.* 1997 Prevalence of child physical and sexual abuse in the community. Journal of the American Medical Association 278 (2): 131–135

Nash C L, West D J 1985 Sexual molestation of young girls. In: West D J (ed) Sexual victimisation. Gower, Aldershot

NSPCC 2000 Prevalence of abuse among young adults in the United Kingdom (provisional title)

Nunno M 1992 The abuse of children in out-of-home care. Paper given at Conference on Institutional Abuse. NSPCC, London

O'Toole R, Turbett P, Nalepka C 1983 Theories, professional knowledge and diagnosis of child abuse. In: The dark side of families. Sage, Beverly Hills, ch 22

Parton C, Parton N 1989 Child protection: the law and dangerousness. In: Stevenson O (ed) Child abuse: professional practice and public policy. Harvester Wheatsheaf, Herts, ch 3

Pieterse J J, Van Urk H 1989 Maltreatment of children in the Netherlands: an update after ten years. Child Abuse and Neglect 13: 263–269

Research Team 1990 Child sexual abuse in Northern Ireland. Greystoke Books, Antrim

Russell D E 1983 The incidence and prevalence of intrafamilial and extrafamilial sexual abuse of female children. Child Abuse and Neglect 7: 133–146

Sariola H, Uutela A 1994 The prevalence of child sexual abuse in Finland. Child Abuse and Neglect 18 (10): 827–835

Schene P 1987 Is child abuse decreasing? Commentary on Gelles and Straus paper. Journal of Interpersonal Violence 2: 225–227

Scottish Executive 1999 Child protection statistics for the years ended 31st March 1997 and 1998. Government Statistical Service, Edinburgh

Sedlak A J 1990 Technical amendment to the study findings: national incidence and prevalence of child abuse and neglect: 1988. Westat, Inc.

Siegal J M, Sorenson S B, Golding J M, *et al.* 1987 The prevalence of childhood sexual assault: the Los Angeles epidemiologic catchment area project. American Journal of Epidemiology 126: 1141–1153

Starr R H 1990 The need for child maltreatment research and program evaluation. Journal of Family Violence 5 (4): 311–319

Stevenson O 1989 Multidisciplinary work in child protection. In: Stevenson O (ed) Child abuse: professional practice and public policy. Harvester Wheatsheaf, Herts, ch 8

Straus M A 1979 Family patterns and child abuse in a nationally representative American sample. Child Abuse and Neglect 3 (1): 213–225

Straus M A, Gelles R J 1986 Societal change and change in family violence from 1975 to 1985 as revealed by two national surveys. Journal of Marriage and the Family 48: 465–479

Straus M A, Hamby S L, Finkelhor D, *et al.* 1998 Identification of child maltreatment with the parent–child conflict tactics scales: development and psychometric data for a national sample of American parents. Child Abuse and Neglect 22 (4): 249–270

Toro P A 1982 Developmental effects of child abuse: a review. Child Abuse and Neglect 6: 423–431

Trocme N, McPhee D, Tam K K, Hay T 1994 Ontario incidence study of reported child abuse and neglect. The Institute for the Prevention of Child Abuse, Toronto

Turner C F, Ku L, Rogers S M, *et al.* 1998 Adolescent sexual behaviour, drug use, and violence: increased reporting with computer survey technology. Science 280 (5365): 867–873

US Department of Health and Human Services 1988 Study findings. Study of national incidence and prevalence of child abuse and neglect. National Center on Child Abuse and Neglect, Washington, DC

US Department of Health and Human Services 1996 The Third National Incidence Study of child abuse and neglect (NIS-3). National Center on Child Abuse and Neglect, Washington

Welsh Office 1999 Child Protection Register: statistics for Wales, 1999. Government Statistical Service, Cardiff

Wind T W, Silvern L 1992 Type and extent of child abuse as predictors of adult functioning. Journal of Family Violence 7 (4): 261–281

Zimrin H 1986 A profile of survival. Child Abuse and Neglect 10 (3): 339–349

3

Child abuse: defining, understanding and intervening

Kevin Browne

INTRODUCTION

Child abuse and neglect is one of the most common causes of death in young children in the UK today. It has been claimed that at least two children under 16 years die of non-accidental injury every week (Home Office 1991) with parents and relatives being responsible for three-quarters of the deaths (Central Statistical Office 1994). These grim statistics highlight the fact that not enough is being done to protect children in our society, as exemplified by the increasing number of families maltreating children without social work support (Browne & Lynch 1994). As a result, many children are growing up physically and emotionally scarred for life.

The extent and definition of child abuse

In the book *Early Prediction and Prevention of Child Abuse* (Davies & Stratton 1988), three major forms of child maltreatment are identified: physical, sexual and psychological or emotional abuse. Each type of maltreatment is characterised into 'active' and 'passive' forms (Table 3.1). Active abuse involves violent acts that represent the exercise of physical force so as to cause injury or forcibly interfere with personal freedom. Passive abuse refers to neglect, which can only be considered violent in the metaphorical sense, as it does not involve physical force. Nevertheless, it can cause both physical and emotional injury, such as non-organic failure to thrive in young children (Browne 1993). However, victims of child maltreatment are unlikely to be subjected to only one type of abuse. For example, sexual abuse and physical abuse are always accompanied by emotional abuse, which includes verbal assault, threats of sexual or physical abuse, close confinement (such as locking a child in a room), withholding food and other aversive treatment. Within each type of abuse there is a continuum of severity ranging from mild to life-threatening (Browne & Herbert 1997).

Since 1989, the Department of Health (DOH) has accurately assessed each year the number of children and young persons on Child Protection Registers in

Table 3.1
Two-way classification of abuse with examples of major forms

	Physical	Psychological	Sexual
Active	Non-accidental injury Poisoning	Emotional abuse Denigration and humiliation	Incest Assault and rape
Passive	Non-organic failure to thrive, poor health care and physical neglect	Emotional neglect Lack of affection	Failure to protect Prostitution

(Adapted from Browne *et al.* 1988, p. 293.)

England. The estimates are based on annual statistical returns from 150 Local Government Authorities. Figure 3.1 shows the rate per 10 000 children for those currently on the register at 31 March 2000 and the number of children registered during the past year, by various age groups (DOH 2000). The overall rate was 27 children per 10 000 under 18 years of age. The highest rates were found in very young children under 1 years (71 per 10 000). The likelihood of being on the registers then decreases with age. Therefore, 70% of children on registers are aged under 10 years. Boys and girls are equally represented in all age groups. However, girls account for 60% of those registered for 'sexual abuse'. Thus, boys on the register are younger and represent 53% of those registered for 'physical injury'. Indeed, NSPCC figures show that over 80% of the physical abuse most likely to cause death or handicap (i.e. head injury) occurs to children aged younger than 5 with an over-representation of boys. Over half of all head injuries occur to infants aged less than 1 year (Creighton & Noyes 1989, Creighton 1992).

The definitions of child abuse recommended as criteria for registration throughout England and Wales by the Home Office, the Departments of Health, Education and Science, and Welsh Office (Home Office *et al.* 1991) in their joint document *Working Together under the Children Act 1989* (pp. 48–49) are as follows.

Neglect

The persistent or severe neglect of a child or the failure to protect a child from exposure to any kind of danger, including cold and starvation or extreme failure to carry out important aspects of care, resulting in the significant impairment of the child's health or development, including non-organic failure to thrive.

Physical injury

Actual or likely physical injury to a child, or failure to prevent physical injury (or suffering) to a child, including deliberate poisoning, suffocation and Munchausen's syndrome by proxy.

Figure 3.1
Rates of registrations to Child Protection Registers during the year ending 31 March 2000 and rates on the Register at that date, by age (rate per 10 000 population in each age group)

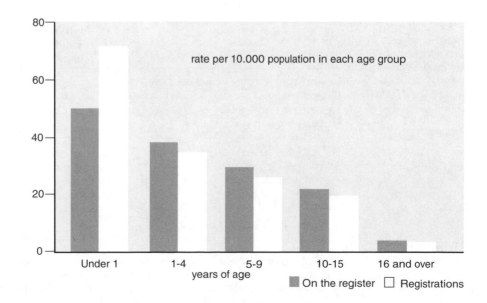

Sexual abuse

Actual or likely sexual exploitation of a child or adolescent. The child may be dependent and/or developmentally immature.*

Emotional abuse

Actual or likely severe adverse effect on the emotional and behavioural development of a child caused by persistent or severe emotional ill-treatment or rejection. All abuse involves some emotional ill-treatment. This category is used where it is the main or sole form of abuse.

All the above categories are used for both intrafamilial and extrafamilial abuse and neglect, perpetuated by someone inside or outside the child's home. Mixed categories are also recorded, which register more than one type of abuse and/or neglect occurring to a child. This is especially important when considering 'organised abuse', which is defined in the same document (Home Office *et al.* 1991, p. 38) as: 'Abuse which may involve a number of abusers, a number of abused children and young people and often encompass different forms of abuse. It involves, to a greater or lesser extent an element of organisation'. For further discussion on the definition of 'organised abuse', see La Fontaine (1993).

Local authorities in England record each child on their Protection Register in only one of the eight categories presented in Table 3.2, choosing the one that provides the most accurate picture of the situation.

Overall, 14 600 girls and 15 400 boys in England were considered to require protection from maltreatment on 31 March 2000, together with 300 unborn children, and nearly one in four (20%) of them were 'looked after' by local authorities (in care). Of the 7 100 children in care on 31 March 2000, 70% were placed with foster parents, 7% were living in children's homes, 18% were placed with parents and 5% in other types of placement (DOH 2000).

Similar registration rates for child abuse and neglect (30 in 10 000) of children were reported previously by the NSPCC (Creighton & Noyes 1989, Creighton 1992). Furthermore, the NSPCC claims that its figures for reported physical and sexual abuse were not increasing (Creighton 1992). The Department of Health also shows a slight decreased in the number of registrations and to a small

Table 3.2
Percentages and rates of registrations by categories of child abuse under which they were recorded during the year ending 31 March 2000 (n = 29 300).

	Number of children under 18	Percent %	Rate per 10 000
Neglect, physical injury and sexual abuse	300	1	<1
Neglect and physical injury	1 900	6	2
Neglect and sexual abuse	600	2	1
Physical injury and sexual abuse	600	2	1
Neglect (alone)	10 100	35	9
Physical injury (alone)	6 700	23	6
Sexual abuse (alone)	3 600	12	3
Emotional abuse (alone)	4 800	17	4
Unknown*	600	1	<1
Total	29 300	100	26

(Adapted from Department of Health 2000)

*'Unknown', refers to categories used but not recommended by *Working Together* (DOH 1991) or no category available.

*Sexual exploitation represents the involvement of dependent, developmentally immature children and adolescents in sexual activities they do not truly comprehend, to which they are unable to give informed consent or that violate social taboos of family roles (Kempe & Kempe 1978).

increase in the number of deregistrations from 1999 to 2000 (DOH 1999). During the year, 14% of registrations involved children who had been previously registered and perhaps taken off the register prematurely.

Thus, it is not surprising that a report of a particularly nasty incident of sexual abuse or cruelty to an infant or a child murder often makes its way onto the front pages of our daily newspapers, then to a special inquiry and back again to the media. After much painful analysis and discussion, an attempt is made to discover where 'procedures' for managing cases have broken down.

There is a need to recognise the fact that it is not the 'procedures' but parents' social circumstances, attitudes and behaviour that need to be changed in order to prevent children being impetuously attacked. If these facts were faced honestly, education and training could be offered to parents who are unable to cope. This might actually prevent the recurrence, if not occurrence, of child maltreatment. A recent study (Hamilton & Browne 1999) has shown that 27% of cases of child abuse referred to police child protection units are already known to the police authorities on account of previous injury to the child under review. Repeat victimisation is a common finding throughout the child abuse literature, yet it is one apparently little appreciated by those who intervene in child-abusing families (Hamilton & Browne 1998). Nevertheless, the prevention of child maltreatment must be based on a comprehensive understanding of the causes of child abuse and neglect.

Causes of child abuse and neglect

In seeking to understand the many causal factors involved in child abuse and neglect, several theoretical models have been proposed. However, some researchers distinguish between acts of physical violence and other forms of abuse because the causes and their potential solutions are different (see Frude 1989, 1991). While all harmful acts have some causes in common, other factors are unique to physical abuse and neglect. It may be suggested that the following outline is related more to physical maltreatment. However, poverty, social isolation, family breakdown and poor parent–child relationships are associated with all forms of child abuse and neglect and have been cited as risk factors for child sexual abuse (Finkelhor 1980, Bergner *et al.* 1994). Furthermore, a third of sexually abused children have been previously physically abused (Finkelhor & Baron 1986), indicating that a number of common factors are involved.

Social and environmental focused models

Social stress perspective

Studies of abusing families (e.g. Garbarino 1977, Krugman 1986, Browne & Saqi 1988*a*) have shown that factors such as low wages, unemployment, poor housing, overcrowding, isolation and alienating work conditions are associated with child maltreatment. Such factors are seen by Gelles (1987) and Gelles & Cornell (1997) as causing frustration and stress at the individual level, which in turn may lead to violence in the home. Gelles concluded from his research that 'violence is an adaptation or response to structural stress'. However, since physical abuse of children is not confined to families in the lower socio-economic groups but is spread across the entire class spectrum, this interpretation may be questioned. Nevertheless, it is suggested that social and environmental stress factors may have a greater influence on child maltreatment in lower class families than in middle-class families. Higher socio-economic groups may be more susceptible to individual factors that influence child abuse and neglect, such as psychological disturbance, alcohol and drug abuse. For all social classes, Gelles' (1983) 'exchange theory' proposes that the private nature of the family home reduces the 'costs' of behaving aggressively, in terms of official sanction. This results in a higher probability of violence in the home, where there are fewer social constraints on aggressive emotional expression. Thus, family 'privacy' makes child abuse less detectable and easier to commit (Browne 1988, Straus *et al.* 1988, Browne & Herbert 1997).

Environmental and cultural perspective

An alternative approach, but one that is also couched in terms of the social position of the people involved, can be referred to as the micropolitical view. This holds that individual violence is a microcosm of the power relations in the wider society. For example, a common feminist explanation of violence towards women and children is to view it as a function of their generally oppressed position in society. Within this framework, the purpose of male violence is seen as to control other family members (Gilbert 1994).

The broadest sociological perspective (Gil 1970, 1978, Straus 1980, Goldstein 1986, Levine 1986) holds that cultural values, the availability of weapons and the exposure to unpunished models of aggression affect personal attitudes towards violent behaviour. These, in turn, influence an individual's acceptance and learning of aggression as a form of emotional expression and as a method of control over others. Within British and American societies, it would appear that violence in the family home is considered to be less reprehensible than violence outside it. There is a general acceptance of physical punishment as an appropriate method of child control, with nine out of ten children being disciplined in this way (Gelles & Cornell 1997, Nobes & Smith 2000).

Individually focused models

This perspective concentrates on individual personality characteristics, often of a psychopathological or deviant nature. This research tradition is characterised by the use of rating scales to measure aggressiveness and hostility (e.g. Buss & Durkee 1957, Novaco 1978, Edmunds & Kendrick 1980) and the study of biological variables which underlie a tendency to be violent.

Other authors have attempted to establish a causal connection between testosterone levels and violence (Persky *et al.* 1971) and the identification of specific pathological conditions, such as alcoholism, which are likely to be predisposing or determining factors in violent behaviour (Gerson 1978, Steinglass 1987).

The psychopathic perspective

This focuses on the abnormal characteristics and psychological dysfunctions of abusing adults. Based on the theories of Freud (1964), Dollard *et al.* (1939) and Lorenz (1966) to explain aggression, the emphasis of psychiatry is on a psychodynamic approach to the abuser's 'abnormal death instinct' or 'excessive drive' for aggressive behaviour. This is seen as the result of genetic make-up and adverse socialisation experiences that produce a 'psychopathic' character with a predisposition to behave violently, especially when 'frustrated'.

One form of this predisposition is referred to as 'transference psychosis' (Galdston 1965). This involves transference from parent to child. For example: the parent often interprets the child as if they were an adult and perceives the child as hostile and persecuting, projecting that part of their own personality they wish to destroy (Steele & Pollock 1968). Thus, the child is seen as the cause of the parent's troubles and becomes a scapegoat towards which all anger is directed (Wasserman *et al.* 1983). However, Kempe & Kempe (1978) suggested that only 10% of child abusers can accurately be labelled as mentally ill. Nevertheless, this model has been useful in recognising certain predispositions of abusive individuals. These include a tendency to have distorted perceptions of their children (Rosenberg & Reppucci 1983), difficulty dealing with aggressive impulses as a result of being impulsively immature, self-centred, often depressed, and possibly having a history of having been abused, neglected or witnessing violence as children (Wolfe 1991).

The social learning perspective

This provides an alternative form of individual explanation to biological or psychodynamic determinism. More than 40 years ago, Schultz (1960) claimed that the source of violence in a family context lies in unfulfilled childhood experiences. Gayford (1975) later carried out research in conjunction with Chiswick Women's Aid and attempted to show the learned character of domestic violence within the family of origin.

This approach is based on the assumption that people learn violent behaviour from observing aggressive role models (Bandura 1973). In support of this argument, Roy (1982) has stated that four out of five abusive men (*n* = 4000) were reported by their partners as either observing their fathers abusing their mothers and/or being a victim of child abuse themselves. In comparison, only a third of the abused partners had witnessed or had been victims of parental violence as a child. Findings from many other studies have supported this observation of the intergenerational transmission of violent behaviour (Browne 1993, 1994).

There is evidence that violence between parents affects the children in a family (Jaffe *et al.* 1990, Carroll 1994). The behaviour and psychiatric problems discovered in children of violent marriages include truancy, aggressive behaviour at home and school, and anxiety disorders (Hughes & Barad 1983, Jaffe *et al.* 1986, Davis & Carlson 1987). It is suggested that such children learn aversive behaviour as a general style for controlling their social and physical environments, and this style continues into adulthood (Gully & Dengerink 1983, Browne & Saqi 1987).

The special victim perspective

In direct contrast with the viewpoints considered so far are suggestions that the victims themselves may be instrumental in some way in eliciting attack or neglect. Friedrich & Boroskin (1976) review the complex reasons why a child may not fulfill the parent's expectations or demands. The child may in some way be regarded as 'special'. For example, studies have found prematurity, low birth weight, illness and handicap to be associated with child abuse (Elmer & Gregg 1967, Lynch & Roberts 1977, Starr 1988). Indeed, it has been pointed out that the physical unattractiveness of these children may be an important factor for child abuse (Berkowitz 1989).

A link between the social learning and special victim perspectives has been suggested by Lewis (1987), who claims that some women learn to accept violent behaviour towards themselves as a result of childhood experiences.

Interaction focused models

Some researchers have advocated a more interactive approach that includes the social relationships of the participants and their environmental setting, rather than seeking to isolate the person or situation. This entails a move from the individual psychological level to a study of social interactions between members of the family.

The interpersonal interactive perspective

Toch (1969), for example, in his study entitled *Violent Men* looked not only at the characteristics of these men but also at the context of their violence and the characteristics of their victims. He concluded that aggressive behaviour was associated with 'machismo' and the maintenance of a particular personal identity in relation to others.

The person–environment interactive perspective

Frude (1980) puts forward the notion of a causal chain leading to 'critical incidence' of child abuse. This is a function of complex interactions between the individual and their social and physical environments. The 'critical incidence model' of child abuse is presented in Figure 3.2 and can be described as follows.

1. Environmental stress situations, which are usually long-term, such as poverty, influence domestic abusers to assess their personal situations differently from non-abusing family members (i.e. as threatening).
2. They perceive a discrepancy between their expectations for life and social interactions and what they actually see happening. This often results in feelings of frustration for the person.
3. Anger and emotional distress are likely as a response to these situations rather than problem-solving strategies for change.

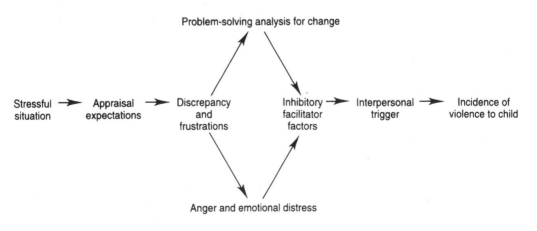

Figure 3.2
The critical incidence model of child abuse (adapted and modified from Frude 1980).

4. Lack of inhibitions with regard to violent expression, together with a lower threshold of tolerance, increases the possibility for violence. This is of course enhanced by disinhibitors such as alcohol or drugs.
5. Under the above conditions, even a facial expression (perceived as a dirty look) can lead to, or trigger, an incidence of violence.

These causal links result in the caregiver being more easily provoked to take violent action. Frude (1991) challenges the assumption that 'abusers' differ from 'non-abusers' and suggested that they might be more usefully considered as points on a continuum. For this reason, he argued that studies of interactions in the family may have much to contribute towards our understanding of domestic violence and child abuse and neglect. Frude's causal chain model demonstrates the need to assess a violent person's understanding of the environment. Their perceptions, attitudes and attributions will all influence the possibility of overt aggressive behaviour. In relation to violent behaviour, Browne & Howells (1996) have developed the work of Novaco (1978) on anger arousal. This work emphasises the role played by cognitive processes, such as appraisal and expectations of external events, in evoking an aggressive response.

Recently, there has been a move away from accounting for violence in the family purely in terms of individual psychopathology towards models that attempt to integrate the characteristics of abusing parents, their children and the situation in which they live. Child abuse and neglect cannot be explained by a single factor, it is a consequence of complex interactions between individual, social and environmental influences (see Belsky 1988, Browne 1989a, Browne & Herbert 1997).

Integrated models

The different explanations for the causes of violence towards children and other family members have been useful in that together they have served to emphasise the diverse nature of the variables involved in child abuse and neglect. Simple explanations make the solution to this pervasive problem appear easy. For example, the 'demon rum' explanation of physical and sexual violence towards women and children is an old and popular one (Gelles & Cornell 1997). It is true that alcohol appears to exacerbate pre-existing impulse control and emotional problems, thus increasing the likelihood of serious injuries (Coleman 1980). This seems to be especially the case in the evening, at weekends and on holiday, when children and couples are alone with their problems and are relaxing with alcoholic drink (Frude 1991).

However, the majority of alcohol-abusing individuals who are violent to members of their family when drinking heavily also admit that they have been violent while not under the influence of alcohol (Sonkin *et al.* 1985). Therefore, alcohol abuse is neither a necessary nor sufficient condition for violent behaviour.

Heavy drinking and drunkenness is not the cause of child abuse and neglect, but rather a condition that co-exists with it, like many other factors. Nevertheless, it is often used as an excuse for violent behaviour personally, socially and legally (Pahl 1985).

Psychosocial perspective

The inadequacies of single factor explanations has led to a psychosocial approach which integrates sociological and psychological explanations for family violence and child abuse. Originally proposed by American researchers (for example,

Gelles 1973), this perspective suggests that certain stress factors and adverse background influences may serve to predispose individuals to violence. As Frude (1980, 1989, 1991) suggested, violence will occur in the presence of precipitating factors, such as a child misbehaving.

It has been claimed that 'predisposing' factors may form a basis for identification of families 'at risk' of violence (e.g. Browne & Saqi 1988*a*, Browne 1989*b*, 1995*a*, 1995*b*). However, a more pertinent question is why the majority of families under stress do not abuse their children. It may be that stress will only lead to violence when adverse family interactions exist. Belsky (1988) and Browne (1989*a*) have taken this approach to child abuse. They conceptualise child maltreatment as a social–psychological phenomenon that is 'multiply determined by forces at work in the individual, the family, as well as in the community and the culture in which both the individual and the family are embedded' (Belsky 1980). Given a particular combination of factors, an interactional style develops within the family, and it is in the context of this interaction that child abuse occurs. This approach may be equally adopted to explain other forms of family violence.

Multifactor perspective

The study of social interactions and relationships can be seen as occupying a central and potentially integrating place in explaining the causes of aggression in the family. In relation to child abuse and neglect, Browne (1988, 1989*a*) presents a multifactor model which suggests that stress factors and background influences are mediated through the interpersonal relationships within the family (see Figure 3.3).

The model assumes that the 'situational stressors' are made up of the following four components:

1. Relations between caregivers – inter-marriage, marital disputes, step-parent/cohabitee or separated/single parent.
2. Relations to children – such as spacing between births, size of family, caregivers' attachments to expectations of their dependants.
3. Structural stress – poor housing, unemployment, social isolation, threats to the caregiver's authority, values and self-esteem.
4. Stress generated by the child – for example, an unwanted child; one who is incontinent, difficult to discipline, often ill, physically or mentally disabled; one who is temperamental, frequently emotional or very demanding.

The chances of these situational stressors resulting in abuse and neglect are mediated by and depend on the interactive relationships within the family. A secure relationship between family members will 'buffer' any effects of stress and facilitate coping strategies on behalf of the family (Browne 1988, 1989*a*). By contrast, insecure or anxious relationships will not 'buffer' the family under stress and 'episodic overload', such as an argument or a child misbehaving, may result in a physical or emotional attack. Browne (1988, 1989*a*) suggests that overall this will have a negative effect on the existing interpersonal relationships and reduce any 'buffering' effects still further, making it easier for stressors to overload the system once again. Hence, a positive feedback ('vicious cycle') is set up which eventually leads to 'systematic overload', where constant stress results in repeated physical and emotional assaults. This situation becomes progressively worse without intervention and could be termed 'the spiral of violence'.

In some cases, violent parents will cope with their aggressive feelings towards their child by physical or emotional neglect, to avoid causing a deliberate injury.

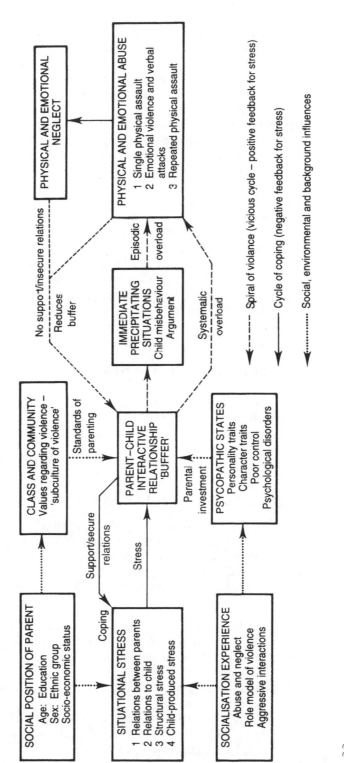

Figure 3.3
The causes of child abuse and neglect. (From Brown 1988 The nature of child abuse and neglect: an overview. In: Browne K D, Davies C, Stratton P (eds) Early prediction and prevention of child abuse. Wiley, Chichester, p. 23 (Figure 1). With kind permission from J Wiley & Sons.)

As indicated earlier, culture and community values may also affect attitudes and styles of interaction in family relationships which, in turn, will be influenced by the social position of individuals in terms of their age, sex, education, socio-economic status, ethnic group and social class background.

According to Rutter (1985), aggression is a social behaviour within everyone's repertoire, and he suggests that it is under control when the individual has high self-esteem, good relationships and stress is appropriately managed. However, the quality of relationships and responses to stress in the family will depend on the participant's personality and character traits and their pathology, such as low self-esteem, poor temperament control and psychological disorders. These may be a result of early social experiences, which may indirectly affect behavioural investment in the family.

Two main features of violent families are a lack of skill in handling conflict and discipline and high rates of aversive behaviour. These coercive family interactions have been previously described by Patterson (1982) and are seen as the primary focus for intervention.

In conclusion, it is suggested that stress factors and background influences are mediated through the interpersonal relationships within the family. Indeed, it is these relationships that should be the focus of work on prevention, treatment and management of family violence and child maltreatment. It is at this level that health and social service professionals can make a significant contribution.

Intervention strategies

Effective intervention strategies to control and prevent family violence have recently been reviewed (Willis *et al.* 1992, Gough 1994). The majority of current intervention techniques operate at the third level of treatment, i.e. after violence to the child has occurred. This is despite the fact that there are three levels of prevention (Browne & Herbert 1997).

Primary prevention: fundamental changes in society and family life

Techniques of intervention which attempt to prevent the problem before it starts are termed 'primary preventions'. These usually operate at the societal level through public awareness campaigns and advocacy groups, and then are realised by social, legal and educational processes of change. Gelles & Cornell (1990) suggest the following actions for the primary prevention of violence in the family:

1. Eliminate the norms that legitimate and glorify violence in the society and the family, such as the use of violence as a form of media entertainment.
2. Reduce violence-provoking stress created by society, such as poverty and inequality.
3. Incorporate families into a network of kin and community and reduce social isolation.
4. Change the sexist character of society by educational development.
5. Break the cycle of violence in the family by teaching alternatives to violence as a way of controlling children.

The above proposals call for fundamental changes in family life and society as a whole. If they are not unrealistic, they are at least long-term solutions.

Secondary prevention: early prediction and identification

In the short-term, intervention techniques aimed at the early identification of potential or actual violence are more realistic. This is considered to be secondary prevention and includes professionals involved in counselling, telephone helplines, home visits and clinic, health centre or hospital care. Such professionals can be instructed to screen routinely all families who come into contact with the service they are providing and identify predictive characteristics.

It is difficult to predict the chances of child abuse and neglect in the family, as some people resort to violence inconsistently while others may do so only under extreme stress. However, studies on the causes of child abuse and neglect have identified factors that are usually present when parents maltreat their children (Browne & Saqi 1988a, Browne 1995a).

Men and women are often reluctant to admit relationship problems and may feel ashamed of their own violent interactions and their abuse and neglect of their children. Predictive characteristics are helpful, therefore, in identifying the possibility of violence for both the family and the health professional. Where there is undue concern about the possibility of violence, the problem should be referred to a more appropriate agency who may fully assess the coercive relationships and adverse factors affecting the family (see Browne 1995b). Indeed, recent research has shown that there is a high association between spouse abuse and child maltreatment, and that spouse abuse is one of the most important indicators for children at high risk of abuse and neglect (Browne & Hamilton 1999).

Tertiary prevention: intervention, treatment and control of the problem

At the tertiary level of prevention, techniques are employed when child maltreatment has actually been determined. Without secondary prevention, this will only be after many repeated episodes of maltreatment have occurred and have become established in the family system. Section III of this book puts forward ideas for intervention in families where a high risk of child maltreatment has been identified, the aim being to ameliorate the adverse effects and to reduce the risk of it recurring. Even for individuals who were maltreated as children, the prognosis may be good with effective intervention (see Hall & Lloyd, Chapter 26, in this volume).

Implications for assessment and intervention

The causal factors of child abuse and neglect must be considered within the context of the family's interpersonal network. Affectionate familial relationships act as a buffer against internal and external stress (Browne & Saqi 1987, Browne 1988, 1989a). An awareness and concern for other family members characterises affectionate relationships (Browne 1986). It is important to consider maltreatment in the light of these family dynamics. Hence, intervention needs to be aimed at any negative interaction or lack of interaction between a child and their caregiver which results in harm to the child's physical and psychological development (Patterson 1982).

For all forms of child maltreatment, physical, sexual, emotional abuse and neglect, views range from the necessity of working with a family together from the earliest point of diagnosis (e.g. Bentovim 1991) to the view that work has to be focused on members of the family separately. For example, Berliner & Wheeler (1987) suggest that the sexually abused victim should be separated from the offender in the family (and the two treated independently), together with the non-abusing family members. Conjoint family work is seen only as a final step in suitable families.

There is a growing body of therapeutic experience, practice and conceptual models to help the clinician, but little empirical data on the time when it is safe and appropriate to return the child to the home of an abusing family. The assessment of families in terms of the danger of repeated physical and sexual assault to the child will be outlined and discussed.

Assessing violent families: how safe is the child?

There are five important aspects to consider when assessing violent parent–child relationships (Browne 1995a):

1. Caretaker's knowledge and attitudes towards child rearing.
2. Parental perceptions of the child's behaviour.
3. Parental emotions and responses to stress.
4. Parent–child interaction and behaviour.
5. Quality of child and parent attachment.

Knowledge and attitudes towards child rearing

Research suggests that abusing and non-abusing families have different attitudes about child development. Martin & Rodeheffer (1976) commented that abusers have unrealistic and distorted expectations about their children's abilities. They are said to have much higher expectations of their children and this influences discipline and punishment. Therefore, a significant proportion of sexual and physical abusive incidents involve senseless attempts by parents to force a child to behave in a manner that is beyond the child's developmental limitations.

Research also suggests that these deficits in parental knowledge or understanding were due to low adult intelligence (Smith 1975), but this has been refuted. The parents know what to expect and do with young children but do not apply this knowledge to their own children. Starr (1982) found that one of the differences between abusing and non-abusing parents is that the abusing group see child rearing as a simple rather than a complex task. Many of them show a lack of awareness of their child's abilities and needs (Hyman & Mitchell 1975).

Parental perceptions of child behaviour

It has been shown that abusing parents have more negative conceptions of their children's behaviour than non-abusing parents. They perceive their children to be more irritable and demanding (Browne & Saqi 1987). This may be related to the fact that abused children are more likely to have health problems, eating or sleeping disturbances. Alternatively, it may be a direct result of the unrealistic expectations often reported for abusing parents (Rosenberg & Reppucci 1983).

It has previously been suggested that the child contributes to its own abuse (Kadushin & Martin 1981). Browne & Saqi (1987) do not support this notion; for example, they found no significant differences in children's health records. The abuse may be attributed to the fact that the parents have unrealistic expectations of their children. They interpret certain age-appropriate behaviours as deliberate or intentional non-compliance, concluding that this behaviour is an indication of the child's inherent 'bad' disposition. Thus, abusive parents may see their child's behaviour as a threat to their own self-esteem, which then elicits a punitive attitude and an insensitive approach to parenting.

Parental emotions and responses to stress

A factor common to many child abusers is a heightened rate of arousal in stressful situations. In a study conducted by Wolfe and colleagues (Wolfe *et al.* 1983), abusive and non abusive parents were presented with scenes of videotaped parent–child interaction, some of which were highly stressful (such as children screaming and refusing to comply with their parents) and some of which were non-stressful (for example, a child watching television quietly). The abusive parents responded with greater negative psychophysiological arousal than did the non-abusive comparison groups. Thus, it may be suggested that poor responses to stress and emotional arousal play a crucial role in the manifestation of child abuse and neglect.

The majority of incidents of physical abuse which come to the notice of the authorities arise from situations where parents are attempting to control or discipline their children. Abusive parents are significantly more harsh to their children on a day-to-day basis and are less appropriate in their choice of disciplinary methods compared to non-abusive parents. It is the ineffectiveness of the abusive parent's child-management styles which contributes to the abuse. If the parent's initial command is ineffective and is ignored by the child, the situation will escalate and become more and more stressful until the only way the abusive parent feels they can regain control is by resorting to violence.

Patterson (1986) described rejecting parents as very unclear on how to discipline their children. They punish for significant transgressions, whereas serious transgressions such as stealing go unpunished. Where threats are given, they are carried through unpredictably. Neglectful parents show very low rates of positive physical contact, touching and hugging, and high levels of coercive, aversive interactions.

In contrast, effective parenting is characterised by a flexible attitude, with parents responding to the needs of the child and the situation. House rules are enforced in a consistent and firm manner, using commands or sanctions where necessary. In most situations, the child will comply to the wishes of the parent and conflict will not arise.

Parent–child interaction and behaviour

Interaction assessments demonstrate that abused infants and their mothers have interactions that are less reciprocal and fewer in number than their matched controls, whether in the presence or absence of a stranger (Hyman *et al.* 1979, Browne 1986, Browne & Saqi 1987, 1988*b*).

Observational studies provide evidence that social behaviours and interaction patterns within abusing and non-abusing families are different. Abusing parents have been described as being aversive, negative and controlling, with less pro-social behaviour (Wolfe 1985). They also show less interactive behaviour, both in terms of sensitivity and responsiveness towards their children. This may result in infants developing an insecure attachment to their abusive caretakers, which in turn produces marked changes in the abused children's socio-emotional behaviour, in accordance with the predictions of attachment theory (Browne & Saqi 1988b). Nevertheless, the consequences of maltreatment are not the same for all children. Findings suggest there are more behaviour problems in children who are both abused and neglected (Crittenden 1985, 1988). Abusing and neglectful parents, together with their children, suffer from pervasive confusion and ambivalence in their relations with each other. This is not the same as simple parental rejection. It reflects rather an uncertainty in the relationship which leaves the child vulnerable and perplexed as to what is expected.

Quality of child and parent attachment

The view that children are predisposed to form attachments during infancy (Bowlby 1969) has considerable importance for the study of child abuse (see Morton & Browne 1998). The literature contains numerous reports regarding the high number of abusive parents who were themselves victims of abuse as children (e.g. Egeland 1988). It has been suggested that, in some cases, the link between experiences of abuse as a child and abusing as a parent is likely to be the result of an unsatisfactory early relationship with the principal caretaker and a failure to form a secure attachment (Browne & Parr 1980, DeLozier 1982, Bowlby 1984).

Ainsworth *et al.* (1978) have examined the relationship between the infant's attachment (as measured by the infant's responses to separation and reunion) and the behaviour of the mother in the home environment. Their findings suggest that matternal sensitivity is most influential in affecting the child's reactions. In the homes of the securely attached infants, the mother was sensitive to the infant's behaviour and interactions. While insecurely attached, avoidant infants were found to be rejected by the mothers in terms of interaction, and it was suggested that the enhanced exploratory behaviours shown by these infants were an attempt to block attachment behaviours which had been rejected in the past. In the home environments of the insecurely attached, ambivalent infants, a disharmonious mother–infant relationship was evident, and the ambivalent behaviours shown were seen as a result of inconsistent parenting.

Maccoby (1980) concludes from the above findings that the parents' contribution to attachment can be identified within the four following dimensions of caretaking style.

Sensitivity/insensitivity

The sensitive parent 'meshes' their responses to the infant's signals and communications to form a cyclic turn-taking pattern of interaction. In contrast, the insensitive parent intervenes arbitrarily, and these intrusions reflect their own wishes and mood.

Acceptance/rejection

The accepting parent accepts in general the responsibility of child care. They show few signs of irritation with the child. However, the rejecting parent has feelings of anger and resentment that eclipse their affection for the child. They often find the child irritating and resort to punitive control.

Cooperation/interference

The cooperative parent respects the child's autonomy and rarely exerts direct control. The interfering parent imposes their wishes on the child with little concern for the child's current mood or activity.

Accessibility/ignoring

The accessible parent is familiar with their child's communications and notices them at some distance, and hence is easily distracted by the child. The ignoring parent is preoccupied with their own activities and thoughts, and often fails to notice the child's communications unless they are obvious through intensification. The parent may even forget about the child outside the scheduled times for caretaking.

The four dimensions above are heavily influenced by parental attitudes, emotions and perceptions of the child, as discussed earlier. The dimensions are inter-related and together they determine how 'warm' the parent is towards the child. Indeed, Rohner (1986) has developed a description of parental warmth and rejection which he terms the warmth dimension. This can be considered as the overall picture when Maccoby's four dimensions are integrated together. A summary of Rohner's warmth dimension is given in Figure 3.4.

It has been suggested that helping to promote secure mother–child attachments may also prevent sexual abuse of the child by another family member(s), but many mothers are also maltreated by the child sex offender (Goddard & Hiller 1993), so this notion has been brought into question. Nevertheless, many sexually abused children (approximately one-third) have been physically abused (Finkelhor & Baron 1986). Therefore, comprehensive approaches to assessment and intervention for emotional/physical abuse and neglect early in the child's life may also help to prevent sexual abuse.

Conclusion

Intervention with potential or actual child-abusing families

The inability of child-abusing parents to interact adaptively with their children is seen by many researchers as being representative of their general lack of inter-personal skills. Abusive parents share a common pattern of social isolation, poor work history and few friendships with others outside the home. This isolation means that child-abusing parents are not willing or able to seek help from outside agencies who could provide assistance or emotional support. If they do interact with other people, abusive parents are most likely to choose people in similar situations to themselves, so they gain no experience of alternative parental styles or coping strategies and continue to be ineffective in controlling their children.

It follows that it is the parent–child relationship that should be the focus of work on the prevention, treatment and management of child abuse and neglect, and that interventions to achieve these goals are most effectively carried out in the homes of abusing families (Olds *et al.* 1986, 1993, 1994, 1997, Wolfe 1993). Therefore, those involved in the treatment of abusive families should be concerned with the development of a 'secure' relationship between parent and child. It is not sufficient to evaluate treatment programmes on the basis of the occurrence or non-occurrence of subsequent abuse. Helping parents to inhibit violence towards their children may still leave the harmful context in which the initial abuse occurred quite unchanged.

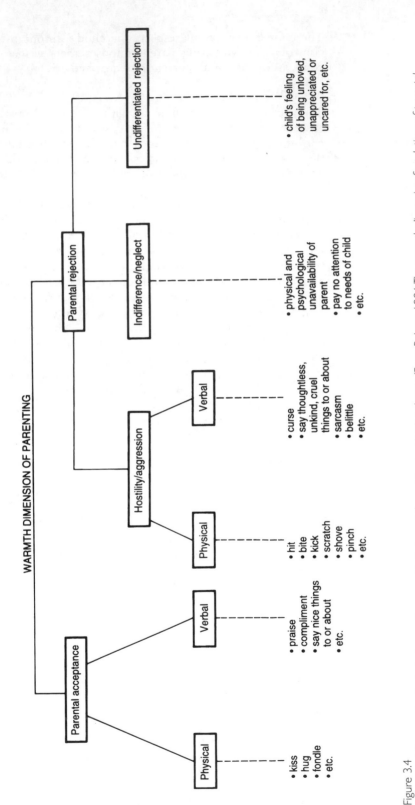

Figure 3.4
Conceptual framework of principal parenting concepts in parental acceptance-rejection theory (From Rohner 1986 The warmth dimension: foundations of parental acceptance–rejection theory. Sage, Beverly Hills, p. 20 (Figure 1). With kind permission of Sage Publications).

References

Ainsworth M D S, Blehar M C, Waters E, Wall S 1978 Patterns of attachment: a psychological study of the strange situation. Lawrence, Erlbaum Associates, New Jersey

Bandura A 1973 Aggression: a social learning analysis. Prentice-Hall, Englewood Cliffs, New Jersey

Belsky J 1980 Child maltreatment: an ecological integration. American Psychologist 35: 320–335

Belsky J 1988 Child maltreatment and the emergent family system. In: Browne K, Davies C, Stratton P (eds) Early prediction and prevention of child abuse. Wiley, Chichester, ch 17, pp. 267–287

Bentovim A 1991 Clinical work with families in which sexual abuse has occurred. In: Hollin C R, Howells K (eds) Clinical approaches to sex offenders and their victims. Wiley, Chichester, pp. 179–208

Bergner R M, Delgado L K, Graybill D 1994 Finkelhor's risk factor checklist: a cross validation study. Child Abuse and Neglect 18 (4): 331–340

Berkowitz L 1989 Laboratory experiments in the study of aggression. In: Archer J, Browne K (eds) Human aggression: naturalistic approaches. Routledge, London, pp. 42–61

Berliner L, Wheeler J R 1987 Treating the effects of sexual abuse on children. Journal of Interpersonal Violence 2: 415–434

Bowlby J 1969 Attachment and loss, Vol. 1, Attachment. Hogarth, London

Bowlby J 1984 Violence in the family as a disorder of attachment and caregiving systems. American Journal of Psychoanalysis 44 (1): 9–31

Browne K D 1986 Methods and approaches to the study of parenting. In: Sluckin W, Herbert M (eds) Parental behaviour. Blackwell, Oxford, ch 12, pp. 344–373

Browne K D 1988 The nature of child abuse and neglect: an overview. In: Browne K D, Davies C, Stratton P (eds) Early prediction and prevention of child abuse. Wiley, Chichester, ch 2, pp. 15–30

Browne K D 1989a The naturalistic context of family violence and child abuse. In: Archer J, Browne K (eds) Human aggression: naturalistic approaches. Routledge, London, ch 8, pp. 182–216

Browne K D 1989b The health visitor's role in screening for child abuse. Health Visitor 62: 275–277

Browne K D 1993 Violence in the family and its links to child abuse. Bailliere's Clinical Paediatrics 1 (1): 149–164

Browne K D 1994 Child sexual abuse. In: Archer J (ed) Male violence. Routledge, London, pp. 210–230

Browne K D 1995a The prediction of child maltreatment. In: Reder P (ed) The assessment of parenting. Routledge, London, pp. 118–135

Browne K D 1995b Preventing child maltreatment through community nursing. Journal of Advanced Nursing 21: 57–63

Browne K D, Hamilton C E 1999 Police recognition of the links between spouse abuse and child abuse. Child Maltreatment 4 (2): 136–147

Browne K D, Herbert M 1997 Preventing family violence. Wiley, Chichester

Browne K D, Howells K 1996 Violent offenders. In: Hollin C R (ed) Working with offenders. Wiley, Chichester, pp. 188–210

Browne K D, Lynch M A 1994 Prevention: actions speak louder than words. Child Abuse Review 3 (4): 240–243

Browne K D, Parr R 1980 Contributions of an ethological approach to the study of abuse. In: Frude N (ed) Psychological approaches to child abuse. Batsford Press, London, ch 6, pp. 83–99

Browne K D, Saqi S 1987 Parent–child interaction in abusing families: possible causes and consequences. In: Maher P (ed) Child abuse: an educational perspective. Blackwell, Oxford, pp. 77–104

Browne K D, Saqi S 1988a Approaches to screening families at high risk for child abuse. In: Browne K D, Davies C, Stratton P (eds) Early prediction and prevention of child abuse. Wiley, Chichester, ch 5, pp. 57–85

Browne K D, Saqi S 1988b Mother–infant interactions and attachment in physically abusing families. Journal of Reproductive and Infant Psychology 6 (3): 163–282

Browne K D, Davies C, Stratton P 1988 Early prediction and prevention of child abuse. Wiley, Chichester

Buss A H, Durkee A 1957 An inventory for assessing different types of hostility. Journal of Consulting Psychology 21: 343–349

Carroll J 1994 The protection of children exposed to marital violence. Child Abuse Review 3 (1): 6–14

Central Statistical Office 1994 Social focus on children 1994. HMSO, London

Coleman K H 1980 Conjugal violence: what 33 men report. Journal of Marriage and the Family 6: 207–313

Creighton S J 1992 Child abuse trends in England and Wales 1988–1990. NSPCC, London

Creighton S J, Noyes P 1989 Child abuse trends in England and Wales 1983–1987. NSPCC, London

Crittenden P M 1985 Maltreated infants: vulnerability and resilience. Journal of Child Psychology and Psychiatry 26 (1): 85–96

Crittenden P M 1988 Family and dyadic patterns of functioning in maltreating families. In: Browne K D, Davies C, Stratton P (eds) Early prediction and prevention of child abuse. Wiley, Chichester, ch 11, pp. 161–189

Davis L V, Carlson B E 1987 Observation of spouse abuse: what happens to the children? Journal of Interpersonal Violence 2 (3): 320–345

DeLozier P 1982 Attachment theory and child abuse. In: Parkes C M, Stevenson-Hinde J (eds) The place of attachment in human behaviour. Tavistock, London

Department of Health (DOH) 2000 Children and young persons on Child Protection Registers year ending 31st March 2000 England. Department of Health Personal Social Services Local Authority Statistics. The Stationery Office, London

Dollard J, Doob L W, Miller N E, Mowrer O H, Sears R R 1939 Frustration and aggression. Yale University Press, New Haven

Edmunds G, Kendrick D C 1980 The measurement of human aggressiveness. Ellis Horwood (Wiley), Chichester

Egeland B 1988 Breaking the cycle of abuse: implications for prediction and intervention. In: Browne K D, Davies C, Stratton P (eds) Early prediction and prevention of child abuse. Wiley, Chichester, ch 6, pp. 87–102

Elmer E, Gregg G 1967 Developmental characteristics of abused children. Pediatrics 40: 596–602

Finkelhor D 1980 Risk factors in the sexual victimization of children. Child Abuse and Neglect 4: 265–273

Finkelhor D, Baron L 1986 Risk factors for child sexual abuse. Journal of Interpersonal Violence 1 (1): 43–71

Freud S 1964 New introductory lectures on psychoanalysis (1932–36). Hogarth Press, London

Friedrich W N, Boroskin J A 1976 The role of the child in abuse: a review of the literature. American Journal of Orthopsychiatry 46 (4): 580–590

Frude N 1980 Child abuse as aggression. In: Frude N (ed) Psychological approaches to child abuse. Batsford, London, pp. 136–150

Frude N 1989 The physical abuse of children. In: Howells K, Hollin C (eds) Clinical approaches to violence. Wiley, Chichester, ch 7, pp. 155–181

Frude N 1991 Understanding family problems: a psychological approach. Wiley, Chichester

Galdston R 1965 Observations of children who have been physically abused by their parents. American Journal of Psychiatry 122 (4): 440–443

Garbarino J 1977 The human ecology of child maltreatment. Journal of Marrriage and the Family 39 (4): 721–735

Gayford J J 1975 Wife battering: a preliminary survey of 100 cases. British Medical Journal 25 (1): 94–97

Gelles R J 1973 Child abuse as psychopathology: a sociological critique and reformulation. American Journal of Orthopsychiatry 43: 611–621

Gelles R J 1983 An exchange/social control theory. In: Finkelhor D, Gelles R, Straus M, Hotaling G (eds) The dark side of the family: current family violence research. Sage, Beverly Hills, California, pp. 151–165

Gelles R J 1987 Family violence, 2nd edn. Library of Social Research No. 84. Sage, Beverly Hills, California

Gelles R J, Cornell C P 1997 Intimate violence in families, 3rd edn. Sage, Beverly Hills, California

Gerson L W 1978 Alcohol-related acts of violence. Journal of Studies on Alcohol 39: 1294–1296

Gil D 1970 Violence against children. Harvard University Press, Cambridge, Massachusetts

Gil D 1978 Societal violence in families. In: Eekelaar J M, Katz S N (eds) Family violence. Butterworths, Toronto, pp. 14–33

Gilbert P 1994 Male violence: towards an integration. In: Archer J (ed) Male violence. Routledge, London, pp. 352–389

Goddard C, Hiller P 1993 Child sexual abuse: assault in a violent context. Australian Journal of Social Issues 28 (1): 20–33

Goldstein J H 1986 Aggression and crimes of violence, 2nd edn. Oxford University Press, Oxford

Gough D 1994 Child abuse interventions. HMSO, London

Gully K J, Dengerink H A 1983 The dyadic interaction of persons with violent and non-violent histories. Aggressive Behaviour 9 (1): 13–20

Hamilton C E, Browne K D 1998 The repeat victimisation of children: should the concept be revised? Aggression and Violent Behavior 3 (1): 47–60

Hamilton C E, Browne K D 1999 Recurrent maltreatment during childhood: a survey of referrals to police child protection units in England. Child Maltreatment 4 (4): 275–286

Home Office, Department of Health, Department of Education and Science, Welsh Office 1991 Working together under the Children Act 1989: a guide to arrangements for inter-agency cooperation for the protection of children from abuse. HMSO, London

Hughes H M, Barad J 1983 Psychology functioning of children in a battered women's shelter: a preliminary investigation. American Journal of Orthopsychiatry 53 (3): 525–531

Hyman C A 1978 Non-accidental injury. A report to the Surrey County Area Review Committee on child abuse. Health Visitor 51: 168–174

Hyman C A, Mitchell R 1975 A psychological study of child battering. Health Visitor 48: 294–296

Hyman C A, Parr R, Browne K D 1979 An observation study of mother–infant interaction in abusing families. Child Abuse and Neglect 3: 241–246

Jaffe P, Wolfe D, Wilson S, Zak L 1986 Similarities in behaviour and social maladjustment among child victims and witnesses to family violence. American Journal of Orthopsychiatry 56: 142–146

Jaffe P G, Wolfe D A, Wilson S K 1990 Children of battered women. Sage, Beverly Hills, California

Kadushin A, Martin J 1981 Child abuse: an interactional event. Columbia University Press, New York

Kempe T S, Kempe C H 1978 Child abuse. Fontana/Open Books, London

Krugman R D 1986 The relationship between unemployment and physical abuse of children. Child Abuse and Neglect 10 (3): 415–418

La Fontaine J S 1993 Defining organised sexual abuse. In: Browne K D, Lynch M A (eds) Special issue on organised abuse. Child Abuse Review 2 (4): 223–231

Levine E M 1986 Sociocultural causes of family violence: a theoretical comment. Journal of Family Violence 1 (1): 3–12

Lewis B Y 1987 Psychosocial factors related to wife abuse. Journal of Family Violence 2 (1): 1–10

Lorenz K 1966 On aggression. Harcourt, Brace and World, New York

Lynch M, Roberts J 1977 Predicting child abuse. Child Abuse and Neglect 1: 491–492

Maccoby E E 1980 Social development: psychology growth and the parent–child relationship. Harcourt Brace Jovanovich, New York

Martin H P, Rodeheffer M 1976 Learning and intelligence. In: Martin H P (ed) The abused child: a multidisciplinary approach to developmental issues and treatment. Ballinger, Cambridge, Massachusetts

Morton N, Browne K D 1998 Theory and observation of attachment and its relation to child maltreatment: a review. Child Abuse and Neglect 22 (11): 1093–1104

National Society for the Prevention of Cruelty to Children (NSPCC) 1985 Child abuse deaths. Information Briefing No. 5. NSPCC, London

Nobes G, Smith M 2000 The relative extent of physical punishment and abuse by mothers and fathers. Trauma, Violence and Abuse 1(1): 47–66

Novaco R W 1978 Anger and coping with stress. In: Forey J P, Rathjen D P, Rathjen D P (eds) Cognitive behaviour therapy. Plenum, New York

Olds D, Henderson C, Chamberlin R, Tatelbaum R 1986 Preventing child abuse and neglect: randomized trial of nurse home visiting. Pediatrics 78: 65–78

Olds D L, Henderson C R, Kitzman H 1994 Does prenatal and infancy nurse home visitation have enduring effects on the qualities of parental care giving and child health at 25 to 50 months of life. Pediatrics 93 (1): 89–98

Olds D L, Henderson C R, Phelps C, et al. 1993 Effect of prenatal and infancy nurse home visitation on Government spending. Medical Care 31 (2): 155–174

Olds D, Eckenrode J, Henderson C, et al. 1997 Long-term effects of home visitation on maternal life course and child abuse and neglect: fifteen-year follow-up of a randomized trial. Journal of the American Medical Association 278 (8): 637–643

Pahl J 1985 Violent husbands and abused wives: a longitudinal study. In: Pahl J (ed) Private violence and public policy. Routledge and Kegan Paul, London, pp. 23–94

Patterson G R 1982 Coercive family process. Castalia Publications, Oregon

Patterson G R 1986 Maternal rejection. Determinant or product for deviant child behaviour. In: Hartup W W, Rubin Z (eds) Relationships and development. Lawrence Erlbaum Associates, Hillsdale, New Jersey

Persky H, Smith K D, Basu G K 1971 Relation of psychological measures of aggression and hostility to testosterone production in man. Psychosomatic Medicine 33: 265–277

Rohner R P 1986 The warmth dimension: foundations of parental acceptance–rejection theory. Sage, Beverly Hills, California

Rosenberg M S, Repucci N D 1983 Abusive mothers: perceptions of their own and their children's behaviour. Journal of Consulting and Clinical Psychology 51 (5): 674–682

Roy M 1982 The abusive partner. Van Nostrand Reinhold, New York

Rutter M 1985 Aggression and the family. Acta Paedopsychiatrica 6: 11–25

Schultz L G 1960 The wife assaulter. Journal of Social Therapy 6: 103–112

Smith S 1975 The battered child syndrome. Butterworths, London

Sonkin D, Martin D, Walker L 1985 The male batterer: a treatment approach. Springer, New York

Starr R H 1982 Child abuse and prediction: policy implications. Ballinger, Cambridge, Massachusetts

Starr R H 1988 Pre and perinatal risk and physical abuse. Journal of Reproductive and Infant Psychology 6 (3): 125–138

Steele B F, Pollock C B 1968 A psychiatric study of parents who abuse infants and small children. In: Helfer R E, Kempe C H (eds) The battered child. University of Chicago Press, Chicago, pp. 103–147

Steinglass P 1987 The alcoholic family. Hutchinson, London

Straus M A 1980 A sociological perspective on causes of family violence. In: Green R (ed) Violence and the family. Bould & Westview, New York, pp. 7–13

Straus M A, Gelles R J, Steinmetz S K 1988 Behind closed doors: violence in the American family, 2nd edn. Sage, Beverly Hills, California

Toch H 1969 Violent men. Aldine, Chicago

Wasserman G A, Green A, Allen R 1983 Going beyond abuse: maladaptive patterns of interaction in abusing mother–infants pairs. Journal of American Academy of Child Psychiatry 22 (3): 245–252

Willis D J, Holden E W, Rosenberg M 1992 Prevention of child maltreatment. Wiley, New York

Wolfe D A 1985 Child abuse parents. An empirical review and analysis. Psychological Bulletin 97: 461–482

Wolfe D A 1991 Preventing physical and emotional abuse of children. Guildford, New York

Wolfe D A 1993 Child abuse prevention: blending research and practice. Child Abuse Review 2: 153–165

Wolfe D A, Fairbank J, Kelly J A, Bradlyn A S 1983 Child abusive parents and physiological responses to stressful and nonstressful behaviour in children. Behavioural Assessment 5: 363–371

4 Characteristics of sexual abusers

Stephen Frosh

Stephen Frosh

INTRODUCTION

This chapter focuses on a specific subgroup of abusers of children, those who abuse sexually. To a considerable degree, there may be overlaps between sexual and non-sexual abusers of children. For example, at least some sexual abuse is associated with physical abuse, and sometimes with extreme abuse such as torture; there may be similarities in attitudes towards children, degree of psychopathology, personal history, social isolation, level of intergenerational continuity and other characteristics (Kaufman & Zigler 1989); Feshbach's (1989) account of lack of 'empathy' in physical child abuse is also reminiscent of many clinical descriptions of sexually abusive behaviour. Browne (1993) notes similarities between those 'who physically and sexually abuse their children, those who abuse their wives, and those who abuse their aged relatives' as including:

a misperception of the victim, low self-esteem, sense of incompetence, social isolation, a lack of support and help, lack of empathy, marital difficulties, depression, poor self-control, and a history of abuse and neglect as a child.

(Browne 1993, p. 152)

More generally, the ambivalent social attitudes and values surrounding children – for example, that they are the property of adults but that they are also entitled to protection, or that they are individuals but must also do what adults demand of them – may be contributory factors to all forms of abuse, seen as a destructive manifestation of adults' power over children.

On the other hand, there are ways in which sexual abusers may be different from those who abuse children physically or who neglect them. In particular, only some sexual abuse involves overt acts of violence towards the child (Glaser & Frosh 1993). The seductive behaviour and degree of planning employed by some paedophiles may also mark them out as different from those non-sexual abusers whose behaviour is characterised more by an inability to respond appropriately to their children's cues or to deal with relatively minor difficulties before they escalate (Rutter 1989). There may also be meaningful differentiations to be made in the identity of the abuser; whereas in the field of physical abuse the roles of abuser and care-giver are very likely to be (but are not invariably) fused, a far greater proportion of sexual abusers of children are not their primary caregivers (Glaser 1993).

From the point of view of understanding the characteristics of abusers, a crucial question bearing on the relationship between sexual and non-sexual forms of child abuse is that of the degree to which sexual abuse is *sexual*, that is, concerned with the sexual gratification of the adult over and above the use of power to assert the adult's will on the child. It will be argued below that this is indeed a component of sexual abuse – that the sexual element is no accident or irrelevance – and that degree of sexual arousal to children is one of the few features reasonably reliably shown to discriminate between sexual abusers and non-abusers. Furniss (1991) goes so far as to suggest that the main difference between physical and sexual abuse is that the 'addictive egosyntonic' aspect of sexual abuse – the 'kick' the abuser gets from it – is generally absent in all but the most severe forms of physical abuse. According to Furniss, this is specifically due to the sexual aspect of sexual abuse – the pattern of arousal and release that creates both dependence and a denial of dependence in the perpetrator.

There are other characteristics which differentiate sexual and non-sexual abusers, the most important of which is gender. The high preponderance of male sexual abusers differs from the pattern amongst non-sexual abusers of children (Meier 1985). As will be seen, recognition of this gender imbalance and its possible connection with sexual socialisation fuels some of the currently existent theories of sexually abusive behaviour. Nevertheless, the overlaps mentioned above should not be lost sight of. All forms of child abuse involve an assertion of adult power over children, a betrayal of trust and dependence, and a disavowal of the protective and nurturing elements in adult psychology upon which children rely for the creation of a stable and supportive developmental context.

Methodological issues

Research in the area of child sexual abuse has always been fraught with methodological difficulties, ranging from divergences in definition resulting in non-comparable studies, to the ethical issues involved in comparing the effectiveness of various forms of therapy or no-treatment for children who have been sexually abused (Haugaard & Emery 1989, Glaser & Frosh 1993). Sample selection has also been a problem, with children identified through social services or mental health facilities probably being a select group of the wider population of abused children – as the differences in incidence and gender distribution suggest (Haugaard & Reppucci 1988; and Creighton, Chapter 2, in this volume). All these factors also apply in research on sexual abusers. There are variations in definition and in usage of terms such as 'abuser', 'offender' and 'paedophile'; there is confusion over the extent to which findings with incestuous abusers can be generalised to non-incestuous abusers and vice versa; there are problems connected with the reliance of research on incarcerated offenders, as most abusive acts probably remain undetected and are certainly unpunished; and there is the possibility that certain types of abuser, e.g. those in the middle-class, may be systematically less likely to be discovered and prosecuted (Bentovim *et al.* 1988, Becker 1994, McConaghy 1998). In addition, the criminal justice system in Britain and in the USA does not encourage abusers to admit their guilt and responsibility for their actions, something which has deleterious effects both on research and on the well-being of victims.

Araji & Finkelhor (1986) propose that it might be possible to differentiate between the various terms employed to describe abusers in the literature on logical grounds, with 'sexual abuse' and 'child molesting' referring to behaviours that can also be regarded as indicators of the existence of the underlying state of 'paedophilia'. With regard to the latter term, they write:

We define paedophilia as occurring when an adult has a conscious sexual interest in prepubertal children. We infer that sexual interest from one of two behaviours: (1) the adult has had some sexual contact with a child (meaning that he or she touched the child or had the child touch him or her with the purpose of becoming sexually aroused), or (2) the adult has masturbated to sexual fantasies involving children. Thus we are defining paedophilia to be a little broader than sexual abuse or child molesting. It includes the conscious fantasising about such behaviour, too. (pp. 90–91)

They also note that paedophilia 'can be a state and not necessarily a trait' (Araji & Finkelhor 1986), thus producing a very broad category, of which the convicted offenders who represent the standard research sample represent only a very small subsection. While one can appreciate the rationale for the distinction between sexually abusive behaviours and the hypothesised or actual underlying state from which they arise, creating the category of paedophilia so that it includes fantasy with no attached activity as well as overt sexual abusiveness towards children, is highly problematic. In the terms associated with Finkelhor's own model of sexual abusiveness (see below), this obscures the important dynamic of inhibition – the barrier between impulse or desire and action. If there are systematic connections between, for example, masculine sexual socialisation in general and sexual abusiveness, the question of why only some men translate their desire into action is an important one, and one that does not seem to be totally answered by stating that only some men have the requisite opportunity.

Given the inchoate state of research into sexually abusive behaviour towards children, it is probably better to follow the advice given by Haugaard & Reppucci (1988) in regard to classifying sexually abused children. They advocate providing as clear and exact as possible an account of the actual behaviour in question, leaving issues of differentiation and classification to be worked out empirically. Hence, 'incestuous' or intrafamilial abusers should be identified separately from abusers who focus on children outside their own family. Those who abuse in the context of a relationship should be categorised differently from those who abduct children they do not know. Those who only have sexual relations with children should be considered independently from those whose sexuality is more promiscuous and undifferentiated, and so on. In particular, given what has taken place in the research literature, generalisations from sexual *offenders* to sexual abusers of all kinds should be treated with the utmost caution – there are all sorts of reasons why some abusers pass through the criminal justice system and others do not. The question of which if any of these or other possible groups is genuinely 'paedophiliac' is not at present an issue of primary significance.

These guidelines are easier to make than to adhere to, given the confusion that prevails in the literature. In what follows, the available data on characteristics of sexual abusers are outlined and some theoretical points are made about how to understand and explain the psychology of sexual abusiveness. However, it should be noted that there is a high level of methodological uncertainty in all reported studies, described repeatedly in reviews in the area, so all integrative and theoretical efforts are more speculative than might be desirable. There is insufficient space here for a full methodological critique of the material employed, even if this would have been helpful, but where possible the strength or weakness of the research evidence is indicated. Unless otherwise noted, however, all quoted research findings in the area should be handled with care, and grandiose claims should be automatically discounted.

Research on abuser characteristics

One of the most notable features of the literature on child sexual abuse is the extent to which men and adolescent boys make up the vast majority of abusers. All studies investigating the question have uncovered only a very small proportion of female abusers, with figures from studies in the 1980s suggesting that women are perpetrators in no more than 4% of instances where the victims are girls (Russell 1983) and 20% where the victims are boys (Finkelhor 1984). Finkelhor (1984) comments that:

> Especially since contacts with female children occur with at least twice or three times the frequency as [those with] male children, the presumption that sexual abusers are primarily men seems clearly supported. (p. 177)

In coming to these conclusions, Finkelhor suggests that the male preponderance is unlikely to be due simply to abuse by women going undetected, because they apply to retrospective non-clinical surveys, and also because they remain even when only sexual 'contacts' rather than 'abuses' are asked about. Nevertheless, there is some more recent evidence that the numbers of female abusers may have been systematically underestimated in the past. For example, Lawson (1993) points out that the majority of documented cases of mother–son abuse are found in the clinical rather than the survey literature. 'These reports indicate that cases of mother–son sexual abuse are more likely to be disclosed in long-term therapeutic treatment, are rarely reported to child abuse authorities (or rarely treated seriously), and are not included in public statistics' (p. 261). Wakefield & Underwager (1991) note the existence of a great range in the estimated frequency of child sexual abuse by females in different studies. According to these researchers, there are widely differing circumstances under which women abuse children, and these may in turn be different from those under which men abuse. Many studies depict female abusers as socially isolated, alienated, coming from abusive backgrounds and having emotional problems, although most are not psychotic. This seems to suggest a more homogeneous group than is the case for male abusers, but the research is still much too unclear to establish this with any degree of confidence.

Despite recognition of the way the number of female abusers may have been underestimated in the past, there remains little doubt that the great majority of abusive acts are perpetrated by men, and it is the characteristics of such men with which the research literature is primarily concerned. Given how much of this literature focuses on incest, it is worth noting first that the stereotypical notion that most abuse is incestuous abuse by fathers or step-fathers is not completely accurate; much of the abuse is by other relatives, family friends (who may concurrently incestuously abuse their own children), or other adults in positions of power over the children concerned. In Baker & Duncan's (1985) study, 49% of abusers were known to their victims and 14% of all reported abuse took place within the family. Girls were more likely to have been abused by parents, grandparents or siblings, while boys were more at risk from people outside the family but known to them. Russell (1983) found that abusers were mostly not relatives, but also were not likely to be strangers; only 11% were total strangers, 29% were relatives and 60% were known to the victims but unrelated to them. Within the extrafamilial abuse group, 40% of abusers were classified as 'authority figures'.

It is quite clear from the literature that sexual abuse of children is often a repetitive act and that it may have 'addictive' components. However, despite the claim by Furniss (1991) reported above, it is uncertain to what extent this is due to the specifically sexual element of the abuse or to other elements such as the exploitation of power. For example, Herman (1981) suggests that some incestuous fathers enjoy the unhappiness of their victim, implying that the power-denigration dynamic is operating; on the other hand, as others such as Finkelhor (1984) have pointed out, this does not mean that the sexual component of sexual abuse is not also bound up with this same dynamic. Whatever the cause, there is good evidence that amongst convicted abusers there are very few 'one off' offences.

Although one cannot be sure that this picture extends to non-convicted abusers, it seems unlikely that an unpunished addictive act should be repeated less frequently than a punished one, even if it is the case that the convicted group are caught in part because of their repetitive behaviour. In the most quoted study in this area, Abel *et al.* (1987) found that the total number of sexual acts against children committed by 561 sexual offenders in their outpatient treatment programme was 291 737. The subgroup of offenders with the largest number of victims were the 155 non-incestuous paedophiles targeting male children – they admitted to a total of 29 981 victims between them. The incestuous paedophiles had a much smaller number of victims (an average of under two each), but as one would expect tended to commit more sexual acts per victim. In a similar study of 129 outpatient child molesters quoted by Murphy *et al.* (1991), the offenders against males averaged 376 victims, the offenders against females outside the home five victims, and the incest cases one victim. Reviewing material of this kind, Conte (1991, p. 26) comments that the findings 'raise questions about the validity of the assumption that the initial referral diagnosis (e.g. father or step-father incest) has any significance in understanding the nature of the incest father or step-father's problem.'

On the face of it, the data suggest a potentially useful distinction between abuse that occurs within the context of a relationship (such as incest) and other kinds of abuse. However, this is called into question by other data demonstrating at least some overlap between these groups of abusers. For example, in a further study by Abel *et al.* (1988), 49% of the incestuous fathers and step-fathers referred for outpatient treatment at their clinics abused children outside the family during the same time period when they were abusing their own children. Eighteen per cent of these men were raping adult women at the same time as they were sexually abusing their own child. Becker (1994) also notes the diversity of abusers in terms of age, occupation, income level, marital status and ethnic group. She describes how it was once believed that sex offenders could be easily categorised along three dimensions:

- offending against either adults or children
- offending against either members of their families or against acquaintances and strangers
- offending in non-contact ways (for example, exhibitionism) or through bodily contact.

However, there is now considerable evidence that many abusers offend across these categories.

In a similar vein to the evidence concerning the widespread nature of abusers' sexual acts, it also appears that a more formal psychiatric evaluation of their sexuality calls into question any claim that paedophilia or incest is a specific and circumscribed disorder. Working with an offender group, Abel *et al.* (1988) found that the average number of sexual disorder diagnoses (paraphilias) elicited from sexual offenders in treatment was 2.02. On the other hand, the number of paraphilias is not unlimited. Marshall *et al.* (1991) interviewed 129 outpatient child molesters (91 non-familial, 38 father–daughter). Fourteen per cent of the non-familiar offenders against boys, 11.8% of the non-familial offenders against girls and 7.9% of the incest offenders had one or more paraphilias additional to their index offence; however, only three individuals in the total sample had more than two additional paraphilias.

Given the frequency with which at least convicted offenders abuse children, and the extent to which their sexual disturbance seems to spread, it is perhaps not surprising to discover that there is a considerable amount of pessimism concerning recidivism. Finkelhor (1986) reviewed the literature available up to the mid-1980s, finding recidivism rates between 6 and 35% for sexual offences, with general agreement that abusers of boys and exhibitionists are most likely to repeat their offences. However, he points out serious problems with most of the studies, undermining the certainty of any conclusions: for example, recidivism is often measured in terms of new convictions, and the studies themselves only apply to convicted offenders, who are a selected group. The finding of lower rates for incest offenders may also be unreliable, as they might need very long follow-up to control for the possibility of intergenerational (e.g. grandfather–grandchild) abuse. In a slightly more recent review, Furby *et al.* (1989, p. 27) comment that, 'The vast majority of existing studies either do not give a breakdown of their sample in terms of offender type or do not present recidivism results separately for each type'. In those that do, recidivism for paedophiles tends to be lower than that for exhibitionists and rapists, and there may also be lower rates for homosexual versus heterosexual paedophiles. The actual recidivism figures in the studies are between 7 and 35%, but variations in samples and follow-up times, as well as in type of treatment received, make these difficult to interpret.

In her review of the characteristics and treatment of sexual offenders, Becker (1994) notes that there are very few controlled therapy outcome studies on the effectiveness of treatment, and that most published studies are marked by methodological problems. This makes it hard to assert that treatment for child abusers can be effective. However, Becker also points out that some recent studies provide reasons for optimism about the effectiveness of current treatment methods for some offenders. Examples here include some behavioural, cognitive and psychosocial interventions with adolescent abusers (e.g. Hoghugi & Bhate 1997) and work carried out in a context that facilitates good, supportive communication between the many professionals usually involved in each case (Griffin *et al.* 1997).

A considerable amount of laboratory-based research has been carried out on the sexual responsiveness of sexual abusers, again focusing primarily on convicted offenders. In their 1986 review, Araji & Finkelhor comment, 'There is a fairly impressive body of experimental evidence suggesting that [child molesters] are indeed unusually sexually responsive to children' (p. 101). However, it was not clear to them whether all molesters are sexually responsive to children under laboratory conditions, with incest offenders being the most likely exceptions. On the whole, amongst contradictory data, it seems likely that whereas non-abusive males seem to show substantial increase in arousal by children 14 years and older, offenders may be more aroused by younger children. For example, Marshall *et al.* (1986), using the favoured penile plesythmographic method, found child molesters to be maximally aroused by 9-year-old children, though they were also aroused by adults. Conte (1991), reviewing the area, notes as follows:

Some studies have found that physiological sexual arousal measures can discriminate between violent and less violent offenders ... In addition, child molesters respond differentially to adult and child stimuli, with more arousal to child stimuli (both male and female children), however a sample of normals selected from the community and non-sexual offenders responded only to adult, consenting stimuli.

(Conte 1991, p. 28)

Quinsey & Chaplin (1988), on whose work Conte bases part of his conclusion, also showed that arousal responses to children and women may involve both sexual and sadistic images of victims, and that physically violent child molesters are more sexually responsive to scenarios involving gratuitous violence (sadism) towards victims than are non-violent offenders.

Some caution needs to be exercised in interpreting these findings, however, as there are contradictory data obscuring any neat divisions between offenders and 'normals'. For instance, Hall *et al.* (1988) suggest that up to 80% of sexual offenders do not respond to supposedly sexually arousing stimuli under laboratory conditions, while Freund *et al.* (1972) found that a group of non-paedophiliac community volunteers showed significant penile tumescence to female children as young as 6 years of age. Frenzel & Lang (1989) showed erotic and sexually neutral movie clips of males and females aged between 6 and 25 years to 62 heterosexual intrafamilial abusers, 57 heterosexual and 25 homosexual extrafamilial abusers, and 47 community controls. Penile volume changes were recorded during the 30-second presentations. Homosexuals in the sample reacted most to pictures of 13–15-year-old boys; this discriminated them from other groups. Intrafamilial abusers overlapped considerably with controls, and only 10% showed a pattern of responses expected for the 'classical paedophile' (i.e. largest responses to female children). This implies that abusers are more heterogeneous in their sexual preference profiles than has previously been suggested. Howes (1998) compared arousal observed in the plethysmographic profiles of 50 males incarcerated for non-sexual offences, 40 males who were convicted of heterosexual rape and 10 convicted male paedophiles. There were strong similarities in the 'arousal profiles' of abusers and controls, indicating that deviant arousal alone did not distinguish sexual offenders from non-sexual offenders. The only marked difference between the groups was in the almost-perfect ability of control participants to inhibit deviant arousal and the weak ability of sexual offenders to accomplish this. Howes suggests from this that a determination of an offender's ability to inhibit deviant arousal may be the only aspect of plethysmographic testing with practical application. Murphy *et al.* (1991) argue more generally on the basis of accumulated evidence that penile plethysmography or phallometry measuring erection responses to deviant stimuli does not give a specific response profile for all sex offenders, or for certain types of offender. Its utility for legal and model-building purposes is therefore limited.

Overall, it is likely that the laboratory studies have exaggerated the difference between abusers and non-abusers. This suggestion is supported by other forms of evidence; for example, Briere & Runtz (1989), in a study of male university students, found that 21% reported sexual attraction to some small children, 9% described sexual fantasies involving children, 5% admitted to having masturbated to such fantasies and 7% indicated 'some likelihood' of having sex with a child if they could avoid detection and punishment. These are higher rates than would be expected from the number of university students who actually are known to abuse children.

Other suggestions concerning the possible personality characteristics of abusers also receive only mixed support from the empirical literature. Araji & Finkelhor (1986, p. 99) comment,

there seem to be a number of investigators who are in general agreement that child molesters are immature or inadequate … However, these investigators have often made broad and unwarranted inferences from test data and we believe that the hypothesis is not much advanced beyond the state of a clinical inference.

This stricture seems to apply quite strongly to more recent studies as well, for example those apparently showing failures of empathy amongst sexual offenders, or tendencies of homosexual paedophiles to prefer to interact with children on the child's level, while incest offenders prefer to elevate their victims to adult status rather than fixating on the child role themselves (Pithers 1999, Wilson 1999).

From clinical accounts, it seems that many sex abusers may have problems relating to women and 'possibly poor social skills and sexual anxiety contribute to this' (Araji & Finkelhor 1986, p. 110). However, when explored empirically it appears that heterosexual and bisexual paedophiles (but not, for obvious reasons, homosexual paedophiles) have average levels of the sexual contact with adult females (Langevin *et al.* 1985). This makes it less likely that paedophiles suffer greatly from what is sometimes tendentiously referred to as 'reduced outlets' for adult sexual gratification. In addition, the meek and unassertive stereotype attached at least to paedophile abusers is undermined by research suggesting that violence may be a more common and integral part of the lives and sexual behaviour of some paedophiles and incest offenders than previously believed (Langevin 1985, Lang *et al.* 1988). For example, Langevin *et al.* (1985) quote data from the late 1970s suggesting that a half to two-thirds of sexual offenders of all types employ violence or serious threats of violence as part of their abusive behaviour. Again, it is uncertain to what extent this finding generalises to non-incarcerated abusers.

The notion that alcohol abuse may be linked to sexual abuse, at least as a disinhibiting influence, is better supported in the literature (Langevin *et al.* 1985, Araji & Finkelhor 1986). Many studies do support another common contention that a high proportion of convicted child molesters were themselves abused in childhood but the majority of these studies report rates well below 50%, making it apparent that this can by no means be seen as a full explanation of sexual abusiveness (Araji & Finkelhor 1986). Rates of under one-third are usually found. For example, Groth & Burgess (1979) report childhood sexual abuse in 32% of their sample, and Abel *et al.* (1984) similarly document rates of 24% (amongst abusers of girls) and 40% (amongst abusers of boys) for past history of sexual abuse. Hanson & Slater (1988), reviewing the literature, suggest that 28% of sexual abusers of children were themselves sexually victimised in childhood – a rate similar to those found in other sexual or non-sexual offender populations. On the other hand, over 50% of Lang & Langevin's (1991) sample of paedophile and incest offenders had themselves been sexually victimised as children, and nearly as many had been physically abused. Therefore, it is likely that there is a raised incidence of sexual victimisation in the histories of sexual offenders against children, but is less clear that this is different from other sexual offenders, and indeed it may be that all 'disturbed' populations show an increase in previous sexual abuse. In addition, the finding is mostly with incarcerated child molesters and it is unclear how much it applies to a more representative group (Finkelhor 1986) or how well it differentiates child sexual abusers from other sexual or non-sexual offender groups. Once again, the absence of studies of non-incarcerated abusers increases the tentativeness of any conclusions.

It should be clear from all that has been reported here so far that there is unlikely to be any simple typological system with which to classify child sexual abusers. Even setting aside the restriction that most evidence derives from work with convicted sexual offenders, there is an enormous amount of uncertainty and heterogeneity amongst the abuser population. Often what appear to be relatively strong findings (such as that available from the sexual preference research) melt away when one looks at them closely. The utility of theoretical systems will be returned to towards the end of this chapter, but this does call into question conventional typologies such as the distinction between 'fixated' and 'regressed' abusers advanced by Groth *et al.* (1982). Fixated abusers are supposed to have a primary sexual orientation to children, beginning in adolescence with no precipitating events and with males as main targets. Regressed abusers reportedly have a primary sexual orientation to age-mates, so that sexual involvement with a child is a clear change in interest and behaviour, occurring usually at times of stress and primarily taking female victims. But there is little empirical evidence supporting the validity of this distinction, which was made on a prison sample, and there is some evidence against it. For example, Simon *et al.* (1992) studied 136 consecutive cases of convicted child molesters who had personality data available for inspection, finding a continuum rather than a dichotomy on the regression-fixation dimension. More generally, Murphy & Peters (1992) have argued that there is no research evidence to suggest that clinicians using all the tools available can profile sexual offenders with sufficient validity and reliability for use in criminal trials. Conte (1991, p. 25) comments that 'reviews of the existing empirical literature have failed to identify a consistent psychological profile or set of characteristics which discriminates between sexual offenders and others.'

If there is unlikely to be a psychological profile of the 'sexual abuser', it may be that what has to be examined is the extent to which contingent factors such as access to vulnerable children and absence of inhibiting forces are the crucial determinants of the likelihood of abuse. This unpalatable idea will be returned to below, but it is worth noting here that at least some offenders would support that view. Conte (1991), for instance, reports earlier research by his group in which a sample of sexual offenders treated in the community were interviewed about the victimisation process. These offenders claimed to have the ability to identify and use vulnerabilities in a potential child victim in order to gain sexual access to and maintain control over the child. Such vulnerabilities were defined in terms of *status conditions* (e.g. living in a single-parent family), *emotional characteristics* (e.g. a child who was needy, unhappy, or shy) and *situational factors* (e.g. the child was alone and unprotected). Such findings do not, of course, demonstrate that *any* man would abuse children given these circumstances (see the finding by Howes 1998, mentioned earlier, that abusers differed from controls on their lack of ability to inhibit arousal to 'deviant' sexual stimuli), but they do indicate that the determinants of abusive behaviour consist of far more than simply the personality characteristics of the abusers themselves. On the other hand, it also appears to be true that at least some paedophiles are extremely skilled at, and invest a great deal of energy and planning in, the task of obtaining access to vulnerable children – for example by becoming responsible for Children's Homes and other institutions to which needy children might be sent. The extent to which the paedophilia predates the acquisition of a position of power, as opposed to being constructed in the context of access to vulnerable children, is an open and currently unanswerable question.

Adolescent abusers

Before discussing theoretical models of abuse, it is important to deal with a topic that has come to be of great interest – the large proportion of sexual abuses that seem to be perpetrated by adolescents (e.g. Becker 1994). Kelly *et al.* (1991) found that 27% of their sample of abused 16–21-year-olds had been abused by adolescents; in the UK, 34% of males convicted for rape in 1985 were under

21 years of age (Lloyd & Walmsley 1989, quoted in Bentovim 1991). Davis & Leitenberg (1987), reviewing the literature on adolescent sex offenders, state:

Arrest statistics and victim surveys ... indicate that about 20% of all rapes and about 30% to 50% of all cases of child sexual abuse can be attributed to adolescent offenders ... In addition, approximately 50% of adult sexual offenders report that their first sexual offence occurred during adolescence. (p. 417)

These arrest rates are probably substantial underestimates of the actual proportion of abusive acts carried out by adolescents, as a number of factors inhibiting legal action operate more strongly with adolescents than with adults (e.g. not perceiving the seriousness of abusive acts). Nevertheless, the arrest rates do give an indication of the scale of the problem, and it is of importance that the largest proportion of victims of adolescent male sexual offenders are younger children – in a study by Feherenbach *et al.* (1986), 62% of victims were under 12 and 44% were 6 or younger. Most of these boys' victims were female, but the proportion of male victims seems higher than in samples of adult abusers. Manocha & Mezey (1998) found a similar pattern in the victims of their British study of adolescent abusers, with the victims' average age being 8.9 years.

The seriousness of adolescent abusive acts is considerable. In a study of substantiated physical and sexual abuse carried out by caregivers and resulting in entery of the child on the Iowa Child Abuse Registry for 1985–6, Margolin & Craft (1990) found that adolescents were the most severely sexually abusive caregivers and represented a significantly higher proportion of those who committed sexual abuse than of those who committed physical abuse.

Not only did adolescents account for 44% of all cases of child sexual abuse among non-parental caregivers, a proportion which was more than twice that of any other caregiver cohort, but ... the sexual abuse they committed was more likely to involve threats, physical injury and intercourse than was true of older caregivers.'

(Margolin & Craft 1990, p. 369).

There are little empirical data bearing on the comparative attributes of adolescents who do or do not sexually abuse children. Davis & Leitenberg (1987) list the following clinical suggestions on possible aetiological factors: 'feelings of male inadequacy; low self-esteem; fear of rejection and anger towards women; atypical erotic fantasies; poor social skills; having been sexually abused; and exposure to adult models of aggression, dominance and intimidation' (p. 421). Of these suggestions, a history of having been abused seems to be the best supported in the general adolescent sexual offender group, although it is not clear how well these findings apply to those adolescents who abuse *children* (a subgroup of the whole). For example, Van Ness (1984) found that 41% of adolescent sex offenders reported histories of physical abuse or neglect, compared with 15% of a matched group of delinquents. Awad & Saunders (1991) conducted clinical assessments of 49 male adolescent sex offenders revealing that most of them were recidivists, had a history of antisocial behaviour predating and coinciding with their sexual offences, and came from a disturbed family background. One-third of the sample had a history of physical abuse in childhood, although sexual abuse could be confirmed in only two cases.

Bentovim (1991), noting the high proportion of adolescent abusers who appear to have been abused themselves, distinguishes between the situation with female abusers (of which almost all seem to have been previously abused) and male abusers, for whom rates of about 50% are more characteristic. More generally, it is clear that many juvenile offenders of various kinds have a past history of physical and sexual abuse (e.g. Brannon *et al.* 1989), so it is unlikely that a specific causal mechanism operates to link abusive experiences with becoming a sexual abuser in adolescence. As Bentovim suggests, a more subtle and yet broad set of factors must be operating, possibly connected with what he calls 'the notion that if during development a child is treated as a thing instead of a person, then he or she will treat the other as a thing'. Again, how closely this refers to specifically sexual forms of abuse is a moot point.

Towards a theory of sexual abusiveness

The material presented in this chapter so far is deeply unsatisfying in relation to its coherence and implications for theory and practice. On balance, the research on male sexual abusers has found little to distinguish them from other offenders, and perhaps little to distinguish them from men in general, other than the possibility of an increased rate of prior history of sexual victimisation and some suggestion of unusually marked specific sexual interest in children. Part of the difficulty derives from the absence of studies of non-institutionalised abusers, which means that generalisations concerning the characteristics of most abusers (who do not get imprisoned) cannot be made. But it may also be that the differences between abusers and non-abusers are rather subtle, residing more in a set of contingencies such as access to vulnerable children and absence of other inhibiting factors, rather than purely to psychological characteristics of the abusers alone. It is on this assumption that the most influential theoretical model of sexual abusiveness, that of Finkelhor (1984) is premised, a model which is described and discussed below. If this is correct, it suggests that there is some systematic component particularly to male sexual socialisation that contributes to the abusiveness of so many men, i.e. that there is something in most or all men which can get triggered into abusive acts given the appropriate circumstances. The next part of this section discusses one possible psychoanalytically and feminist-influenced reading of what these socialisation influences might be.

A major attraction of Finkelhor's 'four-factor model' of child sexual abuse is precisely that it does not claim that abusiveness is the determinate product of any one elemental cause. The mixed and confusing evidence on characteristics of abusers described earlier, is one aspect of the argument that such a multifactorial model is required; more generally, the enormous range of behaviours that might be termed 'abusive' makes it unlikely that any simple descriptive, let alone causal, framework will encompass all the relevant phenomena. An additional attraction of the model is that, even given the poor state of most of the research, the empirical evidence that exists can be incorporated into its claims.

Araji & Finkelhor (1986) describe the model as arising out of a review of the theories of sexual abusiveness, suggesting that most of these theories

> could be categorised as trying to explain one of four factors: (1) why a person would find relating sexually to a child to be emotionally gratifying and congruent (in the sense of the child fitting the adult's needs), (2) why a person would be capable of being sexually aroused by a child, (3) why a person would be frustrated or blocked in efforts to obtain sexual and emotional gratification from more normatively approved sources, and (4) why a person would not be deterred by the conventional social restraints and inhibitions against having sexual relations with a child. (p. 92)

These four factors are then collected in the model to form a series of interconnections which may have sexual abuse as their outcome. For some of these connections there is empirical support; for most there is only speculation or logic, but they still offer the best available framework for conceptualising the complex pathways that may result in abusive acts. In summary, the suggested elements in each factor are as follows (adapted from Araji & Finkelhor 1986, pp. 93–94):

Factor 1: Emotional congruence

- Children attractive because of lack of dominance
- Arrested development/immaturity
- Low self-esteem
- Mastery of trauma through repetition
- Identification with aggression
- Narcissism
- Male socialisation to dominance.

Factor 2: Sexual arousal

- Heightened arousal to children
- Conditioning from early childhood experience
- Modelling from earlier childhood experiences
- Hormonal abnormalities
- Misattribution of arousal
- Socialisation through child pornography or advertising.

Factor 3: Blockage

- Difficulty relating to adult females
- Inadequate social skills
- Sexual anxiety
- Unresolved Oedipal dynamics
- Disturbances in adult sexual romantic relationships
- Repressive norms about sexual behaviour.

Factor 4: Disinhibition

- Impulse disorder
- Senility
- Mental retardation
- Alcohol
- Failure of incest avoidance mechanism
- Situational stress
- Cultural toleration
- Patriarchal norms.

From the overview of research evidence presented above, it will be apparent that many of the subsidiary elements to each factor are not supported by evidence, and that in some instances there is little other than clinical reports to prop up an entire hypothetical factor. For example, few studies offer anything positive on Factor 3, and Factor 4 only really has supportive evidence from recordings of alcohol as a disinhibitor. Factor 2 also has equivocal support from the laboratory studies of sexual arousal, and Factor 1, while seeming very plausible, is again reliant on clinical reports and speculation for support. Once again it has to be noted that research in this area is very insubstantial, and even the best and most cautious of models relies mainly on face validity and clinical appropriateness for its influence. But Finkelhor's approach does offer very specific suggestions for research and is potentially falsifiable and improvable – hallmarks of a move towards something a little less speculative for the future.

As mentioned above, one of the implications of the multifactorial approach is that, given certain circumstances, many men could be abusers. Inspecting the model, it is interesting how many of the suggestions in each factor are couched at a fairly general social level, concerned with masculine dominance, repressive sexual norms, the influence of pornography and so on. This reflects a painful question facing all men working in the area of sexual abuse: to what extent must abusiveness be seen as an element of masculinity, as opposed to an attribute only of some (pathological) men? The difficulty of establishing clear differences between abusers and others suggests that the shared masculine economy of abusive potential might be more general than one might wish. Alongside the influence of feminist thinking on sexual violence in general, this has led to some attempts to piece together a model of masculine sexual socialisation that might have explanatory power and also suggest ways forward for therapy, prevention and even (over-optimistically perhaps) social change. One such theoretical perspective worthy of consideration arises from recent psychoanalytic thinking, coupled with a general project of analysing the components of contemporary masculinity. Here, I shall present the version of this approach given in Glaser & Frosh (1993); interested readers are referred to Frosh (1994) for a fuller account, and to Jukes (1993) for a related description arising out of engagement in therapeutic work with violent men.

In recent years, feminist-influenced analyses of the characteristics of masculine sexuality have converged on the notion that at the core of the problematic elements is a combination of power and fear. Seidler (1985, p. 169) comments:

Masculine sexual identity is established through feeling superior to women we are close to and through establishing our sense of identity in a masculine competitive world. It is as if we only know how to feel good ourselves if we put others down.

Traditional 'masculinity' focuses on dominance and independence, an orientation to the world which is active and assertive, valorising competitiveness and turned away from intimacy. The fear at the heart of this image is of emotion – that which makes us vulnerable and 'womanly'. Emotion is dangerous not only because it implies dependence, but also because (with the important exception of anger) it is alien, a representation of the maternal dimension against which masculinity is contrasted. This fear of emotion in turn makes sex both over- and under-invested in by men. Sex is one of the few socially acceptable ways in which men can aspire to closeness with others and, as such, it becomes the carrier of the unexpressed desires which men's emotional illiteracy produces. However, this same power of sex to produce emotionality makes it dangerous to men whose identity is built upon the rejection of emotion; sex then becomes split-off, limited to the activity of the penis, an act rather than an encounter. It is also a means of taking up a particular place in the world of men: sexual 'conquest' as a symbol of male prowess. The link between such a form of masculinity and sexual abuse is inherent in the rejection of intimacy, producing the possibility of a slide from sex as achievement to sex as degradation of the other.

There are numerous different accounts of the processes that might construct masculinity along these lines, ranging from the sociological 'male sexual drive' discourse to radical feminist readings of masculine psychology as little more than an organisation of force relations to oppress women. The approach deriving from feminist psychoanalytic writers such as Chodorow (1978) and Benjamin (1988) has been particularly influential in its emphasis on the negative impact of gender-differentiated child care on the ability of boys to experience themselves as dependent and emotionally connected to others. In outline, such accounts of masculine development run something like this. At first, there is a tremendously powerful bond between infant and mother, an absorption of the one in the other which is bodily relatively unmediated, perhaps already infused with anxieties and a horror of separation. Girls may have problems arising from this – problems of differentiation, of constructing a feminine self that is both bodily and autonomous, of entering the world of symbols and culture, and of becoming true 'subjects'. For boys, attaining masculinity involves striving towards something unknown and unknowable: a state of difference from the mother, yet grounded in her. The trend of early experience is to suck the boy in, to make him fused with the mother; but fused he can neither become independent of her nor take on the vague but intensely felt promise of masculine mastery. Consequently, his temptation is to repudiate the mother, a repudiation helped by her own fantasy of him as 'other', different from her, and also by the cultural fantasy that the masculine dominates the feminine.

The boy's sense of mastery, however, is far from secure: he knows that he is really dependent, that he cannot survive without help. Consequently, as a defensive manoeuvre against his own emotional needs, reinforced by the cultural derogation of womanhood and the opposition between 'feminine' and 'masculine' qualities, the boy's ability to form intimate relationships is suppressed while his assertive, aggressive and spoiling elements are encouraged: 'the devaluation of the need for the other becomes a touchstone of masculine development' (Benjamin 1988, p. 171). Hence 'successful' masculine socialisation involves effective action in the world at the price of a fragile and underdeveloped emotional capacity, which fuels both an urgent demand for more closeness with the mother and a destructive rejection of her. Sexually, the boy learns to fear his desire, because it brings back the loss of mastery; hence its conversion into conquest and performance.

The common product of this developmental process is an adult male whose capacity to nurture is severely impaired, whose ability to form affectionate relationships is restricted, and whose masculine identity, since it rests upon a repudiation of his identification with the person who first cared for him, is forever in doubt.

(Herman 1981, p. 56)

There are several difficulties with this simplified and partial version of the psychoanalytic theory of masculine development. For instance, it is unclear how some people come to rebel against their traditional gender role, and it concentrates too strongly on the mother–child bond, neglecting consideration of wider social processes (see Frosh 1999). It does one important thing, however, and that is to move discussion of the sources of sexual abuse away from specific traumatic events that occur almost accidentally to particular men, and towards those normative processes in socialisation that make sexual abuse possible. This is not to say that there may not be particular causes that create an abuser out of any particular man: Finkelhor's model supplies examples of just such possible causes, with the experience of being abused oneself being a powerful example. Rather, the point here is that there may be systematic features of masculine sexuality that contribute to sexual abuse. Of course this does not mean that all men abuse children, and the differences between those who do and those who do not are crucial for theory and for therapeutic practice. These differences may in principle arise from a number of sources, e.g. the quality of early relationships as well as those formed during adulthood, challenges to emotional distancing faced during development, differences in patterns of gender socialisation and specific experiences of trauma or reparation. But amongst all the vague and contradictory empirical data, the finding that most abusers are men seems a secure one, requiring explanation. The suggestion in this theoretical material is that the systematic links between masculinity and abuse are not given through biology, nor are they caused only by the organisation of society on patriarchal lines; rather, they are constructed in the specific patterns of relationship and desire which are characteristic of masculine sexual socialisation. The painful mixture of impulse and over-control, of separation and intimacy, of fear and desire – this mixture so common in men – is also something that infiltrates men's relationships with children, sometimes leading to abuse.

Implications for practice

To the extent that the empirical and theoretical material described in this chapter offers reasonably strong evidence of anything, it is that:

- Sexual abusers are an extremely heterogeneous group
- They are a dangerous group in that they are prone to abuse in multiple and repetitive ways and, when prosecuted and punished, their recidivism rate is not particularly low
- Most abusers are male, although more women abuse than was previously thought
- Many abusers are very young themselves, with abusing careers often beginning in adolescence
- The sources of abusive behaviour lie in a mixture of individual history and shared socialisation processes.

Given all this, it is perhaps not surprising that attempts to draw up characterological profiles of abusers are unsatisfactory, and that the work on sexual arousal patterns now looks less powerful than once thought. Sexually abusive behaviour arises out of a particular cultural milieu in which sex is something done *to* another, and in which children are available for exploitation. It is linked with, but not specific to, the experiences of abuse suffered by some who go on to abuse others, and it may be strongly connected with dynamics of power and powerlessness, and fears of intimacy and dependence. Its repetitive nature suggests that it might have addictive components and thus may need to be managed cognitively and behaviourally, but an approach that does not separate 'sex' from sexuality and personality is needed for a fuller account of the meaning and potency of abusiveness. For this reason, and despite the lack of supportive empirical data, it is important that focused psychotherapeutic work with abusers continues alongside more cognitive-behavioural approaches. Currently, there is little evidence to support any one way of working over another – nothing seems to offer any particularly good omens of success. But it may be that intensive therapeutic work across a range of theoretical orientations can lead to better understanding of the nature and vicissitudes of abusive behaviour towards children.

A final point returns us to the problem of working only with incarcerated offenders. It is still extremely difficult to persuade abusers to enter into treatment programmes, because if they do so they are in effect admitting their responsibility or guilt for acts of sexual abuse, and thus may incriminate themselves and receive substantial punishment when they would otherwise not be prosecuted. Unfair though it may seem to some or even many victims of abuse, if any substantial impact is ever to be made on abusers it is going to be necessary to establish legal practices resulting in non-custodial, treatment-oriented interventions. This does not mean that such treatments will necessarily be effective; but prison sentences also do not work particularly well, and therapeutic efficacy cannot develop unless it has a chance.

Conclusion

This chapter contains a presentation of some empirical and theoretical work bearing on the characteristics of sexual abusers of children. It will be clear that the empirical situation is very unsatisfactory, partly for good reasons given the endemic difficulties of researching an area in which secrecy, shame, dissimulation and obscurity are the norm. Most of the research is little more than clinical speculation, and where empirical studies have been carried out the sample populations concerned have usually been varieties of incarcerated sexual offenders, making generalisations to the wider population of non-convicted abusers problematic. It is important that future efforts both in research and in therapy move beyond this narrowly defined group, but it must be acknowledged that, given current legislation, this is going to be difficult to achieve. In particular, more focused studies of, and intervention programmes with, adolescent abusers are needed. It may be that such studies and programmes will also provide clearer documentation of the way in which social mores (especially those relating to the sexual socialisation of males) are linked to the production and perpetuation of sexually abusive behaviour.

References

Abel G, Becker J, Cunningham-Rathner J, Rouleau J, Kaplan M, Reich J 1984 The treatment of child molesters. Unpublished manuscript, quoted in Conte 1991

Abel G, Becker J, Mittleman M, Cunningham-Rathner J, Rouleau J, Murphy W 1987 Self-reported sex crimes of non-incarcerated paraphiliacs. In: Stuart R (ed) Violent behavior. Brunner/Mazel, New York

Abel G, Becker J, Cunningham-Rathner J, Mittleman M, Rouleau J 1988 Multiple paraphiliac diagnoses among sex offenders. Bulletin of the American Academy of Psychiatry and the Law 16: 153–168

Araji S, Finkelhor D 1986 Abusers: a review of the research. In: Finkelhor D (ed) A sourcebook on child sexual abuse. Sage, London

Awad G, Saunders E 1991 Male adolescent sexual assaulters: clinical observations. Journal of Interpersonal Violence 6: 446–460

Baker A, Duncan S 1985 Child sexual abuse: a study of prevalence in Great Britain. Child Abuse and Neglect 9: 457–467

Becker J 1994 Offenders: characteristics and treatment. Future of Children 4: 176–197

Benjamin J 1988 The bonds of love. Virago, London

Bentovim A 1991 Children and young people as abusers. In: Hollows A, Armstrong H (eds) Children and young people as abusers. National Children's Bureau, London

Bentovim A, Elton A, Hildebrand J, Tranter M, Vizard E 1988 Child sexual abuse within the family. Wright, London

Brannon J, Larsen B, Doggett M 1989 The extent and origin of sexual molestation and abuse among incarcerated adolescent males. International Journal of Offender Therapy and Comparative Criminology 33: 161–172

Briere J, Runtz M 1989 Post sexual abuse trauma. In: Wyatt G, Powell G (eds) Lasting effects of child sexual abuse. Sage, London

Browne K 1993 Violence in the family and its links to child abuse. In: Hobbs C, Wynne J (eds) Ballière's clinical paediatrics: child abuse. Ballière Tindall, London

Chodorow N 1978 The reproduction of mothering. University of California Press, Berkeley, California

Conte J 1991 The nature of sexual offences against children. In: Hollin C, Howells K (eds) Clinical approaches to sexual offenders and their victims. Wiley, Chichester

Davis G, Leitenberg H 1987 Adolescent sex offenders. Psychological Bulletin 101: 417–427

Feherenbach P, Smith W, Monastersky C, Deisher R 1986 Adolescent sexual offenders: offender and offense characteristics. American Journal of Orthopsychiatry 56: 225–233

Feshbach N 1989 The construct of empathy and the phenomenon of physical maltreatment of children. In: Cicchetti D, Carlson V (eds) Child maltreatment. Cambridge University Press, Cambridge

Finkelhor D 1984 Child sexual abuse. Free Press, New York

Finkelhor D 1986 Abusers: special topics. In: Finkelhor D (ed) A sourcebook on child sexual abuse. Sage, London

Frenzel R, Lang R 1989 Identifying sexual preferences in intrafamilial and extrafamilial child sexual abusers. Annals of Sex Research 2: 255–275

Freund K, McKnight C, Langevin R, Cibiri S 1972 The female child as a surrogate object. Archives of Sexual Behavior 2: 119–133

Frosh S 1994 Sexual difference: masculinity and psychoanalysis. Routledge, London

Frosh S 1999 The politics of psychoanalysis. Macmillan, London

Furby L, Weinrott M, Blackshaw L 1989 Sex offender recidivism: a review. Psychological Bulletin 105: 3–30

Furniss T 1991 The multiprofessional handbook of child sexual abuse. Routledge, London

Glaser D 1993 Emotional abuse. In: Hobbs C, Wynne J (eds) Balliére's clinical paediatrics: child abuse. Ballière Tindall, London

Glaser D, Frosh S 1993 Child sexual abuse. Macmillan, London

Griffin S, Williams M, Hawkes C, Vizard F 1997 The professional carers' group: supporting group work for young sexual abusers. Child Abuse and Neglect 21: 681–690

Groth A, Burgess A 1979 Sexual trauma in the life histories of rapists and child molesters. Victimology 4: 10–16

Groth A, Hobson W, Gary T 1982 The child molester: clinical observations. Social Work and Human Sexuality 1: 129–144

Hall G, Proctor W, Nelson G 1988 Validity of physiological measures of pedophilic sexual arousal in a sexual offender population. Journal of Consulting and Clinical Psychology 56: 118–122

Hanson R, Slater S 1988 Sexual victimisation in the history of sexual abusers. Annals of Sex Research 1: 485–499

Haugaard J, Emery R 1989 Methodological issues in child sexual abuse research. Child Abuse and Neglect 13: 89–100

Haugaard J, Reppucci N 1988 The sexual abuse of children. Jossey-Bass, London

Herman J 1981 Father–daughter incest. Harvard University Press, Cambridge, Massachusetts

Hoghughi M, Bhate S (eds) 1997 Working with sexually abusive adolescents. Sage, London

Howes R 1998 Plethysmographic assessment of incarcerated nonsexual offenders: a comparison with rapists. Sexual Abuse: Journal of Research and Treatment 10: 183–194

Jukes A 1993 Why men hate women. Free Association Books, London

Kaufman J, Zigler E 1989 The intergenerational transmission of child abuse. In: Cicchetti D, Carlson V (eds) Child maltreatment. Cambridge University Press, Cambridge

Kelly L, Regan L, Burton S 1991 An exploratory study of the prevalence of sexual abuse in a sample of 16–21-year-olds. Polytechnic of North London, London

Lang R, Black E, Frenzel R, Checkley K 1988 Aggression and erotic attraction towards children in incestuous and pedophilic men. Annals of Sex Research 1: 417–441

Lang R, Langevin R 1991 Parent–child relations in offenders who commit violent crimes against children. Behavioral Sciences and the Law 9: 61–71

Langevin R 1985 Pedophilia and incest. In: Langevin R (ed) Erotic preference, gender identity and aggression in men. Lawrence Erlbaum, New Jersey

Langevin R, Hucker S, Handy L, Hook H, Purins J, Russon A 1985 Erotic preference and aggression in pedophilia. In: Langevin R (ed) Erotic preference, gender identity and aggression in men. Lawrence Erlbaum, New Jersey

Lawson C 1993 Mother–son sexual abuse: rare or under reported? Child Abuse and Neglect 17: 261–269

Manocha K, Mezey G 1998 British adolescents who sexually abuse: a descriptive study. Journal of Forensic Psychiatry 9: 588–608

Margolin L, Craft J 1990 Child abuse by adolescent caregivers. Child Abuse and Neglect 14: 365–373

Marshall W, Barbaree H, Christophe D 1986 Sexual offenders against children: sexual preference for age of victims and type of behavior. Canadian Journal of Behavioral Science 18: 424–439

Marshall W, Barbaree H, Eccles A 1991 Early onset and deviant sexuality in child molesters. Journal of Interpersonal Violence 6: 323–335

McConaghy N 1998 Paedophilia: a review of the evidence. Australian and New Zealand Journal of Psychiatry 32: 252–265

Meier J 1985 Definition, dynamics and prevalence of assault against children. In: Meier J (ed) Assault against children. Taylor and Francis, London

Murphy W, Haynes M, Worley P 1991 Assessment of adult sexual interest. In: Hollin C, Howells K (eds) Clinical approaches to sexual offenders and their victims. Wiley, Chichester

Murphy W, Peters J 1992 Profiling child sexual abusers: psychological considerations. Criminal Justice and Behavior 19: 24–37

Pithers W 1999 Empathy: definition, enhancement, and relevance to the treatment of sexual abusers. Journal of Interpersonal Violence 14: 257–284

Quinsey V, Chaplin T 1988 Penile responses of child molesters and normals to descriptions of encounters with children involving sex and violence. Journal of Interpersonal Violence 3: 259–274

Russell D 1983 The incidence and prevalence of intrafamilial and extrafamilial sexual abuse of female children. Child Abuse and Neglect 7: 133–146

Rutter M 1989 Intergenerational continuities and discontinuities in serious parenting difficulties. In: Cicchetti D, Carlson V (eds) Child maltreatment. Cambridge University Press, Cambridge

Seidler V 1985 Fear and intimacy. In: Metcalfe A, Humphries M (eds) The sexuality of men. Pluto, London

Simon L, Sales B, Kaszniak A, Kahn M 1992 Characteristics of child molesters: implications for the fixated-regression dichotomy. Journal of Interpersonal Violence 7: 211–255

Van Ness S 1984 Rape as instrumental violence: a study of youth offenders. Journal of Offender Counselling, Services and Rehabilitation 9: 161–170

Wakefield H, Underwager R 1991 Female child sexual abusers: a critical review of the literature. American Journal of Forensic Psychology 9: 43–69

Wilson R 1999 Emotional congruence in sexual offenders against children. Sexual Abuse: Journal of Research and Treatment 11: 33–48

5 | Consequences and indicators of child abuse

Helga Hanks and Peter Stratton

Helga Hanks and Peter Stratton

INTRODUC- TION

An accurate evaluation of the effects of child abuse is fundamental in the protection of children from maltreatment. It is essential in specific cases to know what level of risk the child is exposed to by being left in the abusive family; what aspects of abuse are most damaging and therefore are the most urgent targets for protection; and what consequences, both short- and long-term, the child may need professional help to overcome. Also, much diagnosis and detection depends on working back from signs, physical and behavioural, in the child to forms of abuse known to produce these signs. At a service level, an estimate of the effects of abuse is needed to plan services, and to specify the training needed by workers. Nationally and internationally, a realistic understanding of the widespread and serious consequences of abuse would indicate the scale of need, the urgency of the problem, and the resources needed to tackle it.

At present there are many factors which work against being able to make even an approximate evaluation of the effects of abuse. This is true both for individual cases, and in the general context. The history of child abuse has been one in which clear medical evidence has been the first, and necessary, indicator before the problem was accepted. Even in physical abuse nearly 40 years after Kempe's seminal article (Kempe *et al.* 1962) medical consequences of abuse are still regarded as more tangible evidence, and are better understood, than the psychological consequences. But the resistance to recognising the full range and severity of the effects of abuse goes much deeper. Abuse is a painful reality and everybody, given the chance, would prefer to avoid the pain of recognising it. Maybe our own relative terrors as children, or our inadequacies as parents are brought closer to awareness as we encounter obvious examples of abuse. And of course, many professionals who work in this field have been victims of earlier maltreatment in their own lives. Finally, by confronting maltreatment we risk becoming aware of our own capacity to abuse and we risk being overwhelmed by the scale and horror of the problem.

Because of the variety of factors working against a clear recognition of the effects of maltreatment, we start this chapter with a consideration of two sources of difficulty: myths about children, and the power of denial. Next we provide a framework for understanding the consequences of maltreatment which is designed to give full weight to psychological as well as physical effects. The core of the chapter uses representative examples from the great volume of research and clinical experience to map out the major consequences in different areas of child maltreatment.

Perceptions of children, or the 'spoilt child' – can we put the record straight

During the twentieth century Western society gave considerable thought and discussion to the issue of how children should be brought up. We entered the so-called 'child centred' era. With hindsight we can easily detect deficiencies in earlier views, and with insight we may even criticise our current beliefs. Two themes that apply both to the past and the present relate to the idea that if children get their way they will become too powerful and the rather contradictory image of the child as a helpless recipient of influence.

For instance, Western societies put great emphasis on sameness, uniformity and, despite what they often say, obedience, compliance and competition at the same time. The competitive struggle was proposed by politicians as an economic one (making money) but has become firmly established in the interpersonal and family sphere, often with destructive consequences. Partly because of this, the accepted way to bring up children is to mind that they are not made too comfortable, don't get their way even when it might be quite sensible, but for the parents always to win. The 4-hour feeding schedule is an example of compliance, sameness and teaching obedience. The child that cries at night must not be picked up and comforted; the child who has not eaten their dinner must not have a pudding; there must be no talking during mealtimes etc. These are just a few examples of what people generally think might spoil a child.

What word do we have for a child who is being treated really nicely, listened to etc.? The only word you will hear is that the child is being spoilt. Mothers are advised not to feed their baby whenever it shows signs of wanting food in case it becomes too powerful, learns how to exploit you, and is spoilt. Though it is not an original idea we would like to draw attention to what we consider to be the true meaning of a 'spoilt' child. Something being spoilt is defined in the dictionary as being damaged or injured, something made useless, valueless … destroyed. The paradoxical juxtaposition of the meaning of 'the spoilt child' in the English language alerts us to a fundamental ambivalence about the rights of children. When attempting to help maltreated children, professionals and parents alike have to take into consideration that these are the children that someone has tried to spoil, in the 'real' (dictionary) sense. The abused, maltreated children are the children that are spoilt.

This issue is important for another reason too. Many children, adolescents and adults who have been maltreated have over the years described how they feel. The cry from those who have been maltreated that they feel and are treated as 'damaged goods' is a stark reminder of what being spoilt really means.

The other myth, which can damage professional attempts to care for maltreated children, is of the child as passive recipient of influence. Our whole approach to child rearing, and to education, reflects this assumption. We are very ready to talk of the effects of education, of child care practices and of maltreatment on the child. It is much more difficult to recognise that children are active participants in creating their worlds. Perhaps we are afraid of blaming the victim; perhaps it is just easier to see things from an adult's point of view. But damage is not primarily something that can be put into a child to be carried around, invisible inside them. Damaging environments are places in which children function and grow. The ways they function and the form of their growth will be affected and that is what we need to understand. It may be helpful to think in terms of the child adapting to the environment. The important effects of abuse are at least as likely to be in the kinds of adaptations the child comes to make as in simple direct consequences. This is an idea we return to after considering the second issue which obstructs the clear recognition of the effects of abuse.

Denial

In every eye there is a spot that is incapable of sight. The optic disc exists as a black hole right next to the central point of clearest vision. Yet anyone who has not learned the trick of finding it would swear that there is no such void.

(Summit 1988, p 51)

Kempe & Kempe (1984) pointed to the stages that society needs to go through in its progressive recognition of the reality of child abuse. These stages are progressive defences of denial to keep out a recognition of something that is unacceptable and at odds with the view we want to have of ourselves and our society. Equally we know very well that abused children may take refuge in denial to avoid the destructive effects of recognising what is being done to them. But, in our experience, even committed professionals still have to use denial in self-protection (Summit 1988).

Denial and the effects of abuse are intricately linked. The reader is referred particularly to Summit (1988) and Furniss (1991). The material that follows about the forms, function and areas of denial of Child Sexual Abuse (CSA) has been taken from Furniss (1991).

Forms of denial

These can be seen in the context of the abuse being denied by the abuser, the non-abusing care giver, the child or other family members. Each of them might deny different aspects of the abuse. It may be total denial that any abuse has taken place or it may be partial denial of:

- abusive circumstances
- damaging effects
- the addictive and repetitive nature of CSA
- the abuser's responsibility.

The function of denial

Denial can relate to anxieties about:

- the legal consequences
- consequences for family and relatives
- psychological consequences
- social consequences
- financial/work/career consequences.

There are several areas of denial to disclaim responsibility for abuse, e.g.:

- primary denial of any abuse
- denial of severity of acts
- denial of knowledge of abuse (perpetrators may say they were drunk, asleep, depressed, tired, etc.)
- denial that the maltreatment was abusive (this may involve pretending that the abuse was a normal/educational activity)
- denial of the harmful effects of the abuse (the abusive act is said not to have harmed the child)
- denial of responsibility (the perpetrator makes the child responsible for the abuse, saying that the child triggered the abuse by their behaviour).

Child maltreatment is linked to denial because the pain, helplessness, worthlessness and rejection that children feel when they are maltreated has to be hidden in

> **Case**
>
> Keely, who is 9 years old, was in therapy because she had been severely maltreated all her life. She had been in care in a stable foster home for a number of months and recently began not only to disclose further specific incidences of her abuse but also to behave in a way that made it difficult to contain and look after her. She began hitting adults and children alike, ran away (the foster parents thought she was with older youngsters and experiencing sex), lied, stole and then felt terribly sorry, sobbing and pleading with the foster parents not to send her away. The discussions between the professionals and foster parents centred on the fact that Keely was going through a very difficult time in coming to terms with her previous abuse. One way of explaining what was happening is outlined below.

some way. We have many examples in Western society which indicate that child abuse is much easier to blame on professionals who identify the children and the problem, than on an acknowledgement that all is not well in society and particularly in the family where unfortunately but undeniably most abuse takes place.

When children are maltreated consistently and severely (though what children can take varies from one to another), they have to build up some defences in order to bear what is happening to them. When there is no help to deal with the psychic pain, the pain becomes encapsulated, as if put into a sealed space. This idea comes from psychoanalytic literature and there is called encapsulation (Ferenczy 1949). The sealed space might be thought of as a nut with a shell that has become harder over time and all the painful, angry, desperate feelings are contained in this nut.

However, when children like Keely have the chance to 'open up', so to speak, and feel secure to let the feelings come out through a crack in the nut's shell, the situation described above might occur.

During one therapy session, when Keely talked about what had been happening in the previous few weeks, the therapist told her the story of the nut and said: 'it feels as if nobody knows the strength of the feelings that are in this nut. It is such a surprise to you to discover some of the terrible feelings of revenge and anger you might have inside that nut. So much so that you feel that you could kill someone. (Keely had taken a broom and tried to hit her foster mother with it during the last week. She had also said afterwards that it was a terrible feeling because at that moment she could have killed her.) The feelings are so strong that at that moment of discovery they are difficult to control.' Keely, who had been sitting very still and listening, burst into tears and wept bitterly.

Becoming very sad is one reaction to abuse that needs to be tackled in therapy; being angry is another. But these children with their strong feelings also need some very practical input. In Keely's case, the therapist had a meeting with the child, the mother and the social worker and discussed with them the fact that Keely needed some help in managing her angry feelings. The issues about setting boundaries, what could be done and what could not be done by Keely were discussed, particularly in relation to feeling and at times when she seemed out of control. It was suggested that she should try not to hurt either herself or others. The foster parents were asked to see Keely through these difficult times and not be afraid to call for help if they needed it from the social worker.

The concept of 'denial' has changed over the years and researchers and clinicians have been preoccupied with issues related to minimisation, how decisions and attitudes are formed and how child abuse can be missed or even ignored both in the public and professional setting. An important example can be found in the research carried out by Hetherton & Beardsall (1998) when they examined the reporting of females as perpetrators of sexual abuse. They discovered that female sexual abuse of children remains so rarely recognised because it seems to deviate both from cultural norms as well as the ideal of women as mother or caregiver and therefore not thought to be capable of such an act. An equally important example relating to the 'backlash' that has reverberated throughout the world in cases of child abuse, is the discovery of children being sexually abused in the Dutch town of Oude Pekela which provoked a significant '... backlash in the Dutch nation. Sceptical people immediately labelled the case as mass hysteria' (Jonker & Jonker-Bakker, 1997, p. 552).

Denial is also touched on in Arnold & Cloke's (1988) paper. Importantly, they talk of the reasons why abuse can keep its momentum to such an extent and see the cause in the fact that society keeps abuse hidden for all manner of reasons personal, political and religious. 'Societal denial' of abuse, they recommend, can be lessened by creating child-friendly communities in which there is a climate where children can be heard, respected appropriately and listened to.

The earlier writings about denial and clear naming of the phenomenon are still an important guide today.

Once it is possible to recognise the range of factors which might make us under-estimate the effects of abuse, we are better able to confront the huge amount of evidence on particular aspects of these effects.

The subject of severity has been a difficult one and has preoccupied different professional groups in various ways. The demand in the legal field for clarity and proof of the extent of the abuse is one requirement. The measurement of emotional and psychological consequences, the medical consequences of injuries and the social issues that are brought into the open about standards of care are other concerns. Margaret Adcock, in her chapter on assessment (see Chapter 12, in this volume) guides us through many of these issues and we will here briefly concentrate only on the issues of severity and how it might be measured.

So far it has been difficult to quantify 'severity' of abuse and particularly the emotional and psychological consequences of child maltreatment. We know from the literature and research into some of the forms of abuse (i.e. emotional and sexual) that when a child is repeatedly abused over a long time the consequences are more severe. However, a caution is raised by research carried out by Barnett *et al.* (1993) who developed a system for measuring severity. They discovered that when they assessed 'mild' abuse of children it nevertheless turned out to have a powerful effect on the children's adjustment. This raised the concern that those children who come out of an assessment as having been abused 'mildly' in comparison to others would be excluded from treatment, their response to what happened not recognised and the psychological consequences ignored. If we follow this line of thinking, we might influence child care and parenting issues in a detrimental way by ignoring the extent to which the individual child in their particular circumstances may be affected detrimentally by child-rearing practices.

Brassard & Hardy (1997) discuss a range of assessment scales and techniques and recognise that a definition of severity in the legal arena is highly complicated. They recommend the *Guidelines for the Psychosocial Evaluation of Suspected Psychological Maltreatment in Children and Adolescents*, which can determine both 'acts' of maltreatment and demonstrate the 'harm' that has either occurred or could occur in the future. However, in many American States, professionals are not permitted to make such a determination until after the evidence has been collected for Court.

So there is a beginning of assessing the extent of harm done and severity. Certain scales can be useful but do not stand undisputed. Sanders & Becker–Lausen (1995) developed the Child Abuse and Trauma Scales (CATS), which measures three subscales – sexual abuse, punishment and neglect. Because the scale seemed to be robust, Kent & Waller (1998) added an emotional subscale to the CATS and had positive results, while admitting that further validation was essential.

Briere (1992) talks of the 'symptoms' of abuse and uses them as a guide or indicator to measure the impact of the abuse on the individual. However, this is not an assessment tool of severity but a tool to recognise what has happened to the person. The literature on resilience may also give us some indication of the ways in which children react differentially to a variety of stressors, including abuse, and Rutter (1999) usefully reviews the issues on resilience and the implications for family therapy.

We have so far talked mainly of the unseen difficulties of child abuse. When a child has been physically abused, bruised, burnt, their bones broken (Hobbs *et al.* 1999), an element of severity can be assessed. Is it a 40% burn? Is there one fracture or several? But even here the severity of the injury and the resulting emotional impact are difficult to assess. It may be quantitatively easier but not anywhere near assessing the emotional cost for the individual, the consequent impact this has on their emotional life and behaviour, now or in the future.

Read (1998) links child abuse and severity of disturbance in an adult psychiatric population and comes to the conclusion that '... child abuse may have a causative role in the most severe psychiatric conditions, including those currently thought to be primarily biological in aetiology' (p. 366).

The main task of this chapter is to review the kinds of effects that different forms of abuse may create.

Severity of abuse

In order not to be overwhelmed by the complexity, we offer three sets of concepts to help coordinate the material: abuse as trauma; the child's adaptation to abuse; and the central issue of attachment.

Fundamental concepts in abuse

Trauma

Recent research on victims (often adult) of a variety of catastrophes has given us an understanding of the effects of trauma which is also very helpful in making sense of events surrounding abuse. Briere (1992) gives a very clear account of the theory, practice and effects. Joseph (1999) has given an insight into the neurology of traumatic dissociative amnesia. He is critical of those denying the damage to certain structures in the brain and the functional integrity of the brain when trauma has occurred. His review of the literature is a helpful guide. He comes to the conclusion that trauma does affect the brain and has consequences indicating that memory loss is only too common, particularly after repeated traumatic events.

Bentovim (1992, p. 24) points out that:

Trauma comes from the Greek word meaning to 'pierce'. In the context of physical injury it implies that the 'skin is broken', that something intact has been breached. It implies a certain intensity of violence, with long-standing consequences for the organism. From the physical notion of trauma, the notion of psychological trauma arises: an event that in a similar intense or violent way ruptures the protective layers surrounding the mind with equally long-lasting consequences for psychic well-being. Helplessness overwhelms, mastery is undermined, defences fail, there is a sense of failure of protection, disintegration, acute mental pain as the memory of the event intrudes and replays itself repeatedly.

The traumatic stress response thus imperceptibly becomes the 'post-traumatic stress disorder'. This type of consequence might be seen in any victim of a traumatic event. A car accident, floods, fires, earthquakes and more personal tragedies will all be included.

The physical pain is closely linked to the psychological experience and pain of the individual. However, there is a difference between an adult's experience of trauma and that of a child. Something additional happens to children because they, by virtue of their age, are in a developmental stage in which they lack the perspectives by which adults can distinguish and make sense of the traumatic event in which they have been involved. Because trauma, and what it means to human beings, is a complex issue it is important to think about two major issues when considering the consequences of such an event:

- Short-term consequences
- Long-term consequences

It also has to be recognised that the effects of child abuse are dynamic and interact with each other; that the experiences and adaptations interweave and become part of the child's developmental process, shaping their view of the world and most importantly themselves.

So childhood trauma is likely to affect the child immediately – during and after the abuse – and this can cause post-traumatic stress, resulting in painful (physical and emotional) effects, and contributing to cognitive distortions (see Bowlby 1988) of all kinds. Abuse will often influence the child's developmental stage and will show itself in arresting or slowing down development, while the child's resources go into coping with the abusive situation.

Many children, sometimes after a brief period of protest, start developing ways of 'coping', as one might describe it, and keeping as safe as possible. Summit (1988) called this 'accommodation', others also described an important developmental process called 'adaptation' (see below). Both these processes are like psychological survival mechanisms and help the child and adult to cope with the continuing maltreatment. The children may develop behaviours they think can keep them safe or lessen the immediate physical and emotional pain. It is as well to note here that children who have been abused by a stranger once and then made safe, will not have to engage in this accommodation to the abusive situation.

Trauma may also affect the child and adult in the long-term. The long-term consequences that will encompass the above two notions set adaptation and accommodation firmly into a defensive pattern from which some victims never return. These patterns become a more intrinsic part of the individual's functioning and are likely to generalise to other aspects of their psychological development throughout life.

Case

Zake, a 5-year-old boy, had witnessed the brutal murder of his father, and had developed a way of existing in the world by abandoning speech and only humming tunes. He said later that he thought that if he only hummed tunes he could stop thinking of what he witnessed around his father's death, and if he could stop thinking about it then he would not feel so terrible.

Thinking of the unthinkable, experiencing and then re-experiencing painful and humiliating episodes is what the children attempt to avoid both in the short- and in the long-term. But such psychological manoeuvres are not accomplished without a price. In order to repress such events considerable psychic energy has to be expended.

The developmental stage might be influenced in such a way that the child is arrested in their development at the time of the abuse. For instance many small children, though not all, who have been maltreated have very little language. Cognitive distortions as a consequence of trauma – misunderstandings, memory loss, blocking and dissociation – may also occur. Any such cognitive distortion carries a cost through distorting subsequent learning, understanding and adjustment.

Adaptations

It is often useful to take behaviour that we might describe as 'symptomatic', and instead see it as an adaptation the person has made. With adults, if we think of, say, depression as a symptom, there is a certain range of things we can think of doing to cure it. If we think of depression as the best adaptation that a person could manage to the circumstances they are in, we can have different ideas about how it helps them; for instance whether they could achieve the same with some alternative adaptation; whether they could change the demands they have felt obliged to meet. The shift is not towards blaming them but to see people as having made the best response they could manage at the time, while opening up the possibility of helping them to make a more useful response in the future. Adaptation is a broader version of the ideas contained in the concept of accommodation.

To a large extent the emotional and behavioural effects we see are the attempts of maltreated children to adapt to the environment surrounding them, including their caregivers (Stratton & Hanks 1991). From this point of view the behaviour of the child is not a 'symptom' but the best response they could make for their own protection. Think of a child who flinches every time someone moves suddenly anywhere near them. Classifying this as a symptom of twitchiness, or as a neurotic behaviour, is not only unhelpful, it disparages the child. Seeing flinching as an adaptive response to an environment in which you might be suddenly assaulted without warning makes more sense and also opens up ideas of what might be done about it.

A child's withdrawal and isolation from peers may be the result of parental rules that wish for a quiet and unassuming child. Other parents may be irritated by a timid, withdrawn child and respond angrily to such a child, who may adapt by putting on displays of aggressive behaviour. Some children find mealtimes traumatic because of emotional tension surrounding eating, or at a more extreme level because they have had burning hot food forced into their mouths. They may adapt by using every way possible to avoid meals (and become labelled as 'poor feeders' as a result). Children who have been sexually exploited may adapt by using the sexual behaviour they have been 'taught' in order to obtain much needed cuddles from adults. Or they may provide the sexual behaviour to avoid punishment. Either way they may be further maltreated by having their adaptation labelled as a symptom of sexual promiscuity.

The ways in which cycles of adaptation to abuse build up, and the implications of these cycles for treatment, have been described in detail by Stratton & Hanks (1991). For the purposes of this chapter we would ask the reader to keep in mind that *all* of the identified consequences of abuse should be thought of as adaptations by the child. The outcome of abuse can then be seen more clearly as following from the adaptation the child is forced into, and not just as a deficit built into the child by the abuse itself.

Attachment relationships of maltreated children

Attachment is a specific relationship and human beings are quite unable to exist without it. For the infant and child it provides a base from which to explore the world and works in a way to ensure that the child's needs are met (Bowlby 1988).

This exploration of the world is recognised as being vital for the infant's development and shows optimal effects when a parent figure is available to provide a secure base. A baby can attach to about five people who are close to the infant and develops the first most important steps of attachment during its first year of life. The role of the attachment figure(s) is to reduce anxiety in stressful situations and provide the infant and child with the confidence to explore and experience unknown and new situations. Attachment to significant adults in infancy is also the foundation for lasting relationships throughout life. So for instance, anxious attachment is often the consequence when a child has to take responsibility for keeping close to an attachment figure (most often the mother).

Infants and young children attach to figures who are their caregivers even when these caregivers are reluctant, neglectful and maltreating towards the child. What it encourages the child to do is to try harder, and stay closer, in their effort to make the situation more tolerable (Crittenden & Ainsworth 1989). It seems also that the children often believe that if only they behaved in a different way, or engaged in more of the same behaviours the adults would stop being maltreating. This issue of the children thinking and believing that somehow this abusive relationship is their fault feeds into the adaptational cycle of trapped attachments. Adults who have been maltreated as children, in later life often puzzle over why and how it was that they would run towards the caregiver or close adult and greet them warmly even though they were fully aware of the painful relationship and afraid of it.

Poor relationships may also occur because of the loss of a primary figure especially if this happens while the infant is between 6 months and 3 years. Also, multiple breaks and separations can have considerable consequences and cause more long-term distress to the child. It needs to be acknowledged that some separations are inevitable and will not harm the child. In a 'good enough' environment, separations can in fact give a child the experience that they are safe even when, say, mother is not there, and also that she will return. However, longer-term separations repeated over this sensitive period between 6 months and 3 years can lead to the child becoming very withdrawn, uncommunicative, agitated and anxious. Or the child may show in their behaviour that they cannot discriminate and are therefore inappropriately friendly and/or overfriendly to any adult, even someone strange to the child. For professionals this may become quickly obvious when a child on a first visit to a clinic for instance offers kisses and demands cuddles from people they have never met before.

The early attachment patterns are the foundation for future development. The pattern is a dynamic one, changes over time throughout the child's growth and development, and depends on the experiences the child has. It is a powerful process and has strong links to the development of how the child and later adult perceive themselves. Children model on their significant caregivers and will react to many situations with the model in their minds. This is particularly relevant when it comes to the maltreated child as a grown-up in a parenting position, when their experience becomes a model for their own parenting. Early attachment patterns influence the adult's way of behaving and form part of a cyclic pattern which has intergenerational consequences.

Morton & Browne (1998) reviewed what is known about attachment in relation to child abuse. They emphasise that patterns of attachment that have been found useful for assessment can also be utilised when children and families are in treatment and for interventions to the family or professional system. They also make an important point about the intergenerational patterns of attachment, and state that '... insensitive parenting (maltreatment can be seen as an extreme form of insensitivity) will produce an insecure attachment relationship in the infant. This will lead to a poor representational model of the self, which in turn will influence the formation of future relationships' (p. 1100). And so the abuse can continue from one generation to the next.

With the three broad potential consequences of abuse (trauma, adaptation and disrupted attachment) in mind we now consider specific forms of abuse in turn.

Physical maltreatment and its consequences

Physical abuse, like all other forms of abuse, has a strong emotional component, and disentangling the specific consequences of the physical and emotional aspect is not possible. Physical abuse can vary from moderate to severe and, in a considerable number of cases, it can be fatal (Hobbs *et al.* 1999). The review of the child abuse inquiries presented by Reder *et al.* (1993) describes the devastating end of the continuum of all forms of child abuse and affords us some insight into the seriousness of the maltreatment of children.

Figures released by the NSPCC in their annual report (Creighton & Noyes 1989) showed that over 8000 cases of physical abuse were placed on the register for England and Wales during 1987. By March 1995 25 000 children were on the Child Abuse Register in Britain (see Creighton, Chapter 2, in this volume). These statistics also highlighted the fact that the birth parents inflicted over 90% of the injuries. Speight (1989) pointed out that diagnosing physical abuse or non-accidental injury is important, not least because the maltreatment can be so severe that the child dies, or that brain damage persists and handicap is the consequence. Wissow (1990, p. 172) states that:

homicide is among the leading causes of death for American children ages 1–14 ... Most of the deaths among children under the age of 3 represent fatal child abuse ... A consequence so grave ... our actions if there were any were too late, thoughts about prevention were either not there or so hesitantly formed they came too late and there is nothing we can make good about it.

Detailed descriptions of the issues can be found in Hobbs *et al.* (1999), Wissow (1990) and Helfer *et al.* (1997) who address the medical issues and link them to psychological and emotional factors.

Bruises are the most commonly encountered injury, followed by fractures and brain injury.
(Hobbs *et al.* 1993)

These authors pointed out (p. 78) that 'abusive fractures usually result from the more extreme forms of violence and represent serious injury. They may co-exist with other signs of trauma: external (e.g. bruises, scratches) or internal injuries. The internal injuries may result in subdural haematoma, retinal haemorrhage or internal injuries to the abdomen.'

Physical abuse results in the physical injuries which leave wounds to heal and scars visible. Such scars can occur from bruises, cuts, bites, kicks, marks from beatings with objects, burns and scalds. The invisible/internal injuries, as in bone fractures, breaks and other internal injuries can also be present. Powerful as these images of physical damage are, it is essential also to consider our three concepts: the trauma for the children in experiencing such assaults; the kinds of adaptations they will have had to make simply to try to survive; and the effects on attachment processes when their parents have maltreated them or failed to protect them. Psychological interventions need to go alongside the physical treatment for any of these injuries.

All professionals have to be vigilant in order to detect the physical injuries children present with, either in hospital and medical centres or in social services offices. Denial can occur when children are brought with obvious physical injuries just as much as with less visible or detectable signs in emotional abuse, sexual abuse or forms of neglect.

The effects of physical abuse are influenced by several factors that can either stand alone or arise in combinations. These factors are:

- the relationship of abuser to child
- the nature of the abuse
- the severity of the assault
- the child's age
- the child's development
- how long the traumatic event lasted
- how often the traumatic event was repeated.

For instance the more often the abusive situations are repeated, the more likely will it become that successive stages of development are affected. The effects are either disruptive to the developmental process of the child or halt it in a certain phase. This is often called being 'stuck', or fixated in a certain developmental stage.

'Flashbacks' (see Case) are not only caused by visible stimuli, but for children with physical injuries such as burns or badly healed breaks, the injury is a constant reminder of what happened. As Bentovim (1992, p. 25) pointed out, when any human being has to 'cope with the uncopeable' the individual devises strategies, often quite unique and individual, to avoid the stress which is caused. Bentovim said:

Case

One of the children presenting for a medical absolutely and resolutely refused to take off his T-shirt to have his chest listened to. The doctor tried to persuade the child and eventually became firm, telling the child that he would not be hurt but that they had at least to lift his shirt and put the stethoscope to his chest. When they lifted the garment the child let out a piercing yell as if he was very badly hurt. What the doctor saw was a chest full of scars from a burn which had occurred 2 years previously. The child became inconsolable and wept for a long time, kicking anyone who tried to come near him. A little later he told his mother that when the doctor lifted his shirt he felt as if he was back in the time and place when he was burnt 2 years ago. He said this happened every time he had to take his shirt off and that he had learned to keep it on. If he could keep a shirt on always, day and night he said, he would not see the scars, not be reminded of what had happened, and therefore not feel the pain over and over again. This phenomenon is called 'flashback'.

The basic response is the replaying and re-enactment of the event thrust into experience, e.g. through flashbacks triggered by reminders, spontaneously, or during play, through dreams or nightmares. There are struggles to overcome these experiences by 'avoidance' or attempts to delete reminders, avoiding places, people, situations that trigger memories; or through dissociation – a form of self-hypnotism which blanks the experience out, creating a hole in the mind. Finally the overwhelming traumatic experience can induce a state of arousal and irritability, and can affect sleep and the ability to relax.

Links between physical and psychological pain

Making links between physical pain and emotional pain is an important step. It is also realistic to recognise that some children are more resilient (Heller *et al.* 1999) than others and that the consequences of physical abuse do not in all cases lead to the same effects. What has to be acknowledged is that some effects are inevitable and that the length of time during which a child has been subjected to abuse, as well as the severity of the injuries, are contributing factors in terms of effects.

Children who have been subjected to deliberate, and sometimes planned, harm have a very different experience of their treatment than children who may have been smacked or even hit hard by their caregivers but have been given explanations, ways of changing the cause which led them to be chastised, and possibly even an apology.

The well known facial expression of frozen watchfulness which can be seen in many maltreated children is there for a very long time if not for life. It relates to the mistrust of others, of feelings about being unsafe in an unpredictable position and the likelihood of being harmed at any time. Threats to the child's basic sense of security can trigger adaptations in the form of emotional responses ranging from anxiety and being withdrawn, to angry and uncontrollable acting-out behaviour.

Major psychological signs of physical maltreatment

There follows a list of signs of physical maltreatment. These provide a basis for estimating the potential consequences of maltreatment and can also be used as indicators that a child may have suffered this form of maltreatment. In the bulleted list, common consequences are listed against ■, while those that are strong indicators of abuse when exhibited by an individual child are listed with →.

- ■ Stress-related symptoms (tension, headaches, psychosomatic symptoms)
- → being very alert and aroused as if in a constant state of readiness of an attack, sudden fear of being injured
- ■ intrusive thoughts appearing as if from nowhere
- → sudden intrusive thoughts and consequent action of being violent often perceived by others as uncontrollable aggressive impulses (see Keely's case)
- ■ flinching as if for no specific reason
- → avoiding any thought or talk of the abusive event(s)
- → dreams and nightmares of the traumatic abusive events.

Simultaneously, delays can include:

- ■ developmental delays
- ■ delayed fine or gross motor development (gross: walking, jumping, climbing; fine: holding a pencil, picking things up, holding feeding implements etc.).

As the children get older the consequences can manifest themselves in:

- angry behaviour
- depression
- anxiety
- dissociation, which includes detachment and numbing effects
- repression (developing a way of not consciously remembering the abusive event).

Unpredictableness of maltreatment and its consequences

The unpredictable nature of maltreatment is often an added strain on the child and later adult, which precludes having the time or energy to concentrate, learn, play and form relationships. Instead it leaves the child with a need to be watchful, careful, predict when an attack might occur, pretend that nothing is worrying the child, etc. This pattern of alertness can be seen in adults who have been maltreated as children, and as in childhood it still prevents the adult from concentrating, learning and forming relationships. Engel (1998) provides a useful guide by taking the reader through the stages experienced by adults who have been abused as children. We are presented with descriptions of people's behaviour and feelings and also with the clinical signs so often present when an adult begins to cope with these issues.

There is also the issue of parental models. Children who have been maltreated often say as adults that hitting and punishing is the right way to bring up children, as if there is no other way.

Emotional abuse and its consequences

Rather than casting psychological maltreatment as an ancillary issue, subordinate to other forms of abuse and neglect, we should place it as the centrepiece of efforts to understand family functioning and to protect children.

(Garbarino *et al.* 1986, p. 7)

Society's response to this form of maltreatment has been slow and lags behind. Wissow (1990) quite rightly reminds us that though it is now much more accepted that parents should pay more attention to their children in every respect, how they should relate to their children remains a controversial issue. He said that 'while a warm and loving parent–child relationship is widely advocated as essential, significant minorities still feel that strict discipline and a certain detachment (especially from fathers) are important elements of child-rearing' (p. 158). This is one area in which cultural differences in definitions of appropriate care must be taken into account (Stratton & Hanks 1991; see also Chapter 5, in this volume). There is still no clear consensus on how to define emotional abuse, not least because there are different opinions of whether the emphasis should be on the abuse of the child or the behaviour of the parent. Brassard & Hardy (1997) offer a useful account of the issues involved in the assessment of emotional abuse.

It is not fully understood why children react differently in the face of maltreatment and why some show more severe consequences than others when they have had abusive experiences. Attention has been paid to the phenomenon of 'resilience' in human beings. How do some children and adults who have been abused manage to lead a less disturbed life despite their abusive childhood experiences? Heller *et al.* (1999) point out that while there are no clear answers at present, there are better understood indicators which link to the abusive situation and how the children are treated during that time. Kagan *et al.* (1978) showed that how children perceive themselves, and how their inner self develops is of crucial importance. The self is influenced by both adults and peers and if a child receives persistently negative feedback then the child's view of themselves will be affected.

There is no such thing as a perfect parent or a perfect child. Every parent will at some time or other behave towards the child in such a way that the child will be upset, maybe frightened or feel rejected and suffer a loss of self-esteem, etc. What happens after this event of commission (an active or cruel behaviour towards the child) or omission (behaviour which neglects or ignores the child even when they are in unsafe or dangerous situations) in the adult's behaviour towards the child is what matters. The parents may manage to acknowledge and 'make good' the situation, giving the child appropriate alternative options for behaving. If reparation is made, the child learns that people/parents/caregivers can make mistakes but that they can recognise them as such. However, even 'the making good' of a poor/hurtful situation to the child is not going to be helpful if the situation occurs repeatedly. When the caregiving is constantly changing (doing hurtful things then making good), it becomes inconsistent and potentially damaging.

Garbarino *et al.* (1986) provided us with a helpful model which distinguishes between the different forms of emotional maltreatment:

- rejecting
- isolating
- terrorising
- ignoring
- corrupting.

These are the categories essential in order to recognise children who are maltreated emotionally. Childhood inevitably includes experiencing some of these patterns at sometime or other, but our capacity to cope with such treatment in an environment where it is repeated over and over again is fairly limited. Such behaviour delivered consistently towards a child is damaging.

Egeland *et al.* (1983) claim from their longitudinal study that emotional abuse has the most serious consequences for a child's social and intellectual development. These researchers showed, for instance, that verbal abuse and psychological unavailability as well as physical abuse and neglect produced children who presented with anxious rather than secure attachments and that they showed frustration, hostility and anger. Developmental skills also declined for the group of children having to live with verbal abuse and the unavailability of their parents. The children in this group were quickly frustrated when attempting tasks and approached new tasks feeling negative towards them and anxious. From this study, it seemed that children who were emotionally maltreated suffered more severe setbacks in their performance skills than those children who were physically abused or neglected. This is particularly important to recognise and gives an insight into the possibility that emotional abuse can be more damaging than physical abuse. The research indicated that this may be because the children who are physically harmed may receive this treatment more sporadically than those children who are emotionally abused, whose maltreatment is much more likely to be a constant feature in their and their parents' lives.

Glaser (1993) developed a model that has enhanced our understanding further. She proposed six dimensions of emotionally abusive or inappropriate relationships. These are:

- persistent negative attitudes (negative attributions and attitudes, harsh discipline and over-control)
- promoting of insecure attachments (through conditional parenting)
- inappropriate developmental expectations and considerations
- emotional unavailability
- failure to recognise a child's individuality and psychological boundaries
- cognitive distortions and inconsistencies.

Crittenden (1988) described different family patterns in maltreating families. For instance, the neglecting families had a pattern of ignoring the children, and these children – who were practically invisible to their caregives – were passive and cognitively delayed before they reached year 1. As they grew older, their behaviours altered and they became 'uncontrolled and seekers of novel experiences'. At that stage, these children need a great deal of looking after and fall into the category of being abused by 'omission' as much as by 'commission'. Claussen & Crittenden (1991) showed that much psychological abuse intercorrelates with physical abuse and other forms of abuse of children and that when this happens the developmental risks increase accordingly. Both Wissow (1990) and Hobbs *et al.* (1999) would endorse these findings.

Non-organic failure to thrive (FTT) and its consequences

Taylor and Taylor (1976) stated what is in essence still accepted today when they said:

The period between the start of weaning and the fifth birthday is nutritionally the most vulnerable segment of the human life cycle. Rapid growth, loss of passive immunity and as yet undeveloped acquired immunity against infection produce dietary needs more specific and inflexible than at later periods. (p. 820)

We would add that special attention is necessary to the infant's needs in the feeding situation from birth onwards. It is recognised that many children, for example, 5% of an inner city population, fail to thrive before the weaning period (Skuse 1985, Hobbs *et al.* 1999).

The consequences for children who fail to thrive for non-organic reasons are better understood now, and detailed discussions can be found in Frank & Zeisel (1988), Boddy & Skuse (1994), Hanks & Hobbs (1993) and Hobbs *et al.* (1999). The overall consequences of FTT relate to developmental retardation and include motor, language, intellectual, social and behavioural components.

A definition of FTT needs to encompass a wide range – from the child not growing fully to their potential at one end, and the situation being life-threatening for the child at the other end of the continuum (Table 5.1). Psychological aspects of development can be delayed, sometimes irreversibly, with emotional and cognitive deficits (Table 5.2).

It is interesting to note where different definitions put their emphasis. Is it something that the child is to be responsible for? 'The feeding interaction in FTT appears to be unsuccessful, because the child does not achieve an adequate nutritional intake' (Boddy & Skuse 1994, p. 407); is it that 'the child refuses to gain weight in an appropriate manner' (Illingworth 1983); or is it that FTT results from caregivers feeding an infant inadequate calories – not enough food or an inappropriate diet? It is important for practitioners to carefully review their assumptions and decide where to put their energies in terms of interventions. FTT

Table 5.1 *The physical consequences of failure to thrive (After Hobbs et al. 1993, Hanks & Hobbs 1993)*	Overall body shape	Thin and wasted, little fat
	Feet and hands	May be swollen, red and cold
	Arms	Thin, mid-upper arm circumference (Hobbs et al. 1993)
	Stomach	Large and swollen
	Hair	No shine, looks wispy, thin, is falling out
	Brain	Can be retarded particularly in early months (Illingworth 1983, Frank & Zeisel 1988)
	Physical growth	Can be permanently damaged including a poor posture

Table 5.2 *Developmental consequences of non-organic failure to thrive*	• Developmental delay • Delayed motor development • Delayed language development • Delayed intellectual development • Delayed social development • Delayed behavioural development

in small children is a potentially life-threatening situation and needs clear thinking which will not be helped by concentrating on deciding who is to blame.

Both parents and professionals alike find it difficult and emotionally taxing to recognise and acknowledge when a child fails to thrive, let alone realise that if nothing is done to remedy this state of affairs the consequences can be severe and at times result in death. Iwaniec *et al.* (1985, p. 251) pointed out that children who fail to thrive can show consequences that can lead to the child having a 'pattern of unmalleable behaviour, resistance to new routines' and that their 'general volatility of mood and behaviour, appeared to make them difficult to rear from early life. Feeding routines, and other training tasks, were made into fraught enterprises for many parents'.

This leads to a further complication in intergenerational terms and warrants detailed research. Understanding how mothers perceive the causes is crucial to any intervention in this relationship and to aiding the ultimate growth of the child. FTT is one situation in which the child's adaptation to mistreatment or mishandling may easily be misconstrued by a parent. The child's avoidance of the (possibly traumatic) mealtime may be interpreted as the child's wilfulness, or just lack of interest in food on the child's part, and so the underfeeding continues.

McCann *et al.* (1994) researched the eating habits and attitudes concerning body shape and weight of 26 mothers who had children who were failing to thrive non-organically. These mothers, none of whom were either bulimic or anorexic, restrained their FTT children from eating, for instance, 'sweet' foods. Thirty per cent of these mothers restricted their children in the consumption of foods they considered fattening or not healthy. Despite the objective measurements of weight and height which were low in the FTT children, 50% of these mothers believed that their FTT children had 'normal' weights and 38% were convinced that their children's shape was the same as that of other ordinary children who did not fail to thrive. They did not seem to be able, for whatever reason, to perceive their children's position. This coincides with our clinical experience (Hobbs *et al.* 1999).

Parents, grandparents and professionals have made the following comments to us while we were working with children who were severely failing to thrive. Such children are well below the third centile in weight, look thin and are visibly much smaller than most children of the same age:

'Not to worry, we are all small in our family.'

'He runs around too much to put on weight, that is why he is thin and little.'

'His dad says he will catch up when he's older.'

Grandmother said in the clinic: 'all my children were small when they were young, he will catch up, just leave him alone.'

'I will not have you think I don't feed him; he is to blame, he won't eat.'

'I think you (doctor, psychologist) are fussy, there are much thinner children on the estate where I work, you should see them and not worry his mother.'

Such statements indicate the difficulties caregivers can have while trying to protect themselves from the psychological distress of a child who does not eat. However, such interpretations have considerable consequences for the child, particularly when the lack of food intake continues because of such beliefs and makes it difficult to achieve change.

Observations of children eating

In an attempt to understand the mutual adaptations of parent and FTT child, we have been observing, or if possible filming, children during a main mealtime. Their eating behaviour and the families' rules about eating have often provided us with the information we needed in order to come up with adequate interventions.

The video recordings have also enabled us to detect some of the interactions that have become established in the pattern of poor feeding and how this has made itself felt in the child's behaviour and development.

Children can become frightened and stop eating when:

- the food is too hot and the child's mouth is burnt during feeding
- the pieces of food are too large and the child cannot chew them adequately
- they are fed roughly and injured during feeding
- they are left alone to eat the food and have no social contact or model of a positive attitude to eating.

Recognising the emotional consequences in FTT

The emotional consequences of FTT need to be assessed for each individual child. We have recognised that a checklist is helpful in determining how the child is emotionally behaving and what the carer's experience is in looking after the child.

Hobbs *et al.* (1999) compiled such a checklist of opposite reactions (Table 5.3).

This checklist is a guideline only. It is not a diagnostic tool but may help the professional and parent to recognise that behaviours like the ones listed in Table 5.3 are often present in children who fail to thrive. Further it may help those involved to be more able to help the child in these areas rather than to ignore them.

Neglect and its consequences

Neglect of children is one of the most obvious aspects of maltreatment where not only the caregives of the children are responsible, but where the issue has to be widened to include society as a whole and a global view has to be adopted. As an example: the neglect of children in the Developing World is the responsibility of

Table 5.3 *Possible behaviours by children with failure be thrive*		
Still	Confused
Expressionless	Insecure
Unresponsive	Anxious
Sad	Demanding
Depressed	Frustrated
Not inquisitive	frantically searching
Minimal or no smiling	Tearful
Little vocalisation	Angry
Detached	Rejecting

the individual country, but also that of the industrialised nations who may exploit a Third World country's natural resources. Poor health care, poor education, drug addiction, crime and starvation are often the consequences on one level in society.

Helfer (1990) stated that it is within the grasp of all of us to understand the consequences of a neglected childhood and how this permeates from one generation to the next. Hobbs *et al.* (1999, p. 126) take this further and point out that 'Childhood is a vulnerable time and needs which are not met during the child's period of growth and development may have irreversible consequences.'

Neglect is defined in *Working Together* (Home Office 1991) as: 'The persistent or severe neglect of a child, or the failure to protect a child from exposure to any kind of danger, including cold or starvation, or extreme failure to carry out important aspects of care, resulting in the significant impairment of the child's health or development, including non-organic failure to thrive.'

Kempe & Goldbloom (1987) defined neglect as 'a very insidious form of mal-treatment. It implies failure of the parents to act properly in safeguarding the health, safety and well-being of the child.' Stevenson (1998) has a unique understanding of the issues of neglect in society and emphasises particularly that small children, all children, do not have time to wait for interventions to be successful. The children's developmental stages are progressing and will be shaped by the abuse. Interventions may either be too late or the children have grown up and adapted into ways of being which make it hard to address the changes.

The consequences of neglect, as in physical abuse, can range from death of a child through neglect (death from cold, starvation, lack of medical and daily care) to children who are dirty and unkempt, not stimulated to learn and left to their own devices. Iwaniec's (1996) description of children and their circumstances when there has been neglect and failure to thrive are recognised as giving the practitioner both practical and theoretical insight into the problem.

Hobbs *et al.* (1999) and Cantwell (1997) describe the various patterns of neglect, including lack of car seat belts, helmets when cycling, lack of medical care, lack of hygiene in the home, clean food, drink and water, physical and emotional care and adequete supervision appropriate to the developmental stage of the child and teenager.

As with FTT, there are cases in which the needs of the child are clearly not being met, but which it would not necessarily be appropriate to label as abuse. For example, if the parents fail to provide the kinds of interaction needed for the child to form attachments. We have suggested that the important task is to decide upon the child's requirements for healthy growth, and not be so concerned about apportioning blame (Stratton & Hanks 1991). To some extent the decision will vary between cultures, and the decision about whose responsibility it is to provide these requirements will also vary. It is appropriate that we should have a progressive debate, and a progressive raising of the level of what we regard as essential requirements. In the year 2000 we would, for example, claim that there is clear evidence about the negative consequences for a child of having inadequate models of attachment relationships. The disruption to both the childhood and long-term development seem to be serious enough to justify a claim that the child who is not given the basics of social development is suffering neglect.

Neglect is closely linked to emotional abuse in that, as a result of their neglect, the children often:

- are very passive in infancy
- are sometimes very active, but totally unfocused when older
- have a limited ability to attend to the behaviour of others
- show significant developmental delay
- have poor speech and learning ability
- have poor ability to interact socially
- are accident prone because they are not properly protected
- may have stunted growth.

Sexual abuse and its consequences

Sexual maltreatment of children is the subject most written about during the last 15 years. It is in this area that more distinct categories of effects can be recognised. There is now considerable evidence (Kempe & Mrazek 1981, Finkelhor 1986, MacFarlane & Waterman 1986, Bentovim *et al.* 1988, Glaser & Frosh 1988, Wyatt & Powell 1988, Furniss 1991, Briere 1992) that child sexual abuse (CSA) is an aversive and damaging experience to children, with often harmful effects in the long term.

Physical consequences

Paediatricians, starting with Henry Kemp, have taken a lead in working in the area of abuse and sexual maltreatment. We recommend that the reader makes themself familiar with the physical aspects of this form of abuse so that they can cooperate with medical staff in such situations. Texts to consult include Wissow (1991), Hobbs & Wynne (1993), Hobbs *et al.* (1999), Meadow (1993) and Helfer *et al.* (1997). What is striking in CSA is that the physical injuries exist along a continuum from severe injury and death to no physical injuries at all.

Psychological consequences

Effects of CSA may be short-term or long-term, and usually the child experiences both forms. Further division may be useful:

1. emotional and behavioural effects
2. educational and learning
3. all forms of interpersonal relationships.

The *short-term effects* of CSA can show in terms of: fear, anxiety, aggressive behaviours, angry outbursts, hostility and feeling got at (persecuted), and developmentally inappropriate sexual behaviour.

The *long-term effects* of CSA have been found in terms of: anxiety, depression, feeling isolated, lack of trust, poor self-esteem, self-harming behaviours (including eating disorders), dissociation, the range of traumatic and post-traumatic effects. Guilt and shame are invariably present.

It is sobering to reflect on the fact that potentially the list of effects on the child in both the short- and long-term can be overwhelming. We give some indication of the consequences below, dividing the most salient effects into three age groups. These effects may stand singly or present in clusters of behaviours, depending on each child's environment and specific situation.

Common consequences, which may also occur following other kinds of abuse or childhood disturbance, are listed against ■; those that are strong indicators of sexual abuse when exhibited by an individual child are listed with →.

For the pre-school child, the effects may show in:

→   sexually explicit play and behaviour
■   wetting and soiling
■   delayed language and development
■   eating and sleeping problems
■   dysfunctional attachment behaviour
■   withdrawn or over-active states
■   aggressive behaviours (to self and others)
■   clinging behaviour and becoming mute.

For children between the ages of 6 and 12 years, the above effects may be recognisable, with further elaborations:

■   poor learning and concentration
→   heightened sexual behaviour and arousal
■   truanting and self-neglecting
■   depression and anxiety
■   psychosomatic illnesses
■   physical risk-taking
■   poor social skills
■   as if out of control at times
→   avoidance of men or women (depending on gender of abuser).

For the older child, the effects include any of the above-mentioned patterns with further escalations:

→   sexually precocious behaviour and prostitution
■   solvent/alcohol/drug abuse
■   self-harming and suicide attempts
■   anorexia and bulimia
■   changes in school performance
■   isolation from peers
→   starting to sexually abuse other children.

Overall, one may view the child's position in the following way. The difficulties of sexually abused children are:

■   lack of individuation
■   poor interpersonal relationships
■   communication problems
→   inappropriate sexual behaviour and confusion about it
■   low self-esteem, feelings of depression and anxiety
■   feelings of shame, guilt and powerlessness
■   feelings of dissociation
→   experiencing something akin to the 'damaged goods syndrome'
■   trauma and post-traumatic stress syndrome.

The behaviours can have both a delayed and immediate impact on a child. What we have witnessed is that it can take a long time before certain behaviours emerge. Some consequences can emerge quickly, some emerge over time and then fade, yet others can be triggered by events such as having a baby, the death of the perpetrator, the death of a non-abusing parent, or a child of the previously abused adult approaching puberty and potential sexual activity.

Vizard (1993) highlighted another dimension when she stated that:

sexually abused children often behave in a confusing way in relation to the abuse experience. This may be because their experience of sexual abuse was itself confusing.

She proposes three levels of experience:

1. bodily experience
2. external world experience
3. inner world experience.

She also postulates that many children who have been subjected to CSA experience physiological arousal at the time of abuse and this results in a body memory. The memory is then lodged both as a thought and as a feeling, sexual and exciting in nature, which can give rise to a memory of sounds or visual images connected to the abusive situation. This feeling memory, so to speak, stands instead of the psychic memory of the actual event. So the intense experience of the act of CSA may have switched off the mind memory but activated the body memory. In children who have been chronically sexually abused this body memory can function quite independently. It also includes passive and active modes. The active body memory can present in physical arousal. The passive body memory may appear like a psychosomatic conversion (headaches, stomach aches, wetting and soiling, being mute). The stress factors related to this dimension are discussed further below.

Most professionals working in this area recognise that CSA has consequences that are difficult to overcome and usually leave the person with lifelong problems. The degree to which these problems rule a person's life can, as with all forms of maltreatment, vary. We have begun to talk to a very small group of people who experienced CSA as children but who feel they are leading a life not dominated by the consequences of this experience. What has made it possible for these people to be different is not quite clear. One of the recognisable factors is that they have been able to tell a trusted adult and that they have been believed and protected from that moment on. Another important factor seems to be that they have not been blamed for the event.

There is considerable evidence that CSA is an aversive experience for children. It has also been recognised that very young children often go through periods when they are not aware that the sexual contact imposed on them is abusive. As the children get older, they do become aware of the fact that they are involved in a relationship(s) which is wrong or disapproved of. Often, this awareness comes about when the child has been given an injunction to secrecy. The issue of secrecy in itself leads to considerable difficulties both for the children and those around them. Should the children attempt to disclose, they often enter into a world of denial, described above, and then into internal confusion.

Even if they have not been warned by the perpetrator, the children are often painfully aware of the consequences of releasing their secret. Not only will they be disapproved of in many cases, but also the turmoil created within their family or institution will be extremely painful to them and often result in the children themselves being blamed. This recognition is often built in to the perpetrator repertoire of both 'grooming' the child and maintaining the abusive situation.

The use of threats to silence children in intrafamilial CSA is common and includes the threat of loss of love, separation or physical harm.

Another important distinction has to be drawn between children who have been sexually abused within the family, and thus experienced incest, and those children who have been abused by someone outside the immediate family.

Incest at any age seems to leave considerable consequences, particularly in the areas of relationships, trust, closeness and dependency. If the incest started early in life and continued over time, the child is shaped into sexualised behaviours which are observable but difficult to overcome. Summit's (1988) 'Accommodation Syndrome' describes the position of the child and leaves no doubt about the consequences of incest and the breaking of the incest taboo. In respect of the sexualised behaviour so often witnessed when children have been abused over a considerable time, Kempe & Kempe (1984, p. 190) pointed out that these children are 'trained to be a sexual object'. They also highlighted how in such circumstances, the children (assumed at that time to be almost invariably girls abused by men) 'try to make each contact with any adult male an overt sexual event'. It is interesting that, in 1985, sexual abuse by women was not discussed, in public at least. However, it can now be said that women do abuse children sexually, and the same behaviour occurs for boys and girls abused by men and women (Mathews *et al.* 1989, Hanks & Saradjian 1991, Elliott 1993, Saradjian 1996).

The effects of post-traumatic stress are described in Finkelhor (1986), Wyatt & Powell (1988), Briere (1992) and Bentovim (1992). Children and adults who experience traumatic responses to their abuse are often in the grip of that experience in a manner which is well outside their control. They may re-enact the events, engage in inappropriate sexual behaviours (hence the often witnessed sexualised behaviour), have visualisations of the event(s), have actual flashbacks and triggering memories which obscure any concentration on ordinary aspects of their lives. The effects may lead to avoiding places, things and people which may trigger memories of the event, and it can also lead to dissociation and sometimes multiple personality and deletion of memories, which further leads to irritability or distractedness.

For the adult, the long-term difficulties can include problems in sexual adjustment or aversion to appropriate sexual contact. Equally, consequences can occur when the abused child grows up and has their own child. As parents, they may become overprotective (thinking 'I will never leave my child with any person because they may be abused'), or they may be neglectful, not having had any experience themselves of being adequately cared for. Boundaries may be blurred and crossed, and closeness may be difficult to achieve. Once again, our increasing understanding of attachment is relevant here, but in sexual abuse in particular it is essential to think in terms of adaptation rather than deprivation. The child who experiences sexual abuse will have to adapt in ways that preserve their psychological and physical integrity as much as possible. Most adaptations will be in a form that leaves them resistant to forming trusting emotionally close relationships. Such adaptations, however sad, are entirely understandable and in some contexts quite functional. The challenge to the professional, and to society more generally, is to provide contexts in which the child can begin to explore alternative adaptations and so start to undo some of the harm that has been done to them.

Conclusion

One further point we wish to make is that there is an important distinction relating to the intergenerational patterns of abuse. What we know about the repeating cycle of abuse is that many of the adults who sexually abuse have been abused sexually as children themselves. This connection is sometimes taken to mean that a sexually abused person automatically abuses sexually when they grow up. Many adult survivors voice this concern and feel as if they are doomed to repeat the pattern. What has to be added to the equation is that not every adult who has been sexually abused will become a perpetrator of abuse. Furthermore, we know of specific factors which can be protective, as discussed above and by Egeland (1988). What we can say is that when the history of those abusing children and adults is examined, it almost always shows that they have been abused as children themselves.

It is the issue of protective factors on which we wish to conclude. Much of the value of knowing about the consequences of abuse is that the knowledge is a first step towards effective protection of children. Knowing the common consequences alerts us to the possibility that abuse has occurred when we see children showing these signs. It indicates the tasks that treatment must undertake. And it enables us to identify maltreated individuals who have managed to avoid these consequences, and to discover what has been protective, or ameliorative for them. Recognising the full extent of the consequences of abuse may look like a dispiriting exercise. But when the positive potential of this knowledge is recognised, there is every good reason to continue to try to understand the significance of the harm that abuse does to children.

Acknowledgements

To our patients – all the people who have entrusted us with their difficulties. The cases quoted in this chapter are composite cases so as not to break confidentiality of any specific individual and to respect people's trust. We would also like to thank Dr Chris Hobbs and Dr Jane Wynne for their support.

Annotated further reading

Adcock M, White R, Hollows A (eds) 1991 Significant harm. Significant Publications, Croydon
This book centres on the 1989 Children Act which has had a profound influence on everyone's practice. It covers all forms of abuse. A must for every practitioner.
Bell M 1999 Child protection: families and the conference process. Ashgate, Aldershot
This is an interesting book for those who are wishing to undertake evaluative research. Though written specifically with social workers in mind, the book describes research and how it can be used when working with families and children in need.
Bentovim A 1992 Trauma organised systems. Karnac Books, London
Another important book by Bentovim discussing all forms of abuse and relating it to trauma organised systems and what that might entail for the child, family and professional involved.
Briere J N 1992 Child abuse trauma. Sage, Newbury Park.
This book describes the theory and treatment of the lasting effects of child abuse examining the inter-relationship between the different forms of abuse and neglect with an emphasis on the trauma such experiences have on the victim of abuse.
Ceci S J, Hembrooke H 1998 Expert witness in child abuse cases. American Psychological Association, Washington, DC
Though the topic of exper witness has not been described in the chapter, this book will help professionals and guide them through the often incomprehensible legal system when they are to appear as expert witnesses. The book is written from an American perspective but has valuable advice for the British reader.
Hobbs C J, Hanks H G I, Wynne J M 1999 Child abuse and neglect – a clinician's handbook, 2nd edn. Churchill Livingstone, Edinburgh
A textbook written with both the medical and therapeutic practitioner in mind. It has been described by reviewers as 'a landmark textbook in the field of child abuse and neglect'. The many tables, diagrams, drawings and the photography make the material accessible to the reader in a way that is quite unique. The 2nd edition of this book includes not only updated references but also a considerable amount of new material.

Hobbs C J, Wynne J M (eds) 1993 Ballière's clinical paediatrics, Vol. 1, Child abuse. Baillière Tindall, London

This is an important collection by some of the most experienced writers in the field. It covers aspects of ritual abuse, the handicapped child and maltreatment, recent advances in radiology with reference to child abuse as well as interviewing children, emotional abuse, the cycle of abuse in adolescents as well as other contributions, 14 chapters in all. All very well written and relevant to the practitioner.

Wissow L S 1990 Child advocacy for the clinician – an approach to child abuse and neglect. Williams & Wilkins, Baltimore

Another important textbook combining physical issues of child maltreatment and psychological issues. A powerful and thorough piece of work combining the medical and psychological.

Wyatt G E, Powell G J 1988 Lasting effects of child sexual abuse. Sage, Newbury Park

Outstanding contributions focusing on the effects of child sexual abuse.

References

Arnold E, Cloke C 1988 Society keeps abuse hidden – the biggest cause of all: the case for Child Friendly Communities. Child Abuse Review 7: 302–314

Barnett D, Manly J T, Cicchetti D 1993 Defining child maltreatment: the interface between policy and research. In: Cicchetti D, Toth S (eds) Child abuse, child development, and social policy. Ablex, Norwood, New Jersey

Bentovim A 1992 Trauma - organised systems – physical and sexual abuse in families. Karnac Books, London

Bentovim A, Elton A, Hildebrand J, *et al.* 1992 Child sexual abuse within the family. Wright, London

Boddy J, Skuse D 1994 Annotation: the process of parenting in failure to thrive. Journal of Child Psychology and Psychiatry 35 (3): 401–424

Bowlby J 1988 A secure base: clinical applications of attachment theory. Routledge, London

Brassard M R, Hardy D B 1997 Psychological maltreatment. In: Helfer M E, Kempe R S, Krugman R D (eds) The battered child. University of Chicago Press, Chicago

Briere J N 1992 Child abuse trauma. Sage, Newbury Park

Briere J 1997 Psychological assessment of adult posttraumatic states. APA, Washington

Cantwell H B 1997 The neglect of child neglect. In: Helfer M E, Kempe R S, Krugman R D (eds) The battered child. University of Chicago Press, Chicago

Creighton S, Noyes P 1989 Child abuse trends in England and Wales 1983–87. NSPCC, London

Claussen A, Crittenden P 1991 Physical and psychological maltreatment: relations among types of maltreatment. Child Abuse and Neglect 15: 5–18

Crittenden P 1988 Family and dyadic patterns of functioning in maltreating families. In: Browne K, Davies C, Stratton P (eds) Early prediction and prevention of child abuse. Wiley, Chichester

Crittenden P, Ainsworth M 1989 Child maltreatment and attachment theory. In: Cicchetti D. Carlson V (eds) Child maltreatment Cambridge University Press, Cambridge

Crittenden P, Claussen A 1993 Severity of maltreatment: assessment and policy. In: Hobbs C, Wynne J (eds) Baillière's clinical paediatrics, Vol. 1, Child abuse. Baillière Tindall, London, pp. 87–100

Egeland B 1988 Breaking the cycle of abuse. In: Browne K, Davies C, Stratton P (eds) Early prediction and prevention of child abuse. Wiley, Chichester

Elliott M (ed) 1993 Female sexual abuse of children. Longman, Harlow

Engel B 1998 Living with the legacy of abuse: how to make your relationship work when your partner is a survivor of childhood sexual abuse. Camden, London

Ferenczy S 1949 Confusion of tongues between the adult and the child. International Journal of Psycho-Analysis 30: 225–230

Finkelhor D 1986 A sourcebook on child sexual abuse. Sage, Beverley Hills, California

Frank D, Zeisel S 1988 Failure to thrive. Paediatric Clinics of North America 35: 1187–1206

Freud S 1914 Remembering, repeating and working through. In: The standard edition of the complete psychological works of Sigmund Freud 1950–1974. Hogarth Press, London

Furniss T 1991 The multiprofessional handbook of child sexual abuse. Routledge, London

Garbarino J, Guttmann E, Wilson Seeley J 1986 The psychologically battered child. Jossey-Bass, San Francisco

Glaser D 1993 Emotional abuse. In: Hobbs C, Wynne J (eds) Baillière's clinical paediatrics. Baillière Tindall, London

Glaser D, Frosh S 1988 Child sexual abuse. Macmillan, London

Hanks H, Hobbs C 1993 Failure to thrive: a model for treatment. In: Hobbs C, Wynne J (eds) Baillière's clinical paediatrics. Baillière Tindall, London

Hanks H, Saradjian J 1991 Women who abuse children sexually. Human Systems Journal of Systemic Consultation and Management 2: 247–262

Helfer R 1990 The neglect of our children in child abuse. Paediatric Clinics of North America 37 (4): 923–942

Helfer M E, Kempe R S, Krugman R D 1997 The battered child. University of Chicago Press, Chicago

Heller S S, Larrieu J A, D'Imperio R, Boris N W 1999 Research on resilience to child maltreatment: empirical considerations. Child Abuse and Neglect 23: 321–338

Hetherton J, Beardsall L 1998 Decisions and attitudes concerning child sexual abuse: does the gender of the perpetrator make a difference to child protection professionals. Child Abuse and Neglect 22: 1265–1283

Hobbs C J, Wynne J M 1993 The evaluation of child sexual abuse. In: Hobbs C, Wynne J (eds) Baillière's clinical paediatrics. Baillière Tindall, London

Hobbs C J, Hanks H G I, Wynne J M 1993 Child abuse and neglect – a clinician's handbook. Churchill Livingstone, Edinburgh

Hobbs C J, Hanks H G I, Wynne J M 1999 Child abuse and neglect: a clinician's handbook, 2nd Edn. Churchill Livingstone, London

Illingworth R S 1983 Weight and height. In: Hobbs C, Hanks H G I, Wynne J (eds) The normal child, some problems of the early years and their treatment. Churchill Livingstone, Edinburgh

Iwaniec D 1996 The emotionally abused and neglected child. Wiley, Chichester

Iwaniec D, Herbert M, McNeish A 1985 Social work with failure to thrive children and their families. British Journal of Social Work 15: 243–259

Jonker F, Jonker-Bakker I 1997 Effects of ritual abuse: the results of three surveys in the Netherlands. Child Abuse and Neglect 21: 541–556

Joseph R 1999 The neurology of traumatic 'dissociative' amnesia: commentary and literature review. Child Abuse and Neglect 23: 715–727

Kagan J, Kearsley R B, Zelazo P R 1978 Infancy: its place in human development. Harvard University Press, Cambridge, Massachusetts

Kempe R, Goldbloom B 1987 Malnutrition and growth retardation in the context of child abuse and neglect. In: Helfer R, Kempe R (eds) The battered child. University of Chicago Press, Chicago

Kempe S, Kempe C 1984 Sexual abuse of children and adolescents. W H Freeman, New York

Kempe C *et al.* 1962 The battered child syndrome. Journal of the American Medical Association 181: 17

Mathews R, Matthews J, Speltz K 1989 Female sexual offenders. The Safer Society Press Orwell

MacFarlane K, Waterman J 1986 Sexual abuse of young children. Holt, Rinehart & Winston, London

McCann J, Stein A, Fairburn C, Dunger D 1994 Eating habits and attitudes of mothers of children with non-organic failure to thrive. Archives of Diseases in Childhood 70: 234–236

Meadow S 1993 ABC of child abuse, 2nd edn BM J Publishing, London

Morton N, Browne K D 1998 Theory and observation of attachment and its relation to child maltreatment: a review. Child Abuse and Neglect 22: 1093–1104

Mrazek P, Kempe C 1981 Sexually abused children and their families. Pergamon Press, Oxford

Read J 1998 Child abuse and severity of disturbance among adult psychiatric inpatients. Child Abuse and Neglect 22: 359–368

Reder P, Duncan S, Gray M 1993 Beyond blame – child abuse tragedies revisited. Routledge, London

Rutter M 1999 Resilience concepts and findings: implications for family therapy. Journal of Family Therapy 21: 119–144

Sanders B, Becker-Lausen E 1995 The measurement of psychological maltreatment: early data on the child abuse and trauma scale. Child Abuse and Neglect 19: 315–323

Saradjian J (in association with Hawks H) 1996 Women who sexually abuse children. Wiley, Chichester

Skuse D 1985 Failure to thrive: failure to feed. Community Paediatric Group Newsletter. (British Paediatric Association) August, pp. 6–7

Speight N 1989 Non-accidental injury. In: Meadow R (ed) ABC of child abuse. British Medical Journal, London

Stevenson O 1998 Neglected children: issues and dilemmas. Blackwell Science, Oxford

Stratton P, Hanks H 1991 Incorporating circularity in defining and classifying child maltreatment. Human Systems 2: 181–200

Summit R 1988 Hidden victims, hidden pain: societal avoidance of child sexual abuse. In: Wyatt G E, Powell G J (eds) Lasting effects in child sexual abuse. Sage, Newbury Park

Taylor C, Taylor E 1976 Multifactorial causation of malnutrition. In: McClaren D (ed) Nutrition in the community. Wiley, Chichester

Varia R, Abidin R R 1999 The minimizing style: perceptions of psychological abuse and quality of past and present relationships. Child Abuse and Neglect 23: 1041–1055

Vizard E 1993 Interviewing sexually abused children. In: Hobbs C, Wynne J (eds) Baillière's clinical paediatrics. Baillière Tindall, London

Wissow L S 1990 Child advocacy for the clinician. Williams & Wilkins, Baltimore

Wyatt G, Powell G 1988 Lasting effects of child sexual abuse. Sage, Newbury Park

6 Gender and child abuse

Brid Featherstone

Brid Featherstone

INTRODUC-TION

What is meant when we invoke concepts such as gender? Is it relevant to understanding that contested notion 'child abuse' and if so how? This chapter initially explores how I understand both gender and child abuse and then goes on to argue that an understanding of how gender relations operate and are changing can help facilitate the welfare of children in the widest sense, as well as contributing important insights into the phenomenon of child abuse.

Biology or culture or beyond both?

The term gender was popularised by second-wave feminists (the name commonly given to the generation of women who emerged in the late 1960s/early 1970s to contest their situation). They were careful to distinguish between sex and gender, taking the view that sex is biological and gender is a social construction which refers to the 'culturally-shaped group of attributes and behaviours given to the female or to the male' (Humm 1989, p. 84). Although concerns have emerged about this distinction it directs us to an important insight. Gender can no longer be treated as a simple, natural fact (Flax 1990).

However, over time the majority of feminists have moved away from earlier assumptions that we are simply socialised into being men or women by something called society and that we can therefore be re-socialised if given the correct information. Psychoanalytic insights have been employed to explore how we develop and internalise our identities as men and women, and to emphasise that change is not simply a rational process (Hollway 1989). Changes in the meanings attached to masculinity and femininity, and the relations between them, are frequently accompanied by feelings of anxiety and vulnerability, and this will be expanded on further in this chapter.

One of the most important insights theoretically and practically to emerge in the last period is the recognition that gender is a social relation. 'Gender, both as an analytic category and a social process is relational. That is, gender relations are complex and unstable processes ... constituted by and through interrelated parts. These parts are interdependent, that is, each part can have no meaning or existence without the others' (Flax 1990, p. 44). Putting this simply, a notion of man does not make sense without having a notion of woman. This is clearly demonstrated in everyday life when boys are exhorted not to cry because it's girlish and similarly girls are chastised for being tomboyish. Consequently, when what it means to be a woman changes, this has a knock-on effect on what it means to be a man. For example, if the majority of married women work, this potentially questions a traditional and central aspect of men's identity, that of economic provider.

Another important insight is that gender relations are power relations that are unequal in that men are generally more powerful than women. There is, however, considerable controversy among feminists about the nature and extent of these power relations. Early analyses proposed the radical, but quite simple, notion that all men exercised power over all women, frequently supported by the use of sexual violence (see Segal 1987 for a critical account of early debates). However, other feminists have pointed to the importance of questioning universalist notions such as 'all men' or 'all women', pointing out how differences between women and men in terms of class, 'race' and sexuality matter considerably in terms of who has power over whom and when.

The recognition of difference has been inspired by both political and theoretical developments. Politically, for example, black women have pointed out that they are oppressed by racism as well as sexism and that racism implicates white women as well as white men (hooks 1984). Theoretically, the increased interest by some feminists in ideas emanating from post-modernism and post-structuralism has also encouraged the deconstruction of categories such as men or women, as well as scepticism about whether there is one central imperative governing men's relations with women. They have argued for drawing attention to the local and the specific in terms of analysing who gets oppressed by whom and how (Featherstone & Fawcett 1994–5).

Psychoanalytic feminists and pro-feminist men have also added another dimension to attempts to understand power. They have cautioned against perspectives which see men's or women's behaviour solely in rational terms. For example, as I have indicated, men's sexual violence has been seen as motivated by their desire to assert their power over women and children. Psychoanalytic approaches, as we shall see later, point to the importance of exploring men's feelings of vulnerability, anger, rage and powerlessness (see Frosh 1994).

Today, feminists from a range of perspectives recognise that we cannot assume that what it means to be a man or a woman, or a mother or a father, is straightforward, as there have been considerable transformations in the lived practices of men, women, mothers and fathers. For example, the involvement of many more women, including mothers, in the paid labour force has meant a challenging of the assumption that motherhood is the sole source of women's identity. There has been an increase in the numbers of women either not bearing children or delaying child bearing. Again, this also fractures the assumption that woman equals mother.

There has been a considerable growth in the divorce rate in the UK. Whilst this cannot be attributable in any straightforward way to feminism, it does appear that it is frequently women who are leaving unsatisfactory marriages despite the often very adverse consequences for them and their children, particularly economic. When large numbers of women are mothering on their own, or fathers are not living with their children, this in turn fractures notions of family, mother and father.

These changes inform how everyday lives are lived at every level from the psychic to the material. It is therefore important to remember that such processes arouse great anxiety since they are concerned with how we understand and think about ourselves and our relationships, and involve feelings such as love, loss, anxiety and vulnerability. Given that it is widely perceived that women in the West initiated and are propelling many of the contemporary developments, an important outcome has been the varied and complex reactions of men. Bewilderment, fury and welcome are some of the responses which can be discerned currently.

What has all this got to do with child abuse?

Clearly, the term child abuse itself not straightforward. What it is and who defines it are all the subject of ongoing debate, particularly in the UK (see Parton,

Chapter 1, in this volume), where for many years child abuse appears to have been constructed solely in terms of the action/inactions of caregivers or other adults towards children, which manifest themselves in physical symptoms on a child's body. However, there have been ongoing critiques of this particular perspective and the associated emphasis within practice on risk and danger. Writers have argued for a move away from individualism towards a recognition of the role structural factors play in the lives of individuals in terms of influencing their actions/inactions (Frost & Stein 1987). For example, the role of poverty in relation to physical abuse and neglect has been stressed. In recent years, *Child Protection: Messages from Research* (Department of Health (DOH) 1995) has suggested that abusive actions always need to be located in context and this has continued to broaden the debate. There has been an increased recognition of the importance of emotional abuse, which cannot always be measured by signs on the child's body. This shift is most apparent in the Government's document *Framework for the Assessment of Children in Need and their Families* (DOH 1999*a*).

There is also a broader policy context currently in which issues like child poverty, racism, domestic violence and the mental health needs of parents have come on to the agenda (see, for example, *Working Together to Safeguard Children*, DOH 1999*b*). Feminists have brought gender to the fore largely by emphasising the harm suffered by children and women from violent and abusive men. They have been particularly active in highlighting the prevalence of child sexual abuse and its links with other forms of male violence. Indeed, the notion of a continuum has been coined to underscore the linkages between a range of activities from pornography, rape and domestic violence to child sexual abuse (Kelly 1988), a notion which serves to highlight the continuities between what have been previously treated as discrete activities. The key continuities cohere around the evidence of men's disproportionate involvement in such activities and the underlying rationale for all such behaviour, which is deemed to be men's desire to maintain their power over women and children.

Feminists have made explicit connections between the welfare of children and the welfare of women, for example, by pointing out the links between domestic violence and child abuse (of all varieties). They have pointed out most valuably that a man's physical violence towards his partner should be considered a risk factor in assessing the safety of any children involved (Stark & Flitcraft 1988). They have also been critical of the 'systems' set up to deal with child abuse generally, pointing out, for example, how often the generic term 'parent' is deployed to obscure the reality of men's violence (Campbell 1988). In particular, they have been concerned at how often policy and practice appear to focus on mothers and ignore fathers/men. Furthermore, they have pointed out how often mothers are held responsible for the protection of their children but are left without adequate resources (Hooper 1992).

Whilst overall the above critiques have been invaluable in placing sexual violence on the social work map and in 'naming' much of the oppression suffered by women and children at the hands of men, these feminist positions are open to criticism. Most do not address adequately the complexities of men's, women's and children's positions. There is a tendency to portray men as an homogenous group who rationally and consciously abuse women and children as part of an overall power strategy. The differences *between* men and what they do are seen as irrelevant. In contrast, the complexities of women's positions are acknowledged to some extent. Differences between women are seen as important in terms of, for example, the differential resources which may be available to women who wish to leave violent men. Kelly (1996) argues that the evidence of women's involvement in abusive activity cannot be ignored by feminists and requires a general rethinking. However, there is a tendency on the part of some feminists to assume that abusive behaviour by women is solely attributable to their oppression by men. This reproduces the fantasy of the 'perfect mother' who, if given the right circumstances, will both know how to and desire to be a good mother. Such a fantasy leaves little space for considering some of the more difficult and uncomfortable emotions which may be evoked by the mothering process.

In terms of understanding children, Wise (1995) has argued that a hierarchy of oppression approach has been developed by feminists. Women's oppression is accorded the highest priority, which can result in a failure to address properly the vulnerability of children at the hands of abusive or neglectful mothers. Moreover, there can be a tendency to assume that mothers' and children's interests are synonymous.

A general problem with dominant feminist critiques is that a gendered perspective has, generally, been conflated with documenting men's violent and abusive activities and the subsequent injustices suffered by women and children. However, as indicated in the first section, the notion of gender encompasses much broader developments and processes. Whilst a consideration of all of these is beyond the scope of this chapter, I would like to address some of the key issues which I see as relevant to child abuse in today's climate.

The elements I want to consider are as follows.

1. What meanings are attached to children today?
2. What impact have changes in gender relations had upon these?
3. How are changes in the relationships between men and women and in mothering and fathering affecting the welfare of children more broadly as well as in terms of specific abusive activities?
4. What issues are raised for contemporary social work practices in the light of the changes in gender relations which are occurring?

The meaning of the child

First, what do children mean to parents today? Do they signify differently from other periods in history? Beck & Beck-Gernsheim (1995) argue that:

> The sort of change evident in the marital relationship, as society moved from pre-industrial to modern times is also apparent in the relationship between parents and child. In both, the common cause – the survival of the family unit – has disappeared; in both the relationship between the persons involved is less economic and more personal and private, with all the hopes and interests this involves; in both the relationship depends largely on the growing, not to say hypertrophic emotional needs of all parties in an individualized world (including all the rewards and horrors inherent in intense feelings). (p. 105–106)

More generally, Jenks (1996) locates the meanings attached to children within an analysis of post-modernity. He argues that the child has become the site of discourses concerning stability, integration and the social bond. Children, in a period where partners come and go, are seen not so much as promise but as primary and uncontested sources of love in 'the most fundamental, unchosen, unnegotiated form of relationship. The trust that was previously anticipated from marriage, partnership, friendship, class solidarity and so on, is now invested more generally in the child' (p. 107). Children are now seen as dependable and permanent, perhaps the only thing reliable and permanent in a world of such rapid change. He argues that because we need them, we watch them and develop a range of mechanisms to oversee them. 'We have always watched children, once as guardians of their/our future and now because they have become the guardians. Our expanded surveillance has, needless to say, revealed more intrusions into their state of wellbeing. Child abuse ... has clearly "increased" through the magnification and breadth of our gaze' (p. 108).

According to Jenks, the dramatic increase in the reported occurrence of child abuse in recent times is attributable not solely to the improved technology of scrutiny or our diligence but also to the collective response to contemporary conditions. To abuse a child today is to strike at the one remaining vestige of the social bond embodied in the child. The manner in which we have come to organise our social relationships is vital here. What Beck & Beck-Gernsheim and Jenks are addressing seems to me to be the way in which the changes in the relationships between adult men and women, and particularly the stability of marriage, has impacted on the meanings invested in children.

Certainly a striking feature of the contemporary policy climate is a concern with the welfare of children, a concern that is central to the current policy context in the UK and which appears to unite otherwise quite diverse forces (see, for example, Etzioni 1993, Giddens 1998). Giddens (1998) is particularly interesting in that he appears to accept, if not celebrate, many of the changes that are occurring in and to contemporary families. He argues, for example, that 'First and most fundamentally we must start from the principle of equality between the sexes, from which there can be no going back. There is only one story to tell about the family today and that is of democracy' (p. 93). He then goes on to argue that the protection and care of children is the single most important thread that should guide family policy, an argument which would be shared by those who decry many of the contemporary changes and would indeed wish to roll the clock back. This emphasis on the protection and care of children has a different impact on men and women. Women are often perceived, or indeed perceive themselves, as selfish if they jeopardise the welfare of children. Men increasingly are seen as losing out or becoming marginalised.

However, it is important to acknowledge that children are increasingly promoting themselves and being promoted as subjects in their own right, as well as the objects of adults' concerns/projections, and furthermore that they do not form a homogenous group. There has been a considerable development in initiatives which open up possibilities for children to articulate their concerns and difficulties (for example, see MacLeod's (1999) account of the use of help-lines such as ChildLine). In terms of the concerns of this chapter, important differences in relation to gender are emerging and there is, for example, an increased recognition that boys and girls may have differing needs in terms of assessment and intervention.

Changing gender relations, the welfare of the child and child abuse

In terms of changes in the relationships between men and women and the welfare of children, the post-war rise in the number of divorces (often initiated by women) and the rise in lone parenthood (primarily motherhood) are both phenomena which are complexly related to the changing nature of gender relations and the changing aspirations of women. Whilst most women are not in any sense straightforwardly rejecting marriage or male involvement in their lives, matters have changed for both men and women. Beck & Beck-Gernsheim (1995) write of the rise of the 'female biography', arguing that one property of contemporary society has been an extended process of individualisation, a key aspect of which is that it is a process open to women.

They identify three general phases: in the first, the family was essentially an economic unit, with neither partner possessing an individual biography; in the second, men were expected to take the initiative in organising their own lives, family cohesion remaining intact at the expense of women's rights; and in the third, roughly since the 1960s, both men and women have been faced 'with the blessings and burdens of making a life of their own' (Beck & Beck-Gernsheim 1995, p. 76), Scrambler & Scrambler 1997, p. xvii).

This emphasis on individual biography militates against stable monogamous relationships at a time when individuals are actually searching ever more anxiously for stability in such relationships.

As a consequence of contemporary changes, many 'families' who come to the attention of social services today are complex in structure, with women either living on their own or with a partner who is not the biological father of any or some of the children. Consequently, in engaging with such families, assumptions cannot readily be made about the attachments involved. This has not been adequately taken on board in the literature directed at practitioners, where notions of 'supporting families' or 'working with parents' continue to be used in a way which assumes that we all know who the family or the parent is. The recent *Framework for the Assessment of Children in Need and their Families* (DOH 1999*a*) appears to recognise contemporary changes to some extent but does not, in my view, deal adequately with the potential ramifications.

An interesting finding, for example, from some of the research studies points to the adverse consequences of divorce for adults in terms of their economic, physical and emotional well-being (Day Sclater 1998). Yet, how often is this considered in terms of assessing the ability of a parent to protect a child? How aware are social workers in working with separated parents of the complex emotional processes they may be going through and the consequences this may have in terms of caring for their children?

The possibility that divorce may have an adverse impact upon children is much better recognised generally but how well is this recognition integrated into contemporary child care practice? Indeed, in relation to much practice the focus can be quite appropriately on facilitating the break up of a parental relationship where one party is the abuser. However, understandable as this may be in practice, frequently little support is given to either the divorcing/separating partner or the child(ren) in terms of the practical or emotional dynamics involved. For example, mothers of children who have been sexually abused and who are assessed as protective frequently find no resources available to them to help them to work through the impact of the separation and associated consequences.

The dangers violent men can pose to both women and children when post-divorce contact is insisted upon have also increasingly been acknowledged in the child protection literature (Hester & Radford 1996). Johnston & Campbell (1993) have deconstructed such violence in terms of assessing the risk such men pose, however, and have concluded that separation itself can precipitate violence by previously non-violent partners of either gender. This is not surprising if one accepts Day Sclater's (1998) argument that separation and loss evoke elemental feelings which the current emphasis on conciliation and mediation obscures, with potentially very damaging consequences for all concerned, including children.

These are just some of the areas of overlap between changing gender relations, family forms, the welfare of children and child abuse. I now want to look at some aspects of the changing faces of contemporary motherhood and fatherhood.

'Changes' in mothering

It would appear that the current Government has adopted a very pragmatic attitude to the 'realities' of the contemporary labour market and clearly accepts and supports a situation where the majority of women, including mothers, are in the paid labour force. It has also promoted the desirability of the 'paid worker' identity for mothers on state benefits. Indeed, their emphasis has led to a general perception that they are valorising the worker role over the carer role.

The changing aspirations of women have combined with labour market realities to 'alter' the contemporary landscape within which mothering occurs. I use the word 'alter' advisedly here, however. For example, black African-Caribbean mothers have been consistently in the paid labour force full-time and equate being a good mother with working (Duncan 1999). White mothers are more likely to work part-time, therefore combining the two identities rather than rejecting or embracing one or the other. However, young women with few economic opportunities continue to invest heavily in mothering as an identity. Furthermore, mothers generally continue to invest in notions of 'good motherhood' although there appears to have been a shift in the content of such notions. Coward (1993) found in her research that most mothers did not identify the good mother as the 'stay at home' mother but rather as someone who enjoyed mothering. This ideal in itself was the source of much anguish for those who did not enjoy motherhood in the way they felt they should.

Kaplan (1992) has pointed out that a 'new' (as in historically unprecedented) discourse has emerged which enjoins women to find self-fulfilment in mothering. Previous discourses stressed sacrifice and duty. The corollary of such a discourse is that they may not find what they are seeking – an unsettling possibility for all concerned.

Therefore, the pragmatism of the current policy context could give a misleading picture in that it obscures the practical and emotional conflicts that mothers currently can experience. Moreover, the emphasis on the welfare of children can leave little space for mothers to articulate what may be perceived as their own 'selfish' desires. For example, in research with women and men on post-divorce contact arrangements, women experienced a conflict between 'welfare of the child' and 'independence' discourses. Thus, they recognised that the welfare of the child was served by continued contact between their ex-partner and the children but this was often in conflict with their own need to make a clean break (Day Sclater & Yates 1999).

The current policy context poses a specific set of conflicts for both workers and mothers in child abuse cases. These may concern the availability of the mother to attend meetings, therapy, or more generally attend to the well-being of her child. In the USA, where welfare reform has resulted in the imposition of time limits on welfare eligibility and a requirement that welfare recipients engage in work outside the home, commentators have noted some of the problematic implications for mothers of abused children who are seeking to be protective. Mothers may find themselves subject to conflicting advice and demands from the different systems. One agency may require that she enter employment, whereas another might insist that she is at home to protect her child from an abusive partner (Pearce 1999).

In terms of potential changes in practice these could include child protection plans having to include specific provisions in terms of appropriate child care in mothers' absence and the re-scheduling of services to fit in with mothers' work patterns. As Ferguson (1998) has noted, one factor which may have contributed to the failure by practitioners to engage fathers who are in paid work has been the timing of services and this could now begin to apply to mothers. The 'available' mother is now potentially under threat in the current policy context. There are other more theoretical developments which also undermine the desirability of this construction of motherhood (see Benjamin 1995). This work contradicts earlier assumptions that mothers were there primarily to facilitate their children's development and points to the importance for both mothers and children of mothers being subjects in their own right and the role of paid work in facilitating this.

As I have indicated, constructions of the 'available' mother which underpin contemporary child protection practices are now under threat. Other constructions also need to be challenged. As mothers increasingly articulate their own stories rather than being subject to the prescriptions of others, particularly experts, it is becoming clearer that mothering evokes quite complex feelings which are not always acknowledged in child protection practice. Here, the general assumption is that they are either protective or collusive, an assumption that fails to capture the potential range of feelings that may be around. The necessity to make assessments within very quick time frames is significant here.

However, according to Parker (1995), maternal ambivalence is the experience shared variously by all mothers in which loving and hating feelings for their children co-exist. She argues against regarding this as a problem in itself. Indeed, it can be creative as the conflict mobilised by both sets of feelings forces a mother to think about her relationship with her child. If a mother only regarded her child with either hostile feelings or untroubled love, she would not 'think' about the relationship. In psychoanalytic perspectives, the capacity to 'think' is seen as vital as it helps us avoid either unhelpful acting-out in relation to others or merely being passive reactors to others. Crucially, ambivalence allows the mother to experience both herself and her child as separate, and as subjects rather than as intertwined and objects. She argues, however, that ambivalence can become unmanageable and this can lead to violence and abuse on the part of the mother.

The widespread societal taboo on the expression of ambivalence in Western culture is one of the central factors in rendering such ambivalence unmanageable for particular women. Other factors contribute, although Parker (1995) is undeterministic about these. They include the support of partners, physical health, economic pressures, the availability of emotional support and the contribution of the individual child. However, this is not an approach that lends itself to checklists that can unproblematically identify risk factors. For example, in terms of emotional support, Parker found that some mothers found others a lifeline, whilst for others they activated their deepest insecurities and anxieties. Equally, a partially absent father can be more problematic than one who is not available at all, in the sense that some fathers provide no space for mothers to express ambivalence and indeed can actively repress such expressions.

The notion of ambivalence also alerts us to the dangers of assuming any simple correspondence between a mother's and child's needs. It obliges us to recognise that both mother and child are engaged in separate as well as connected journeys. Moreover, Parker's work obliges us to recognise that mothers are not just 'origins' who impact upon children. They are often assessed solely in terms of their impact upon children, but having a child changes a woman too as she sets off on her journey. This has implications for assessment and intervention practices. In terms of assessment, allowing the expression of ambivalence in defensive climates is difficult. However, as I have indicated, there is possibly a more hopeful climate being ushered in.

In terms of intervention there is currently a restricted menu, which usually involves work with mother and child together or requires attendance at parents' groups (in practice, usually mothers' groups). What about time off, money for a babysitter and so on?

In terms of mothers who engage in violent and sexually abusive behaviour, contemporary writings would indicate that mothers are strongly implicated in physically abusive behaviour towards children but much less likely to engage in sexually abusive behaviour (Featherstone & Fawcett 1994–5). Using a gendered perspective to understand this means not denying or obscuring the potential of mothers to be abusive, but recognising that there may be differing meanings attached to such behaviour by mothers themselves, children and workers, than those attached to men's behaviour. For example, women who kill children are much more likely to be seen as mad and men as bad (Wilczynski 1995).

To summarise, some of the challenges today for practitioners cohere around the following:

- Mothering today may be carried out in the context of other identities/options.
- Whilst the welfare of children and their mothers overlaps, it does not coincide.
- Current constructions are premised either on assumptions about mothers' lives that no longer may pertain, such as availability, or assumptions that are being challenged by the voicing of feelings such as ambivalence.

I want to look now at some of the contemporary debates and writings on fathers and the implications for practice.

Changing fathers

Who or what is a father? These questions take on particular resonance when many men do not live with their biological children or are living with children who are not biologically related to them. Technological developments, particularly in terms of donor insemination, reinforce the importance of attending to the rupture that has occurred between biological and social conceptions of fatherhood.

What this means is that we need to attend to and distinguish between fatherhood as a status and fathering as a set of practices. In terms of the latter, considerable attention has been paid to what men do or do not do in terms of the domestic division of labour and child care. In terms of the former, there is a substantial literature on the problem of absent fathers and the assumed implications of this for children's well-being. More recently, a research paradigm around father presence has emerged which explores the contributions fathers can make to children's development irrespective of living arrangements.

There is no consensus among feminists about the role of fathers, however. Whilst some high profile feminists argue for measures that facilitate the involvement of fathers in family life, others emphasise the dangers violent fathers can pose to women and children (Featherstone 1999). There is also a wider ambiguity, not confined to feminists, relating to the question of what is a 'good father'. Is a 'good father' someone who is interchangeable with a mother, or does he contribute something distinctive and if so, what is this? The current literature on fathers and fathering is replete with notions of crisis and redundancy. This is echoed in men's own accounts. For example, research with men on post-divorce contact notes that a sense of loss and injustice pervaded these accounts, irrespective of whether this was confirmed by the actual realities of particular men's situations (Day Sclater & Yates 1999).

How are fathers and fathering discussed in contemporary discussions about child abuse? The dangers of violent men have been well documented and the failure by professionals to engage with such men is becoming well documented (Milner 1996). There is little discussion of fathers as resources or assets. The focus on violence, whilst understandable, is not adequate, however, in my view. We need to address broader issues in order to develop a gendered perspective to take us into the next millennium.

What does this mean? It requires engaging with broad questions around the meaning of fathering today for men themselves as well as women, children and workers. This involves dealing with fathers in terms of status and fathering as practice. Who engages with children on an everyday basis and what conflicts emerge as a result are important issues, as we shall see illustrated in the case study in the next section.

Thinking through what is meant by a good father and acknowledging that this is not straightforward, is required. For example, Lewis (1999) found that many fathers identified being a good father with being a provider, as did the women they were involved with. Consequently, those who were unemployed or disabled and unable to provide, had little confidence in their ability to be good fathers. Ferguson (1998) argues that practitioners need to pay particular attention to those whose traditional identities have been thrown into turmoil through long-term unemployment. Such men can get stuck in grief, mourning the loss of the productive self, and experience major problems in finding meaning in domestic roles and intimacy. Can or should such men change? How should such change be achieved?

The links between changing notions of masculinity and violence and abuse need to be interrogated. Feminist understandings of the links between power and abuse are useful but are overly rational, in my view. Much of men's violence and abuse needs to be explored in a way that recognises that many men today may actually *feel* and indeed *be* powerless, particularly in terms of their ability to engage in intimate family relations. This may be contributing to the way they act out and frequently objectify women and children. However, this is difficult territory as approaches to why men act violently which look at men's vulnerability and powerlessness are often assumed to be exercises in excusing such men. Ferguson (1998), for example, draws a distinction between vulnerable men and abusive men, advocating quite different strategies for both. Thus, he advocates personal development work for vulnerable men but sees this as entirely inappropriate for violent men, who need to acknowledge that they have power and are abusing it.

In practice, I am not sure that this distinction is quite so clear cut. Frosh (1994) argues that much of men's violence has its origins in the sense that masculinity is built on emptiness, including disavowal of the capacity to link with others in a mode of reciprocal neediness and intimacy.

Under contemporary conditions, the traditional masculine defence of flight into rationality and repudiation of the feminine can no longer bolster the fragility of masculine identity. This is both welcome and problematic. Men's domination has always been supported by violence; this violence is no less present as domination is called into question. It is observable all the time, particularly as sexual violence but also in other paranoid exchanges within family life. It arises from a mixture of rage at the dissolution of the fantasy of masculine rationality and power and of employment as a strategy to hold on to this power. (p. 230)

As Frosh acknowledges, the vulnerability of men has not been high on many agendas. Certainly, workers in child abuse find their resources stretched to the limit and do not often give adequate support to victimised children or women, never mind men. But we do need to think about this in the broadest as well as the narrowest sense and, as I have indicated, it is increasingly evident on the policy agenda.

To summarise this section, the key points are:

- There is no current agreement on what is required from fathers or what a 'good father' is.
- For many of the fathers who come to the attention of social services, the role of economic provider may not be available and they may have considerable problems with finding an alternative role.
- The links between contemporary changes in men's lives and violence need to be recognised.

In the next section I want to use some case studies to illustrate some of the themes I have been attempting to get across in preceding sections.

Stories of today

John's story

John came to see social services with concerns about the care of his children, who were being looked after by his ex-wife. They had split up acrimoniously 2 years previously when she had acquired a new boyfriend. A pattern of contact had been established, though not without difficulties. His concerns were not specific. He just had a general sense that the children were not 'happy' and that they talked of not liking the new boyfriend when he got angry with them.

Currently, this kind of referral is dealt with under child protection procedures although a change of emphasis in relation to this is being signalled most strongly in the new consultation documents produced by the Department of Health (DOH 1999a, 1999b). However, understandably, the emphasis will still be on the children's rather than the adult's needs. Given the vagueness of John's allegations this referral would not be perceived as high priority at all and there might be a suspicion that the referral was malicious in that John was using the children to 'get back' at his wife.

Given the time and resource constraints under which social workers operate, it is not surprising that John's needs as an individual are not assessed. However, one sensitive initial interview might look at not only trying to specify his precise concerns about the children but also try and ascertain how he himself was coping since the divorce and how he felt about his current life and the man who was 'fathering' *his* children. The contact with the children could also be explored in terms of how equipped he felt as a caregiver. This not only deals with his, and indeed the children's, needs but could act preventatively in terms of future referrals. In a case similar to John's the divorce had coincided with job redundancy and the man in question had focused a lot of his anxieties around the children rather than facing up to the reality of constructing a new life.

As I have indicated, a divorce or relationship break up forces an engagement with complex processes, including reassessment of the past as well as constructing a present and imagining a future. If that coincides with other crises such as a job loss then the consequences can be very difficult indeed. There is evidence that middle-aged men cope less well with unemployment and divorce than women.

Jeannie's story

Jeannie is bringing up three children largely on her own. Her partner, who is not the father of the children, does not live with her and is not involved in the day-to-day care of the children. The three children have different biological fathers. Two have contact with their fathers and the other does not. Jeannie is on income support and struggles financially. She admits to getting very frustrated with the children and has hit one of them (the oldest, who is 10) quite hard on the arm on more than one occasion.

Currently, an initial assessment in this situation would be likely to concentrate on assessing the risks to the particular child in terms of age, the overall relationship with mother and her degree of recognition of how inappropriate her behaviour was. Depending on the degree of risk assessed, little input might be offered here.

There are, however, a range of issues which could and arguably should be considered even in an initial assessment. What does mothering mean to Jeannie? What does this specific child? How do they all cope with the complexities of the attachment figures around? Do the men in her life support her or undermine her? What do she and her children want from the fathers in terms of concrete involvement or support? How do they see their roles?

Neither of these cases would be classified as high priority at all in the current climate. The resources available would also be extremely limited. Furthermore, social workers have become increasingly aware in recent decades of the delicate balancing act they must perform between the welfare of children and adults.

Recent governmental guidance supports a shift towards assessing need rather than risk but the focus still remains firmly on the needs of the child. However, the framework does allow for the possibility that focusing on the needs of the adult may, at times, be beneficial to the child(ren) concerned. It also recognises, to some extent, the complexity of family life today, with its recognition that significant adults may not live with children and absent parents need to be included in assessments. The framework, however, pays no attention to how constructions of mothering and fathering may be changing with the changes in expectations and roles that are occurring.

Conclusions

Taking gender seriously requires acknowledging that we are engaging with men and women, mothers and fathers, boys and girls, but these categories are neither straightforward nor fixed. Mothering is an important, but not the only, aspect of women's identities today, and fathering is the subject of much anxiety and uncertainty. At the same time, the instability of adult relationships is altering the meanings attached to children.

To understand relationships between adults and children, including those that are abusive and neglectful, we need to engage with some key questions around what is happening to mothers and mothering, fathers and fathering today, and to recognise that we are living in a period of considerable transition for all concerned.

References

Beck U, Beck-Gernsheim E 1995 The normal chaos of love. Polity Press, Cambridge

Benjamin J 1995 Like subjects, love objects: essays on recognition and sexual difference. Yale University Press, London

Campbell B 1988 Unofficial secrets, child sexual abuse: the Cleveland case. Virago, London

Coward R, 1993 Our treacherous hearts: why women let men get their way. Faber and Faber, London

Day Sclater, S 1998 The psychology of divorce: a research report to the ESRC. University of East London, London

Day Sclater S, Yates C 1999 The psycho-politics of post-divorce parenting. In: Bainham A, Day Sclater S, Richards M (eds) What is a parent? A socio-legal analysis. Hart Publishing, Oxford

Department of Health (DOH) 1995 Child protection: messages from research. HMSO, London

Department of Health (DOH) 1999a Framework for the assessment of children in need and their families. The Stationery Office, London

Department of Health (DOH) 1999b Working together to safeguard children. The Stationery Office, London

Duncan S 1999 Personal communication

Etzioni A 1993 The parenting deficit. Demos, London

Featherstone B 1997 What has gender got to do with it? Exploring physically abusive behaviour towards children. British Journal of Social Work 27: 419–433

Featherstone B 1999 Taking mothering seriously: the implications for child protection. Child and Family Social Work 4 (1): 43–55

Featherstone B, Fawcett B 1994–5 Feminism and child abuse: opening up some possibilities? Critical Social Policy 42: 61–81

Ferguson H 1998 State services and supports for fathers. In: McKeown K, Ferguson H, Rooney D (eds) Changing fathers? Fatherhood and family life in modern Ireland. Collins, Cork

Flax J 1990 Thinking fragments: psychoanalysis, feminism and postmodernism in the contemporary West. University of California Press, Oxford

Frosh S 1994 Sexual difference: masculinity and psychoanalysis. Routledge, London

Frost N, Stein M 1987 The politics of child welfare. Harvester Wheatsheaf, Hemel Hempstead

Giddens A 1998 The third way: the renewal of social democracy. Polity Press, Cambridge

Gordon L 1989 Heroes of their own lives: the politics and history of family violence. Virago, London

Hester M, Radford L 1996 Domestic violence and child contact arrangements in England and Denmark. Policy Press, Bristol

Hollway W 1989 Subjectivity and method in psychology. Sage, London

hooks b 1984 Feminist theory: from margin to center. South End Press, Boston

Hooper C-A 1992 Mothers surviving child sexual abuse. Routledge, London

Humm M 1989 The dictionary of feminist theory. Harvester Wheatsheaf, Hemel Hempstead

Jenks C 1996 Childhood. Routledge, London

Johnston J, Campbell L 1993 A clinical typology of interpersonal violence in disputed-custody divorces. American Journal of Orthopsychiatry 63: 190–199

Kaplan E A 1992 Motherhood and representation: the mother in popular culture and melodrama. Routledge, London

Kelly L 1988 Surviving sexual violence. Polity Press, Cambridge

Kelly L 1996 When does the speaking profit us?: reflections on the challenges of developing feminist perspectives on abuse and violence by women. In: Hester M, Kelly L, Radford J (eds) Women, violence and male power. Open University Press, Milton Keynes

MacLeod M 1999 Don't just do it: children's access to help and protection. In: Parton N, Wattam C (eds) Child sexual abuse: responding to the experiences of children. John Wiley, NSPCC, Chichester

Milner J 1996 Men's resistance to social workers. In: Fawcett B, Featherstone B, Hearn J, Toft C (eds) Violence and gender relations: theories and interventions. Sage, London

Parker R 1995 Torn in two: the experience of maternal ambivalence. Virago, London

Pearce D 1999 Doing the triple combination: negotiating the domestic violence, child welfare and welfare systems. In: Brandwein R (ed) Battered women, children and welfare reform. Sage, London

Scrambler G, Scrambler A 1997 Foreword. In: Scrambler G, Scrambler A (eds) Rethinking prostitution: purchasing sex in the 1990s. Routledge, London

Segal L 1987 Is the future female? Troubled thoughts on contemporary feminism. Virago, London

Segal L 1990 Slow motion: changing men, changing masculinities. Virago, London

Stark E, Flitcraft A 1988 Women and children at risk: a feminist perspective on child abuse. International Journal of Health Services 18 (1): 97–118

Wilczynski A 1995 Child killing by parents: a motivational model. Child Abuse 4 Special Issue: 365–371

Wise S 1995 Feminist ethics in practice. In: Hugman R, Smith D (eds) Ethical issues in social work. Routledge, London

7 Issues of ethnicity and culture

Melanie Phillips

Is it a social service to steal our culture
Is it a social service to take the fruit from the trees
Which our families grew
    Our ancestors knew
    That the fruit from the trees
    Which our families grew
    Is being stolen, social worker,
    By you.

(Sissay 1988)

These are the powerful words of Lemn Sissay, a black poet and writer who grew up in care. They describe the anger and bitterness of many black children who experience the care system at first hand, and they are a powerful lesson to all professionals who work in child protection because they pose the uncomfortable question: what are we protecting children from?

The child abuse debate often centres on better ways of protecting children who are suffering or likely to suffer significant harm as a consequence of the care that they are receiving from their parents. In fact, the legal preconditions for statutory intervention to protect children from abuse in the Children Act 1989 are based on this concept of harm. There is no doubt that there needs to be a system of State protection which exists to safeguard the welfare of children. However, 'harm' also has a wider meaning in a broader social context, as discrimination and social inequality are in themselves harmful to the welfare of children and their families.

For black families (for the purposes of this chapter, black refers to peoples of Asian, African or African-Caribbean origin) this social reality has tangible consequences, since there is clear evidence that, in this country, the colour of your skin is a determining factor in your access to resources and life opportunities:

Children's skin colour is a strong determinant of their life chances and so black children fare worse on the whole range of social and economic indicators in comparison to whites.
(Popple 1986, p. 187)

Discriminatory treatment on the basis of skin colour is a component of racism, and it is racism which institutionalises the power imbalance between black and white communities to produce socially reinforced inequality.

Racism refers to the construction and institutionalisation of social relationships based on the assumption of the inferiority of ethnic minority groups, their customs, lifestyles and beliefs. As a result they experience marginalisation in the economic and social spheres. Prejudice and crude racial stereotypes reinforce and legitimate such divisions. While there is a range of ethnic minority groups, the major division is in terms of black and white.
(Channer & Parton 1990, p. 106)

An understanding of the impact of racism on the lives of black communities is a vital adjunct to any discussion of culture and ethnicity in child protection services because it is impossible to adequately respond to the needs of black children without taking into account the social consequences that this power differential has on the lives of black families.

As definitions of abuse have become increasingly 'professionalised' in legislation and professional guidance to welfare agencies, the impact of racial inequality and racial injustice has been largely ignored. Abuse and protection are not so much discussed within a social and economic context as within an individual and pathological framework, which sees the child's family and carers as the targets for intervention.

In looking at the effect of local authorities' intervention on black children and their families, it is evident that they have not only failed to promote equality but their own practices and procedures have discriminated against black families.

Experience sustained by members of black communities suggests that there is a deep and ingrained racism that perceives them as more threatening than whites, and, accordingly, metes out harsher measures to them. It seems that the strengths of black families and communities are not recognised.

(Channer & Parton 1990, p. 108)

The report of the Black and In Care Group to the NSPCC (1992) summarises the views of large numbers of black families:

While black children, like white children, need to be protected from harm and helped to overcome the effects of abuse, the way in which both the social services and the NSPCC have professionalised the issues has left many people feeling powerless and victimised.

(Black and In Care Group 1992, p. 4)

The message from the black communities is clear: State intervention in family life can in itself leave children vulnerable to other forms of abuse, some of which are as a direct consequence of the intervention itself.

This does not mean that welfare agencies cannot and should not intervene to protect children from harm. It means that welfare agencies in general, and social services in particular, need a wider perspective when looking at child abuse rather than diagnosing individual or family pathology. They need to keep in mind the personal and social consequences of racism, and adopt models of assessing families that are inclusive of these factors rather than exclusive of them.

Culture, ethnicity and social policy

In social work in general, and child protection in particular, race, culture and ethnicity have appeared only comparatively recently on the professional agenda in this country. This reflects the developing political climate of race relations which has shaped social policy in this country over the last 40 years.

For the purposes of this chapter, race refers to the social categorisation of people defined by skin colour and physical characteristics. Culture represents the shared behaviours, attitudes and traditions of a group of people which are characterised by similar language, symbols, food, dress, history, etc. Ethnicity describes geographic origin and heritage which is acquired by birth.

Following the arrival of black migrants to this country in the 1950s there was increasing concern about potential racial conflict. Many white communities expressed open hostility towards black immigrants, and black people were organising resistance to the racism that they were experiencing.

In this uneasy racial climate, it was politically important that the impact of black communities in British society was underplayed as much as possible. It is not a coincidence, therefore, that from the 1960s to the 1980s the notion of 'assimilation' or 'integration' underpinned most political debate about race relations at a national and local level.

Assimilation was a useful term for the public and politicians alike, portraying a more comfortable concept of future relationships between the races in which black migrants adapted to the requirements of British society by assimilating into the British way of life. It contained none of the perceived threats of separateness or difference.

The policies of the personal social services during this period are a reflection of this. Up until the 1980s, the general practice of social services and other child welfare agencies was to adopt a 'colour blind' approach to the organisation of services for families in which a 'same for all' policy operated. This was represented as the fairest way of providing services, since it meant that there was no special treatment for any particular family or community. Child welfare legislation, central government and local departmental guidance all presented this view. Race and culture were not mentioned, and the illusion was created that black families were being treated equally within the systems of welfare provision.

However, the reality was very different. From 1970 onwards, there was an ever-increasing body of evidence revealing a widespread pattern of discrimination on the basis of colour. It was clear that local government institutions were no less guilty than any other social institution, since they were not only treating black people differently from whites but their policies and procedures were in themselves discriminatory. In 1973, the Race Relations Board highlighted this point by arguing that 'racial discrimination was less a matter of "active discrimination against individuals" than the reproduction of "situations in which equality of opportunity is consciously or unconsciously denied"' (Solomos 1989).

In 1976, the Government responded by passing the third Race Relations Act. Unlike the two previous Race Relations Acts in 1965 and 1968, the 1976 Act was a public recognition that racism was not only about hostile and individual acts of discrimination, but that it was also institutionalised in employment and the provision of services to black communities.

Section 17 of this Act places a specific duty on local authorities to tackle the effects of racism:

It shall be the duty of every local authority to make appropriate arrangements with a view to securing that their functions are carried out with regard to the need;
a) To eliminate unlawful racial discrimination; and
b) To promote equality of opportunity and good relations, between persons of different racial groups.

(Race Relations Act 1976)

Enshrined in the Act was the concept that local authorities were the key agents of change, and that it was through their intervention that discrimination and disadvantage could be tackled.

However, the response from local authorities was poor. A study conducted by Jones in 1977 (*Immigration and Social Policy in Britain*) reported that most social services departments had not responded to the needs of black clients, either in service provision or in staff training and ethnic record-keeping. According to the Community Relations Commission Report of 1977, 'It was very rare for Social Services Committees to have even discussed the needs of minorities' (Husband 1989, p. 10).

It was evident that the Race Relations Act was making little difference to service provision, and that local authorities were largely reneging on their responsibilities. Services continued to be offered on the same basis as before, with scant attention being paid to the needs of the varied communities in their localities. The 1980s sparked a shift in policy, however, as a consequence of the urban resistance of 1981. The demands of the black communities could no longer be ignored and even the Scarman report (Scarman 1981) had highlighted a desperate need for change.

During this period, two influential schools of thought began to emerge about the best way of tackling racial inequality. They both had their origins in education, but they rapidly gained popularity in social services. The first of these was multi-culturalism. In the late 1970s and early 1980s a number of articles began to appear in social work journals about the importance of culture and language in service provision to families who were not a part of the majority culture (Powell 1978, Reynolds 1978, Roskill 1979).

Multi-culturalism, as outlined in the 1985 Swann Report *Education for All* was essentially a recognition that assimilationist and colour blind approaches to service provision were grossly inappropriate ways of responding to the needs of black communities, whose cultures and lifestyles were different from white cultures (Rattansi 1992). At the heart of the multi-cultural perspective was the concept that racism was based on ignorance and prejudiced beliefs about cultural practices. Recognition of, and respect for, cultural difference was an important step in tackling racism and disadvantage, as it allowed cultural diversity to be seen positively as an asset rather than negatively as a threat. It essentially challenged the assimilationist position:

The expectation that the Afro-Caribbean and Asian minorities would simply blend into a homogeneous British or even English stew, perhaps adding some harmless spice, was revealed as not only hopelessly unrealistic but symptomatic of a form of racism which regarded 'Britishness' and 'Westernness' as the only touchstones of cultural value.

(Rattansi 1992, p. 13)

At the same time, the second school of thought, anti-racism, was also gaining ground as the solution to racial disadvantage: 'The 1980s was … an important decade with a move away from multi-culturalism and towards the more strategic approach of anti-racism and equal opportunity' (Phillips 1992, p. 16).

Like multi-culturalism, anti-racism emerged in the wake of the civil unrest of the early 1980s. Its precise roots are hard to trace, but its origins represent the collective impact of black youth, black communities, black professionals and supportive white radicals. It manifested itself in different forms, ranging from youth protest and community action to political and professional debate, but it was essentially a political, intellectual and social opposition to racism. Anti-racists saw race, and not culture, as the central issue in tackling racial disadvantage. Racism was about unequal access to jobs, housing and education. It was based on social and institutional discrimination on the basis of colour, and not just on prejudiced views about lifestyles and traditions.

As these two approaches identified different causes for racism and racial disadvantage, they both offered differing solutions for the problem. Multi-culturalists essentially saw education and cultural sensitivity as the solution, whereas anti-racists saw the need for a more fundamental political change that tackled disadvantage through the policies and practices of State and Government institutions rather than focusing on attitudinal change.

Whilst multi-culturalism was often seen to represent a tokenistic approach to tackling inequality which left the roots of the problem untouched, anti-racism gained popularity with black and white radicals alike. It provided an opportunity for a political unity between black and white professionals to launch a collective assault on the racist practices of State institutions.

During the early 1980s, at the height of local authority intervention in the area of racial equality, much hope was placed in the role of local authorities, as an agent of change, particularly in the context of the neglect of racial equality by the Thatcher administrations.

(Solomos 1989)

Change, however, was short-lived. In the face of a media 'backlash' about the 'loony left' policies of local authorities such as Hackney, Lambeth and Haringay, many local authorities saw race as a political hot potato to be avoided at all costs. Anti-racism was a vote loser, and local authorities backtracked on their earlier promises in the hope that they would avoid the glare of media attention: 'During the late 1980s there have been signs that even previously radical local authorities are now adopting a lower profile on issues concerned with racial equality' (Solomos 1989).

In the face of this inaction and backtracking on the part of local authorities, many black professionals became increasingly disillusioned. The promises of the early 1980s had proved to be hollow, and change was seen to be slow and tokenistic. For many, being a cog in the anti-racist wheel was unsatisfactory and exploitative. They wanted the opportunity to define their own models of practice. They wanted a black perspective.

From the mid – 1980s onwards, there was an increasing body of social work literature written from a black perspective. This was not a new phenomenon, for black professionals had been active in writing about their experiences and demanding change from the time of their entrance into the profession. It was only that the concept of a black perspective gave these collective experiences a name and an identity that represented a sense of solidarity and of achievement.

The factors that prescribe a black perspective have a long history of subjugation and subordination. The circumstances that shape a black perspective stem from the experience of racism and powerlessness, both past and present. The motivation that energises a black perspective is rooted in the principle of racial equality and justice.

(Ahmad 1990)

Whilst black perspectives in social work have often been marginalised within mainstream social work theory, policy and practice, the assimilationist, multi-cultural and even the anti-racist approaches have had varying degrees of impact on social work education and training. In the field of child protection in particular, however, it is evident from research that the perspective has not had a significant impact on practice with black families.

Review of literature and research

Race ethnicity and culture in research

Despite attempts to make social work practice with black children and families more sensitive and relevant, research undertaken in the last 30 years has raised questions about the way in which professionals respond to black children and their families.

A central concern about child welfare practice relates to the number of black children who are 'looked after' by local authorities. Many of the studies undertaken into the number of children in the care system concentrate more on the actual numbers in care rather than the reasons for their admission. There are also difficulties in interpreting the research in that it is the *proportion* of black children from particular black minority ethnic groups in the care system relative to the profile of the local black child care population which is significant, and not just the numbers of black children in care. Due to difficulties in the detail, accuracy and reliability of demographic information available on black communities it is often hard to interpret the statistics available to us.

However, three decades of research has highlighted the need for careful monitoring in relation to the number of black children entering the care system. The first study on children in care was conducted in the 1960s and found that children of 'mixed origin' were eight and a half times more likely to come into care than 'white indigenous' and 'Afro-Caribbean and Asian' children (Barn 1990).

In 1975, a similar study conducted by Batta *et al.* showed a similar pattern, indicating that, 'the number of Afro-Caribbean and Asian children coming into care had increased much faster than the other two groups since the study was done' (Barn 1990).

'The Soul Kids Campaign' in 1977 was a response to growing concern about this issue: 'the picture that gave rise to the steering group's concern (was) a large number of black children coming into and remaining in care, usually growing up in a predominantly white, institutional environment' (Soul Kids Campaign 1977).

Two studies in the 1980s also reflected the high proportion of black children in the care of local authorities: 'The Lambeth study (Adams 1981) selected a random sample of children in care and found that 49 of the 90 children were black (54%). The Tower Hamlets study stated that over 50% of the children in their care were black (Wilkinson 1982)' (Barn 1990). In their 1989 study, Rowe *et al.* also state that:

Black children were over-represented in admissions to care of all six project authorities, although the extent to which this was happening varied considerably.

(Rowe *et al.* 1989, p. 14)

As many of these studies are small scale and localised, it is not appropriate to draw conclusions about the national picture from these findings. However, local authorities do need to consider the extent to which the ethnic profile of the numbers of black children in care from particular black minority ethnic groups reflect the demographic characteristics of their locality since evidence suggests that skin colour is a significant factor in admission rates into the care system.

Children of dual heritage (particularly where one parent is African-Caribbean and one is white European) are over-represented in the care population. There are also indications that they have different patterns of admission in comparison to white children. Thoburn *et al.* (1995) found that there was an over-representation of referrals to social services for children of dual heritage, relative to the national percentage of black children in this country who have a white parent. Barn (1998) found that a significant number of children of mixed parentage with white mothers referred themselves to social services. Batta *et al.* (1975) also found that children of mixed parentage came into care at an earlier age and tended to stay in care for longer periods. Rowe *et al.* (1989) found the same to be true in her study of six London authorities, and also found that children of mixed parentage were the most likely to have multiple admissions.

In contrast, however, a number of studies have indicated that there are a comparatively low number of Asian children in the care system. In Rowe *et al.*'s (1989) study Asian children made up 8% of the care population, whilst in Barn's (1993) study Asian children made up only 2% of the population of black children in care. However, in recent research undertaken by Barn *et al.* (1997), Asian children made up 14% of the care population. Relative to the local Asian child care population, this represented an over-representation of Asian children in the care system. This study also highlighted an over-representation of children of African-Caribbean origin, as well as an over-representation of children of dual heritage.

As well as the numbers of Asian children in care, recent research has also highlighted differences in the types of referrals made in respect of Asian families. Gibbons *et al.*'s study (1995) indicated a higher referral rate for Asian families in respect of physical injury to children and a lower rate of referrals for sexual abuse in comparison to white families. They explain these disparities in terms of cultural differences in child rearing and punishment between white families and Asian families, with the inference that Asian families are more physically punitive of their children because of cultural norms.

Apart from the inaccuracy of such generalisations, the assumption that referral rates are an accurate reflection of the level of abuse within a given community is a dangerous one, as it leads to myths about the prevalence of sexual abuse within the Asian community. If professionals assume that high rates of physical injury and low rates of sexual abuse are cultural norms in the Asian community, they are less likely to identify sexual abuse and more likely to make assumptions about discipline in the Asian community.

Although there is a dearth of British research on the link between ethnicity, culture and child abuse, studies from America have shown that rates of abuse are consistently similar across different ethnic groups, and that black children are at no greater risk of abuse or maltreatment than their white counterparts: 'across the board studies have consistently failed to find any black–white differences in rates of sexual abuse' (Finkelhor 1986, p. 69). The same is also true of physical and emotional abuse: 'Race stands out due to the similarities between blacks and white' (Jones & McCurdy 1992).

Not all child abuse is referred to statutory agencies, however, and whilst incidence of abuse may be similar across communities, the number of incidences referred to statutory agencies may vary from community to community. Race, culture and ethnicity do not only have an impact on the numbers of children known to social services but are also significant in terms of the circumstances under which admission into the care system takes place. Thus, for example, Barn (1993) found a link between race and rapidity of admission into care:

The Wenford research was able to ascertain that black children came into care much more quickly than white children. For example, in the first 4 weeks of referral, 28% of black children were admitted into care compared to 15% of white children.

(Barn 1990, p. 101)

She also found that 'black children were much more likely than white children to come from higher socio-economic groups. For example, 47% of the black children's mothers were in white collar and skilled manual occupations compared to 22% of white children' (p. 102).

Whilst economic and social factors are significant contributory factors in admission rates to care and black families are economically disadvantaged through racism, it is also apparent from this that an explanation of the statistics based purely on economic and social disadvantage is inadequate.

This is supported by Barn's (1993) examination of case files and interviews with social workers and natural parents, where 'it became apparent that preventative work was less likely to be done with black families' (p. 104). She also found that although the majority of black children entered care via the voluntary route, they were as likely as white children to be made subject to compulsory care and that they were much more likely to be made subject to parental rights resolutions than white children.

Whilst there are no published national statistics about child protection registration and ethnicity, NSPCC research indicates that ethnicity may be a significant determinant in registration of children as well as entry into care: 'it would appear that ethnic minorities are over-represented amongst the parents of the registered children' (Creighton 1992, p. 28).

Thus, although there is some information about black children and the child care system, there are still many gaps in our knowledge, particularly in relation to the national picture. Most local authorities do collect ethnic monitoring information, but very little of this is used to inform policy in relation to service provision to black children and their families. If changes are to occur, local authorities will need to be much more systematic and focused about what information they collect, and more particularly, how they act on this information.

Race, ethnicity and culture in child protection literature

Until the late 1970s, social work literature adopted a broadly 'colour blind' approach to explanations of psychosocial problems. Most theoreticians came from the assimilationist school, whereby race and culture were largely seen as irrelevant to the debate. Child protection was no exception to this rule.

In British society, the recognition of child abuse as a social problem is a surprisingly recent phenomenon. In 1961, child abuse was 'discovered' by Henry Kempe in America and, in 1963, two British orthopaedic surgeons, Griffiths and Moynihan, published an article in the *British Medical Journal* entitled 'The battered baby syndrome' (Parton 1985).

With the 'discovery' of abuse emerged theories about the causes and effects of such abuse (see preceding chapters in this section). Causal theories ranged from the concept of individual family pathology to the concept of society as the abuser, originating from psychological perspectives, on the one hand, to sociological analysis on the other.

One of the core principles of psychological theory to be applied to child protection is that individuals and families are a product of their past experiences. The work of Bowlby in the 1960s paved the way for this view, his concept of 'maternal deprivation' providing a theoretical link between early childhood experience and psychological development (Bowlby 1965).

If individual and family pathology was identified as the cause of abuse, then it followed that particular families were more likely than others to abuse their children. The task for social workers, therefore, was to identify which families were potentially abusive: 'The proportion of "high risk" cases out of all proved cases of persistent child abuse will be small, and the task of identifying may not be easy. But the attempt to isolate such cases from the majority of child abuse must always be made' (London Borough of Brent 1985). There were a variety of methods suggested to facilitate this, ranging from individual to family assessment, but all shared a common assumption – that there is a normative standard of family functioning against which pathology can be measured. From this the level of risk could be established.

'Good enough parenting' was the key phrase in this type of assessment. It was based on the work of Margaret Adcock and Christine Cooper (Adcock & White 1985), amongst others, in the mid-1980s. It essentially set out the standards of care necessary for a child to grow into a healthy adult. The task of the social work assessment was to establish how far the family were short of the required standards of parenting.

The notion that there are characteristics present in families which predispose them to abuse their children, and which can be detected and acted upon, led to the concept of 'dangerousness' in families. Checklists for dangerousness were produced based on retrospective studies of families where abuse had taken place – early family history, social and economic status, and family composition were all factors that were given weighting (Parton & Parton 1989).

Theories about family dynamics also offered explanations for abuse which were linked to the nature of family functioning. There are various schools of family therapy, but they all share the essential belief that the family is a system which is reliant on its component parts for it to work effectively. For family therapists, abusive families are ones in which parts of the family system are dysfunctional, which may be either the cause or the effect of the abuse. The task of the therapist is to restore normal or effective functioning to the family through realigning and strengthening parts of the family system whose weakness has contributed to the dysfunction.

Despite the differences between such theories, all theories of family pathology share certain characteristics. The first is that the family itself is the focus of attention, and that problems inherent in the family have a role to play in creating preconditions for the abuse. The second is that they identify characteristics that are present in the family as dysfunctional or dangerous, and that need to be changed if the child is to be protected. Identifying the deficiencies that exist requires that a benchmark of normative family functioning is applied to an assessment of family behaviour. This enables the level of dangerousness or the level of unhealthy functioning in a given family to be established. It is here that the drawbacks of these approaches can be identified in relation to working with black families. These models have all the inherent problems of an assimilationist or 'colour blind' approach to child protection. It is not simply that they ignore race, culture and ethnicity, but that they require that families are judged according to a white (and middle class) view of normality. In making such a judgement, black families will not just be seen as different, but as negatively different. Factors which are environmentally or socially determined will be pathologised and racist stereotypes perpetuated:

> Many texts simply ignore the existence of black families. Discussion is framed in terms of 'families' as if all families are white. There is an assumption that the concepts and methods set out are applicable to all families.
>
> (Gambe *et al.* 1992)

The sociological view of child abuse, on the other hand, does include an analysis of social and environmental factors. One of the first sociologists to research this link was Gil, whose study of physically abused children in the 1960s emphasised the social context of abuse: 'by looking at a broad sample of child abuse cases Gil widened the parameters of the subject and pointed to major structural changes in society as the means of tackling child abuse' (Corby 1987).

Essentially, the sociological view of child abuse is that it is a social problem, which requires a social and political solution. In terms of race, ethnicity and culture therefore, the sociological perspective does consider the impact of structural inequality on the lives of families. However, few sociologists have considered the impact of racism and cultural stereotyping in the context of child abuse. Discussions of race within sociological texts have normally confined themselves to discussions of race policy and ethnic relations, rather than child protection practice. Along with psychological theories, sociological theories have often ignored the relevance of race, culture and ethnicity to social work theory, and most theoreticians have taken an essentially assimilationist stance.

One further theoretical perspective that has been influential in child protection practice, and work with child sexual abuse in particular, is feminist theory. It does not fit into a broad psychological or sociological niche because it developed as a critique of theories of child abuse for failing to take into account the relevance of gender to the debate. Feminists saw child sexual abuse as simply an extreme of the continuum of sexual violence that is a consequence of a patriarchal society (McLeod & Saraga 1988). Their position was to challenge the 'orthodoxy' of male theorists and therapists, whom they regarded as blaming women and holding them responsible for abuse perpetrated by male abusers. Whilst the feminists recognised the oppressiveness of sexist ideology, however, they made only fleeting reference to race and culture (Knowles & Mercer 1992). Whilst sexism is a feature of black family life, as it is in white family life, a universal formula based on the experiences of white women only serves to subsume the impact of racism and deny the experiences of black women.

The central problem with many of the theoretical perspectives on child abuse is that they tend to ignore the social and environmental context in which black families live and represent external pressures that affect family functioning, such as racism, economic disadvantage, poor housing and unemployment as if they are inherent deficiencies in that family's ability to cope.

A more effective approach to the assessment of black families is one which recognises the inherent strengths that are present in black families who are struggling to deal with the effects of racism. Rather than using normative models of white, middle class family functioning to assess how far the family is falling short of this goal, the aim of professional intervention should be to help the family better to care for their children in the context of the social reality for that family. This approach focuses on strengths, as well as weaknesses, and allows the family to engage in a much more meaningful debate about protection that is based on a realistic plan for change.

Analysis of policy issues

The death of Maria Colwell in 1973 provided the impetus to develop local government structures and procedures for dealing with cases of child abuse, but it was not until 1988 that the Department of Health and Social Services (DHSS) published the first: *Working Together: A Guide to Arrangements for Inter-agency Co-operation for the Protection of Children.*

Also in 1988, *Protecting Children* was published by the DOH in response to a growing level of concern about child protection assessments. It followed a number of inquiry reports in the 1980s into the deaths of children and an inspection by the Social Services Inspectorate (DOH 1988), all of which had highlighted the need for a higher standard of child protection assessments.

Protecting Children was one of the first publications produced by the DOH which had not taken a 'colour blind' approach to child care work as it specifically referred to the need for 'cultural sensitivity' in child protection:

Although no culture sanctions extreme harm to a child, cultural patterns in child-rearing patterns exist. A balanced assessment must incorporate a cultural perspective, but guard against being over-sensitive to cultural issues at the expense of promoting the safety and well-being of the child.

(DOH 1988, p. 13)

The Children Act 1989 was the first piece of child care legislation which conveyed specific requirements upon local authorities in relation to religion, race, culture and language for children who are 'looked after'. Section 22 5(c) of the Act states that, 'In making any such decision (in respect for a child who is looked after) a local authority shall give due consideration ... to the child's religious persuasion, racial origin and cultural and linguistic background.'

In 1992, the *Memorandum of Good Practice on Video-recorded Interviews with Child Witnesses for Criminal Proceedings* was published. This took the same position in relation to the need to be 'culturally sensitive'.

The joint investigating team should consider whether there are any special factors arising from the child's cultural and religious background which are relevant to planning an effective interview. In some cases it will be necessary for the team to seek advice about particular customs or beliefs. Consideration of race, language and also gender may influence the choice of interviewer.

(Home Office 1992, p. 10)

Whilst this guidance acknowledged the relevance of cultural difference to social work practice in protecting children, the 'culturally sensitive' model contained many of the flaws present in its multi-cultural origins. Multi-culturalism suffers from an over-simplisitic and often tokenistic view of cultural difference. It also assumes that all cultures, whether black or white, are equally regarded. The historical legacy of slavery and colonialism in the UK has produced a society in which black cultures are not simply viewed as different, but as negatively different: 'For black children growing up in this country this means that their traditions, languages, lifestyles and social mores may be viewed negatively in comparison with English culture' (Phillips 1993).

Within every society there are sanctions operating to control the excesses of individuals, there are taboos operating to protect the integrity of the society, and there are mechanisms operating to protect the vulnerable. This does not prevent individuals from transgressing these unwritten codes of behaviour, nor does it ensure that all the vulnerable are protected. However, these situations arise in spite of the checks and balances, and not because of them:

While cultures differ in their definitions of child maltreatment, all have criteria for behaviours that fall outside the range of acceptability, and some individuals in all cultures exceed the boundaries of their society's standards.

(Korbin 1991, p. 69)

It is when these safety mechanisms break down, or do not come into operation, that institutional protection in the form of social services involvement is required. The decision about when and how intervention is required must involve a process of fine judgement, based on assessment of what protective factors exist in the situation relative to the risk factors that are present. Social work is not and cannot be an exact science, however. As it is socially constructed, so is the protective task of the social worker. Child protection assessments cannot be value-free.

Opinions and values derive from a personal belief system that is socially constructed and culturally defined. They reflect the dominant ideology for the community from which they originate. In this society, since racism is a part of that dominant ideology, racism itself is socially constructed and culturally defined. Thus, 'although child abuse occurs in all races and cultures workers must guard against viewing suspected abuse through the norms and values of their own background. Different cultural/racial groups organise their own traditions, religions, community of origin and history' (British Association of Social Workers 1989).

When black families are assessed, these cultural differences provide a backdrop to the views and values held by white professionals about black families and distort the assessment in the process. In practice, this means that widely held assumptions about black families can have a direct impact on assessment of risk that are made by child protection professionals. An examination of these stereotypes and their consequent effect on decision-making can help to unpack the dynamics of racism in professional practice.

Implications for practice

The stereotypes that exist in this society often present us with conflictual and confusing ideas about black family life. Thus, for example, the Asian family

is seen as strong but the very strength of Asian culture is seen to be a source of both actual and potential weakness. The hierarchical family structure is said to produce 'stress-ridden relationships'; Asian women are seen to be isolated because of their traditional customs and views of the world.

(Fernando 1988)

However, African – Caribbeans in Britain:

are seen as having suffered 'cultural stripping' during slavery leaving them with a 'weak' version of European culture ... Afro-Caribbean family life in contemporary Britain is seen as weak and unstable, with the lack of a sense of parental responsibility towards children (Pryce 1979), a failure by the family to apply adequate social control over its youth (Cashmore 1979) and a negative personal self-image.

(Fernando 1988)

This negative view of African-Caribbean culture is sometimes juxtaposed with an over-idealised view about the strength and resilience of African-Caribbean women, resulting in an unrealistic and unhelpful approach to working with African-Caribbean families. 'Culturally racist' views such as these can have a powerful impact on social work practice with black families. They can lead to over intervention in black families as a result of pathologising black family life, or they can also lead to a lack of intervention to protect a child, based on an idealised and over-optimistic view about a black family's potential to protect.

The case examples below illustrate the dangers of making assumptions about families which are rooted in cultural stereotypes rather than actualities.

Case example 1

Mr and Mrs P were of Asian origin. They had a daughter aged 8. Mrs P was seen by any professionals who had contact with her (such as the child's school and the housing department) as a 'traditional' woman who always wore saris and spoke little English. Mr P had a blue collar job and spoke good English. As a consequence, most contact which professionals had with the family prior to the referral to social services was with Mr P.

The younger child made an allegation to her teacher that Mr P had been sexually abusing her at night by touching inside her genital area. The teacher contacted social services, and a joint investigation involving the police and social services was undertaken. Mr P was interviewed by the police and denied the allegation.

Case example 1   *Cont'd*

The initial response from social services and the police to the referral was one of concern that cultural pressures on Mrs P, as an Asian woman dependent upon her husband, would prevent her being able to offer protection to her daughter. However, an interview with Mrs P revealed that she was a very strong woman who, although finding it hard to believe that her husband would do something like this, was prepared to work with professionals to keep her daughter safe. She agreed that her daughter would stay with a relative pending the conclusion of the joint investigation.

The outcome of the investigation was that there was evidence to suggest that Mr P had sexually abused his daughter, but not sufficient for criminal charges to be brought. Because of the level of cooperation from Mrs P, and because she had responded so differently to what had been expected of her as an Asian woman, it was decided at the child protection conference that the child could be returned home, even though Mr P was still in the household, as Mrs P had guaranteed the child's protection.

This case illustrates the power of gender-based cultural stereotyping. Because Mrs P had initially been seen as oppressed and subservient, her strength and decisiveness took the professionals by surprise, and led to a false optimism about her capacity to protect her daughter from a suspected sexual abuser.

Case example 2

In the Tyra Henry case (London Borough of Lambeth 1987), Tyra's grandmother, Beatrice Henry, was seen as capable of providing protection for her granddaughter, Tyra, in the face of concerns about the care she was receiving from her mother and step-father, without adequate back-up being provided from social services to assist her in this task. The *Report of the Public Inquiry into the Death of Tyra Henry* makes it clear that practice in this case was influenced by cultural stereotypes about black families:

There is a 'positive', but nevertheless, false stereotype in white British society of the Afro-Caribbean mother figure as endlessly resourceful … essentially unsinkable … it may have been an unarticulated and unconscious sense that a woman like Beatrice Henry would find a way to cope no matter what that underlay the neglect of … social services to make adequate provision for her taking responsibility for Tyra.

(London Borough of Lambeth 1987)

The essential irony of the culturally sensitive approach to child protection work with children and their families is that over-reliance on an inaccurate notion of culture can actually produce a discriminatory rather than a sensitive style of practice. Assessments that are informed by prescriptive and stereotypical views of families will reinforce, rather than challenge, racist practice with black children and their families:

the issue is not simply that some form of 'cultural knowledge' can be superimposed upon the working practices of social workers to equip them to deal adequately with black families. It is that those working practices themselves need to be reviewed as to their relevance to the assessment of black families.

(Dutt & Phillips 1990)

The way forward

There is still a great deal of confusion about the part that race and culture have to play in the diagnosis of and response to child abuse. Current difficulties in professional practice are often characterised by a 'fragmented' or 'hierarchical' approach to the needs of black children where professionals *either* focus on identity needs *or* care needs. Just as race, culture, language and religion are a part of the child's developmental needs, so identity has to be understood in terms of its connection with other aspects of the child's development and not in isolation from them. In current practice there is often a superficial understanding of the nature of racial and cultural identity and its impact on the child's whole development.

As identity is acquired throughout the lifetime of an individual by means of a lived experience (Dutt & Phillips 1999), it forms an integral part of an individual's personality which cannot be divorced from the other component parts of individuality. For example, each child's particular attachments are formed within the context of their racial, cultural, ethnic, religious, linguistic and cultural identity. A 'fragmented' approach, which seeks to isolate identity from other aspects of development such as attachment, emotional, social and behavioural development will give a distorted picture as to need.

The hypothetical case example 3, based on an amalgam of a number of actual cases, offers two alternative approaches to how a referral of alleged child abuse might be dealt with and provides an illustration of how two contrasting approaches to a situation could result in different outcomes. Both of these approaches are based on a 'fragmented' approach to black families.

Approach 1: 'Culturally-based explanation'

The social worker accepts Mr N's explanation that the abuse was culturally motivated, and that he was acting out of the best motives. The worker also attempts to understand his cultural perspective by asking him his views about child rearing and African culture. She comes to the view that Mr N's behaviour

---

Case example 3

Mr and Mrs N are of African origin and have two children, Steven aged 10 and Mary aged 16. Mrs N is in Africa for an extended holiday, visiting relatives. Mr N is caring for the two children.

Following an incident at school, where Mary N got into a fight with another girl over a boy, she was given detention after school. When she returned home her father was extremely angry with her. Mr N said that she had brought disgrace upon her family by her behaviour and pulled her over his knee. He hit her very hard with his hand on her buttocks, causing bruising.

The next day at school, Mary told her teacher about the incident. The school informed Social Services. When the social worker visited Mr N at home and asked him about the incident, Mr N said that it was a cultural issue as the expectations within his community were that girls behaved respectably, took their education seriously and did not 'mess about' with boys and get into trouble.

Mr N said that the trouble with English society was that girls were given too much freedom, and that this was why there were so many teenage pregnancies in this country. He said that he wanted better things for his daughter, but that this required discipline. He was attempting only to effectively discipline his child before the authorities started to intervene. He said that African parents were no longer in charge of their children because Social Services were trying to take their power away from them, and that this was racism. Mary N says that she does not want to give a statement to the police. A medical examination of Mary N shows that the bruising is consistent with the explanation given by both Mary N and Mr N of the incident.

was unacceptable if understandable in the circumstances. It is agreed with the police that a criminal prosecution for assault would only inflame a sensitive situation with this family in this community. Mr N agrees to cooperate with Social Services.

Approach 2: 'Culture is not relevant'

The social worker does not accept Mr N's explanation that the abuse was culturally motivated. The worker says that culture is not relevant in this situation, as what Mr N has done is abusive to his daughter and constitutes assault. The worker discusses the possibility of prosecuting Mr N with the police. The police agree to do so, but there are complaints from the African community of racism on the part of the police and social services.

An alternative approach: holistic assessments

Both of these cases illustrate the difficulty of polarities. Race and culture are relevant to the N case, in that the whole of the context of this African family's life will have developed within a specific cultural framework. From the food they eat to the customs and traditions that they follow, all will have been influenced in some way by their racial, cultural, religious and linguistic background.

Both black or white families are influenced by their racial and cultural context, but all families are unique in the way in which they interpret customs, traditions and social mores. No two families from the same cultural background will behave in the same way in response to grief, loss or trauma. Equally, individuals within the same family have their own personalities and patterns of behaviour.

Although Mr N has described his behaviour as 'cultural', it is obvious that not all African families would discipline a child in this way for getting detention. Many African parents abhor the physical punishment of children, just as many white parents do. Culture explains Mr N's values in terms of his social and educational aspirations for his daughter, but culture does not explain his actions. Many other parents would share the same aspirations for their children, but would not physically assault a child to achieve these.

A fundamental tenet of good child care practice with black families is that the assessment framework for assessing black children and their families is holistic and three-dimensional, providing for an understanding of how all of the factors in a child's life contribute to the child's specific circumstances. It is not only that an holistic framework for need helps provide for more accurate assessments, it is also that it is likely to produce better outcomes for children and their families. Up until December 1999 no national frameworks existed to help workers adopt such inclusive practice, but the *Framework for the Assessment of Children in Need and their Families* (DOH 1999) has provided a mechanism for considering race, ethnicity, culture, language and religion within an holistic model of identity.

Whilst the intentions of the guidance are to improve the inclusiveness of assessments, translating these intentions into action requires a good standard of professional practice. Both black and white workers need to feel confident of their attitudes, values and skills in working with black families. Although the issues are different for black workers working with black families from those for white workers, there is evidence that the ethnicity of the worker is a factor which affects outcomes for black families.

Ethnicity of workers

There has often been the assumption in social work practice that providing black workers will ensure that black families will receive a more relevant service. In some cases this originates from the belief that the experience of racism will help black workers to more effectively understand and relate to black families than will white workers, in other cases it develops from a desire on the part of white organisations to shift the responsibility for race issues onto the shoulders of black workers.

Some research has suggested that 'matching' the ethnicity of workers to families can result in positive outcomes for families. In their study of family involvement in the child protection process, Thoburn *et al.* (1995) identified that there was a greater level of involvement with black families if the social worker was black (78% as compared to 41% if the main social worker was white).

However, there is also research to suggest that there are difficulties posed by matching, both for families and for workers. Brandon *et al.* (1999) make reference to concerns being expressed by black families in one area about being 'spied' upon by members of their own community, and Farmer & Owen (1995) identify that black workers are sometimes rejected by families. Butt (1994) and Jones & Butt (1995) highlight the difficulties for black workers, particularly over joint working with white workers. Their concerns centre on the fact that black workers are often expected to provide advice on culture and racism and not challenge professional practice.

The effective deployment of black workers to work with black families can produce real benefits for children and their families when decisions to match the ethnicity of worker and family are made on the basis of matching skills and expertise provided by particular black workers to particular black families, and facilitating black workers in using these skills and expertise creatively. However, the responsibility for service provision to black families must not rest with black workers. White workers need to develop both the skills and confidence in assessing black families. There is evidence that some white workers have avoided intervention in black families out of fear of being accused of racism, as well as evidence that some have been too hasty in their intervention by failing to recognise and build on the strengths of black families.

The antidote to such polarised practice is to undertake a balanced assessment of the child's needs in which race, ethnicity, culture, language and religion are considered throughout the process of intervention. The chapter by Phillips & Dutt on 'Assessing the Needs of Black Children and their Families' in the *Framework for the Assessment of Children in Need and their Families* (DOH 1999) can provide some practice guidance for white workers in undertaking balanced assessments with black families, but in addition there are some key questions that white workers can use to evaluate their own practice.

- What are the needs of this black child and to what extent are they similar to or different from those of a white child in a similar situation?
- Have any stereotypical assumptions been made about the parenting capacity of the child's parents or carers because of the race, culture or ethnicity of this family?
- Are there any concerns in relation to safeguarding the welfare of the child, and to what extent are these connected with the race, culture or ethnicity of the child, if at all? (Consider how judgements have been made, and question stereotypical assumptions about 'cultural practices'.)

■ Are there any specific factors in relation to the family's financial, social or environmental situation which have arisen as a result of the family's race, culture, language or religion? (Consider factors such as racial harassment, access to employment, social and family structures and support.)

■ What specific intervention or support would this family benefit from, and to what extent might this differ from or be similar to a white child in a similar situation? (Consider the relevance and accessibility of mainstream services and availability of specialist resources for black families in the area.)

The challenge to professional practice is how to appropriately take account of race and culture in assessments, but not allow myths and stereotypes to distort the reality of a situation. Agencies need to take their responsibilities to black children and families much more seriously by setting up mechanisms to evaluate their practice and making targeted interventions to achieve change.

If the changes in agency practice do not result in real benefits for Black people, then there have been no real changes.

(Black and In Care Group 1992, p. 6)

Annotated further reading

Ahmad B 1989 Protecting black children from abuse. Social Work Today, 8 June
Provides a pertinent comment on the outcome of professional intervention with black families.
Ahmad B 1990 Black perspectives in social work. Venture Press, London
Outlines a positive black critique in relation to social services practice, including child care and child protection, with case study illustrations.
Ahmed S, Small J 1986 Social work with black children and their families. Batsford, London
Contains an invaluable critique of cultural racism within social work practice.
Barn R 1990 Black children in local authority care: admission patterns. New Community, January
Barn R 1993 Black children in the public care system. Batsford, in association with British Agencies for Adoption and Fostering, London
Outlines detailed research undertaken in a London authority on black children within the care system, and draws important conclusions in relation to the care paths of black children.
Black and In Care Group 1992 Saying it as it is. Report of the Black and In Care Group to the National Society for the Prevention of Cruelty to Children. NSPCC, London
Presents the view of black children and young people, who themselves have been a part of the care system.
Bridge Child Care Consultancy Services. Sukina – an evaluation report of the circumstances leading to her death
Includes an analysis and recommendations as to the impact of race and culture on the decisions made in relation to Sukina.
Butt J, Box L 1998 Family centred: a study of the use of family centres by black families. REU
A research study which identifies the extent to which family support is provided to black families, and identifies ways in which it could be provided more effectively.
Channer Y, Parton N 1990 Racism, cultural relativism and child protection. In: Taking child abuse seriously. The Violence against Children Study Group. Unwin Hyman, London
Gives a useful perspective on racism within the child protection services, and the impact of cultural relativism on child protection assessments.
Dutt R, Phillips M 1990 Towards a black perspective in child protection. Race Equality Unit. Personal Social Services
Looks at the impact of personal views and values on assessments in child protection with black families, and offers some checklists for improving practice with black families.
Dutt R, Phillips M 1996 Race, culture and the prevention of child abuse: report of the National Commission of Inquiry into the Prevention of Child Abuse, Vol. 2. Background Papers. The Stationery Office, London
Identifies the issues in relation to child protection and black families and presents a model for strategic intervention to address these issues.
Dutt R, Phillips M 1999 Working with black and minority ethnic children and families. In: The needs led framework for assessing children and their families practice guide. The Stationery Office, London

Provides guidance to professionals as to how to implement the Department of Health Needs Led Framework with black children and families.

Fernando S 1988 Race and culture in psychiatry. Routledge, London

Although this book focuses on the mental health services, it provides a very useful analysis of the way in which racist stereotypes influence social work assessments with families.

Jones A, Butt J 1995 Taking the initiative: a report of a national study assessing service provision to black children and families. NSPCC, London

This study looks at the extent to which services are meeting the needs of black children and their families. It includes the views of black children and young people, and provides a black perspective in child protection.

Race Relations Act 1976. HMSO, London

This needs to be read, as it outlines our responsibilities in promoting equalities in the personal social services.

Rattansi A 1992 'Race', culture and difference. In: Donald & Rattansi A (eds) Open University Press, Milton Keynes

Contains some very thought-provoking essays that challenge the orthodoxy of current approaches to race relations.

Rouf K 1989 Black girls speak out. The Childrens Society, London

A powerful book of poems and writings by black young women who have experienced sexual abuse.

Sissay L 1988 Tender fingers in a clenched fist. Bogle-Ouverture,

Sissay provides us with a challenging insider view of the experiences of a black young person growing up in care.

Skellington R, Morris P 1992 'Race' in Britain today. The Open University and Sage, Newbury Park

A useful source of annotated statistical information about race and racism in Britain, including information on health, housing, education and social services.

The London Borough of Lambeth 1987 Whose child? A report of the public inquiry into the death of Tyra Henry. London Borough of Lambeth, London

One of the few inquiry reports on a black child that includes an analysis of the impact of race on the case.

References

Adams N 1981 Lambeth directorate of social services. London Borough of Lambeth, London

Adcock M, White R 1985 Good enough parenting: a framework for assessment. British Agencies for Adoption and Fostering, London

Ahmad B 1990 Black perspectives in social work. Venture Press, London

Batta, McCulloch Smith 1979 Colour as a variable in Childrens' Sections of Local Authority Social Services Departments. New Community 7: 78–84

Barn R 1990 Black children in local authority care: admission patterns. New Community January

Barn R 1993 Black children in the public care system. Batsford in association with British Agencies for Adoption and Fostering, London

Barn R, Sinclair R, Ferdinand D 1997 Acting on principle. British Agencies for Adoption and Fostering, London

Black and In Care Group 1992 Saying It as it is: report of the Black and In Care Group to the National Society for the Prevention of Cruelty to Children. NSPCC, London

Bowlby J 1965 Child care and the growth of love, 2nd edn. Penguin, Harmondsworth

Brandon M, Thorburn J, Lewis A, Way A 1999 Safeguarding children with the Children Act 1989. The Stationery Office, London

British Association of Social Workers 1989 A guide to policy and practice in the management of child abuse. British Association of Social Workers

Channer Y, Parton N 1990 Racism, cultural relativism and child protection. In: The Violence against Children Study Group (eds) Taking child abuse seriously. Unwin Hyman, London

Corby B 1987 Working with child abuse. Open University Press, Milton Keynes

Creighton S J 1992 Child abuse trends in England and Wales 1988–1990. NSPCC, London

Department of Health (DOH) 1988 Protecting children: a guide for social workers undertaking a comprehensive assessment. HMSO, London

Department of Health (DOH) 1999 Framework for the assessment of children in need and their families. The Stationery Office, London

Department of Health and Social Security (DHSS) 1976 Local Authority Social Services Letter (76), (2)

Department of Health and Social Security (DHSS) 1980 Child abuse: Central Register Systems. Local Authority Social Services Letter (80)

Department of Health and Social Security (DHSS) 1982 Child abuse: a study of inquiry reports 1973–1981. HMSO, London

Dutt R, Phillips M 1990 Towards a black perspective in child protection. Race Equality Unit, Personal Social Services,

Dutt R, Phillips M 1999 Working with black and minority ethnic children and families. In: The needs led framework for assessing children and their families practice guide. The Stationery Office, London

Farmer E0, Owen M 1995 Child protection practice: private risks and public remedies. HMSO, London

Fernando S 1988 Race and culture in psychiatry. Routledge, London

Finkelhor D 1986 A sourcebook on child sexual abuse. Sage, London

Gambe D, Gomes J, Kapor V, *et al.* 1992 Improving practice with children and families: a training manual. CCETSW, Northern Curriculum Development Project, Leeds

Gibbons J, Conroy S, Bell C 1995 Operating the child protection system. HMSO, London

Home Office in conjunction with Department of Health 1992 Memorandum of good practice on video-recorded interviews with child witnesses for criminal proceedings. HMSO, London

Home Office, Department of Health, Department of Education and Science, Welsh Office 1991 Working together under the Children Act 1989: a guide to arrangements for inter-agency cooperation for the protection of children from abuse. HMSO, London

Husband C 1978 Racism in social work. Community Care 241: 39–40

Husband C 1989 Racism, prejudice and social policy. In: Williams F (ed) Social policy: a critical introduction. Polity Press, Cambridge

Jones A, Butt J 1995 Taking the initiative: a report of national study assessing service provision to black children and families. NSPCC, London

Jones C 1977 Immigration and social policy in Britain. Tavistock, London

Jones E, McCurdy K 1992 The links between types of maltreatment and demographic characteristics of children. Child Abuse and Neglect 16: 201–215

Kempe C H, Silverman F N, Steele B F, *et al.* 1962 The battered child syndrome. Journal of the American Medical Association 181: 17–24

Knowles C, Mercer S 1992 Feminism and anti-racism: an exploration of the political possibilities. In: Donald J, Rattansi A (eds) 'Race', culture and difference. Open University Press, Milton Keynes

Korbin J 1991 Cross-cultural perspectives and research: directions for the 21st century. Child Abuse and Neglect 15 (Supp 1): 61–77

Lee C C 1978 Child abuse: a reader and sourcebook. Open University Press, Milton Keynes

London Borough of Brent 1985 A child in trust: the report of the panel of inquiry into the circumstances surrounding the death of Jasmine Beckford. London Borough of Brent, London

London Borough of Lambeth 1987 Whose child? A report of the public inquiry into the death of Tyra Henry. London Borough of Lambeth, London

McLeod M, Saraga E 1988 Towards a feminist theory and practice. Feminist Review Spring

Parton N 1985 The politics of child abuse. Macmillan, Basingstoke

Parton C, Parton N 1989 Child protection: the law and dangerousness. In: Stevenson O (ed) Child abuse: professional practice and public policy. Harvester Wheatsheaf, Hemel Hempstead

Phillips M 1992 The abuse of power. Social Work Today 23 (25): 16–17

Phillips M 1993 Investigative interviewing: issues of race and culture. Investigative Interviewing Training Pack Resources Booklet. Open University Press, Milton Keynes

Popple 1986 Black childrens' rights. In: Franklin B (ed) The rights of children. Blackwell, Oxford

Powell D 1978 The out of step services. Community Care 191: 41–42

Rattansi A 1992 Racism, culture and education. In: Donald J, Rattansi A (eds) 'Race', culture and difference. Open University Press, Milton Keynes

Reynolds 1978 Leicester: between two cultures. Community Care 241: 27–29

Roskill C 1979 A different social work. Social Work Today 10 (25): 17–20

Rowe J, Hundleby M, Garnett L 1989 Child care now. BAAF Research Series 6

Scarman Report 1981 The Brixton disorders 10–12 April 1981: report of an inquiry by the Rt. Hon. Lord Scarman OBE. HMSO, London

Sissay L 1988 Tender fingers in a clenched fist. Bogle-Ouverture

Solomos J 1989 Race and racism in contemporary Britain. Macmillan, Basingstoke

Soul Kids Campaign 1977 Report of the steering group of the Soul Kids Campaign. Association of British Fostering and Adoption Agencies, London

Thoburn J, Lewis A, Shemmings D 1995 Paternalism or partnership: family involvement in the child protection process. HMSO, London

Wilkinson A 1982 Children who come into care in Tower Hamlets. London Borough of Tower Hamlets, London

8   Disability and child abuse

Margaret Kennedy

INTRODUC-TION

As a starting point for this chapter it is important to put the lives of disabled children into context. Theresia Degener, of Germany (disabled herself, and a disability activist and lawyer), says, 'any child born with a disability growing up today has to survive and overcome discrimination and stigmatisation' (Degener 1992). She describes a political process of the oppression of disabled children and adults. When disability is equated with illness or with something or someone being wrong (therefore not right) (medical model), no concept of oppression or discrimination is or will be entertained. When the condition or impairment becomes the person, and the person becomes the condition, then there is widespread devaluation. The disability movement uses the word 'disabled' not to describe a physical or learning impairment but to *dis*-abling and *de*-valuing by society (social model).

Being different in a way that is negatively valued can trigger a powerful process of rejection, segregation and stigmatisation of which abuse is just one outcome (Wolfensberger 1987). Garbarino (1987) talks of a 'licence' to abuse disabled children in a society in which they are repeatedly stigmatised. Sullivan *et al.* (1987) contend that 'depersonalisation' is also a contributing factor. 'When disabled children or adults are assumed to be less human because of their disability, then abuse is not that inhumane' (Sullivan *et al.* 1987). For children who have been abused, a similar process emerges. We have pathologised disability, and children thus become objects of the medical profession to be put right, to be made more 'normal'.

Sobsey (1994) offers a way to counteract this pathologising of disabled children and sets the context of abuse of them within an ecological framework. Figure 8.1 shows Sobsey's use of the ecological model which he terms 'The integrated Ecological Model'.

The integrated ecological model of abuse provides the structural framwork for understanding abuse of disabled people. It moves away from the dependency-stress model, which has become the most dominant view. This model states that due to the stress on caregivers of a child with impairment, abuse results. Sobsey calls this a 'victim-blaming' model. Indeed it is comparable to saying a woman gives stress to her spouse and that is why he beats her – a view we do not tolerate in the domestic violence field but do in the disability and abuse field!

Table 8.1 lists some of the factors associated with the Integrated Ecological Model.

We also pathologise the child who is abused. Instead of acknowledging and recognising the discrimination (by virtue of being a child) and the oppression they experience, we now label them sick, disturbed, ill. Professionals 'treat' them and, indeed, in the child protection field phrases such as 'symptoms' and 'treatment' are taken directly from the medical model. When we view the child only in terms of their presenting 'symptoms' and outside the political context of oppression, we again devalue the child's experiences. Pathologising is a weakening process, not an empowering one.

Figure 8.1
The integrated ecological model of abuse. Physical and psychological aspects of the interacting individuals are considered within the context of environmental and cultural factors

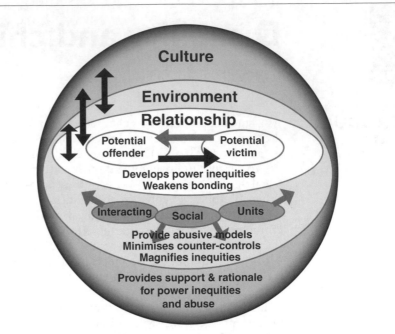

Table 8.1
Individual, environmental, and cultural aspects of the integrated ecological model of abuse

Potential victim	Potential offender	Environment	Culture
Impaired physical defenses	Need for control	Emphasises control	Devalues victims
Impaired communicative functioning	Authoritarian	Attracts abusers	Objectifies victims
Lacks critical information	Low self-esteem	Isolated from society	Teaches compliance
Learned helplessness	Displaced aggression	Provides awarded models of aggression	Emphasises vulnerabilities
Learned compliance	Exposed to abusive models	Covers up allegations	Disinhibits aggression
Undeveloped sense of personal space	Little attachment to victim	Many caregivers	Denies problems
Dependency	Devaluing attitudes	Transient caregivers	Discourages attachment
	Impulsive behaviour	Dehumanises potential victims	Discourages solutions
		Eliminates non-abusers	
		Clusters risks	
		Discourages attachment	

Because disabled children are negatively valued, we neglect to consider their child protection requirements. When I asked a senior policy-maker what she was including in her child protection policies for disabled children (she was writing a new draft), she pondered and then said, 'let me sort out the *normal* child *first*' (Kennedy & Kelly 1992). In another instance, a counsellor said to a mother whose disabled child had been abused, 'well it would have been worse if it had been one of your other (non-disabled) children.' A QC said of a disabled child who had been abused and was applying for criminal injuries compensation, that as the child would obviously (!) not be engaging in sexual relationships in adulthood the harm of the sexual abuse was likely to be less, and refused criminal injuries compensation. Such examples of professionals seeing disabled children as 'worthless' are unfortunately not uncommon.

Cumulative effects of negative perception and myths concerning abuse and disabled children

Other factors also contribute. Marchant (1991) explores the frequent myths surrounding abuse and the disabled child (see Table 8.2).

Because of the myths that surround these issues, professionals working with disabled children and adults have been reluctant to believe that disabled children are abused at all. Myths about abuse are not particularly unique, but there are unique ones relating to disability and abuse. Empirical evidence clearly shows that every one of these myths is false. All of them are dangerous. They must be challenged.

Some people really do believe abuse of a disabled child doesn't matter. A man with cerebral palsy illustrated Myth no. 2 (Table 8.2) for me very eloquently when he gave as his reason for being abused, 'why bugger up a normal child, when I am defective already?'

It was a personal testimony of a most profound kind, and I meet shades of this reasoning very often. It contributes towards the very dangerous and potent 'backdrop' to the abuse disabled children experience which allows us to ignore child protection issues:

- Discrimination, segregation and oppression
- Devaluation and depersonalisation
- Myths about disability and abuse.

Alternatively, disabled children are perceived as rather sad, unfortunate children who *do* require 'over-protection' and 'missionary-like' care and consideration. Patronising attitudes are very unhelpful and in fact lead to disempowerment. In relation to child abuse this disempowerment is positively dangerous. Such attitudes are enshrined in the Children Act 1989, which places children who are disabled under the category of 'children in need'. This seems to fit in with the popular image of disabled children as recipients of charity (e.g. television appeals). This is an unfortunate development at a time when the disability movement is strenuously discussing the theme of rights, not charity (Kennedy & Cross 1993).

Far from disability protecting disability rather protects the abusers (Kennedy 1990). Senn (1988) says, 'in the situation of sexual abuse it does not seem to be the actual disability which creates the vulnerability, but rather the training received and the type of education (or lack thereof) and the environment in which children who are disabled find themselves, that put them at higher risk of sexual abuse.' In other words, society has created a situation in which children who are disabled have been taught to be good 'victims'.

Table 8.2 *Myths concerning abuse and children with disabilities*		
Myth 1	Disabled children are not vulnerable to sexual abuse – they simply would not be targeted
Myth 2	Sexual abuse of disabled children is OK, or at least not so harmful as abuse of other children
Myth 3	It is impossible to prevent abuse of disabled children
Myth 4	Disabled children are even more likely to make false allegations of abuse
Myth 5	If a disabled child has been abused, it is best to leave well alone once the child is safe

The missing research

Very few British/UK studies have been undertaken to determine the prevalence or incidence of abuse of physically disabled children. Most attention (at least in the published literature) appears to have focused on sexual abuse and on victims who have learning disabilities (Westcott 1993). There are no data on disability contained in the long-awaited Department of Health (DOH) national figures of children on at risk registers (1990), and indeed this information is not a requirement of the at risk registration process. It would nonetheless be invaluable, for we need this information in order to assess:

1. whether abuse may be implicated in the creation of impairment
2. whether children with impairments may be differentially targeted for abuse (Kelly 1992).

What we know largely comes from America and Canada. Tables 8.3 and 8.4 outline some of the studies summarised by Westcott & Cross (1995) covering physical and sexual abuse of disabled children.

In the main it is not the researchers who have highlighted and informed practice but the activists, advocates and disabled people themselves. When research is undertaken it is worrying to find that the few studies we can look at are not based

Table 8.3
Physical abuse of disabled children

Study	Children	Source of information	Findings
Frisch & Rhoads 1982 (US)	430 children and young people referred for an evaluation of learning problems during the year 1977–1978	Assessment records	29 (6.7%) children reported for child abuse and neglect (3.5 times that reported for all children)
Cohen & Warren 1987 (US)	1. 2771 children under 5 years in pre-school programmes of 42 United Cerebral Palsy (UCP) affiliates. Children having different physical impairments	1. Questionnaire survey of UCP staff	1. 94 (3.4% children reported as known physically abused with 209 (7.5%) suspected physically abused/neglected. Of 94 children known abused/neglected, 57 (61%) had been physically abused
	2. 435 children under 5 years in respite care programmes of 14 UCP affiliates. Children having different physical and/or learning impairments	2. Questionnaire survey of UCP staff	2. 4 (0.9%) reported as known physically abused
Ammerman *et al.* 1989 (US)	148 children aged 3–19 years, psychiatrically referred and having multiple impairments of varying severity	Medical, psychiatric, nursing and social work records	1. 39% of children showed evidence of past or current abuse (19% definite, 20% probable/possible) 2. Of these 39%, 69% were physically abused 3. Increased risk

Table 8.4
Sexual abuse of disabled children

Study	Children	Source of information	Findings
Ammerman et al. 1989 (US)	148 children aged 3–19 years, psychiatrically referred and having multiple impairments of varying severity	Medical, psychiatric, nursing and social work records	1. 39% of children showed evidence of past or current abuse (19% definite, 20% probable/ possible) 2. Of these 39%, 36% were sexually abused 3. Increased risk
Kennedy 1992 (UK)	Deaf children known to professionals	Survey of 156 teachers and social workers for the deaf	1. Over 50% 1989 returns reported abuse 2. 70 children were suspected victims of sexual abuse, and 50 children were confirmed sexually abused
Sinason (undated) (UK)	40 children with learning impairments and emotional problems referred to Tavistock clinic 1991–92	Psychotherapist seeing children	1. 30 (50%) returns reported abused 2. Of 30, 21 (70%) were girls and 9 (30%) were boys
Sullivan et al. 1987 (US)	1. All members of 9th grade at residential school for deaf children	1. Questionnaire survey	1. 50% children reported sexual abuse
	2. 150 pupils at residential school for deaf children	2. Individual interviews	2. 50% children reported sexual abuse
	3. 322 students at further education college for hearing-impaired students	3. Questionnaire survey	3. 13 students (4%) reported sexual abuse and 24 students (7%) reported both sexual and physical abuse
	4. 100 deaf children attending either residential or mainstream schools	4. Individual interviews	4. Of 64 children attending residential schools, 40 (63%) were sexually abused at school, 10 (16%) were sexually abused at home, and 15 (23%) were sexually abused at both school and home. Of 35 children in mainstream schools, 21 (60%) were sexually abused at home, 9 (26%) were sexually abused at school, and 5 (14%) were sexually abused at both home and school

on direct contact with children/young people/adults who are disabled. This is because research methods fail to accommodate the requirements of these children and young people, by using, for example, questionnaires in Braille, or researchers who can use Sign Language or other augmentative communication systems. The research and what we think we know is based primarily on clinicians', practitioners' and parents' perceptions – the vast majority of whom are not disabled. Nor is there much awareness of the additional factors of oppression due to race, class, gender or sexuality (Kelly 1992).

What is abuse?

Definitions describing physical, sexual and emotional abuse and neglect are 'standard' until we look at the life of disabled children. In a study undertaken by a British Association for the Study and Prevention of Child Abuse and Neglect (BASPCAN) Working Party, professionals were asked what abuse they had experienced or come across. This revealed a catalogue of 'abuses' that would rarely be considered under statutory provisions, including:

- Force feeding – children with cerebral palsy
- Over-medication – the learning-disabled or hyperactive child
- Medical photography – children with physical impairments
- Deprivation of visitors – anorexic children
- Opening mail – children in residential care
- Lack of privacy, and personal clothes, toys being used communally – children in residential care
- Financial abuses – depriving children of rightful access to own money
- Segregation to special schools (many disabled adults felt this to be abusive)
- Open days where adults would come in and view the children at school
- Behaviour modification programmes
- Physical 'therapy' (some felt that aspects of the Peto and Doman methods of physiotherapy were abusive).

It was disturbing to discover that many disabled children had basic human rights infringed for example, access to their *own* clothes and toys, their *own* mail, their *own* money, and yet we are still powerless to prevent such abuses given the present legislation under which we might take action (BASPCAN Working Party on Disability and Abuse).

It is therefore important to realise again that even *before* we entertain the forms of abuse (as described by DOH definitions), children who are disabled have experienced both discrimination *and* the other subtle 'abuses' and infringements of human rights described above. These other forms of 'abuses' or infringements of human rights need to be borne in mind when designing safety and prevention programmes for disabled children. If disabled children are already in an atmosphere/environment which condones even these more subtle abuses, then disabled children may not be able to disclose more extreme forms of physical or sexual abuse.

In child protection, we need to be more proactive, so before I discuss disclosure I will look closely at safety and prevention programmes.

Communication

Large numbers of disabled children use alternative forms of communication and a large range of methods to communicate. Children do feel frustrated when adults cannot communicate with them, and, as I shall discuss in relation to investigative interviews, interpreters or facilitators are required to enable children who wish to disclose abuse to communicate this. The principal systems used are listed below.

Signs

- Makaton (learning-disabled children)
- See and Say

- Paget Gorman (language-disordered children)
- British Sign Language (BSL) (deaf children)
- Sign Supported English (SSE) (deaf children).

Symbols

Augmentative communication systems using communication boards:

- Blissymbolics (children with cerebral palsy)
- Makaton (children with cerebral palsy and/or learning disabled children)
- Sigsymbols
- Rebus
- Icons, written words, etc.

Technology-aided

- Light writers
- Liberator/Touch Talkers
- Possum, etc.

Many child protection workers who cannot sign may provide a pen and paper, thinking that the deaf child may write down what it is they need to say. Here is what a young girl wrote to me during an initial assessment for counselling. Her signing had been extremely difficult to 'read'. (She had an idiosyncratic signing system and my signing system was Sign Supported English (SSE); hers was a form of British Sign Language (BSL). They are very different.)

My aunt thought me 2 days ill not school but so she still angry with me much go school I'm not want to school.

This is, in fact, how some profoundly deaf people write English, since it is a second language for signing deaf children and adults. Asking them to write things down may not necessarily clarify the situation! What it demonstrated to me was that I was not the right person to help in this situation. I was able to refer her to a counsellor with BSL signing skills. The communication assessment was vital before undertaking any child protection work, and this will be true of all disabled children who use alternative means of communication. Interpreters may need to be employed who are qualified and skilled in particular language systems.

Safety and prevention programmes

Safety and prevention programmes are the main platforms of empowerment for all children.

These were developed following the many concerns connected with the sexual abuse of children. They are helpful provided we aim to 'give children enough information to be able to respond to a sexual abuse situation before it becomes serious, *not to make them responsible for protecting themselves*' (Mayes *et al.* 1986).

What of the disabled child? Senn (1988) suggests that such children lack the effective education necessary to empower them, since many teachers are reluctant to implement any programme even vaguely connected to sexual assault or incest in schools.

In addition, since choosing and decision-making is a fundamental element of any safety programme, and since for many disabled children this has never been an aspect of their lives, the implementation of such programmes may sometimes prove problematic.

Principles of various programmes

Many safety and prevention programmes use similar principles to try to help children tackle difficult situations.

Children are often taught to say 'no' to things they do not like, particularly touch, and then to get away and find someone they can trust to tell. For non-disabled children, such advice has sometimes been used to good effect, but in the case of disabled children these principles do not take into account their specific impairments. Many may use different forms of communication of a non-verbal kind (see above). To say 'no' therefore may be very difficult, and to tell someone even more so.

This is compounded by the fact that many forms of augmentative communication systems, particularly symbol systems (where children use fingers or eyes to point to boards to indicate what they wish to convey), censor all use of words/symbols to describe genitals or sexual acts. What is required for even very young children using communication boards is that they include, as a matter of course, symbols which show anatomical body parts and genitals, so that if required they may discuss their worries and concerns. Some residential institutions (for example, Chailey Heritage, Sussex) are already changing policies concerning access to sexual symbols from an early age (Fig. 8.2). Producing them at a later stage, for example, when required for investigative purposes, can be construed by defence barristers as 'leading' in the investigative interview.

Children who use symbols boards and access these by either finger-pointing or eye-pointing may furthermore only be understood by one or two key people. The potential danger for children who use alternative means of communication and who have a limited number of people whom they can tell needs to be borne in mind, since these same people may be the abusers.

Children may not be able to find someone who can understand what they are saying, since even some teachers cannot understand the children they teach. This can be true of some deaf children who have a greater fluency in signing than their teachers. Deaf children who do not sign but who are being taught by the oral/aural method can be particularly difficult to understand, as they may have poor speech and intonation skills and limited grasp of language and words.

Children are often taught in safety programmes to try and get away from the harmful situation. Here we need to ask – how? For blind children, going might mean running into a road, wall or door, particularly if they have just been hurt or terrified by abuse, or taken to a strange place. Children with cerebral palsy may be able to leave, but at a slower pace using crutches or walking sticks. Children using wheelchairs may find it difficult to leave if the room in which they are being threatened opens onto, say, two steps down, or if the door opens inwards. They may have muscular dystrophy and may not have the strength to propel their own wheelchair.

Children with learning disabilities often find these principles of safety and prevention programmes difficult to grasp. They may understand them within the

Figure 8.2
Chailey Heritage PHSE symbols

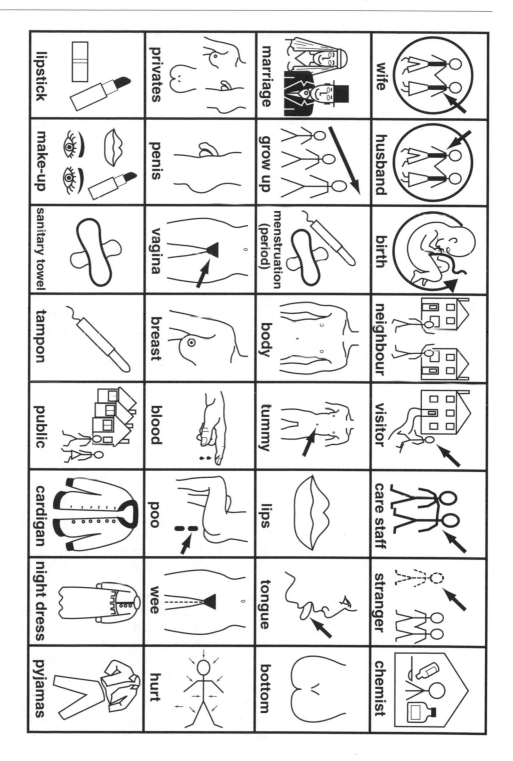

classroom setting, but outside may not be able to apply them. We need to be more aware of the fears and ambiguities these children may be prone to and to be more careful about explaining concepts and debriefing sufficiently. Excellent materials for these children have been produced by the Ann Craft Trust, Nottingham

University, and by the Shepard School, Nottingham, which take into consideration the cognitive abilities of learning-disabled young people.

Role plays can be helpful, but often children who are disabled find it scary if a teacher they know and trust becomes a 'baddie' in a role play. The idea of acting and pretending can be a concept beyond their grasp and may prove more frightening than helpful. Children who role play 'baddies' also need to know they are not in fact bad, but only acting. Equally, the audience will need to know this child actor is not bad either, only acting. Whilst aspects of such programmes may be 'easy' to explain to the non-disabled child, the experience, knowledge and understanding of disabled children may require a completely different approach.

Children are helped to understand touch they like and touch they do not like, and how to handle, especially, the unwanted, scary, hurtful touch. For many children with severe physical impairments, touch is a constant feature in their lives. Their body space has been invaded so many times for care and hygienic purposes that it seems in fact that their own body does not belong to them. A woman who had polio describes how constant invasion had confused her by the time a hospital porter abused her:

The medical *experiences* I had made me very vulnerable to being abused; it just seemed the same as everything else that had been done to me, so I wasn't able to discriminate. There's no way you can say no to what a doctor does to you, they just damn well do it when you're a kid and you don't have any choice about it. I didn't say no to any doctor, the porter actually was to me doing absolutely nothing different at all that every doctor or nurse had ever done.

(Westcott 1993)

Marchant, however, found that children she cared for could discriminate between the sort of touch which was for personal hygienic necessity and the abusive touch. The child protection team at Chailey Heritage (a residential school for multiply disabled children where Ruth Marchant works) has designed both a children's rights charter, to help children understand their rights, and an intimate care policy so that staff can be more aware and careful about the intimate care they give to disabled children. The disabled children in Chailey are helped to overcome this confusion of touch by clear education concerning the different sorts of touch which are necessary, and what to do if there is touch which falls outside the remit of intimate care for hygienic/medical purposes.

Prevention and safety programmes can only work if the child receives sufficient information which will enable him or her to understand that their abusive experience need not be tolerated and that they have permission to tell.

Provided we are aware that some of the safety and prevention programmes and the principles taught to non-disabled children have their limitations and difficulties for disabled children, these programmes can still be utilised when adapted by skilled teachers or parents who understand the disabled children's particular requirements. To supplement programmes designed for non-disabled children, new material is being produced for the disabled child which is more relevant and appropriate. These include:

- *You Choose* by the National Deaf Children's Society, which utilises English, Sign Supported English and Signed English (Fig. 8.3).
- A set of books by the Shepard School, Nottingham which utilises Makaton and English for learning-disabled young people (Fig. 8.4).
- A set of books for learning-disabled young people called *Jenny speaks out* and *Bob tells all* (Sinason & Hollins).

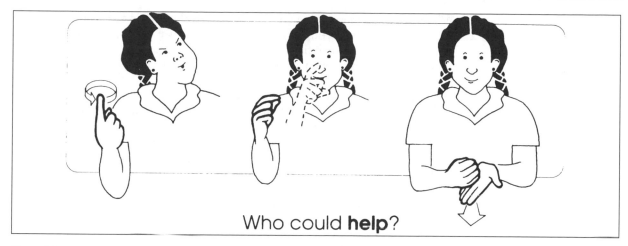

Who could **help**?

Figure 8.3
You Choose *Sign Supported English, Signed English and English (The National Deaf Children's Society)*

Figure 8.4
Paul Plays Football,
Makaton over English
(Shepard School,
Nottingham).

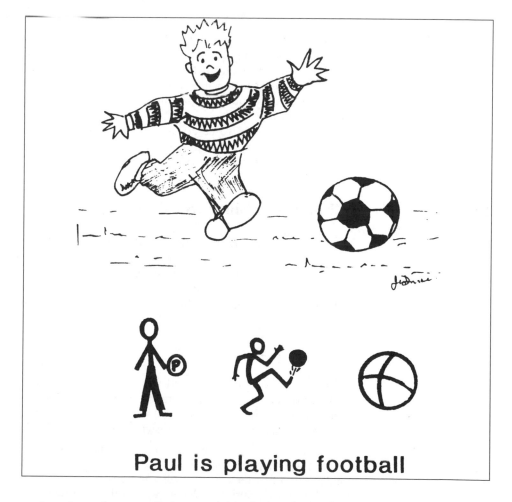

Paul is playing football

At a time when very little material is designed specifically for disabled children, we can at least ensure that when we adapt existing materials we ask ourselves relevant questions. Marchant (1993) suggests a number of such questions:

1. Why might this message be confusing for a child who is disabled?
2. What kind of safety 'code' would make more sense for children who are disabled (or have a specific disability)?
3. What difficulties might there be in using these materials with children who are disabled?
4. How could these materials be made more inclusive?
5. *Representation.* Are children who are disabled included in the text and illustrations? Are they represented positively?
6. *Accessibility.* Is the material itself accessible? (For example, for children with sensory impairment; learning disability; physical impairment, etc.) *Points to consider.* Complexity of language; use of signs; Braille; audio; large print; computer presentation; sub-titling or video, etc.
7. *Content.* Does the message make sense for children who are disabled? Does it rely on abilities that they have? Does it talk about experiences they are familiar with? Does it tackle all forms of infringements of disabled children's rights? Does it confuse issues of intimate care? Can the advice given be acted upon? Does it address issues of oppression due to race, culture and disability?

We discovered in using *You Choose* that deaf children more readily absorbed the safety messages for one reason: there were more pictures of deaf children in the book. It seems that if the children in the books do not represent them, they do not believe the messages are for them. This has profound implications. Safety books which exclude visual representation of disabled children are regarded by them as 'not for us'.

Although access to safety and prevention programmes is a disabled child's right, it will take commitment by agencies and policy-makers to ensure that appropriate materials are available and that these rights are fulfilled.

Children's ability to tell of abuse

I have previously discussed how disabled children's lack of knowledge and access to safety and prevention programmes means that they may not readily be able to tell others about situations of abuse due to inappropriate or absent educational input. There are, however, other factors which may make it difficult for children to tell and for adults to be receptive to what they are indicating or saying.

Isolation and risk

Children isolated in segregated residential schools are at far more risk of abuse (Marchant & Page 1993, Westcott 1993). There may also be a greater collective pressure not to tell in a residential situation. Ruth Moore (Morris 1991) describes her experience in a hospital following the onset of Still's disease:

I think I began to realise then how I was an object. I felt that for years, it was very very strict. I never dared to tell my parents what was going on, all our letters were censored and at the visits which we were allowed the staff were always around. My father gave me a doll for my eleventh birthday – I wanted this because I never had my own toys. I wasn't allowed to keep it.

(Morris 1991)

Using a different form of communication, having no access to a telephone (use of which may, indeed, be difficult due to physical impairment) and the isolation from family and friends provides fertile ground for abusive practices to go unchecked (Table 8.5). A new minicom text telephone line has recently been installed in 'ChildLine' for deaf children to use, a major step forward for at least one group of children.

Disabled children's trust of adults

Children may be inhibited from disclosing depending on whether or not the adult is disabled and on their ethnic origin. Children who are disabled are more likely to have been abused by a non-disabled adult, and there will be a clear power and status imbalance. Disabled children who have been abused may believe that *all* non-disabled adults are not to be trusted and therefore would want to disclose to a disabled adult.

The issue of race and ethnic group of the abuser is important. I knew of 16 boys all from ethnic minority groups who had been abused by a white adult. These children had been multiply abused through disabilism, racism and sexual abuse. Many of them did not trust other white people, and the situation required very sensitive handling from the child protection team. It is difficult to know how to overcome these issues because an appropriate person may not readily be available, but it remains important to determine from the child who they want to be involved: a male or female worker, a black or white worker, a disabled or non-disabled worker. Many disabled children are not asked or given this choice.

Receptive skills of adults

Adults may also be less receptive to disclosure from disabled children because denial about abuse of disabled children is very much stronger than it is for non-disabled children. No one wants to know that a disabled child has been hurt. We have these feelings with non-disabled children, but they are greater when the child is disabled. There is also a great fear of not knowing what to do in such a situation, and it becomes easier to ignore than to face the issue.

Confusion of signs and indicators

Many children do not disclose by verbally telling their story, they are 'picked up' by adults who see behaviours or signs and indicators which worry them. Watching for certain behaviours, signs and indicators in disabled children which will alert to possible abuse is a more difficult task, since adults may be inclined to attribute all signs and indicators to the child's impairment. It is important when we see bedwetting, fear of the dark or withdrawn behaviour also to consider the possibility that the child is being abused. Many workers with disabled

Table 8.5
Blocks to disclosure for disabled children

- They receive less information on safety and prevention programmes
- They may use other forms of communication such as British Sign Language, Sign Supported English, Makaton Rebus, Blissymbolics, Paget Gorman
- They may be isolated in segregated schools and residential care
- They may not have access to telephone helplines
- Their disclosure may be disbelieved or misunderstood
- Their communication system may be 'censored' of the words and phrases crucial to disclosure

children have not had child protection training (as it is believed that disabled children are not abused, and therefore training is not necessary). So when any signs of possible abuse occur, workers do not know how to make sense of them and attribute them automatically to behaviour stemming from impairment.

It is precisely because we may be able to justify another construction based on 'signs and indicators' that signs from the abused disabled child may be missed because we attribute signs and indicators to the wrong cause. To be disabled and to be abused is to experience oppression, powerlessness, stigmatisation and traumatic sexualisation.

It could be argued that some of the more explicit signs of sexual abuse could never be confused with the effects of disability or a disabling society. Unfortunately, experience shows that even the more explicit signs have been so attributed (BASPCAN Working Party on Disability and Abuse).

What is necessary within training programmes is for workers to begin to recognise the fact that they may confuse signs and indicators of abuse with those of disability. To overcome this tendency, workers need to be directed to explore all signs and indicators fully rather than making assumptions too quickly.

The investigative interview

The *Memorandum of Good Practice on Video Recorded Interviews with Child Witnesses for Criminal Proceedings* (Home Office *et al.* 1992) lays down the protocol for interviewing children suspected of being abused. The *Memorandum of Good Practice* states, 'each child is unique and the effective interview will be … tailored to the child's particular needs and circumstances' (p. 2). It also notes, 'if the child has any disabilities, for example speech or hearing impediment (*sic*), or learning difficulties, particular care should be taken to develop effective strategies for the interview to minimise the effect of such disabilities' (para 2.10).

Certainly, the *Memorandum of Good Practice* has recognised the presence of disabled children, but in actual fact the document does not really provide the help needed by those who will undertake the interview with disabled children. Throughout the document, reference is made to 'hearing' the child's evidence, indicating that verbal communication is assumed. They do know about deaf children using sign language, but there is no guidance on the level of skill, training or qualifications necessary, in spite of the fact that there is official training that can been undertaken (Council for the Advancement of Communication with Deaf People, CACDP). There is an alarming suggestion that, exceptionally, it may be in the interests of the child to be *interviewed* (this is not interpreting, but interviewing itself) by an adult in whom they have already put confidence (Home Office *et al.* 1992, para 2.24). Although it adds, 'provided that such a person is not party to the proceedings, is prepared to co-operate with appropriately trained interviewers and can accept adequate briefing'. This may lead to adults who are actually party to the abuse being used or to inappropriate people being used simply because 'they can sign'.

The lack of clear guidance here means that when children use other forms of communication virtually anybody can be used to 'interpret', 'facilitate' or actually carry out the interview itself. There is no acknowledgement or guidance concerning children using Blissymbolics, Rebus or other augmentative communication systems. Invariably, the child protection team turns to teachers to fill this role (a practice quite common with signing deaf children). There are many

Table 8.6
Contraindications for using teachers in the investigative interview

1. The child may fear being punished if they speak out
2. Blurred boundaries
3. Teachers have limited signing skills/understanding of child abuse and no training in counselling
4. Teachers lack knowledge of deaf culture
5. The child may identify school life with abuse
6. The child may want school to be the place where they can 'get away' from implications of assault
7. Teachers not aware of legal implications
8. An easy option for professionals – little choice for child
9. Difficult to separate pedagogic and therapeutic rules
10. The child feels 'watched', 'guilty', 'bare' and vulnerable
11. Child may receive differential treatment and/or expect it
12. Confound learning situations
13. Contaminates relationships with teacher
14. The child may not disclose fully, to save teacher embarrassment
15. The child fears teacher's relationship with parents
16. Difficult for teacher/child to put issues aside during school day
17. Use of teacher may 'taint' evidence
18. Can never be sure teacher not involved in abuse (if suspected in school setting)
19. The child has a right to an independent worker

Source: Kennedy 1992

contraindications for using teachers in this role (Table 8.6). These contraindications could also apply to any person who is in a position of authority and known to the child in another capacity.

What is seriously missing in training is guidance on how to interview disabled children using non-voiced methods such as Blissymbolics, Makaton, BSL and computer-aided systems, and other augmentative systems. This seems to result in the Crown Prosecution System (CPS) vetoing all disabled children who do not use voice from going to court.

Provided that certain ground rules are observed, the use of qualified (CACDP) interpreters in child abuse investigations is essential. There are a number of factors involved in the role of interpreters in this context which I shall now consider. (The reader is also referred to an excellent book by Baker *et al.* 1991, which explores the role of interpreters of foreign languages in public services and sets out principles that can be usefully transferred to the situation of children who use sign language or other augmentative communication systems such as Bliss, Rebus and Makaton.)

The interpreter's and facilitator's role is to convey the *meaning* of everything which is said or indicated. This does not mean literal word-for-word translation since it is impossible to word-for-word translate from British Sign Language to English or to translate from Bliss Board to English.

(Kennedy 1993)

The lack of guidance about interviewing disabled children under *Memorandum* guidelines is reflected in the very inadequate training of police officers who are mandated to interview such children.

The Aldridge & Wood (1999) study sent 400 questionnaires to police forces in Wales and England. A total of 104 were completed: 54% of respondents had interviewed a disabled child, 46% a learning disabled child, 30% a deaf child, 12% a Down's syndrome child, 8% a child with cerebral palsy and 4% a visually impaired child. Only 11% of the respondents had some training regarding disabled children. Looking at the breakdown of 'training', this included a deaf awareness course, i.e. a 1-day course, part of a 4-day course and a conference. It is my view that none of these so called training days was in fact a *training to interview disabled children*.

In the *Abuse and Children who are Disabled (ABCD) Pack*, Kennedy (1993) has drawn up checklists (see below) for setting up interviews with disabled children and interpreters.

What the child protection workers (interviewers) will need to know of the interpreter/facilitator:

1. The extent of the training the person has received in that communication system.
2. The qualification the person holds.
3. The experience of that person working in the investigative context.

What the child protection workers (interviewers) will need to know of the child:

1. The level and understanding the child has reached regarding language (receptive and expressive).
2. The use and extent of vocabulary the child has acquired.
3. Whether the child has words for body parts and sexual activity. (Some systems exclude these words and the child may not be able to name body parts.)
4. How the child communicates.
5. How the child accesses their augmentative signing/symbol system (finger points, eye points).
6. The implications of that communication system (how it functions) on the investigative process and whether it will allow for language and concepts that may arise at interview.
7. Whether the child favours male/female interpreters/facilitators.
8. Whether the child favours a white or black worker/interpreter or facilitator.

The investigative team should make clear to the interpreter or facilitator:

1. The identity of the people involved and their relationship with each other.
2. The purpose of the conversation to be interpreted. This may include relevant background information about the case.
3. The worker's own objectives and desired outcomes, where appropriate.
4. How long the interpreting process is likely to last.
5. Any difficult language or concepts which are likely to arise.
6. Any difficult behaviour that may be encountered (e.g. anger, tearfulness, withdrawal) and how the interpreter should respond.
7. Any difficulties or misunderstandings that might arise between interviewer and interpreter/facilitator and how to overcome these (Kennedy 1993).

Much work has been done in child protection for learning-disabled children (Craft), deaf children (Kennedy) and children with complex disabilities (Marchant). Readers are directed to the relevant agencies at the end of this chapter for further advice and guidance. Marchant & Page (1993), in *Bridging the Gap*, show very clearly the dynamics of using a facilitator for children using augmentative communication boards. It is worth reproducing here what they observed:

Over the course of several interviews we observed how the flow of communication between the interviewer, the child and the interpreter appeared to move through several stages as the interview progressed. We have found it most helpful to conceptualise these stages as progressing through different 'triangles' of communication, as follows.

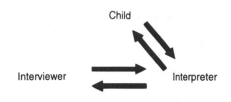

Stage 1

In the first stage all communication tends to be routed through the interpreter. The interviewer may find it difficult to address the child directly for a variety of reasons and the child is unlikely to direct his or her responses towards an unfamiliar adult who clearly does not yet know about his or her communication systems.

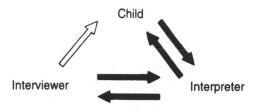

Stage 2

In the second stage some communication begins to move directly between the interviewer and the child, as the interviewer begins to have confidence that the child is understanding what is being said, and begins to address the child directly. The child is likely to continue to address his or her responses to the interpreter at this stage.

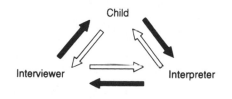

Stage 3

The third stage seemed to mark a turning point in most interviews: this is the point at which the interviewer begins to understand the child's 'yes' and 'no' responses for him/herself. At this point the child begins to address his or her responses directly to the interviewer and the first two-way direct communication is established.

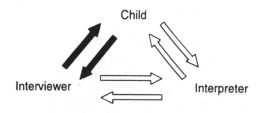

Stage 4

The final stage may not be reached in every interview. At this stage the interviewer has understood enough about the child's language ability and 'yes' and 'no' responses to have the confidence to communicate directly with him or her, and the child responds directly to the interviewer. The role of the interpreter becomes more of a fallback loop for clarification or if there are difficulties.

The main lesson for practice must be to place a very high priority on the interviewer learning and understanding the child's 'yes' and 'no' responses, as this seems to mark a point at which the interview can 'change gear' and enable direct, two-way communication to get underway. This also has an impact on the interviewer's ability to adjust his or her language and approach to the level of understanding of the child. We found that some interviewers tended to adjust their approach 'down' to their perception of the child's understanding, and would unnecessarily speak slowly and simply until they were receiving direct feedback that the child was understanding them.

(Marchant & Page 1993, p. 27)

Unlike the above, where the child protection interviewer may establish direct communication with the child, communication with deaf children will always require going through an interpreter. The gender of the interpreter is crucial. Recently, a woman police officer telephoned me to tell me a 14-year-old girl failed to tell her everything because a male interpreter had been present. She wrote on a piece of paper after the interview, 'not all – could not tell all – man'. The police officer was rightly upset and concerned since the prosecution may fail because of this.

Interviewing disabled children who have been abused is fraught with difficulties not only because of communication issues. The CPS is loath to take such cases to court, because in a great many cases the credibility of the child's statement is regarded as less reliable simply on the grounds of disability. The logic seems to be:

- this child must be 'disturbed' due to disability
- this child may be lying due to lack of attention because of disability (attention seeking)
- this child is probably also learning-disabled.

This is discrimination and yet common practice. Recently, an excellent pack (Plotnikoff *et al.* 1993) was produced for child witnesses going to court which, although I would recommend it for non-disabled children, includes only three sentences of guidance – for parents – on disabled child witnesses:

Being a witness at court is an experience no child finds easy. For children with a learning disability or other disability it can be even more difficult, especially if the disability affects the child's speech or hearing. Remember that you child may need extra encouragement and support both before and on the day of the trial.

(Plotnikoff *et al.* 1993)

It would have been useful to have given more consideration to the needs of children who are disabled. Disabled children may have the following fears and worries.

- What if I know I'm about to have an epiletic fit?
- What if my hearing aid battery goes flat in the middle of my testimony?
- What if the lighting is poor and I can't lip read?
- What if I don't understand the interpreter?
- How will I know who everyone is? (blind child)
- What if I cannot get into the toilets? (child using wheelchair)

We know of instances where disability has been used to discredit a child's testimony. A partially deaf child who said he couldn't hear the defence barrister was brutally shouted at: 'Can't hear or don't want to answer my question?' The child burst into tears. This same barrister, with a child who was incontinent of urine and faeces due to emotional disturbance, said, 'Who would want to abuse a smelly, shitty child like you?' Such questioning of the child's integrity is damaging, and some preparation for the possibility of this occurring needs to be made. Children who are disabled should be able to give their account in open court, but more work is required to enable this to be an empowering process, not a disempowering one.

'Therapeutic' services

The terms relating to services for disabled children following abuse are not helpful. There is a tendency to medicalise/pathologise the child who has been abused. For this reason, the ABCD training pack on disability and abuse (Kennedy 1993) uses the term 'survival process' in place of 'therapy/treatment'. This term will be used here too.

Survival services are often denied to disabled children because, especially if they do not use speech, they are considered unable to benefit from counselling following abuse. Disability workers know little about issues of abuse, and child protection workers know little about the experience of disability. Often, instead of acknowledging that there are difficulties with the services offered, the problem is located in the child. Lack of commitment, time, knowledge or confidence on the workers' part becomes, 'she wouldn't have the understanding to cope with counselling'. Inadequacies in toilet facilities are translated into, 'he can't use our toilets'.

Before looking at the themes of survival work, one must look at the practicalities of doing this work. Workers need to ask themselves whether they can do the work on their own, or whether they need specialist help.

Workers can gain much help from co-working with speech and language therapists and/or specialist social workers in disability (e.g. social workers with deaf people or with learning-disabled people). There is advice available from Craft (NAPSAC) and the Keep Deaf Children Safe Project (deaf children). Sinnason of the Tavistock can offer advice on psychodynamic work with abused, learning-disabled people. Merchant of Chailey Heritage is available where multiply disabled children are concerned.

Intepreters or facilitators may be necessary for children who use other forms of communication, but their skills will need to be considered in relation to their experience in interpreting, and their awareness and ability to work in the area of child abuse. Some facilitators or interpreters could find the work too painful or stressful and may not have the training to support them through this. Sometimes it might even be necessary to use non-abusive family members as co-workers, or a person the child knows well (but this should be considered with utmost care for the reasons given previously in using teachers as interpreters and should only be considered as a last resort with the approval of the child).

For children who are disabled, the creative therapies such as art therapy, play therapy and drama therapy can be especially helpful, particularly for children who find voice/language a real difficulty. At the end of the day, the most appropriate worker is one who is able to be creative and take risks in trying new ways of implementing techniques previously used. The person who is imaginative and persistent is ideal.

Survival work with disabled children

Children who are disabled and have been abused often ask, 'Was I abused because I am disabled?' The sad reality is that this is often the case. Even though we know many children are abused, we equally know disabled children are more likely to be targeted. The child is therefore faced with two very painful realities: they are disabled and they have been abused. It is vitally important that the worker appreciates both these aspects of the child's life.

For work to be truly empowering, one must acknowledge both the experience of being impaired in a disabling society, and the oppression of child abuse and how the child has been harmed, used and devalued. They cannot be separated (Table 8.7).

A service offered by a disability worker may tend to focus more on the aspects of impairment, that offered by the child protection worker may focus more on the abuse. There is a very clear need for dual specialists (Kennedy 1990). Until that time, co-working is essential where disability worker and child protection worker cooperate and offer services together to facilitate the empowerment/ survival process.

New developments

Quality Protects. This initiative has been designed by the DOH to enable local authorities to develop their services to a more appropriate level and to better standards. The first analysis of Management Action Plans (MAPs) with reference to disabled children has been studied by the DOH. The results of this analysis are available on the Internet: *www.doh.gov.uk/qualityprotects/exec.htm*

From 88 MAPs, a number of concerns have arisen which clearly show services to disabled children in some disarray. These include the remit of the Children Act to ascertain the wishes and feelings of disabled children. Concerns include:

■ How best to include disabled children and young people within wider consultation processes with children and young people in the area.
■ Limited awareness of how best to support children and young people with communication or other special needs (this confirms the Aldridge & Wood (1999) study on interviewing disabled children by police. This means that both social services and police are unable to communicate with their client group!).
■ Concerns about potential clashes of interest between children and parents.
■ An absence of reliable planning data for working with disabled children from ethnic minorities.

The DOH analysis of the 88 MAPs seems to make no reference to child protection for disabled children. Given that the basic services are in such disarray, as evidenced by this analysis, then it is unlikely that an overview of child protection for this group will be very much better. What is encouraging is an ADSS (Association of Directors of Social Services) group chaired by Matt Bukowski; '*Agenda for disabled children*' is addressing the grave concerns of services to disabled children.

A Children-in-need funded research project undertaken by Pam Cooke of the Ann Craft Trust will give us some idea of the state of play for disabled children. Preliminary findings were presented at the Kennedy/Wonnacott Conference: 'From the Cradle to the grave – violence against disabled children and adults' in October 1999 (see website *www.prodisca.com*). A crucial finding was that there was a real anxiety expressed by most of the social workers in the research about a need for training and a lack of knowledge. Social workers noted a tendency not to 'see' abuse of disabled children due to lack of knowledge and support but also

	Disabling society/disability	Possible responses	Abusing society/abuse
Table 8.7 *The worker must understand the possible responses of two separate experiences*	'I've caused all the family problems by *being disabled*'	Self-blame	'I've caused all the problems by being abused'
	'My fault'	Anger	'My fault'
	Against: family, educational system, society, God for being disabled		*Against*: abuser, family, professionals, siblings
	About: missing information, feeling: ineffective		
	Hate: hearing aids, special schools, hospital visits, speech therapy	Hatred	For abuser, family, sex/sexuality
	'I can't hear' (deafness)	Frustration	'How do I stop it?'
	'I don't understand'		'How do I get away?'
	'I'm useless, stupid'	Suicidal	'I'm bad, useless'
	'I've had enough – struggle is too great'		'I've had enough'
			'The pain is too great'
	Disability becomes the focus, not education	Poor concentration	Can't study in school, distracted, preoccupied by abuse and possibility of future abuse
	'I'm bad'	Lack of confidence	'I'm bad'
	'I'm faulty'		'I'm dirty'
	For being rejected because disabled	Bitterness	For being 'used'
	For being deaf		For 'loss' of family care/protection
	For 'failing'		
	Of social situations	Fear	More abuse
	Of not hearing (deafness)		Touch/closeness
	Of appearing stupid		Injury/harm
	Of making a mistake		Pregnancy
	Of failing		Someone finding out
	No control over events, no choice	Powerlessness	No control over events
	'I can't keep up and I'm keeping away'	Withdrawal	'I don't want anyone to know what's going on'
			'I don't want to be noticed by abuser'
	'I'm not the child my parents wanted'	Guilt	'I've caused it'
			'I'm abused because I'm disabled'
			'I liked it'
	'They don't want me to be disabled – I have to be normal' (rejection of true identity)	Rejection	'I'm only good enough for this'
			'They don't love me'
	'I'm not like everyone else'	Isolation	'I'm not like everyone else'
	Feeling 'left out'		
	I'm useless'	Depression	'I hate myself'
	'I'm stupid'		'I'm bad/dirty'
	'I'm defective'		
	'Nobody can help me'	False belief	'Nobody can help me'
	'Will I make bad/stupid mistakes? Confusion'	Anxiety (constant)	'When will it happen?'
	'Will I go completelydeaf?'		'Will I be harmed?'
			'Will he kill me?'
	'What's happening?'	Confusion	'What's happening?'
	'Why am I disabled?'		'Why is this happening?'
	'Am I deaf or hearing?'	Conflict (identity)	'Am I child or partner?'
	'Am I normal/abnormal?'		
	Pretending to be 'normal'	Fatigue	Pretending all is okay
	Lip reading		Keeping going
	Concentrating (deafness)		

Source: Kennedy 1990

because of complications that might arise in such cases, including the cost in terms of time and resources, i.e. lack of resources.

New assessment framework (Fig. 8.5)

This new framework will supersede the old framework: *The Orange Book*. Comprising 'domains' and 'dimensions', it would appear to offer a more integrated and holistic framework. If properly implemented, this framework should fit nicely with Sobsey's Integrated Ecological Model of abuse of disabled children. What is encouraging is that the disabled child's developmental needs will be addressed and given equal weight to parental capacity. This is being interpreted by social workers as a mandate to work more equably with the disabled child and not to concentrate solely on working with the parents, which has been an historic tendency hitherto, particularly in the field of disability.

There is, however, continuing confusion over whether to rate the disabled child's development against a non-disabled child or a 'like child', i.e. another, similar disabled child. The dangers of assessing against a non-disabled child would be to put too much pressure on the disabled child to match a benchmark of 'normalcy'; conversely, assessing against a disabled 'similar' child could lower the benchmark of achievement if it is assumed that all disabled children are being 'held back' developmentally by a discriminatory practice and poor services. The constant dangers of this assessment framework will be apparent if assessors concentrate too much on the medical side of *impairment* (the child's physical or learning condition) and not enough on the child's *disability* (the child's oppression within a prejudiced society). The dimension of 'identity' will allow all social workers to assess how a disabled child feels about both their impairment *and* their disability. This aspect will be most interesting to watch and could prove an extremely positive development, but will only happen if and when social services adopt the social model of disability and not the medical model.

Figure 8.5
Assessment framework

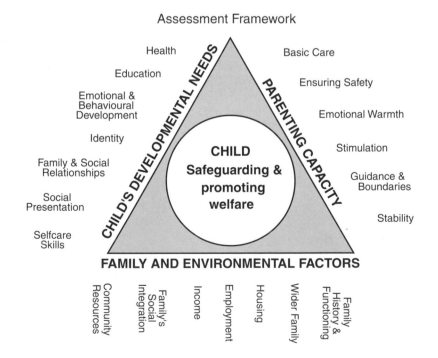

Conclusion

This chapter has, in a sense, catalogued the deficiencies and the discrimination towards disabled children in the child protection domain. It reflects the general level of society's devaluation of disabled people and the low priority given to a group considered to be of less importance.

Child protection services, as they are structured at the moment, often do not suit the requirements of disabled children. Safety and prevention programmes, survival/empowerment facilities and investigative and criminal proceeding have never considered this group of children. Children who are disabled cannot be offered the same services as are offered to the non-disabled child. This is because they often have very different needs in relation to communication, mobility, dexterity, physical strength and cognitive abilities. Adapting the current ways of working with non-disabled children seldom works, for it fails to grasp the fact that disabled children's experiences are unique and sufficiently different to necessitate a new approach to service provisions. This new approach must take as its starting point the fact that a disabled child is not simply a child who happens to be disabled (and so we only need to adapt our current ways of working with non-disabled children), but a disabled child who requires a completely different input.

Requirements for disabled children include:

1. Intimate care policies which promote confidentiality and privacy and safety for disabled children.
2. Disabled children's rights policies which encourage and enable choice and decision-making.
3. Training which will challenge workers' stereotypes, disabilist attitudes and prejudices.
4. Assertion training for disabled children which promotes self-respect, high self-esteem and confidence.
5. Self-defence training for disabled children which addresses the issues of fight or 'flight' appropriately.
6. Safety and prevention programmes relevant to the additional requirements for children who are disabled.
7. Programmes for disabled children which explore and address issues of racism and disabilism.
8. Programmes for disabled children which explore issues of sex, sexuality and gender.
9. Area child protection policies which address the specific needs of these children in relation to safety·and prevention programmes, investigative interviews, empowerment/survival work and criminal proceedings.
10. Programmes which take account of alternative forms of communication.
11. Programmes which take account of the child's physical strength, mobility, dexterity and impairments (visual or hearing impairment) and cognitive abilities.

To undertake any child protection work with disabled children demands that we as workers address our stereotypes, prejudices and attitudes towards disability. It also requires that we begin to value and promote the confidence and self-esteem in disabled children which have been eroded by oppressive practices, disabilism and now abuse, and that we begin to develop a truly personalised service tailored to the exact requirements of disabled children.

References

Aldridge M, Wood J 1999 Interviewing child witnesses with disabilities: a survey of police officers in England and Wales. The Police Journal January

Ammerman R T, Hersen M, Van Hassett V B, *et al.* 1989 Abuse and neglect in psychiatrically hospitalized multi handicapped children. Child Abuse and Neglect 13 (3): 335–343

Baker P, Hussain Z, Saunders J 1991 Interpreters in public services. Venture Press, Birmingham

Degener T 1992 The right to be different: implications for child protection. Child Abuse Review 1: 151–155

Department of Health (DOH) 1990 Children and young persons on Child Protection Register. Year ending 31 March 1989, England. A/F 89/13. Government Statistical Office, London

Department of Health *et al.* (DOH) 2000 Quality protects: Framework. The Stationery Office, London

Doucette J 1986 Violent acts against disabled women, Toronto, Canada. Dawn quoted in Westcott.

Garbarino J 1987 The abuse and neglect of special children: an introduction to the issues. In: Garbarino J, Brockhauser P E, Authier J (eds) Special children – special risks: the maltreatment of children with disabilities. De Gruyter, New York

Home Office, Department of Health 1992 Memorandum of good practice on video recorded interviews with child witnesses for criminal proceedings. HMSO, London

Kelly L 1992 The connections between disability and child abuse: a review of the research evidence. Child Abuse Review 1 (3): 157–167

Kennedy M 1990 The deaf child who is abused. Is there a need for a dual specialist? Child Abuse Review 4 (2):

Kennedy M 1992*a* Not the only way to communicate: a challenge to voice in child protection work. Child Abuse Review 1: 169–177

Kennedy M 1992*b* The case for interpreters – exploring communication with children who are deaf. Child Abuse Review 1 (3): 191–193

Kennedy M 1993 Language and disability: a guide through the terminology maze. Abuse and Children who are Disabled (ABCD) Pack.

Kennedy M, Kelly L 1992 Inclusion not exclusion. Child Abuse Review 1 (3): 147–149

Marchant R 1991 Myths and facts about sexual abuse and children with disabilities. Child Abuse Review 5 (2): 22–24

Marchant R 1993 Safety and prevention programmes. Abuse and Children who are Disabled (ABCD) Training and Resource Pack.

Marchant R, Page M 1993 Bridging the gap: child protection work with children with multiple disabilities. NSPCC, London

Mayes *et al.* 1986 Child sexual abuse: a review of the literature and educational materials. Psychology Department, University of Lancaster, Lancaster

Morris J 1991 Pride against prejudice. Transforming attitudes to disability. Women's Press, London

Plotnikoff J *et al.* 1993 The child witness pack, helping children to cope.

Senn C Y 1988 Vulnerability, sexual abuse and people with learning disabilities. G. Allan Roeher Institute, quoted in inter-agency information and awareness programme in child sexual abuse, Subiaco, Western Australia 1991

Sobsey D 1994 Violence and abuse in the lives of people with disabilities; the end of silent acceptance? Paul Brookes, Baltimore

Sobsey D, Varnhagen C 1988 Sexual abuse and exploitation of people with disabilities. Unpublished manuscript quoted in Westcott 1993

Sullivan P M, Vernon M, Scanlon J M 1987 Sexual abuse of deaf youth. American Annals of the Deaf 3: 256–262

Westcott H 1991 Institutional abuse of children – from research and policy, a review. NSPCC, London

Westcott H 1993 Abuse of children and adults with disabilities. NSPCC, Policy Practice and Research Series, London

Westcott H, Cross H 1995 Thus far and no further: towards ending the abuse of disabled children. Venture Press, London

Wolfensberger W 1987 The new genocide of handicapped and afflicted people. Syracuse, New York

Useful addresses and information

Kennedy M, Gorden R, Marchant B, Cross M 1993 ABCD (Abuse and Children who are Disabled). DOH, London A training pack produced by the National Deaf Children Society, NSPCC, Chailey Heritage and Way Ahead Disability Consultancy. Comprises Trainer pack (exercises) and Reader pack (specialist papers). The reader can be purchased separately. Pack can be ordered from Caroline Riley, Training Department, ABCD Pack, c/o NSPCC National Training Centre, 3 Gilmour Close, Beaumont Leys, Leicester LE4 1EZ.

Ann Craft Trust, Centre of Social Work, University of Nottingham, University Park, Nottingham NG7 2RD

British Association for the Study and Prevention of Child Abuse and Neglect (BASPCAN), 10 Priory Street, York YO1 1EZ

Council for the Advancement of Communication with Deaf People (CACDP), Pelaw House, School of Education, University of Durham, Durham DH1 1TA (provides a list of qualified sign language interpreters)

Margaret Kennedy, 5 Albion Works, Sigdon Road, Hackney, London E8. Freelance Trainer/Consultant on Disability and Child Protection. Previously Founder and National Co-ordinator of the National Deaf Children Society's 'Keep Deaf Children Safe Project'. email: MK@emkay-disab.demon.co.uk

Ruth Marchant, Child Care Manager, Chailey Heritage, North Chailey, Nr Lewes, East Sussex BN8 4EF

Website: *www.prodisca.com* Prodisca–Protecting Disabled Children and Adults. A site of information and trainers who specialise in this important field

9

Abuse in institutional settings

Ian Butler

In 1836 the Clerk of the Bedford Union wrote to the Poor Law Commissioners seeking permission to have

...writing omitted as part of the schoolmaster's instruction in the workhouse, and that he teach reading only. The Board do not recommend this on the score of economy, but on that of principle, as they are desirous of avoiding a greater advantage to the inmates of the workhouse than to the poor child out of it, withdrawing thereby as much as possible any premium or inducement to the frequenting of the workhouse.

(Pinchbeck & Hewitt 1973, p. 503)

This historical anecdote can be made to illustrate several themes that find echo in this chapter. Firstly, it serves as a reminder that residential care in particular, but also other extra-familial forms of care, have their origins in very specific forms of Poor Law provision for children, which were characterised by insensitive, neglectful, deliberately stigmatising and punitive regimes that carried some degree of official sanction. Thus it makes the point that the institutional abuse of children is not a new phenomenon.

Secondly, it demonstrates that the particular experiences of children living away from home have to be understood in the context of the general experiences of children of the time. Whilst one of the defining characteristics of institutional care might be the degree to which children and young people are removed from the wider community, institutional practices are embedded in the prevailing social construction of childhood and in the dominant professional cultures of the period.

Thirdly, it illustrates how individuals in positions of authority can devise schemes and strategies within the boundaries of particular institutions which, however misguided or malicious, nonetheless have a plausibility and even a logic to those with a motive to pursue them.

The main value of setting contemporary concerns over children living away from home in a broader historical perspective, however slight, is in order to contextualise and to limit the current sense of crisis which characterises debate in this area. This is not to argue for complacency but simply to suggest that taking a longer view may help to offset the 'special pessimism', a phrase used by the Department of Health and Social Security (DHSS) to describe the attitude that many social workers and parents have towards residential care (DHSS 1985), which has built up in this area over many years and which can seem to defy any hope of achieving positive and sustainable change.

This chapter examines what is meant by 'institutional abuse' before considering the form and content of recent policy responses. Together, these considerations then form the basis for an exploration of some contemporary practice issues and how these might be addressed.

Review of the literature/research: a catalogue of abuse?

Despite the well-documented experiences of generations of children living away from home (Heywood 1969, Pinchbeck & Hewitt 1973, Hendrick 1994, Department of Health (DOH) 1998), the concept of 'institutional abuse' has only recently entered the discourse of child protection. As recently as 1992, Bloom reported just a handful of papers dealing with the subject in the American social work literature since 1980 (Bloom 1992). Perhaps not surprisingly therefore, much of the literature in the field remains concerned with attempts to define the term and to describe the phenomena to which it refers. There is no universally accepted definition as yet and both elements of the phrase remain problematic.

In its everyday sense, the term 'institution' tends to conjure up the regimented, impersonal and large scale provision of residential care for children developed in the asylums, 'barrack schools' and workhouses of the eighteenth and nineteenth centuries. This sense of the term as referring to specific *sites* of abuse, despite the virtual disappearance of these particular forms of provision, is still reflected in the literature. With the exception of a relatively small number of studies describing the experiences of children attending boarding schools of their own or their parents' choice (Campbell-Smith 1983, ChildLine 1997), the phrase is most commonly invoked to refer specifically to establishments for children in the public care. It has been noted, however (Doran & Brannan 1996), that this reflects a 'bias' in professional and political discourses towards institutions for working class and vulnerable children. They suggest that institutions are viewed through a 'lens of social class, filtering out certain establishments' (p. 155). The bullying of some young army recruits, for example, is not routinely categorised as an example of institutional abuse.

One could argue further that the contemporary debate on the institutional abuse of children in public care is confined only to a sub-set of 'sites', namely children's homes, residential schools and, more recently still, to foster homes. For example, the abuse of children and young people in penal establishments, despite clear evidence of the existence of neglectful and brutalising regimes (Liebling & Krarup 1994), is virtually untraceable in the social work literature (but see Howard League 1995, 1996, Utting *et al.* 1997).

By identifying particular sites, however, a useful distinction is made between familial and extra-familial forms of abuse. Gil (1982), in still the most frequently cited account, defines institutional abuse as (p. 9):

any system, programme, policy, procedure or individual interaction with a child in placement that abuses, neglects or is detrimental to the child's health, safety or emotional and physical well-being, or in any way exploits or violates the child's basic rights.

(see also Shaughnessy 1984, Moss 1990, Stein 1993). She goes on to define system abuse as 'perpetrated not by any single person or programme but by the immense and complicated child care system, stretched beyond its limits and incapable of guaranteeing safety to all children in care' (p. 11).

In relation to such system abuse, the literature on residential care in Britain, both academic and administrative, since the 1980s (DHSS 1985, Milham *et al.* 1986, DOH 1991, Parker *et al.* 1991, Brown *et al.* 1998; Sinclair & Gibbs 1998) provides too many illustrations of how, through 'drift', under-resourcing, inadequate planning and poor decision-making processes the social, educational, health and life chances for children looked after away from home have been diminished. In foster care too, evidence is emerging (NFCA 1995, NSPCC 1995) of how poor relationships with carers, a high number of unplanned moves from placement to placement (which interrupts schooling and weakens parental and community links), as well as poor patterns of communication and inadequate complaints procedures, have a detrimental effect on children whilst in care and afterwards. However, it is important to remember, noting the caution over 'special pessimism' made earlier, that despite such failures, overall outcomes for children in residential and foster care are generally favourable (DHSS 1985, DOH 1991, Bullock *et al.* 1993, Berridge & Brodie 1996).

Against a background of major structural inadequacies within the wider child care 'system', at the level of the individual institution, particular regimes or practices (an approximation of Gil's 'programme, policy or procedure') may also be constituted as abusive. Examples include the mis-use of medication to manage challenging behaviour (Shaughnessy 1984) and the development of idiosyncratic and ill-founded 'therapeutic' regimes, such as the 'regression therapy' practiced by the convicted paedophile Frank Beck in Leicestershire children's homes in the 1970s and 1980s (Kirkwood 1993). The practice of 'Pindown' operated in Staffordshire children's homes (Levy & Kahan 1991) is another example of the abuse of 'expert' knowledge used to justify harsh and abusive regimes, in this case imposing severe restrictions on children's liberty through subjecting them to humiliating and degrading forms of containment (p. 9):

Susan was required to wear pyjamas and kept in a sparsely furnished room. She was not allowed contact with other children or non-Pindown staff and was not permitted to attend school. She was required to knock on the door before going to the toilet.

Thomas (1990), however, has cautioned against understanding institutional abuse simply as a function of wider system or regime-specific abuse in that these are 'inert structures awaiting human operationalisation' (p. 10). In recognising the centrality of human agency in any abusive practice, the concept of institutional abuse begins to overlap with what is usually referred to as 'organised abuse', another elusive category.

Bibby (1996, pp. 5–6), after eschewing the 'official' definition of organised abuse given in *Working Together* (Home Office *et al.* 1991) as 'circular', defines organised abuse as:

- … the systematic abuse of children, normally by more than one male.
- It is characterised by the degree of planning in the purposeful, secret targeting, seduction, hooking and silencing of the subjects.
- Institutional and ritual abuse are but specialised forms of organised abuse.

By implication, Bibby associates organised abuse primarily with sexual abuse. His subsuming of institutional abuse into the broader category of organised abuse is arguable, but should be understood in the context of the specific meaning he attaches to the idea of 'systems':

Organised abuse is therefore not, in essence, a matter of numbers and systems relationships among the perpetrator(s) and the subject(s). It is a matter of process rather than systems. This fits in with the experience of most practitioners that the techniques used by single perpetrators are similar to those used by multiple perpetrators. The core of the definition above, therefore, is in the second item. It directs our thoughts towards the *systems* used by the perpetrators. (p. 6)

By this reading, the systematic, covert and predatory abuse of children by Frank Beck in Leicestershire would constitute organised abuse, whereas the practice of 'Pindown' would not. Accordingly, it would follow that it may be reasonable to consider organised abuse as an instance of institutional abuse rather than vice versa. This may be no more than a matter of semantics. What is common to both positions are the enduring characteristics of any formal provision made for children looked after away from home, namely its relative 'invisibility' and the endemic inequality of power relations between children and adults. It is these factors in particular that permit abuse to take place and to remain undetected. Both residential and foster care are essentially 'private' activities that tend not to come to wider public attention other than through the reports of 'scandals'. Children in care are accordingly relatively isolated (Ayres 1989, Sobsey & Varnhagen 1988). Largely unobserved, children placed in care are also uniquely vulnerable for other reasons in that they will already to some degree have had their self-esteem and support networks weakened by whatever experiences have brought them into institutional care (Solomons *et al.* 1981, Kelly 1992). This may be acutely so in the case of children with disabilities (Crosse *et al.* 1993, Jones 1994). These factors accentuate the powerful positions of adults in whose care children are placed. Such adults are routinely in a position to make life-changing decisions for the young people they are looking after. As Westcott (1991) has observed, children in institutions are a

...voiceless population, having no control over decisions affecting their current and future placements, and no influence over the quality of care they receive. (p. 12–13).

How far general or specific failures in the provision of out-of-home care can be said to constitute abuse is, of course, debatable. If one takes the view that 'abuse in institutions comprises any system which violates the rights of a child to a healthy physical and psychological development' (Doran & Brannan 1996, p. 156), then any failure to provide effective and compassionate care would constitute abuse. If one takes a position further along the spectrum of what might be regarded as abusive, by introducing the concept of 'significant harm' (Children Act 1989), for example, then a narrower range of activities and experiences would fall within the category of child abuse.

It is in this sense that both elements of the concept of 'institutional abuse' are problematic. Both in terms of the site of the abuse and in terms of the form it takes and the manner in which it is pursued, any definition runs the risk of being either too wide or too narrow in its scope. If on the other hand, institutional abuse is regarded as a complex phenomenon, multi-causal and appearing in a variety of forms, then Stein's (1993) conclusion, extended to include all forms of substitute care, is a useful starting point for further action. He argues that we should discard at the outset, any idea of finding a crude homogeneity in the abuse of children living away from home and discard an implicit standard or single response in addressing such abuse.

Definitions of abuse that derive from the actions of the adults involved, rather than from the experiences of children, are perhaps inevitably inadequate and unsatisfying. La Fontaine (1993) in the context of organised abuse has noted that 'even the best constructed definition is a poor substitute for acquiring systematic knowledge' (p. 230). Where such knowledge derives from the documented experiences of children (Butler & Williamson 1994, Butler 1996), consequent definitions may be of more conceptual and practical value.

One further difficulty remains, however. Without a more precise, or at least consensual definition, calculations of both the type of abuse perpetrated upon children living away from home and the questions of its incidence and prevalence become almost impossible to address. There have, perhaps for this reason, been few systematic surveys of incidence or prevalence reported in the literature. American studies (Rindfleisch & Rabb 1984, Powers *et al.* 1990, Blatt 1992) and studies in the UK (Westcott & Clement 1992) would suggest that abuse in institutions is common and that much goes undetected. Hence any extrapolation, particularly from American studies where forms of provision and constructions of abuse differ from those found in the professional and administrative literature in the UK, must be considered as tentative (e.g. Westcott 1991, pp. 11–12).

In the absence of any more definitive accounts, perceptions of the incidence and prevalence of abuse in residential care in the UK have been mediated by the several reports of various 'scandals'. More will be said of these below but in summarising the findings of these inquiries (into the 'Pindown' regime in Staffordshire 1991, Castle Hill School 1991, Ty Mawr School 1992; Leicestershire's children's homes 1993; Kincora Boys Hostel in Belfast 1989, Crookham Court Independent Boarding School in Berkshire 1988), the National Commission of Inquiry into the Prevention of Child Abuse (1996) concluded that:

> The catalogue of abuse in residential institutions is appalling. It includes physical assault and sexual abuse; emotional abuse; unacceptable deprivation of rights and privileges; inhumane treatment; poor health care and education. (p. 19)

In relation to foster care, there is perhaps more cause for optimism but little more solid a foundation of systematic knowledge on which to base it. Thomas (1995), in his review of the largely North American literature, found that 'estimates of the incidence of abuse in foster care vary considerably, not least according to the measures and definitions used' (p. 35). The same observation is made in an earlier study by Benedict *et al.* (1994). This comparative study of foster families and non-fostering families, found that although only 1.1% of all reports of abuse made involved foster families, 15% of foster families were likely to be the subject of an allegation of abuse compared to 4.1% of non-fostering families. Substantiation rates for allegations involving foster families were established at 20% overall (consistent with other studies reported by Benedict *et al.*) compared to 35% for the general population. In the UK, where no such comparative study has been undertaken, the National Foster Care Association (NFCA 1999) has resorted to quantifying the risk of sexual abuse in foster care by relating it to the proportion of adult males in the population with criminal convictions for sexual offences and noting that 'it is not unreasonable to suppose that the incidence of abuse amongst applicants [to foster] may be higher than in the general population, since it is known that vulnerable children are targeted' (p. 21). An earlier NFCA study (1995) has reported that allegations of abuse were made in 4% of foster homes, of which 22% were deemed founded but which in a further 20% of cases it was not possible to decide either way.

The apparent differential between the incidence and prevalence of abuse in foster care as opposed to residential care is also found in ChildLine's analysis of calls made to its help-lines. Of all calls received during 1996 (ChildLine 1997), 2% were from children looked after by local authorities although they make up only 0.4% of the child population of England and Wales. ChildLine estimates that this amounts to 2.3% of the population of looked after children whilst only 0.64% of the whole child population makes contact during the course of a year. Not all such calls relate to incidents of abuse, of course, and there is no corroboration of the matters reported.

From the fragmentary data available, it could be argued that child abuse is more frequent amongst children living away from home than amongst the population of children as a whole but the evidence, particularly in relation to residential care, is not strong. Whilst there remains a degree of uncertainty, or possibly even because there remains a degree of uncertainty, about how many children suffer at the hands of their carers, the case for further research, continued vigilance and direct action remains a persuasive one.

Policy issues – new optimism?

Berridge & Brodie (1996, p. 188) list no fewer than 15 'initiatives' to address problems in institutional care undertaken either by central or local government or national voluntary organisations between 1991 and 1994. Their list includes the reports of several inquiries into child abuse in children's homes but not the 18 Circulars that the DOH and Welsh Office issued between 1992 and 1996 nor the four Circulars published by the Department for Education and Employment (Utting *et al*. 1997). To this growing list should be added at least four other central government initiatives, one Act of Parliament and another White Paper and yet still more inquiry reports with an important one into child abuse in Wales (the 'Waterhouse Report') expected imminently. By any measure, the care of children looked after away from home has been a very active concern of policy-makers over the last decade. The degree of overall coherence of the policy response or its effectiveness remains in question, however.

All of these various initiatives have been taken, in the words of the *Review of Safeguards* (Utting *et al*. 1997), 'against a background of continuing contraction, fragmentation and stress' (p. 13) in residential care services (DOH 1998) and profound changes in the nature and organisation of foster care (Butler & Owens 1993, Butler 2000). It is beyond the scope of this chapter to explore in any depth how the population of looked after children has changed over recent years, or to enumerate in detail all of the areas that have been subject to scrutiny as part of this extraordinary policy interest. Our focus is on institutional *abuse* rather than institutional *care* although, taking the widest possible definition of the former, the distinction may be considered to be one without a difference.

For our purposes, particular attention will be paid to matters of staffing, strategic planning across the range of child care services and to the question of regulations. The staffing of children's homes has perhaps received the most concentrated attention of policy-makers since the renewal of interest in institutional care in the early 1990s. Utting (Social Services Inspectorate 1991) addressed 10 of his 37 recommendations to ensuring a better motivated, rewarded, trained and managed workforce than that which he found to be actually looking after children 'in the public care'. Following the report of the activities of Frank Beck, a subsequent report, *Choosing to Care* (the 'Warner Report') (DOH 1992), recommended particular procedural safeguards in relation to the recruitment, selection and appointment of staff to residential institutions. The DOH wrote to all local authorities urging them to implement 22 of the Report's recommendations immediately and the remaining 19 in the following year. Six years later, the 'Safeguards Review' (Utting *et al*. 1997) urged their adoption by all organisations caring for children away from home. It also recommended the wider publication and adoption of the *Code of Practice for the Employment of Residential Workers* (DOH 1995) produced by the Support Force for Children's Residential Care that was set up as a result of the first Utting Report.

The importance of these and other policy initiatives aimed specifically at training (see Lane 1994) and at pay and conditions (Local Government Management Board 1992) in producing a more capable and effective workforce should be self-evident. Where staff are ill-prepared, lacking in professional status and deficient in the necessary skills, not only is the general standard of care they are able to provide likely to fall below the required level, but so too are they likely to respond inappropriately in stressful situations or to be influenced by the 'expert knowledge' of others.

Similarly, one might anticipate that by filtering out those who pose an obvious threat, children in institutional settings are safer from their predatory attentions. One should note, however, that Frank Beck was the subject of several complaints against him whilst in post and yet received a positive reference from one of his line managers, even after his conduct had become a cause for concern. Hence in 1997, three of the six chapters dealing with staffing in the 'Safeguards Review' (Utting *et al.* 1997) are aimed at refining the process of 'dealing with unsuitable people'. The implementation of the Protection of Children Act 1999, almost a decade after Kincora and Crookham Court, and just ahead of the Waterhouse Report, should ensure that information about 'unsuitable people' is better coordinated and communicated.

As well as finding themselves in the care of 'unsuitable people', children may also find themselves in unsuitable homes which seek to serve too many purposes and which try to accommodate too wide a range of needs. The infrastructure of residential care has been steadily eroding (DOH 1998) as a consequence of the lack of any effective strategic planning. Utting's original report (Utting 1991) and the contemporaneous Welsh Office equivalent (Welsh Office 1991) made a strong case for retaining and developing a broad range of placement provision to ensure adequate choice. In the 'Safeguards Review' he describes such choice as a 'fundamental safeguard' (Utting 1991, p. 2). It is only in the context of a range of provision, differentiated by purpose and function, that individual homes meet individual needs and thus become 'safe places for children' (Utting 1991, p. 2). As well as providing opportunities for raising the quality of care overall, the development of placement choice reduces the risk of mixing abusing and abused young people (see Utting 1991, p. 35, DOH 1999*b*, pp. 85, 92) and allows for the targeted training of appropriate staff.

As with matters of staffing, progress towards a broader range of provision has been slow. Revisiting children's homes previously visited in 1985, Berridge & Brodie (1998) found inter alia:

...the numbers of residential places in the three local authorities had dwindled by three-quarters ... Few of the homes in the new study had Statements of Purpose and those that had been written were often general and out of date. Most homes had not developed any strategy to meet the needs of girls, ethnic minorities or care leavers ... compared to the 1985 sample, there were fewer homes in the 'good' and 'poor' categories and more that were average ... (p. 69)

Both staffing matters and strategic planning, as well as other substantive areas of policy scrutiny (line management; organisational structures; quality of care matters such as health and education; working relationships with parents etc.), have found expression in the form of various sets of guidance and regulations governing the practice of institutional care. Indeed, the amount of such regulation and guidance, described in the 'Safeguards Review' as 'formidable in volume and complexity' (Berridge & Brodie 1998, p. 172), is now recognised as a problem in itself and in need of synthesis and simplification. Far from being a 'tool for practitioners', guidance and regulation is more a 'subject for their research' (Berridge & Brodie 1998, p. 172). Nonetheless, there are some very clear examples of how legislation, regulation and guidance can focus and improve practice (see for example Chapter 4, Utting *et al.* 1997 and the effect on the regulation of boarding schools of improvements to the Children Act 1989 s. 87 requirements). Indeed, Utting's final view (Utting *et al.* 1997) is a positive, if not necessarily wholly unambiguous one. He notes that (p. 17, my emphasis):

Regulations, statutory guidance and other forms of advice provide a full and detailed *web* of safeguards.

Undoubtedly, much progress has been made in establishing a framework to protect children living away from home over recent years, as the above examples show, but that progress has been uneven and there is still some way to go. In part, that is a consequence of the way in which such policy initiatives have arisen. Essentially they have been reactive, incremental and managerialist (see Dyson, Chapter 28, in this volume). This is an echo of how the child protection agenda generally has been driven by the revelations of poor practice contained in the various public inquiries into child care and the 'scandals' that they describe. The role of the public inquiry report in simplifying complex phenomena and compressing them into a single, linear, narrative and of locating structural deficiencies in the failures of individuals or local systems, is too broad a topic for this chapter (see Hallett 1989, Corby *et al.* 1998, Butler & Drakeford 2000) but one must acknowledge that they provide a very particular filter through which institutional life has been viewed. They serve, even in aggregate, to reinforce the idea that the problems of institutional care are sporadic, acute and somehow peculiar to the institutional world. This separation of the institutional abuse of children from the wider societal context in which it appears mirrors the separation of specific institutions and their residents from their wider communities.

One should note also that most of the above policy developments took place in a political climate that was inimical both to the interests of children and to the development of public welfare provision (Lister 1990, Oldfield & Autumn 1993, Oppenheim & Harker 1996). Some of this may now be changing. Recent policy initiatives, specifically, the 'Quality Protects' agenda, *Modernising Social Services* (DOH 1998*b*) and the *Government's Objectives for Children's Services* (DOH 1999*a*) do provide evidence of a degree of 'joined-up' thinking, based on the idea of social inclusion.

The *Government's Objectives for Children's Services* specifically links *prospective* targets for improvement in areas relevant to the better care of children living away from home to broader policy initiatives to tackle poverty, educational disadvantage and health inequalities (paras 9–12). These targets, incorporating elements from the 'Quality Protects Programme' and from *Modernising Social Services*, carry the prospect of increased resourcing and strict accountability based on performance. They include:

- reducing the number of changes of placement for children (para. 1.2)
- improving the educational achievements and health outcomes of looked after children, especially those from ethnic minorities (paras 4.1, 4.2, 4.4)
- improving leaving care services (paras 5.1, 5.2)
- improving assessment processes (para. 7)
- ensuring effective complaints mechanisms (para. 8)
- ensuring compliance with regulations (para. 9)
- ensuring that all residential workers are adequately trained for the job (para. 10.1).

It is too early to say whether such an approach gives grounds for any 'new' optimism.

Implications for practice – quantity protects?

The revised version of *Working Together* (DOH 1999*b*) will be enormously influential in setting out the practice agenda that follows both specifically from the latest policy initiatives and from the experience of the last 10 years. This core guidance, at least in its draft form, devotes a whole section to 'child protection in specific circumstances', including children living away from home. *Working Together* recognises the importance of locating the safety of such children in the wider context of other child protection measures and in terms of the overall quality of care provided (DOH 1999*b*, 6.2–6.4). It also sets out 'basic safeguards' (p. 84) against which any specific child protection measures might be set. These basic safeguards include several elements already familiar from the literature and recent policy developments. For example, a safe placement is one where:

- children feel valued and respected and their self-esteem is promoted
- there is an openness on the part of the institution to the external world
- staff and carers are trained in all aspects of safeguarding children
- recruitment and selection procedures are rigorous.

The revised *Working Together* also provides a useful protocol for managing the various strands of an investigation (child protection enquiries, any police investigation and the employer's disciplinary proceedings) into any allegation of abuse where the child is living away from home. But in order for any investigation to commence, the abuse has to be recognised or at least suspected and there are aspects of the dynamics of institutional care that can inhibit this.

Westcott (1991) identifies four such barriers: the lack of procedures/policies for reporting and investigating a complaint of institutional abuse; a tendency to see institutional abuse as the failure of an individual member of staff, not the institution; the 'closed' nature of institutions and the belief system surrounding institutions which rest on the assumption that out-of-home care is, almost by definition, of a higher standard of care than children would otherwise receive in their parental homes. Although they now appear a little dated, to a degree such barriers to the discovery of institutional abuse may still exert an influence and practitioners will need to be mindful of them. To this list might be added the difficulties staff who 'blow the whistle' have to face (Durkin 1982, Hunt 1998); the studied deviousness of the paedophile (Wyre 1996); the insidious effects of institutional racism (Marrett 1991); and the de-motivating effect of the kind of dysfunctional cultures that can develop in an institutional setting (Whitaker *et al.* 1998; see also Glisson & Hemmelgarn 1998 for an account of the positive advantages of well-functioning organisational cultures). By way of a balance, however, one might note also the devastating consequences that can arise for staff who are wrongfully accused of being an abuser. These can be particularly acute for foster carers (Carbino 1991, 1992). One possible practice response to the inadequate support they usually receive from social workers in such circumstances might be for carers to establish their own network of personal support in anticipation of such an event (Nixon 1997).

The greatest challenge facing practice, however, is one that lies at the heart of the abusive process and which is so easily accentuated in the semi-closed world of out-of-home care. Central to the very concept of abuse is the relative powerlessness of children. It is their relative powerlessness that makes them vulnerable to abuse and which prevents them acting for themselves or engaging others to end it. This powerlessness is deeply embedded in prevailing contemporary constructions of childhood, which generally conceive of childhood in transitional or deficit terms (see James & Prout 1991, Archard 1993). Child protection practice is uniquely prone to regarding children and young people *only* as vulnerable. They are, but they are also capable of being effective authors of their own biographies. Any practice initiative that seeks to truly protect children must seek also to empower them. Any convention, declaration, policy, procedure or protocol that does not have both as its means as well as its ends, increasing the capacity of children and young people to speak and act for themselves is unlikely to prove as effective as one that does (Cloke & Davies 1995).

Butler (1997) and Butler & Williamson (1999) have noted how it is perfectly possible for child protection processes to be entirely driven by adults' priorities without the active involvement of children themselves. Butler & Williamson (1999) have described a model of child protection practice which seeks to place the child as the focus of activity and attention. This model is built on paying close attention to the child's own account of their experiences and the meanings that they attach to them, ascertaining and differentiating between the reasons children seek help from adults, checking out the adult's mandate to take action from the child and communicating openly, honestly and fully with children in the context of a reliable and compassionate professional relationship. It is perhaps in these long-established core components of the social work task that there lies the only real basis for optimism. On its own, quantity of regulation does not protect, only quality of practice.

Summary

The abuse of children living away from home is a complex phenomenon. It includes a wide range of behaviours that take place in a variety of settings, from large boarding schools to the private homes of foster carers. It is difficult to set clear conceptual boundaries between discrete forms of institutional abuse and wider deficiencies in the quality of care provided for children and young people. It has been held that the wider child care system, once extended beyond its capacity to deliver, can directly be abusive or create the circumstances in which abuse can take place. Certain regimes or practices can also be abusive, and institutional abuse can sometimes involve the organised activities of multiple or individual abusers.

Certain characteristics of institutional care, of whatever type, make children particularly vulnerable to abuse, namely the children's relative isolation, invisibility and powerlessness.

Perhaps in part because of the difficulties in defining the phenomenon, there is no structured knowledge base in this field and current estimates of incidence and prevalence are unreliable. Nonetheless, sufficient evidence has been revealed through inquiries into identified abuse, particularly in relation to residential care, for the phenomenon to be recognised as significant and to have created a substantial policy interest over recent years. Most often in the light of evidence refracted through the very particular prism of a scandal, policy and practice initiatives have lacked overall coherence. There is some evidence that a more proactive and integrated approach to policy formulation is now being pursued.

Practice initiatives which challenge prevailing contemporary constructions of childhood as merely a transitional phase, or which counter professional ideologies that rest on deficit models of childhood, can help reduce the likelihood of abuse in the first instance and manage the consequences in the interests of the child when it occurs.

Conclusion

The Poor Law Commissioners did not allow the Bedford Union to proceed in the way in which they had planned. They recognised that providing the workhouse child with every means possible, including the ability to write, was the only way to enable them to grow up and play a full and productive part in the life of the community. In fact, the Poor Law Commissioners worked assiduously and with some considerable success to improve the conditions of the pauper child.

Indeed, the lasting lesson of history is that the best protection against institutional abuse is an unequivocal political commitment to provide the best care for children and young people who have to live away from home. Beyond that, regulation and guidance have an important part to play and there is a momentum in policy circles at the moment that could make irreversible changes in the way provision for such young people is made. Forms of practice are being revised, as they always will be. But there are dangers too in investing all our ambitions in the actions of others. As the poet T S Eliot has noted, one should not put one's faith in 'systems so perfect that no one will need to be good' (*Choruses from the Rock*, 1934).

At the heart of any healthy system, as much as at the heart of a neglectful or abusive system, are the actions and beliefs of individual practitioners. Institutional abuse begins and can only be ended there.

Acknowledgement

Special thanks to Pat Smail for her invaluable help in searching for and finding much of the material on which this chapter is based.

Annotated further reading

Utting W, Department of Health, Welsh Office 1997 People like us – the report of the review of the safeguards for children living away from home. The Stationery Office, London

Department of Health (DOH) 1998 Caring for children away from home – messages from research. John Wiley, Chichester

Both of these, taken together, provide a contemporary and comprehensive account of out-of-home care, particularly residential care. The first provides a general context as well as some specific accounts of the phenomenon of institutional abuse and has been very influential in the development of subsequent policy. The second provides a more detailed account of some of the practice issues that need to be addressed in order to improve the overall quality of out-of-home provision.

National Commission of Inquiry into the Prevention of Child Abuse 1996 Childhood matters. The Stationery Office, London

This provides a general context in which to locate the phenomenon of institutional abuse as a form of abuse and focuses particular attention on the development of the 'child-friendly community' and 'child-centered professional'.

ChildLine 1997 Children living away from home. ChildLine, London

Kirkwood A 1993 The Leicestershire inquiry 1992. Leicestershire County Council, Leicester

Levy A, Kahan B 1991 The pindown experience and the protection of children. Staffordshire County Council, Stafford

Any one of these would serve to illustrate the process and the consequences of institutional abuse. The two inquiry reports are also useful in demonstrating how the public inquiry produces a very particular version of the 'truth' of abuse.

Cloke C, Davies M (eds) 1995 Participation and empowerment in child protection. Pitman, London

This edited collection contains some useful examples of how children and young people can be successfully engaged in their own protection as well as some theoretical account of the importance of doing so.

References

Archard D 1993 Children: rights and childhood. Routledge, London

Ayres M 1989 Sexual abuse in institutional care. Sexual Abuse Newsletter 6 (1): 7

Benedict M I, Zuravin S, Brandt D, Abbey H 1994 Types and frequency of child maltreatment by family foster care providers in an urban population. Child Abuse and Neglect 18 (7): 577–585

Berridge D, Brodie I 1996 Residential child care in England and Wales – the inquiries and after. In: Hill M, Aldgate J (eds) Child welfare services – developments in law, policy, practice and research. Jessica Kingsley, London

Berridge D, Brodie I 1998 Children's homes revisited. In: DOH Caring for children away from home – messages from research. John Wiley, Chichester

Bibby P 1996 Definitions and recent history. In: Bibby P (ed) organised abuse – the current debate. Arena/Ashgate, Aldershot

Blatt E R I 1992 Factors associated with child abuse and neglect in residential care settings. Child and Youth Services Review 15: 493–517

Bloom R B 1992 When staff members sexually abuse children in residential care. Child Welfare LXXI (2): 131–145

Brown E, Bullock R, Hobson C, Little M 1998 Making residential care work – structure and culture in children's homes. In: DOH Caring for children away from home – messages from research. John Wiley, Chichester

Bullock R, Little M, Milham S 1993 Residential care for children – a review of the research. HMSO, London

Butler I 1996 Safe? Involving children in child protection. In: Butler I, Shaw I (eds) A case of neglect? Children's experiences and the sociology of childhood. Avebury, Aldershot

Butler I 1997 Used and abused? Engaging the child in child protection. In: Pithouse A, Williamson H (eds) Engaging the user. Venture Press, Birmingham

Butler I 2000 Foster care. In: Howe D (ed) Encyclopaedia of social work. Blackwells, London

Butler I, Drakeford M 2000 Making public policy – scandal and the public inquiry. MacMillan, London

Butler I, Owens D 1993 Canaries among sparrows: ideas of the family and the practice of family care. Community Alternatives: International Journal of Family Care 5 (1): 25–43

Butler I, Williamson H 1994 Children speak: children, trauma and social work. Longman, London

Butler I, Williamson H 1999 Children's views of their involvement in child protection processes. In: Shemmings D (ed) Involving children in family support and child protection processes. The Stationery Office, London

Campbell-Smith M 1983 The school – liberator or censurer? Child Abuse and Neglect 7: 329–337

Carbino R 1991 Advocacy for foster families in the united states facing child abuse allegations: how social agencies and foster parents are responding to the problem. Child Welfare LXX (2): 131–149

Carbino R 1992 Policy and practice for response to foster families when child abuse or neglect is reported. Child Welfare LXXI (6): 497–509

ChildLine 1997 Children living away from home. ChildLine, London

Cloke C, Davies M (eds) 1995 Participation and empowerment in child protection. Pitman, London

Corby B, Doig T, Roberts V 1998 Inquiries into child abuse. Journal of Social Welfare and Family Law 20 (4): 377–395

Crosse S B, Kaye E, Ratnofsky A C 1993 A report on the maltreatment of children with disabilities. National Centre on Child Abuse and Neglect, Washington DC

Department of Health (DOH) 1991 Patterns and outcomes in child placement: messages from current research. HMSO, London

Department of Health (DOH) 1992 Choosing with care – the report of the committee of inquiry into the selection, development and management of staff in children's homes. HMSO, London

Department of Health (DOH) 1995 Code of practice for the employment of residential workers. HMSO, London

Department of Health (DOH) 1998a Caring for children away from home – messages from research. John Wiley, Chichester

Department of Health (DOH) 1998b Modernising social services: promoting independence, improving protection, raising standards. Cmnd 4169. The Stationery Office, London

Department of Health (DOH) 1999a The Government's objectives for children's social services. The Stationery Office, London

Department of Health (DOH) 1999b Working together to safeguard children – a guide to inter-agency working. Consultation Draft. The Stationery Office, London

Department of Health and Social Security (DHSS) 1985 Social work decisions in child care: recent research findings and their implications. HMSO, London

Doran C, Brannan C 1996 Institutional abuse. In: Bibby P C (ed) Organised abuse – the current debate. Arena/Ashgate, Aldershot

Durkin R 1982 No one will thank you – first thoughts on reporting institutional abuse. Child and Youth Services Review IV (1–2): 109–113

Gil E 1982 Institutional abuse of children in out-of-home care. In: Hanson R (ed) Institutional abuse of children and youth. The Haworth Press, New York

Glisson C, Hemmelgarn A 1998 The effects of organizational climate and interorganizational coordination on the quality and outcomes of children's service systems. Child Abuse and Neglect 22 (5): 401–421

Hallett C 1989 Child-abuse inquiries and public policy. In: Stevenson O (ed) Child abuse: professional practice and public policy. Harvester Wheatsheaf, Hemel Hempstead

Hendrick H 1994 Child welfare in England 1872–1989. Routledge, London

Heywood J S 1969 Childhood and society 100 years ago. National Children's Home, London

Home Office, Department of Health, Department of Education and Science, Welsh Office 1991 Working together under the Children Act 1989: a guide to arrangements for inter-agency cooperation for the protection of children from abuse. HMSO, London

Howard League 1995 Banged up, beaten up, cutting up. Howard League, London

Howard League 1996 Lessons for policy and practice on 15-year-olds in prison. Troubleshooter Project Report. Howard League, London

Hunt G (ed) 1998 Whistleblowing in the social services: public accountability and professional practice. Arnold, Aldershot

James A, Prout A 1991 A new paradigm for the sociology of childhood? Provenance, promise and problems. In: James A, Prout A (eds) Constructing and reconstructing childhood: contemporary issues in the sociological study of childhood. The Falmer Press, London

Jones J 1994 Towards an understanding of power relationships in institutional abuse. Early Childhood Development 100: 69–76

Kelly L 1992 The connection between disability and child abuse: a review of the research evidence. Child Abuse Review 1 (3): 157–167

Kirkwood A 1993 The Leicestershire Inquiry 1992. Leicestershire County Council, Leicester

La Fontaine J S 1993 Defining organized sexual abuse. Child Abuse Review 2 (4): 223–231

Lane D 1994 An independent review of the residential child care initiative. CCETSW, London

Levy A, Kahan B 1991 The Pindown experience and the protection of children. Staffordshire County Council, Stafford

Liebling A, Krarup H 1994 Suicide attempts in prison. Home Office Research Bulletin No. 36. Home Office, London

Lister R 1990 The exclusive society – citizenship and the poor. CPAG, London

Local Government Management Board 1992 The quality of care: report of the residential staff's inquiry. LGMB, London

Marrett M 1991 Raw deal for black children in care. Community Care (Inside) 28 February vii–viii

Millham S, Bullock R, Hosie K, Haak M 1986 Lost in care: the family contacts of children in care. Gower, Aldershot

Moss M 1990 Abuse in the child care system – a pilot study by the National Association of Young People in Care. NAYPIC, London

National Commission of Inquiry into the Prevention of Child Abuse 1996 Childhood matters. The Stationery Office, London

National Society for Prevention of Cruelty to Children 1995 So who are we supposed to trust now? Responding to abuse in care: the experiences of young people. NSPCC/Safe and Sound Partnership, London

Nixon S 1997 The limits of support in foster care. British Journal of Social Work 27: 913–930

Oldfield N, Autumn C S 1993 The cost of a child. CPAG, London

Oppenheim C, Harker I 1996 Poverty – the facts, 3rd edn. CPAG, London

Parker R, Ward H, Jackson S, *et al.* 1991 Assessing outcomes in child care. HMSO, London

Pinchbeck I, Hewitt M 1973 Children in English society. Routledge & Kegan Paul, London

Powers J L, Mooney A, Nunno M 1990 Institutional abuse – a review of the literature. Journal of Child and Youth Care 4: 81–95

Rindfleisch N, Rabb J 1989 How much of a problem is resident mistreatment in child welfare institutions? Child Abuse and Neglect 15: 249–260

Shaughnessy M F 1984 Institutional child abuse. Children and Youth Services Review 6: 311–318

Sinclair I, Gibbs I 1998 Children's homes – a study in diversity. In: DOH Caring for children away from home – messages from research. John Wiley, Chichester

Sloan J 1988 Professional abuse. Child Abuse Review 2: 7–8

Sobsey D, Varnhagen C 1988 Sexual abuse and exploitation of people with disabilities: a study of the victims. Unpublished paper cited in Westcott H L 1991 Institutional abuse of children – from research to policy – a review. NSPCC, London

Solomons G, Abel C M, Epsley S 1981 A community development approach to the prevention of institutional and societal child maltreatment. Child Abuse and Neglect 5: 135–140

Stein M 1993 The abuses and uses of residential care: surviving childhood adversity. Social Services Press, Dublin

Thomas G 1990 Institutional child abuse – the making and prevention of an un-problem. Journal of Child and Youth Care 4 (6): 1–22

Thomas N 1995 Allegations of child abuse in local authority care. Practice 7 (3): 35–44

Utting W, Department of Health, Welsh Office 1997 People like us – the report of the review of the safeguards for children living away from home. The Stationery Office, London

Utting W, Social Services Inspectorate 1991 Children in the public care – a review of residential care. HMSO, London

Westcott H L 1991 Institutional abuse of children – from research to policy – a review. NSPCC, London

Westcott H I, Clement M 1992 Experience of child abuse in residential care and educational placements: results of a survey. NSPCC, London

Whitaker D, Archer L, Hicks L 1998 Working in children's home, challenges and complexities. In: DOH Caring for children away from home – messages from research. John Wiley, Chichester

Wyre R 1996 The mind of the paedophile. In: Bibby P C (ed) Organised abuse – the current debate. Arena/Ashgate, Aldershot

2 MANAGING THE PROCESS OF CHILD PROTECTION

Working Together to Safeguard Children (Department of Health (DOH) 1999) identifies a series of stages in child protection cases: initial assessment and enquiry; further assessment and planning; and implementation of planning for the child. The boundaries between these stages are flexible, but the chapters in this section can mainly be said to address aspects of the structures and processes of the first two stages which have been put in place in the UK in order to try and ensure the protection of children. Thus, the chapters analyse the frameworks (such as that provided by the law), the structures (such as joint investigations or case conferences) and the processes (such as assessment, the involvement of other professionals, and inter-professional cooperation) which have been developed for managing the stages of intervention in cases involving the protection of children.

In no other country in the world, with the possible exception of North America, have the legal and policy structures involved in child protection been so closely scrutinised as they have in this country. The discussion in the chapters in this section therefore reflects the rapid changes that have taken place in recent years, the detailed policy guidelines that have emerged, and the considerable amount of research that has been, and is still being undertaken.

In the first edition of the *Handbook* (1995) we commented that partly as a result of this unprecedented level of scrutiny, practice in many of the areas of child protection considered in this section was changing rapidly, and that this posed certain problems for those attempting to give a 'state of the art' account. However, where this was the case, the authors indicated areas in which they considered practice most likely to alter in the foreseeable future. The ensuing period, leading up to this second edition, has, we judge, seen fewer changes than the preceding one. Nonetheless, two major revisions to practice guidance have recently been produced, *Working Together to Safeguard Children* (DOH 1999) and *Framework for the Assessment of Children in Need and their Families* (DOH 2000). These incorporate some of the lessons learned and some of the modifications which experience of working for nearly a decade under the Children Act 1989 suggest are necessary for effective practice. Many of the chapters, including new ones by Bell on case conferences and Rouse on the role of the health visitor in child protection, have been written in the light of this new guidance.

The ordering of the chapters loosely reflects the sequential stages of the child protection process, beginning with two chapters concerned with the frameworks of child protection. In the opening chapter, Christina Lyon focuses on the civil legal framework for protecting children, considering in some detail the provisions available to protect children under Parts IV and V of the Children Act 1989 and the chapter has been brought up to date by incorporating the most recent cases. Importantly, however, she outlines the main differences between the law in

England and other jurisdictions in the UK. She also highlights some of the potential implications of the Human Rights Act 1998, which is likely to have an increasing impact on family law in the future.

In Chapter 11, Corinne Wattam presents a critical review of policy and practice in relation to making referrals and conducting joint investigations. She reviews some of the research which should inform decision-making in the process of making enquiries, discusses six areas of policy which are relevant to the investigative process, including the new version of *Working Together* (DOH 2000), before considering the practice implications of research and policy.

In Chapter 12, Margaret Adcock discusses the complex issue of assessment in child protection, describing the investigation and assessment model recommended in the statutory guidance, both *Working Together to Safeguard Children* (DOH 1999) and the *Framework for the Assessment of Children in Need and their Families* (DOH 2000) which replaces the original 'Orange Book' guidance on assessment. She considers some of the practice issues involved in the process, linking these to relevant research findings.

A rather different kind of framework is that considered by Brian Corby in Chapter 13. He discusses inter-agency coordination, the merits and demerits of current inter-agency arrangements and reflects on the broader issues to be considered about this type of coordinated activity, such as the little that is known about the effectiveness of our current systems.

Following the likely sequence of child protection intervention, Margaret Bell's chapter on case conferences comes next. In it she considers the role of the initial case conference, which the new *Working Together* guidance (DOH 1999) continues to see as pivotal within the child protection system. Although she highlights certain encouraging developments (for example the development of frameworks for pre- and post-registration practice which may be more welfare-based than hitherto), she is concerned about the ambiguous nature of the tasks and functions of the conference. Her conclusions are perhaps rather less positive than Olive Stevenson, whose original chapter in the *Handbook* Bell's replaces and who commented then that inter-professional work in child protection case conferences is 'light years ahead of other comparable situations that require cooperative endeavour across agencies'. It may be worth reminding ourselves of the achievements, as well as the limitations, of current policies and practice.

We have added in this edition a new chapter on the role of health visitors, which, considering their important role in child protection work, seemed an omission from the first edition of the *Handbook*. Sue Rouse examines their role within the broader remit of public health nursing practice, and explores the nature and extent of health visitors' involvement together with some of the difficulties and dilemmas involved.

In Chapter 16, Anne Peake addresses the concerns of teachers, whom she considers to have a key role in monitoring situations where there are concerns that a child may be the subject of abuse, and sets out a detailed monitoring schedule that teachers in primary and secondary schools could adapt for use in their own schools. She also presents a pro forma that has been developed for use by teachers to ensure that standardised information is collected and provided for initial referrals of cases where child abuse is suspected.

The three remaining chapters in this section focus on that point in the process where court proceedings are being implemented. Ann Head, in her chapter, considers developments in the role of the guardian under the Children Act, recent research studies on the role of the guardian, policy issues arising from these and finally, the implications for practice. Mary Lane and Terry Walsh focus predominantly on court craft in their chapter, considering the preparation of evidence, the role of the expert witness, the use of research findings in evidence and the skills involved in giving evidence in court proceedings. In the final chapter in this section, John Williams considers the impact of the criminal justice process on child victims of crime and the policy issues behind the law, and he explains the implications of these for the various professionals and individuals who have contact with child witnesses in the criminal courts.

10

Child protection and the civil law

Christina M. Lyon

INTRODUC-TION

This chapter considers the legal provisions in England and Wales with occasional notes on the relevant provisions in Scotland and Northern Ireland, all of which are intended to provide the UK jurisdictions with the frameworks within which a range of State and voluntary agencies are expected to work together to prevent children suffering or being at risk of suffering significant harm at the hands of those looking after or caring for them. As far as England and Wales are concerned, these provisions are currently contained within one piece of legislation – the Children Act 1989 (and its consequent Rules of Court, Regulations and Guidance) – although it remains to be seen whether the Welsh Assembly, as constituted by the Government of Wales Act 1998, will in due course enact comparable legislation specific to Wales. The Children Act 1989 was implemented in full in both England and Wales on 14 October 1991.

The relevant provisions for Scotland are principally contained within the Children (Scotland) Act 1995 and its consequent Rules, Regulations and Guidance, although some parts of the Social Work (Scotland) Act 1968 remain relevant. The whole of the Children (Scotland) Act 1995 is now in force, with the private law provisions mainly coming into force on 1 November 1996 and the provisions relating to child protection on 1 April 1997 (see Part II Children (Scotland) Act 1995). Scotland, of course, has a completely different process known as the 'children's hearing system' in which it deals with all aspects of public law relating to the welfare of children including therefore both civil and criminal law. In this respect, the Scottish system is therefore very different. Many of the provisions, however, contained in the Children (Scotland) Act 1995 are very similar to those contained within the Children Act 1989 for England and Wales and the Children (Northern Ireland) Order 1995. The principal way in which the Scottish system differs is in the use of different names for some of the orders, e.g. 'Child Protection Order' instead of 'Emergency Protection Order', and also, and very importantly, in the range of disposals in relation to the child which the Scottish children's hearing system may make (see s.70 Children (Scotland) Act 1995).

The Children (Northern Ireland) Order 1995, which came into force in Northern Ireland on 1 October 1996, contains almost identical provisions with regard to the range of orders which may be made and uses the exact same terminology for the orders. The principal difference with regard to Northern Ireland is that the responsibilities, which in England, Wales and Scotland are exercised by local authority social services departments, are in Northern Ireland exercised by Health and Social Services Boards and Trusts under the direction of the Northern Ireland Department of Health and Social Services. The Northern Ireland Order uses exactly the same terminology and references to orders as does the comparable legislation for England and Wales. As was the case with the Children Act 1989 in England and Wales, detailed Rules of Court, Regulations and Guidance have been introduced as a result of the Children (Northern Ireland) Order 1995 (see Department of Health and Social Services for Northern Ireland 1999).

Inevitably in this chapter, primary attention will focus upon the explanation of the relevant statutory provisions contained in the Children Act 1989 as it applies in England and Wales, and on judicial interpretation of the provisions by courts in England and Wales. Since so many of the relevant provisions relating to child protection in the three different pieces of legislation are so similar, however, it is to be hoped that such analysis will inevitably throw some light on the interpretation of comparable provisions in each of the (currently) three different jurisdictions. Hereafter in this chapter therefore, as well as making reference to the relevant provisions in the Children Act 1989, reference will also be made to the comparable provisions in the Children (Scotland) Act 1995 and The Children (Northern Ireland) Order 1995.

When the Children Act 1989 was first introduced into the House of Lords by the then Lord Chancellor, Lord Mackay of Clashfern, it was described as 'the most comprehensive and far-reaching reform of child law, which has come before Parliament in living memory'. Such has certainly turned out to be the case, not only with that Act, but also with the comparable provisions for Scotland and Northern Ireland. Nevertheless, if that was an apt description of that piece of legislation, it applies even more to the implications of the enactment of the Human Rights Act 1998, and its consequent implementation across the whole of the UK from 2 October 2000. Because of the relevant Acts of Parliament devolving government to both Wales and Scotland, the potential huge impact on the laws of the UK effected by the Human Rights Act 1998 have already been felt. The Scotland Act 1998 and the Government of Wales Act 1998, respectively, introduced the Scottish Parliament and the Welsh Assembly into those two countries on 1 July 1999. Both Acts took effect on that date and both contained provisions, in s.106 Government of Wales Act 1998, and s.100 Scotland Act 1998 providing that Welsh and Scottish citizens may bring actions pursuant to the European Convention on the Protection of Human Rights and Fundamental Freedoms within the Welsh and Scottish Courts. Scotland has already experienced a flurry of activity in its courts related to the European Convention, including, as this chapter goes to press, a challenge to the legality of child protection legislation. The challenge has apparently been made on the basis of a breach of Article 6 of the European Convention which guarantees an individual a right to a fair trial in respect of any determination of his or her civil rights and obligations as well as a right to a fair trial within any criminal process.

The Human Rights Act 1998 extends to all UK citizens the right to rely upon the European Convention in any proceedings which come before any British courts and further requires various agencies including health authorities, social services departments and the police to act in accordance with the rights conferred by that Convention. Space does not permit a lengthy explanation here but various Articles of the Convention will assume critical importance in child protection cases. These will include: Article 3, 'a right to be protected from cruel, inhuman or degrading treatment or punishment'; Article 5, 'a right to liberty and security of person'; Article 6, 'the right of every person to a fair and public hearing within a reasonable time by an independent and impartial tribunal established by law of any determination of an individual's civil rights and obligations or of any criminal charge against him'; Article 8, 'the right of every person to respect for his private and family life, his home and his correspondence, and further that there shall be no interference by a public authority with the exercise of this right except such as in accordance with the law and is necessary in a democratic society in the interests of national security, public safety or the economic well-being of the country for the prevention of disorder or crime, for the protection of health or morals, or for the protection of the rights and freedoms of others'; Article 9, 'the right to freedom of thought, conscience and religion; which includes the freedom to change one's religion or belief and freedom, either alone or in community with others and in public or private, to manifest one's religion or belief in worship, teaching, practice and observance, such right being subject to the same limitations as those governing the right to respect for private and family life'; and finally, Article 14 provides that 'the enjoyment of the rights and freedoms set forth in this Convention shall be secured without discrimination on any grounds such as sex, race, colour, language, religion, political or other opinion, national or social origin, association with a national minority, property, birth or *other status*'.

As can be seen from a very brief perusal of just a few of the Articles which may be deemed to be relevant to the issue of child protection, the implication of the guaranteeing of these rights by the implementation of the Human Rights Act 1998 on 2 October 2000 means that any agencies involved in the sphere of child protection must henceforward ensure that their actions do not breach the fundamental rights secured to citizens, including, it must be emphasised, all children, under the Convention as implemented by the Human Rights Act 1998. Those therefore who are working in the child protection arena would be well advised to access the Core Guidance for Public Authorities: A New Era of Rights and Responsibilities, published by the Home Office on the Home Office Government website and they should be aware that all Government departments are currently reviewing legislation and procedures for which they are responsible in order to check their compliance with the relevant Convention rights. The Core Guidance indicates that all staff will need to be trained in an awareness of the Convention Rights (see para. 81, Human Rights Act – Core Guidance for Public Authorities: A New Era of Rights and Responsibilities). Wherever possible therefore, readers will be alerted to situations in which current law and procedures may conflict with the rights guaranteed under the Convention and where practitioners will have to be particularly alive to the issue of checking that their own individual practice complies with the demands of the Convention.

The Children Act 1989 and the comparable provisions in Scotland and Northern Ireland, have, in almost 10 years in the case of the Children Act 1989, generated much mythology around their provisions and interpretation in law and in practice. The Children Act 1989 deals with a great deal, though by no means all, of the civil family law relating to children in England and Wales. The same is true of the comparable pieces of legislation in Scotland and Northern Ireland. Adoption law, although amended by small parts of the Children Act 1989 (see s.85 and Sched. 10), remains a separate civil code, as it does in the other jurisdictions, and children are subject to a vast plethora of other civil law statutory provisions and case law which impinge upon their lives in many different ways, again in all three jurisdictions, such as Education, Child Abduction and Child Support legislation.

Except for minor provisions amending the orders which may be made in respect of children in criminal proceedings under the Children and Young Persons' Act 1969 (s.90 and Sched. 15), and the criteria that must be satisfied before secure accommodation orders may be made (s.25), the Children Act 1989 does not deal in any way with the criminal justice system. Where, pursuant to a joint police and social services investigation in England and Wales, a child is believed to have suffered or to be at risk of suffering significant harm, within the meaning of the Children Act 1989 (s.31(2)(a) and (b), the decision whether or not to prosecute the adult or juvenile perpetrator is one for the public authority charged with making such decisions within the criminal justice system, the

Crown Prosecution Service. (The position of the child victim in the criminal justice system is considered in detail by John Williams in Chapter 16). There is, however, now a relationship between the provisions of the Crime and Disorder Act 1998 in England and Wales and the Children Act 1989, as a result of new orders introduced by the 1998 legislation. Thus the old criminal 'care orders', abolished by the Children Act 1989 reappear in the Crime and Disorder Act 1998 as the new 'supervision orders with a residence requirement', and there are further inter-relationships between civil care orders made under the Children Act 1989 on the basis of the child being beyond parental control and orders such as the new parenting order, the new child safety order, anti-social behaviour orders and sex offender orders available under the Crime and Disorder Act 1998 (see Gelsthorpe & Morris 1999).

This chapter therefore focuses entirely on the civil legal framework in the three jurisdictions for protecting children. It would, however, be wrong to confine ourselves to thinking in this area solely of the civil justice system, since the three pieces of legislation go much further, at least in their underlying philosophies, than merely to define the terms upon which access to the courts may be sought (see Department of Health (DOH) 1989). Thus, as will be seen, there are provisions expressly designed to foster the development of preventive strategies and approaches, principally by local authority social services departments, but also by other agencies (see s.17 and Sched. 2, Part I, para. 1, Children Act 1989, s.22 Children (Scotland) Act 1995 and Art. 18 and Sched. 2 Children (Northern Ireland) Order 1995). (Note that it is intended to use the description 'local authority social services department' as a general term to embrace social services and agencies and authorities within local authority areas in Scotland which describe themselves variously as well as the Health and Social Services Boards and Trusts in Northern Ireland.) There are also very important provisions in Parts VI–XII of the Children Act 1989, Part II Children (Scotland) act 1995 and Parts VI–XI Children (Northern Ireland) Order 1995, governing the duty of local authority social services departments to secure the welfare and protection of children in whatever environment they are being looked after away from their own parents, whether this is in: local authority children's homes; homes run by voluntary organisations or private bodies; day nurseries or child-minding facilities; private foster places; independent boarding schools; residential health facilities run by private individuals; or in hospitals.

The legal framework provided by each of the respective pieces of legislation is contained not only in the provisions of the statutes but also in Rules of Court and in a large number of Regulations, often referred to by lawyers as 'secondary legislation'. Such Rules of Court and Regulations are as binding as the statutes themselves upon those to whom they relate and in respect of those whom they seek to protect (see, for example, the Family Proceedings Court (Children Act 1989) Rules 1991, the Children's Homes Regulations 1991 for England and Wales, the Family Proceedings Rules (Northern Ireland), the Review of Children Cases Regulations (Northern Ireland) 1996). In addition, the legal framework provided by the Acts, the relevant Rules of Court and Regulations, is further supplemented by Guidance issued by the government departments most closely involved with issues of child protection, that is to say the Department of Health, the Home Office, the Department for Education and Employment (formerly the Department of Education) for England and now also the Welsh Office and the relevant Scottish government departments.

Guidance in the three jurisdictions on the applicable Acts now runs to many volumes, including most crucially for those working in the field of child protection, *Working Together to Safeguard Children: A Guide to Inter-agency Working to Safeguard and Promote the Welfare of Children*, published in 1999 for England by the Home Office, the Department of Health, and the Department for Education and Employment (Home Office 1999) (and see comparable guidance issued in Scotland, *Protecting Children: A Shared Responsibility* (Scottish Office 1998) and in Northern Ireland, *The Children (NI) Order 1995: Regulations and Guidance, Volume 6: Co-operating to Protect Children* (Department of Health and Social Services for Northern Ireland 1996). This guidance, which was issued for England in 1999 must be part of the working Bible of any professional working in the field of child protection in England. Such guidance from government departments is issued pursuant to section 7 of the Local Authority Social Services Act 1970, which requires local authorities in their social services functions to act under the general guidance of the Secretary of State. As such, the guidance does not have the full force of legislation, but it *must* be complied with, unless local circumstances indicate exceptional reasons, which would justify a variation. It should also be noted at this stage that Circulars issued by government departments concerning the implementation of the provisions of statutes or regulations occupy a similar position. Comparable revised guidance is being prepared for Scotland at the present time and for Northern Ireland comparable guidance was issued in 1996 entitled *Cooperating to Protect Children*, which was issued as part of the series of Regulations and Guidance issued by the Northern Ireland Department for Health and Social Services pursuant to the Children (Northern Ireland) Order 1995. Again, the guidance for Scotland and Northern Ireland occupies the same status in law as the comparable English guidance *Working Together*. Responding to a number of concerns about issues of child protection affecting those children who are looked after by local authorities, the Government issued a series of Circulars through the Department of Health in 1999 associated with its *Quality Protects Programme* and a considerable number of new initiatives are being developed by local authority social services departments in response to money being made available under the *Quality Protects Programme* (see DOH 1999a).

Court structures and proceedings

England, Wales and Northern Ireland all provide for the relevant child protection proceedings to be commenced first in their lowest courts, namely the courts of summary jurisdiction, the magistrates' court. In each of these jurisdictions, proceedings for the relevant emergency orders and for care and supervision orders must initially be commenced in the magistrates' courts. If a decision is made by these courts to retain the proceedings against arguments made to have them transferred to higher courts, then there is an appeal from the magistrates' court to the district judge sitting in the county court care centres by any of the parties to the proceedings seeking the transfer of the case to a county court care centre, or alternatively to the High Court, where the party is seeking to argue that difficult issues may be advanced in the course of the case. The judge in the county court care centre can accede to the request to transfer, can substitute their own discretion and allocate the case accordingly, or may in fact decide to re-direct the case to the magistrates' court if the judge determines that the issues being raised in the case are such as can be dealt with appropriately by the magistrates and that the case is unlikely to last longer than 2 days, which is the maximum period of time the higher courts have determined a magistrates' hearing should last (see

Essex County Council v *F* [1993] 1 FLR 847). Whilst, therefore, an emergency protection order, a child assessment order and initial proceedings for an interim care or supervision order have to be begun in the magistrates' courts, once the initial stages are over, the case may be transferred up, or even down at any stage in the proceedings. Usually, where a case does raise difficult issues, the case will be transferred at an earlier stage to the appropriate level, namely the county court care centre, or the appropriate nearest High Court Family Division base (see ss.92 and 93, Children Act 1989 and the relevant Rules of Court and ss.164 and 165, Children (Northern Ireland) Order 1995). Appeals against the making or refusal to make an order in the magistrates' court lie to the High Court in England and against the order made by the country court care centre or the High Court, to the Court of Appeal (see s.94, Children Act 1989). In Northern Ireland, appeals lie against the making or refusal to make an order by the magistrates to the county court and then the High Court, and from the county court and High Court to the Court of Appeal (see s.166, Children (Northern Ireland) Order 1995). In Scotland, by contrast, applications for orders for the emergency protection of children under s.57 are made to the sheriff's courts, as are applications for child assessment orders under s.55, whereas once it has been determined that further resolution of the child situation is necessary, then a children's hearing will be arranged subject to the requirements as to the constitution and running of such hearings laid down in Part II, Chapter 2 Children (Scotland) Act 1995.

The Children Act 1989, the Children (Scotland) Act 1995 and the Children (Northern Ireland) Order 1995, together with their consequent Rules of Court, Regulations, Guidance and Circulars therefore provide the skeleton or framework for protection of children under the law in the relevant jurisdictions. Putting the flesh on the bones of the skeleton is the task of the practitioners working together to achieve the greater protection of children, ranging from the field social worker struggling within limited resource allocations to support a family close to breaking point, down to the judges making orders under, or seeking to interpret the meaning of phrases in, the relevant legislation for their jurisdiction, be it England, Scotland or Northern Ireland.

Review of literature and research

Research on the impact of the various new civil legal frameworks on aspects of child protection is now highly developed. From the earliest days of implementation in England, the Department of Health was quick to respond to concerns about local authority social services departments failing to use the newly-available court orders. It commissioned a study by the Social Services Inspectorate (SSI 1992) from which it was quick to draw out lessons to be learned by local authorities seeking both to work within the new prevailing philosophy of the legislation, that is to say partnership, whilst at the same time continuing to emphasise that children should be and feel properly protected. The message extracted from this study was sent out in the first report on the Children Act entitled the *Children Act Report 1992* (see para. 2.21, DOH 1993). The DOH in England and Wales further funded a number of research projects looking at the effect of the Children Act 1989 on child protection practices generally and these were all finally published by the DOH in *Child Protection: Messages from Research* (DOH 1995a). Very many useful issues emerged from the range of research studies commissioned by the Department of Health and which contributed to the findings published in this document. Despite the tabloids seizing on the document as indicating that 'social workers should intervene less', the more measured response of the Department has led to important evaluation of the research as indicative of the impact of a piece of legislation and its procedures on the practice not only of all the professionals involved in the system, but also and most importantly on the lives of the children and their families whom the professionals are seeking to protect. A whole range of important guidance has been developed as a result of careful research instigated pursuant to the implementation of the Children Act 1989. These have included a number of guides to different aspects of different professional practices in the arena of child protection. These are identified in other chapters and will not be repeated here save to emphasise that in addition to the *Working Together* document produced by the Department of Health in 1999, in order to assist with the process of assessment of children and their families, a publication entitled the *Framework for the Assessment of Children in Need*, was produced in 2000.

Theoretical analyses of the 'political influences' shaping the civil legal framework of child protection developed in the Children Act 1989 can be found in the work of Fox-Harding (1991), but much more importantly in the work of Parton (Parton 1991, Parton *et al.* 1997). An analysis of the legal framework from the perspective of the many professionals who must work within it is provided by the socio-legal work of Lyon & de Cruz (1993, 2001). In addition, very importantly, the Children Act Advisory Committee established by the Lord Chancellor's Department and the Department of Health published Annual Reports, up to 1997 and 1996 respectively, upon the practical effects of implementation of the Act, the former Department from the courts' perspective and the latter from the perspective of the government department in overall charge of social services responsibilities under the Act in England and Wales. The passing of the Children Act Advisory Committee was much lamented by all those working within the legal system in England and Wales, since its Annual Reports had become established as the most authoritative guides not only to current practice and procedures pursuant to the Children Act 1989 but also as a source of recommendations for potential future reform. That Committee published its last report in 1997 and its activities have now been subsumed within the responsibilities of the new Family Law Advisory Board in the form of a Children Act Sub-Committee of that Board chaired by the energetic and enthusiastic Family Liaison Judge for the northwest of England, Mr Justice Nicholas Wall. For Northern Ireland, the first report on the operation of the Children (Northern Ireland) Order 1995 was issued by George Howarth, Minister for Health and Social Services for Northern Ireland in late 1999. This is, so far, the first and only report to be produced for Northern Ireland but, as with its counterparts for England and Wales, it provides extremely interesting and useful information on the operation of the 1995 Order and is strongly recommended (Department of Health and Social Services for Northern Ireland 1999).

The civil legal framework

Prevention

Local authority social services departments are placed under very wide-ranging duties by s.17 Children Act 1989 (s.18 Children (Northern Ireland) Order, s.22 Children (Scotland) Act 1995) to safeguard and promote the welfare of children within their area who are in need; and, so far as is consistent with that duty, to promote the upbringing of such children by their families by providing a range and level of services appropriate to those children's needs. Pursuant to that, s.17(2) Children Act 1989, goes on to provide that for the purpose of facilitating the discharge of their general duty under s.17, local authorities must have specific regard to their duties and powers set out in Sched. 2, Part I Children Act 1989 (see s.18(2)) and Sched. 2, Children (Northern Ireland) Order 1995 and s.22 Children (Scotland) Act 1995).

Under the provisions of Sched. 2, para. 1, Children Act 1989, a duty is imposed upon local authorities to take reasonable steps to identify the extent to which there are children in need within their area, and it is further provided that local authorities must publish information about services provided by them and by voluntary organisations, pursuant to their duty under Part III, Children Act 1989, and that they must take such steps as are reasonably practicable to ensure that those who might benefit from the services, receive the information relevant to them (see corresponding provisions in Sched. 2 Children (Northern Ireland) Order 1995 and ss.23, 24 and 93 (defining 'children in need') in Children (Scotland) Act 1995). (Note hereafter the Children Act 1989 for England will be abbreviated to CA 1989, the Children (Northern Ireland) Order 1995 will be abbreviated to C(NI)O 1995 and the Children (Scotland) Act 1995 will be abbreviated to C(S)A 1995.) In England and Wales, the CA 1989 was further amended to include an additional paragraph 1(A) in Sched. 2, Part I requiring local authorities to devise Children's Services Plans, which had to be made available in public places such as libraries and town halls in order that members of the public could identify the sorts of services to children in need which were being made available by local authorities. As part of the *Quality Protects* initiative, the Government has required that further very detailed programmes are put forward by local authorities to demonstrate that they are taking seriously the issues of providing services to children in need and for the greater protection of those children whom they are required to look after. In addition, local authorities' social services departments all over England and Wales have published a whole series of information leaflets setting out details of those children who they regard as being 'in need', and what services are available to support the families of those 'children in need', supplementary to the relatively new requirement obliging them to publish their Children's Services Plans.

The CA 1989 provides in s.17(10) and (11) a very wide definition of children in need. Thus, a child shall be taken to be 'in need' if they are unlikely to achieve or maintain, or have the opportunity of achieving or maintaining, a reasonable standard of health or development without the provision of services for them by a local authority under the Act; if their health or development is likely to be significantly impaired, or further impaired, without the provisions to them of such services; or if they are disabled, and for these purposes a child is disabled if they are blind, deaf or dumb, or suffers from a mental disorder of any kind, or is substantially and permanently handicapped by illness, injury or congenital deformity or such other disability as may be prescribed. (See for comparable provisions C(NI)O 1995, Art. 17, although note that the Northern Ireland legislation does not define disability in the same way as the English and Welsh statute, and see also s.93(4) C(S)A 1995.) S.17(10) CA 1989 goes on to provide that development under the Act encompasses physical, intellectual, emotional, social or behavioural development and health encompasses both physical and mental health. (Comparable definitions are provided in Art. 2(2) C(NI)O 1995; and s.93(4) C(S)A 1995.) As was noted above, s.17(10) is indeed a very wide definition and many social services departments' information leaflets and Children's Services Plans, as well as the more recent Management Action Plans, seek to restrict the all-encompassing definition in order to 'gatekeep' limited resources available to departments for prevention. In many of the information leaflets, as well as in the Children's Services Plans, a high profile is given to the local authority's duty to safeguard children, and it is made clear that children in need of protection will be given a high priority in the provision of services. (See variously Chapter 2 of successive copies of the *Children Act Report* (DOH 1992, 1993, 1994, 1995*b*, 1996); and see also Chapter 4 *Children Order Report 1999* (Department of Health and Social Services for Northern Ireland 1999).)

Building on this 'preventive' approach, the CA 1989 goes on to provide in para. 5 of Sched. 2 that local authorities must take reasonable steps, through the provision of services under Part III, to prevent children in their areas suffering ill-treatment or neglect (see also para. 5, Sched. 2, C(NI)O 1995). As if to emphasise the point that children who abuse are, potentially, equally to be viewed as children in need as those children who are abused, the local authority is also required to take reasonable steps under the CA 1989 to reduce the need to bring criminal proceedings against children within its area and to take reasonable steps to encourage children in its area not to permit criminal offences (para. 7(A)(B) Sched. CA 1989 and see also para. 8, Sched. 2, C(NI)O 1995). Comparable provisions to paras 5 and 7 in the English, Welsh and Northern Irish legislation is not to be found in the C(S)A 1995. (For a thorough-going analysis of the concept of the 'child in need', see Bedingfield 1998.)

One of the underlying philosophies of the Children Act 1989 was its emphasis on partnership with families with children in need and further a reinforcement of the emphasis on preventive support through services to families. In the Department of Health's own guidance it is clearly stated that 'it would not be acceptable for an authority to exclude any of the three categories describing children in need – for example, by confining services to children at risk of significant harm which attracts the duty to investigate under s.47' (DOH 1991*a*). A study conducted by Aldgate & Tunstill (1995), conducted for the Department of Health into the implementation of s.17 was directed at determining whether the Act's emphasis on preventive support, rather than simply protecting children from the risk of abuse had changed the way in which local authorities performed their duties towards children in need. Aldgate & Tunstill's study revealed that local authorities have had varied success in achieving the goals laid down in s.17. Problems stemmed from basic lack of resources to fund appropriate provision of computers and filing systems so that social workers were unable to properly assess need in their areas, but in a number of situations problems have stemmed from a reluctance to involve other agencies as envisaged by Part III, CA 1989. Aldgate & Tunstill (1995) point out that:

There still remains a distinction between developing a wider partnership in relation to a general corporate strategy for implementation of s.17 and consultation on specific issues, such as the register for disabled children, with more authorities engaging in the latter at present. (p. 54).

As *Child Protection: Messages from Research* (DOH 1995*a*) revealed, child protection work has to be combined with relevant family support services. The editors of the Report 'question whether the balance between child protection and the range of supports and interventions available to professionals is correct ... The research study suggests too much of the work undertaken comes under the banner of child protection'. The clear message from this report is that the editors and researchers involved in the various studies believe that 'a more useful perspective would be where early work is viewed as an enquiry to establish whether the child in need might benefit from services' (DOH 1995a, p. 54). Practitioners working in the field of family support and child protection would be well advised to read this report very closely for

> ... psychological evidence suggests that while children suffer in an environment of low warmth and high criticism, the intervention of professionals in these situations is seldom necessary or helpful. If ... family problems endure, perhaps using s.17 services will be required to ensure that the health and development of the child is not significantly impaired ... the research suggests that, for the majority of cases, the need of the child and family is more important than the abuse, or, put another way, the general family context is more important than any abusive event within it. This message applies when defining maltreatment, designing interventions or assessing outcomes.
>
> (DOH 1995a, p. 54)

As has already been identified, the methods by which local authorities establish which children require safe-guarding services will depend upon the measures for inter-agency collaboration in the identification process laid down by the LACPC (the Local Area Child Protection Committee) pursuant to the guidance provided in Chapter 3 of *Working Together to Safeguard Children* (DOH 1999c). As *Working Together* points out,

> The welfare of children is a corporate responsibility of the entire local authority, working in partnership with other public agencies, the voluntary sector, and service users and carers. All local authority services have an impact on the lives of children and families, and local authorities have a particular responsibility towards those children and families most at risk of social exclusion. Local authorities have a duty to plan services for children in need, in consultation with a wide range of other agencies, and to publish the resulting children's services plans. (Chapter 3.2)

A coherent prevention policy and plan is therefore necessary if local authorities are to take seriously their duty to safeguard the welfare of children within their area. (For a more detailed examination of this, see Lyon & de Cruz 2001, Chapter 4.2.) Other preventive measures can also be identified within the provisions of the CA 1989 and in the comparable legislation for Northern Ireland and Scotland. These include the provisions in s.17(3) that any service provided by an authority in the exercise of its functions may be provided for the family of a particular child in need, or for *any member of his/her family*, if it is provided with a view to safeguarding or promoting the child's welfare (see Art. 18(3) C(NI)O 1995; and s.22(3)(a) C(S)A 1995). It is important to realise, therefore, that where an abused child is suffering at the hands of a family member, whether this is a parent, an older sibling or some other relative living in the family, it may be the case that the local authority will seek to provide services for those family members in order to attempt to safeguard the child who has suffered, or is at risk of suffering significant harm.

Where it is felt desirable that an abusing member of the family should move out of the family home, Sched. 2, para. 6, CA 1989, could be used to encourage the perpetrator to move out of the premises and to provide accommodation for them. (For comparable provisions see Sched. 2, para. 6 and Art. 21 C(NI)O 1995; s.22 (3)(iii) C(S)A 1995.) Use of this provision, of course, depends upon the cooperation of the perpetrator, and where one is considering the case of child perpetrators, who may well have been abused themselves, it may be more appropriate to consider the provision of accommodation under s.20 CA 1989, together with other necessary services such as psychiatric, psychological or social work assessment (see also Art. 21 C(NI)O 1995 and s.25 C(S)A 1995).

The use of both the service of accommodation under the legislation and other support services for such children will, of course, depend upon the level of cooperative partnership achieved between parents and workers. The necessity for the local authority social services to resort to s.20 type provision maybe obviated in situations where the department feels confident that the non-abusing parent will obtain relevant necessary protective measures in the form of domestic violence injunctions or orders, including exclusion orders or ouster orders, under the relevant provisions of the domestic violence legislation. (See Part IV, Family Law Act 1996 for England and Wales, the Family Homes and Domestic Violence (NI) Order 1998; and the Matrimonial Home (Family Protection) (Scotland) Act 1981.) The relevant ouster and anti-molestation orders obtainable under these different pieces of legislation are available to partners of perpetrators of domestic violence where they or their children have experienced such violence. Both types of orders can be obtained in an emergency and also provide for longer-term orders to be granted in a variety of different circumstances.

In recognition of the fact that children in such situations may need the benefit of protection provided by social services to support the parents in whose care they might otherwise remain, amendments to the CA 1989 were made by Sched. 6, Family Law Act 1996. These amendments effected the insertion of a new s.44(A) and 44(B) and s.38(A) and 38(B) into the Children Act. These provisions enable the courts to include exclusion requirements in both emergency protection orders (s.44(A)) and interim care orders (s.38(A)). Under the new power to include an exclusion requirement in an emergency protection order, the court must be satisfied that the criteria for making an emergency protection order are satisfied (see s.44(1)(A), (B) or (C)), and the court must further be satisfied that the conditions mentioned in s.44(A)(2) are also satisfied. These conditions are that there is reasonable cause to believe that if 'the relevant person' (the perpetrator of violence or the threat of violence) is excluded from the dwelling house in which the child lives, then the child will not be likely to suffer significant harm and that another person living in the dwelling house (whether a parent of the child or some other person) is able and willing to give to the child the care which it would be reasonable to expect a parent to give to him, and that thatperson consents to the inclusion of the exclusion requirements (s.44(A)(2)(A) and (B)).

There are comparable provisions in Northern Ireland and Scotland – see Art. 63(A) and 63(B) C(NI)O 1995 and s.76–80 C(S)A 1995 – although it should be noted that the Scottish provisions do not allow for such exclusion orders to be made in the same way as in England, Wales and Northern Ireland. The provisions in s.76 make it unlikely that exclusion orders providing emergency protection for children on a short-term basis would be granted since s.76(9) provides that the sheriff shall not make an exclusion order if to do so would be unjustifiable or unreasonable and it is argued that it is likely to be so considered if one is proposing to exclude a person from their own home on the basis of unproven allegations alone, even when such allegations are sufficient to activate the other protection mechanisms in the Act (see Norrie 1995).

In addition to the provisions relating to emergency orders, social workers could also seek to apply for the insertion of an exclusion requirement into an interim care order. The court in this situation must be satisfied that there are reasonable grounds for believing that the threshold criteria mentioned in s.31(2)(a) and (b)(i) have been met, and must further be satisfied as to the fulfilling of the same conditions with regard to the fact that the child will cease to suffer or be likely to suffer from significant harm as a result of the exclusion of the relevant person and that some other person living in the dwelling house is able and willing to give to the child the care which it would be reasonable to expect a parent to give to them, and that person consents to the inclusion of the exclusion requirement. (See s.38A CA 1989, and comparable provisions in Art. 57(A) C(NI)O 1995 as amended by the Family Home and Domestic Violence (NI) Order 1998, which is now in force.)

It has long been recognised, although it only seemed to be officially acknowledged for the first time in the *Cleveland Report* (Butler-Sloss L.J. 1988), that removal of the perpetrator is far better than seeking to remove the child, and thus every support should be given to the non-abusing parent if they are prepared either in the immediate- or long-term to seek remedial action using the domestic violence legislation or alternatively by using the provisions relating to emergency protection and interim care orders set out above, in an effort to keep the child in the family setting. In those situations where police action has resulted in the removal of either an adult or child perpetrator, the necessity for the local authority to use any of the empowering provisions such as s.20 or Sched. 2, para. 6, or even the additional protective measures linked to emergency protection and interim care orders, will have been removed, either because the perpetrator has been remanded in custody or by the imposition of bail conditions in respect of an adult perpetrator, or in a remand to local authority accommodation in the case of a child perpetrator.

Given that the overriding philosophy in each of the three pieces of legislation is that children are best brought up by their families, the provision of services under s.17 and Sched. 2 (and their corresponding provisions) in order to prevent children suffering from or perpetrating abuse is clearly the most desirable policy. A major tool in achieving the prevention of abuse must also be the education of children in adopting preventive strategies within settings in which they may be susceptible to such abuse. One of the principal defects of the CA 1989 and the corresponding legislation in Scotland and Northern Ireland is that none of the provisions are directed towards providing resources for children to be educated in adopting such preventive strategies. In an era of ever-increasing scarce resources, even under a 'new' Labour government, it would seem that we are probably mis-directing many of our resources to cure rather than prevention in partnership, and this is a major area yet to be tackled by the combined forces of the relevant departments of health and departments for education in the different jurisdictions. It is noteworthy that if one considers the United Kingdom's *Second Report to the UN Committee on the Rights of the Child* (DOH 1999*b*), no reference is made at any stage in that report, which covers all of the UK, to the development of any education programmes for children aimed at their developing such preventive approaches. The only references which are made at different points in the report are to Circulars which have been issued in England by the Department for Education and Employment and in Wales by the Welsh Office. Circular 10/95 *Protecting Children from Abuse: The Role of the Education Service* (DfEE 1995) contains advice to those working in all schools, including the independent sector, on child protection. The Circular makes it clear that children have a fundamental right to be protected from harm and points out that primary responsibilities as such rest with social services departments, whilst the police and the NSPCC have responsibilities for investigating allegations of abuse. The Circular makes it clear that education staff should not investigate allegations or suspicions of abuse, but should refer cases to the local social services department. The guidance, however, recognises that teachers are in a good position to identify signs, or hear allegations of abuse. The report to the UN Committee notes that the main recommendations of Circular 10/95 are that: all staff should be alert to signs of abuse and know to whom they should report their concerns or suspicions; all schools and colleges should have protection policies which should include procedures to be followed if a member of staff is accused of abuse; and all schools and colleges should have a senior member of staff with designated responsibility for child protection, who should receive appropriate training. The report notes that similar guidance has been issued in Wales (Welsh Office 1995) and whilst there is a further Circular, namely Circular 11/95, dealing with issues where staff in schools are accused of abuse by children, laying down procedures for education staff to follow is hardly the same as providing for education programmes for children enabling them to adopt appropriate preventive strategies when put in situations of potential abuse.

Much work still needs to be done in this area, particularly if we are to comply with Article 19 of the United Nations Convention on the Rights of the Child, hereafter UNCRC, but more particularly, in view of the implementation of the Human Rights Act 1998, with Articles 3, 5 and 8 of the European Convention on the Protection of Fundamental Human Rights and Freedoms (see Introduction above). Article 19 UNCRC interestingly provides that

States Parties shall take all appropriate legislative, administrative, social and *educational measures* to protect the child from all forms of physical or mental violence, injury or abuse, neglect or negligent treatment, maltreatment or exploitation, including sexual abuse, while in the care of parents, legal guardians or any other person who has the care of the child.

Arguably, UK legislation has everything the wrong way round in failing to provide suitable educational measures designed to enable children to adopt preventive strategies but this may partly arise out of the difficult position adopted by the UK Government in relation to the issue of corporal punishment of children by their parents. Since the Government has argued, in its Consultation Papers issued in UK jurisdictions in January and February 2000, that parents should retain the right to hit their children, providing educational programmes enabling children to adopt appropriate preventive strategies when put into abusive positions could provoke physical problems to be faced by all concerned.

Nevertheless it is interesting to note that *Working Together to Safeguard Children* (DOH 1999c, para. 2.4) provides that physical abuse may involve hitting a child. It seems inconceivable that this same Department can then be responsible for issuing a Consultation Paper on the issue of 'modernising the law relating to the physical punishment of children, so that it better protects children from harm' (DOH 2000). The Consultation Paper for England, then poses the questions, 'First, within the context of a modern family policy in a responsible society, where should we draw the line as to what physical punishment of children is acceptable within the family setting? Second, how do we achieve that position in law?' (DOH 2000, para. 1.6). It seems inconceivable that a government which has committed itself to the observation of the rights laid down in the UN Convention on the Rights of the Child, and more particularly to Article 19, should then declare that the Consultation Paper proposing the continued legality of physical punishment should be set 'in the context of the Government's wider policy aims in support of families' (DOH 2000, para. 1.7). In Part I, the Government goes on to state a principle which is totally irreconcilable with the provisions of the UN Convention on the Rights of the Child, Article 19, but also it is submitted with the principles of Articles 8 (1) and (2), European Convention on the Protection of Fundamental Human Rights Freedoms, as implemented by the Human Rights Act 1998 (from 2 October 2000). The Government states (DOH 2000, para. 1.8) that it needs 'to achieve a balance between the right of parents to exercise their parental responsibilities and to bring up their children as they think best, without undue interference from Government, the responsibility of parents to bring their children up safely, *and the right of children to be protected from harm*.'

The process of consultation on the issue of parental rights to physically chastise children has been brought to the fore by the ruling of the European Court in *A v UK* [1998] 2 FLR 218. In that case, an application had been made on behalf of Child A by his natural father to the European Commission on Human Rights on the basis that the injuries sustained by his son at the hands of his stepfather were in breach of Article 3 of the European Convention on Human Rights, which provides that 'no-one shall be subjected to torture, or to inhuman or degrading punishment or treatment' (see Introduction above). The European Court concluded that there had been a breach of Article 3 in this particular case and that domestic law in the UK did not give adequate protection to the child. It further ruled that the UK should immediately consider reform of its laws and that damages should be paid to Child A for breach of his human rights under the Convention. The government for England is currently proposing that the law on physical punishment of children by their parents should be changed but only so far as to render the defence of 'reasonable' chastisement, which is available to all charges of assault under English law, clearer. Thus criteria are proposed which will assist courts in determining whether a particular punishment of a child is 'reasonable' and further reforms are suggested with regard to the potential outlawing of hitting a child around the head (DOH 2000, Part 5).

The Scottish Executive Justice Department (SEJD) issued a similar Consultation Paper for Scotland in February 2000 entitled *The Physical Punishment of Children in Scotland: A Consultation* (Scottish Executive Justice Department 2000) which adopts a similar approach to the English Consultation Paper except that it does actually ask a more open question of the Scottish population namely 'do you agree with the Scottish Executive that parents should continue to be allowed to use reasonable physical punishment for their children' (para. 2.16). Whilst this Consultation Paper at least asks Scottish parents the question, it can nevertheless be described as being a loaded one, in that it is implying that the Scottish Government already approves and endorses the practice of parents hitting their children. As far as Wales and Northern Ireland are concerned, it is stated in the English Consultation Paper that 'the Secretary of State for Wales will, with the assistance of the Welsh Assembly, carry out a similar Consultation in Wales, and that Northern Ireland will produce its own Consultation document, adapted to suit the Northern Ireland context' (DOH 2000, para. 1.9). The Department of Health in England and the Scottish Executive Justice Department thus seem to be totally unaware of the mixed message which they are providing to their populations at large as much as to the social work practitioners who have to work within the context of guidance issued by those self-same departments. It would seem totally incredible that a modern government moving into the 21st century could suggest on the one hand that hitting a child may amount to physical abuse whilst on the other hand declaring that it is a process which it not only endorses but thinks should be part of a Government's wider policy aims in support of families! (see further Lyon 2000).

The impact of resources

As has been noted above, the main problem with regard to the achievement of the goal of prevention is that it depends upon available resources which, following the implementation of the 1989 Act in England were felt to be in very short supply. This has continued to be the case with ever-increasing demands being placed upon social services in all the jurisdictions to produce children's services plans and in response to *Quality Protects* (DOH 1998) to produce Management Action Plans, all of which have to provide for better responses by social services to the demands placed upon them. Although some additional government money has been announced to support the Quality Protects programme, in reality this is short-term additional money and does not therefore inspire confidence in social work practitioners that the programmes will continue beyond the remit of the current available funding (see further Lyon & de Cruz 2001, Chapter 4.2). The principal intention behind the supportive measures contained in the relevant Act and high-lighted in the supporting guidance, whether these result in services being provid-ed by local authorities, social services, health, education or voluntary organisations, is to improve both the position of children and the lot of families under stress so that the potential for the child suffering significant harm is dimin-ished, if not totally eroded. Since it is now clearly recognised, that even in the most severe examples of child abuse, one is dealing with a continuum of abuse which may be becoming more and more serious rather than in general with single iso-lated incidents, even limited resource input by social services and the other agen-cies may prevent a situation turning into a case of serious child abuse (see Dale et al. 1986 and DOH 1995a). Local authorities, in particular, must therefore devote far more attention to prioritising resources in the direction of supportive services for children in need and their families. Building upon the points made above in relation to the current lack of education for children on the sort of preventive strategies that they might adopt in potentially abusive situations, it is strongly urged that such supportive services should include relevant education programmes for children, since, in the words of the old adage, 'prevention is better than cure'.

The process of identification and investigation

Suspicions about whether a child is suffering or likely to suffer significant harm, which is the first of the threshold criteria which need to be satisfied in relation to a range of orders under the different pieces of legislation, may arise in a variety of different ways. It should, however, be noted that where concern surfaces about whether a child is suffering or likely to suffer significant harm in family proceed-ings, which are already before the court, the court has the power under s.37 of the CA 1989 to direct a local authority to investigate whether there is a need to bring care or supervision order proceedings in respect of such a child (see also Art. 56 C(NI)O 1995 and s.56 C(S)A 1995). While the local authority is con-ducting such an investigation, the court can consider whether it is necessary to make either an interim care or supervision order.

In the case of *Re H* [1993] 2 FLR 541, a lesbian couple had been refused approval as local authority adoptive or foster parents and had entered into an arrangement with another couple to bring up that couple's baby girl as the les-bian couple's own. The child's natural parents apparently had one child and had previously reached a firm decision that they would have one child only. Accordingly when the child, a baby girl, was born she was handed over to the les-bian couple and they had then applied for a residence order in respect of the child in order that they might have parental responsibility for her. Since the lesbian couple had been refused approval as potential adoptive parents for any child by the local authority, they knew that they would not be able to apply for an adop-tion order in respect of the child, but also knew that they would require parental responsibility for the child in order to give effective consent to such important issues as medical treatment, vaccinations and issues associated with schooling. Although there was no criticism of the applicants' care over the previous 8 months during which they had looked after the child, there were concerns in the longer-term about one of the partner's mental health, the issue of the proximity of the natural parents and the applicants' lack of insight into the difficulties which the child would face as she grew up so close to her own natural family. It appeared to the judge that no-one had assessed the future emotional risk to the child, or how far such risks might be remediable. Accordingly, bearing in mind the 'welfare checklist' in s.1(3) the judge ordered the local authority to undertake an investigation of the child's circumstances under s.37(1) CA 1989 and further set out in detail what it should cover. Scott-Baker, in this first reported decision on the scope of the court's powers under s.37, adopted a wide and liberal interpretation of the section. He stated that in his view 'the child's circumstances' should be widely construed and include any situation which might have a bearing on the child being likely to suffer significant harm in the future. As intended by s.37(2) and (3) of the CA 1989, the consequence of making such an order would be to force the local authority to consider whether a care or supervision order were necessary. He further ruled that the court was not limited only to looking at the present and the immediate future and that if a court were to conclude that a parent, or a carer, was likely to be unable to meet the emotional needs of a child in the future – even if years hence – the condition in s.31(2) would probably be met.

It should be emphasised that while a local authority is conducting such an investigation under s.37, the court can consider whether it is necessary to make either an interim care or supervision order. Indeed, in the case of *Re H*, Scott-Baker J. made an interim supervision order together with an interim residence order in favour of one of the lesbian couple (see further below). The judge in that case also made a prohibited steps order under s.8 CA 1989, forbidding the natural parents from seeking to assume possession of, or contact with, the child without the court's further order (see also *Re CE (s.37 direction)* ([1995] 1 FLR 26). Note that a s.37 direction must not be used as a means of appointing a guardian *ad litem* to represent the child where there is no real prospect of a care or supervision order being made, and it should further be noted that a local authority must not be made a party to private law proceedings if it decides, following its investigations, not to seek a care or supervision order (see further *F v Cambridgeshire County Council* [1995] 1 FLR 516).

More often than not, in situations where it is suspected that a child is suffering or likely to suffer significant harm, the child is a member of a family with whom social services are already working, or the child may already be on the Child Protection Register (see below), or concerns about the child have already surfaced with a number of different professionals, all of whom are working with the child and the family (see Farmer & Owen 1995). Dale *et al.* (1986) reported that in well over 75% of cases which ultimately found their way into the courts, the family or the child was already known to the various helping agencies and was already the subject of considerable concern.

Pursuant to s.47 of the CA 1989, a local authority, in particular, is under a duty to investigate whenever it is provided with information that may suggest that a child living or found within its area is suffering or likely to suffer significant harm, or where it is informed that such a child is already the subject of an emergency protection order obtained by some other person (for example, the National Society for the Prevention of Cruelty to Children (NSPCC), or where the child is in police protection (see below) (see Art. 66 C(NI)O 1995, and s.53 C(S)A 1995). Where, in England, information is passed to the NSPCC, a local authority may also undertake appropriate enquiries and investigations (see e.g. s.44(1)(C) and s.31(1)(9)). To undertake such investigations the local authority, in particular, is required to consult with a range of other agencies to enable it to decide what action it should take to safeguard or promote the child's welfare. The local authority social services may also request other agencies to assist them in such enquiries and investigations (see s.47(5)(9)(11) and (12). (See also Art. 66(5)(9)(11) and (12) C(NI)O 1995 and s.53(1)(a).) These processes are described in much fuller detail in Lyon & de Cruz (2001, Chapters 4 and 5).

The meaning of 'significant harm'

The basis for deciding to embark upon an investigation or to invoke any of the procedures to be described hereafter is that the child about whom one is concerned is suffering or is likely to suffer 'significant harm'. This concept is therefore the trigger for much of what may follow in the way of an investigation, and it is also the ground to which the various concerned agencies and the relevant courts must look when deciding whether to apply for orders, to exercise any special powers, or in the case of the courts, to make orders.

Harm is defined by s.31(9) CA 1989 as meaning 'ill treatment or the impairment of health or development'; development is defined as meaning 'physical, intellectual, emotional, social or behavioural development'; health is defined to include 'physical or mental health' and, finally, ill treatment is defined as including 'sexual abuse and forms of ill treatment which are not physical' (see for comparable provisions, Art. 2(2) C(NI)O 1995; and s.93 C(S)(A) 1995). When looking to satisfy the criterion of 'significant harm', it would appear to be the case that the court may be satisfied that the child is suffering from 'significant harm' if any one of the three types of harm envisaged in s.31(9) and the comparable provision is present. This is indeed the guidance offered by the Department of Health, which states that each of these different elements has been associated with the suffering of significant harm by a child. It also points out that sometimes the process of suffering such harm is a continual process but that 'sometimes, a single traumatic event may constitute significant harm, e.g. a violent assault, suffocation or poisoning' (DOH 1999, para. 2.17).

The grounds for intervention in each of the three jurisdictions can thus be seen to be very wide and, indeed, the Court of Appeal in the English case of *Newham London Borough Council* v *AG* ([1993] 1 FLR 281 at 289) has emphasised that the words of the CA 1989 must be considered but are not meant to be unduly restrictive when the evidence clearly indicates that a certain course of action should be taken to protect a child, a point reiterated by Thorpe J. in *Re A* [1993] 1 FCR 824.

The condition as to 'significant harm' in all the jurisdictions is drawn with reference to the child concerned, so that those conducting the investigations, and the courts who may be called upon to make orders, must look at the position, characteristics and needs of each particular child. The criteria which may trigger off an investigation and the subsequent making of orders are intended to cover both situations, where the child has suffered, or is likely to suffer significant harm and the two may be linked together. Clearly, an investigation relating solely to past events is unlikely to proceed much further unless it is being linked in some way to the evidence that the harm is likely to continue (see *Re M* [1994] 2 FLR 577). It was stated very clearly in that case that a court could make a care order on the grounds that the child had been suffering significant harm at the point at which the local authority had initiated protective action in respect of the child.

As to looking at the likelihood of the future possibility of harm, as indicated by the words 'likely to suffer significant harm', the investigating agency, in consultation with other professionals concerned with the child, must seek to establish that there would be a greater risk to the child in leaving them in their current situation and by seeking to provide the services to ameliorate the situation or, in the worst case, by seeking the child's removal through an application for court orders. Were an application to be based on the issue of the future possibility of harm by reference to past events, then the House of Lords has determined in (*Re H and R* [1996] 1 FLR 80) that the standard of proof required of the likelihood of past events is proof on the balance of probabilities, except that where the allegation is an extremely serious one the evidence required to satisfy the court that there was a real possibility of harm to a child must be even stronger. The basic message of this case somewhat controversially therefore was that the more serious the allegations made in respect of past events then the stronger the evidence would need to be to establish that it had actually occurred. In *Re H and R* itself the risk to the original complainants' younger sisters could only be established by accepting the evidence of the eldest girl that she had in fact been abused by her step-father. Her evidence was the only evidence to suggest that she had been sexually abused by the step-father and, although the judge at first instance had felt that the girl was telling the truth, he had not felt that he was sure 'to the requisite high standard of proof' that her allegations were true. The House of Lords in the case ruled that 'likely' in the context of the relevant section was being used in the sense of a real possibility, a possibility that could not sensibly be ignored, having regard to the nature and gravity of the feared harm in the particular case. The Lords went on to state that the standard of proof in cases involving the care of children was the ordinary civil standard of the balance of probability but the more improbable the event, the stronger must be the evidence that it did occur before, on the balance of probability, its occurrence would be established. They further went on to emphasise that the rejection by the court of a disputed allegation as not proved on the balance of probability might leave scope for the possibility that the non-proven allegation might be true after all. But, they stated 'those unresolved doubts and suspicions could no more form the basis of a conclusion that the likelihood of suffering significant harm had been established than they could form the basis of a conclusion that the criteria relating to the issue of "is suffering" had been established'. The House of Lords went on to emphasise that unproved allegations of maltreatment could not therefore form the basis for a finding by the court that either issue relating to significant harm had been established. They stated that it was, however, open to a court to conclude that there was a real possibility that the child would suffer harm in the future although harm in the past had not been established. They stressed that there would be cases where, although the alleged maltreatment had not been proved, the evidence before the court nevertheless established a combination of profoundly worrying feature affecting the care of the child within the family who was before the court. They emphasised that in such cases, it would be open to a court in appropriate circumstances to find that, although not satisfied the child was yet suffering significant harm, on the basis of such facts as had been proved to the requisite standard of proof there was a likelihood that the child would do so in the future.

The harm suffered or apprehended must be 'significant' and, where this turns on the issue of health or development, the child's health or development will be compared with that which could reasonably be expected of a similar child (s.31(10) CA 1989; and for comparable provisions see Art. 50(3) C(NI)O 1995; and note that the phrase 'significant' is not defined in any way in the Scottish legislation). As far as the word 'significant' is concerned, *Working Together to Safeguard Children* (DOH 1999) states that

there are no absolute criteria on which to rely when judging what constitutes significant harm. Consideration of the severity of ill-treatment may include the degree and the extent of physical harm, the duration and frequency of abuse and neglect, and the extent of pre-meditation, degree of threat and coercion, sadism, and bizarre or unusual elements in child sexual abuse. Each of these elements have been associated with more severe effects on the child, and/or relatively greater difficulty in helping the child overcome the adverse impact of the ill-treatment ... More often, significant harm is a compilation of significant events, both acute and long-standing, which interrupt, change or damage the child's physical and psychological development. Some children live in family and social circumstances where their health and development are neglected. For them, it is the corrosiveness of long-term emotional, physical or sexual abuse that causes impairment to the extent constituting significant harm. In each case, it is necessary to consider any ill-treatment alongside the families' strength and support.

See para. 2.17 for a fuller consideration of the concept of 'significant harm' (Adcock & White 1998; see also Adcock, Chapter 12 in this volume). It is clear therefore that minor shortcomings in the health care provided, or minor deficits in physical, psychological or social development, should not give rise to compulsory intervention unless they are having or likely to have serious and lasting effects upon the child. Prior to implementation of the CA 1989 the Lord Chancellor, Lord MacKay of Clashfern, also stated that, 'Unless there is evidence that a child is being, or is likely to be, positively harmed because of failure in the family, the State whether the guise of a local authority or a court, should not interfere' (Lord MacKay 1990).

The comparison to be made with a similar child is not without problems, however, since one is required to compare this subjective child with that hypothetically similar child. There has been very little reported case law on this particular issue of 'the similar child' before the English courts. The issue did, however, come up for early consideration by the court in the case of *Re O* [1992] 2 FLR 7 where Ewbank J. took a very robust view of what constituted a similar child. In this particular case he was dealing with a young girl aged 15 who had been truanting from school and the issue was whether she had suffered harm compared with the hypothetically similar child. In Ewbank's view, a similar child in this case meant 'a child with equivalent intellectual and social development, who has gone to school, and not merely an average child who may or may not be at school' (p. 12). Clearly, if a child is disabled in some way and this has affected their health and development, the investigating agency must ask itself what state of health or development could be expected of a child with a similar disability.

As to whether 'similar' involves any consideration being given to the child's background has been a matter of debate. According to the Lord Chancellor at the time of debates on the Children Bill, it could be suggested that background as opposed to attributes, should be left out of account. He observed that 'the care that a parent gives to his child must be related to the circumstances attributable to that child in the sense of physical, mental and emotional characteristics' (House of Lords, Hansard 1989). The Department of Health, however, in its *Guidance and Regulations, Volume 1 – Court Orders* (DOH 1991*b*) states that 'account may need to be taken of environmental, social and cultural characteristics of the child' (para. 3.20). There has also been much debate amongst academic commentators as to the relevance of cultural issues. According to Freeman, consideration ought to be given to cultural issues since the legislation itself expresses an ideological commitment to this (see s.22(5)(c) CA 1989) (Freeman 1997), whilst Bainham has argued that 'allowances for cultural background ought not to be made, except at the welfare stage of the court process, since by definition, the threshold criteria for care and supervision orders set minimally acceptable limits of behaviour towards children'. Bainham continues to argue that, as such, society has a right to expect everyone from whatever cultural background to comply and, in any event, he suggests that allowances for ethnic background take insufficient account of the widely divergent attitudes towards child-rearing held amongst the indigenous population (Bainham 1993). While the child protection agencies, when investigating issues of significant harm, will obviously have to be sensitive to racial, cultural and religious issues (see more on this in Lau 1991), what the Lord Chancellor was clearly indicating himself in debates upon the Children Bill was that the agency should focus clearly on the needs of the particular child when contrasting his or her development with that of a similar child.

Processing the investigation further

The provisions in s.47 of the CA 1989, which go on to deal with processing the investigation by social services, provide that enquiries must in particular be directed towards establishing whether the local authority should make any application to the court or exercise any of its powers under the CA 1989, which could include the provision of services pursuant to s.17 of the Act (see Art. 66 C(NI)O 1995; s.53 C(S)A 1995). Such alternative action may well be considered in the context of an initial child protection conference (see below).

S.47 provides for a range of measures to be taken to enable the local author-ity to pursue its investigation, including provisions to allow it to gain access to property in order to see the child (although it should be noted that such provisions do not authorise the local authority to gain access by force) or in terms of engaging the assistance of other agencies to help it further carry out the investigation.

Where the local authority's investigation under s.47 is impeded or frustrated in any way by the unreasonable refusal of access to the child, it should be noted that such refusal may constitute grounds for a local authority seeking an emergency protection order (under s.44 Art. 63 C(NI)O 1995, and ss.57 and 61 C(S)A 1995 and see below) or invoking the assistance of a police constable either to exercise police powers of protection (s.46) or simply to exercise the police powers under s.17(1)(e) Police and Criminal Evidence Act 1984, which allows the police to enter any premises, if need be by force, in order to protect any person believed to be under threat to their life, limb, or liberty.

It should be noted that by this stage of the investigation, as many details as possible relating to the child should have been gathered, including the child's name, address, names of parents, names of others in the household, name of the family's general practitioner (GP), details of any nursery or school which the child attends, and details of the family's or child's social worker, if there is one. The next step will be to check with the Child Protection Register. The purpose of this register is to provide a record of all children in the area who are currently the subject of an inter-agency child protection plan and to ensure that the plans are formally reviewed every 6 months at least. All social services departments normally maintain such registers and the key information to be held on the Child Protection Register is detailed in paragraphs 5.99–5.101 of *Working Together to Safeguard Children* (DOH 1999c).

Wherever there is time, as well as checking the Child Protection Register, the agency involved may also check with the health visitor, school, education welfare department, the probation service, family GP, the police and the NSPCC. All such checks provide essential information, but it might be that speed is of the essence and therefore action is required without being able to make all the desired enquiries.

The initial child protection conference (see paras 5.53–5.89 Working Together to Safeguard Children)

It may therefore be the case that while the next step in a non-urgent situation would be discussions within an initial child protection conference setting, such discussions may actually have to be postponed until after the taking of emergency action. In a non-emergency situation where there is felt to be a risk of harm that has not yet materialised, there may well ongoing work within the family which has identified a looming, potential crisis. In such circumstances, it may be possible to convene an initial child protection conference with all the relevant personnel. An opportunity is thus provided for giving measured consideration to taking further legal steps, such as obtaining a Child Assessment Order (s.43 CA 1989; Art. 62 C(NI)O 1995 and s.55 C(S)A 1995) or the institution of proceedings for an interim care or supervision order (see ss.31 and 38 CA 1989; Art. 50 and 57 C(NI)O 1995 and ss.52 and 65 C(S)A 1995).

Where more measured consideration is possible, the initial child protection conference may have recommended that it is more appropriate to engage in informal social worker involvement with the family together with the provision of additional services from a range of other agencies. The provision of such services is made possible by s.17 CA 1989, and if services from other agencies are to be provided this may require the invoking of s.27 CA 1989 (Art. 18 and 46 and 47 C(NI)O 1995 and ss.22 and 21 C(S)A 1995).

Under s.27 and its comparable provisions, a local authority may request the help of one or more other agencies including health, education and housing in performing duties to provide services under the relevant provisions of the Act, and those agencies must comply with such requests unless they can prove that it is not compatable with their own statutory or other duties, or it unduly prejudices the discharge of any of their functions. The recommendation to provide services and the monitoring of the provision of such services in terms of the effects on the family does, of course, leave open the option of taking more formal legal action through the institution of proceedings for a care and supervision order if and when this might be required.

Placing a child's name on the child protection register and a written child protection plan

It should be noted that the initial child protection conference's only decision-making power is to place a child's name on the local Child Protection Register and, if registration is agreed, to allocate the key worker (DOH para 5.68). The key worker must be a worker from either the Social Services Department or, less usually, the NSPCC (DOH para. 5.75). *Working Together* emphasises that where a child's name is placed on the register, the act of registration itself confers no protection on a child, and should always be accompanied by a child protection plan. The plan must be in writing and may be dependent upon a full assessment of the child and the family having been undertaken. *Working Together* states that the outline child protection plan should:

- idxentify risks of significant harm to the child and ways in which the child can be protected through an inter-agency plan based on assessment findings
- establish short-term and longer-term aims and objectives that are clearly linked to reducing the risk of harm to the child and promoting the child's welfare
- be clear about who will have responsibility for what actions – including actions by family members – within what specified timescale
- outline ways of monitoring and evaluating progress against the plan (para. 5.69).

Working Together emphasises that the conference should agree a date for the first child protection review conference, and under what circumstances it might be necessary to convene the conference before that date.

Working Together also emphasises that

the child protection plan should take into consideration the wishes and feelings of the child, and the views of the parents, in so far as this is consistent with the child's welfare. The key worker should make every effort to ensure that the children and parents have a clear understanding of the objectives of the plan, that they accept it and are willing to work to it. The plan should be constructed with the family in their first language and they should receive a written copy in their first language. If family members' preferences are not accepted about how best to safeguard the child, the reasons for this should be explained. The family should be told about their right to complain and make representations, and how to do so.

The document also stresses that all members of the core group responsible for implementation of the plan have equal ownership of, and responsibility for, the child protection plan, and should cooperate to achieve its aims. It should be emphasised that whilst a decision to register a child and formulate a child protection plan is a formal administrative process it is not a process laid down in the legislation but one designed to supplement it. As such, child protection conferences do not themselves have any status in legal provisions but the Guidance issued in *Working Together* is once again issued under s.7 of the Local Authority Social Services Act 1970, which requires local authorities and their social services functions to act under the general guidance of the Secretary of State (see above). As such, *Working Together* does not have the full force of statute, but as noted above should be complied with unless local circumstances indicate exceptional reasons which justify a variation. In any later legal action therefore, it must be emphasised that detailed explanation would have to be offered as to why any part of the guidance issued in *Working Together to Safeguard Children* has not been complied with and acted upon. Nevertheless, despite all the best endeavours of those involved at the initial child protection conference where a child protection plan has been drawn up, or in those situations where the recommendation was merely more informal social worker involvement and the provision of services, things can go wrong and emergencies may intervene. Thus consideration may have to be given to a more formal legal approach by invoking the provisions relating to the initiation of care or supervision order proceedings, applications for child assessment orders, or in more urgent situations, the invoking of the emergency powers relating to emergency protection orders.

The invoking of formal legal proceedings in relation to the issue of child protection is not an easy issue for the relevant government departments in each of the jurisdictions to provide Guidance. Whilst such Guidance in relation to the use of court orders has been issued in all the relevant jurisdictions, further consideration now needs to be given to the impact upon the relevant processes of the implementation of the European Convention on the Protection of Fundamental Human Rights and Freedoms brought about by the Human Rights Act 1998 (see Introduction). The problems which the courts in the various jurisdictions face upon the coming into force of the European Convention have been highlighted by Wall (1999). Wall quotes from Lord Templeman in the House of Lords in a pre-Children Act case (*Re KD* [1988] AC 806). Wall observes that Lord Templeman in the House of Lords set the tone for what Wall believes remains the judicial attitude to care proceedings. Wall observes that comparing the welfare criteria under what is now s.1 Children Act 1989 with Article 8 of the European Convention for the Protection of Fundamental Human Rights and Freedoms, which, of course, provides for the right to respect for private and family life, and also provides against unlawful interference with the exercise of that right by a public authority, Templeman said this.

The English rule was evolved against an historical background of conflicts between parents over the upbringing of their children. The Convention rule was evolved against an historical background of claims by the State to control the private lives of individuals. Since the last war, interference by public authorities with families for the protection of children has greatly increased in this country. In my opinion there is no inconsistency of principle or application between the English rule and the Convention rule. The best person to bring up a child is the natural parents. It matters not whether that parent is wise or foolish, rich or poor, educated or illiterate, provided the child's moral and physical health are not endangered. Public authorities cannot improve upon nature. Public authorities exercise a supervisory role and interfere to rescue a child when the parental tie is broken by abuse or separation. In terms of the English rule, the court decides whether and to what extent the welfare of the child requires the child shall be protected against harm caused by the parent, including harm which could be caused by the resumption of parental care after separation has broken the parental tie. In terms of the Convention rule, the court decides whether and to what extent the child's health or morals require protection from the parent and whether and to what extent the family life of a parent and child has been supplanted by some other relationship which has become the essential family life for the child.

Wall also observes in his article that the thrust of Part III Children Act 1989 is undoubtedly to emphasise the duty of the local authority to work with the family and to try to keep children within the families wherever possible, and yet he goes on to recognise that early intervention to protect a child may be absolutely crucial if the child's own welfare is not to be displaced by efforts which are far more focused on the needs of the adults or parents. Wall questions how we resolve this tension between the need to act swiftly to determine the child's future and the need to ensure that before placement outside the family occurs there is no realistic prospect of a placement within it. It is therefore the case, that a delicate balance has to be struck between the rights and needs of the child and the rights and needs of the parents, but arguably under both the Convention and the relevant legislation in the different parts of the UK, the overriding principle is the paramountcy of the welfare of the child and it may be that delay in reaching difficult decisions is positively inimical to this. Social work practitioners have therefore to bear in mind not only the messages to be derived from the Department of Health's own publication *Child Protection: Messages from Research* (DOH 1995a) and other research done subsequently, but also the overriding imperatives prescribed by the legislation and the Convention that one must act to safeguard the child's health.

Emergency action

Where, therefore, there is reasonable cause to believe that a child is likely to suffer significant harm if either the child is not removed to accommodation provided by or on behalf of the applicant, or does not remain in a place in which they are then being accommodated, *any person* may make an application for what is termed under the CA 1989 s.44 an 'emergency protection order' (see Art. 63 C(NI)O 1995 and s.61 and 57 C(S)A 1995). Such an application may be made by any person pursuant to s.44(1)(a) CA 1989, and may be made *ex parte* (i.e. without the other parties being present) to a single magistrate. Such *ex parte* applications for emergency protection orders may also be made by any of the relevant child protection agencies using s.44(1)(a) (generally see also Art. 63 C(NI)O 1995 and s.61 C(S)A 1995).

Local authority social services and the NSPCC in England are given additional rights to apply for orders under s.44 in case of emergencies. Thus, in the case of an application made by a local authority, s.44(1)(b) provides that where enquiries are being made with respect to the child in pursuance of an investigation, and those enquiries are being frustrated by access to the child unreasonably refused to a person authorised to seek access, and the applicant's social worker has reasonable cause to believe that access to the child is required as a matter of urgency, the court may make an emergency protection order authorising the removal of the child to accommodation provided by social services or the child's detention in the place in which they are being accommodated, such as for example, a hospital. Almost identical provision is made with respect to officers employed by the NSPCC (see s.44(1)(c)). In Northern Ireland the provisions of Art. 63 are almost exactly the same, and in Scotland the provisions allowing for magistrates to issue emergency protection authority are supplementary to powers possessed by the Sheriff to issue child protection orders under the provisions of s.57 C(S)A 1995.

A great deal of detail with regard to the duration of emergency protection orders, conditions which may be attached to them, and provisions regarding applications to be made for discharge of the orders is provided in ss.44 and 45 CA 1989 and Art. 63 and 64 C(NI)O 1995. In addition to the provisions for any person or local authority or the NSPCC in England or other authorised persons in Northern Ireland, being able to seek court orders authorising the removal or detention of a child from or in a specified place, the Acts also provide the police with the ability to exercise police powers of protection without resort to the courts. These powers are exercisable by any police officer under the provisions of s.46 in England and Wales, Art. 65 C(NI)O 1995 and s.61(5) C(S)A 1995. In England, Wales and Northern Ireland the police powers may be exercised for up to 72 hours (see s.46(6) CA 1989, Art. 65(8) C(NI)O 1995), whereas in Scotland the maximum period of time for which the police may keep the child is not more than 24 hours from when the child is removed (see s.61(6) C(S)A 1995). These powers confer upon the police a very wide power to remove children from dangerous situations in which they might find them on being called out to cases involving domestic violence, disturbance or in response to any other information being laid before them. The police further have a role in assisting with the execution of emergency protection orders, where the applicant feels that it is necessary to obtain a warrant to be able to enter the premises on which a child might be if need be by force. (See s.48(9) CA 1989 and Art. 67(9) C(NI)O 1995.)

It should be noted that the general principles governing the making of decisions by the courts concerning the upbringing or welfare of children apply to the making of emergency protection orders (see s.1(1) CA 1989, Art. 3(1) C(NI)O 1995 and s.16(1) C(S)A 1995). Thus, the courts' primary consideration has to be the welfare of the child, although the court is not required to have regard to the welfare checklist provided in s.1(3) CA 1989 and Art. 3(3) C(NI)O 1995, as these are not applicable to orders for emergency protection. It should be pointed out, however, that no court should make an order under the Act unless it considers that doing so would be better for the child than making no order at all (s.1(5) CA 1989, Art. 3(5) C(NI)O 1995 and s.16(3) C(S)A 1995) – termed by the author the 'positive advantage' principle.

It must be remembered that in addition to obtaining an emergency protection order or its equivalent and the additional powers concerning warrants obtainable under the Acts, all of the relevant pieces of legislation contain the power for the applicant to ask for exclusion requirements to be linked to the emergency protection orders as described in more detail above (see p. 199 above).

As has been noted, emergency protection orders are provided to be made *ex parte*. Although the Guidance states that whilst the court has power to direct an *inter parte*'s hearing, 'the very fact that the situation is considered to be an emergency requiring immediate action will make this inappropriate or impracticable in most cases' (DOH 1991*b*, para. 4.46). Generally, such applications will be made in the magistrates family proceedings court and there is no provision for a hearing to take place in any of the higher courts. Since these orders are specifically to deal with emergencies, in many cases applications may have to be made to a single magistrate because such emergencies generally arise when the courts are not sitting, for example, at night or over the weekend. The Guidance also warns that, 'in certain situations, giving parents notice of the application might be to place the child in great danger' (DOH 1991*b*, para. 4.46). Where, as is generally the case, such applications are heard *ex parte* the rules demand that the applicant serve a notice of the application and a copy of the order within 48 hours on the parties to the proceedings, usually the parents, anyone else with the care of the child and the local authority where it is not the applicant. The rules stress the critical requirement of informing parents of their rights and responsibilities under the order and clearly spell out such conditions as to medical, psychiatric or other assessment as may have been provided for in the directions accompanying the order. It should be noted that the various provisions providing for emergency protection orders and their duration without right of appeal for 72 hours and their equivalent in the various jurisdictions potentially breach Article 6 of the European Convention which guarantees the right to a fair hearing by a court when it is determining anyone's civil rights and obligations. Since the granting of emergency protection orders and their duration crucially affect the enjoyment of the parents' rights and exercise of their obligations towards their child(ren) it may be argued that these provisions breach the requirements of the Convention.

Practitioners should ensure wherever possible that they identify the child who is to be made the subject of an emergency protection order but s.44(14) does provide that where this is not possible the applicant should nevertheless provide such identifying information as will enable the lawful execution of the order.

Finally, it should be noted that there is no appeal to a High Court judge against the magistrates' refusal to grant an emergency protection order. If the magistrates have not been satisfied as to the grounds required to the issuing of an emergency protection order therefore there is no appeal against this decision. In the case of *Essex County Council* v *F* [1992] Family Law 569, a local authority had applied for an emergency protection order to the local family proceedings court later on the same day as a review meeting held between the mother and the social workers where the mother had indicated that she wished to remove the child from hospital. The child had been in hospital as a result of a number of serious medical problems with which the mother had been unable to cope. Since the social workers were of the view that the mother would not at that stage be able to cope with the especially vulnerable child, they had decided to go ahead with an application for an emergency order. However, the mother did not receive notice of the application until the Saturday and then arrived at court on the Monday without a solicitor and in great distress. Although arrangements were made for a solicitor to appear, the mother was not in a fit state and had insufficient time to give proper instructions. The magistrates in this case determined that since the mother had not had one clear day's notice of the proceedings they would not proceed despite the fact that the requirement of the rule as to one clear day's notice did not apply. They refused an alternative application to grant an emergency protection order *ex parte* and the local authority appealed against those two decisions under s.94 CA 1989. Mr Justice Douglas Brown dismissed the local authority's appeal stating that s.45(10) CA 1989 provided that no appeal could be made against the making of, or refusal to make, an emergency protection order or against any direction given by the court in connection with such an order.

Acting on suspicions that the child is suffering or likely to suffer significant harm

Where there are merely concerns or suspicions that a child is suffering or likely to suffer significant harm, the local authority in all the jurisdictions and the NSPCC in England may seek an order, usually from a Family Proceedings Court in England, Wales and Northern Ireland and from the sheriff in Scotland, known as the Child Assessment Order (s.43 CA 1989, s.55 C(S)A 1995 and Art. 62 C(NI)O 1995). In all the jurisdictions, before granting such an order, the court or the sheriff must be satisfied that the applicant has reasonable cause to suspect that:

1. the child is suffering or is likely to suffer significant harm
2. an assessment of the child's state of health or development or the way in which they have been treated is required to enable the applicant to determine whether or not the child is suffering or is likely to suffer significant harm
3. it is unlikely that such an assessment will be made, or be satisfactory in the absence of a Child Assessment Order.

Since an application for such an order is likely to be a planned response to concerns, the various court rules provide that the application must be made on notice and this underlines the fact that the order should not be made in emergencies (see for example in England, the Family Proceedings Court (CA 1989) Rules 1991, r.4(1)). The Child Assessment Order must specify the date by which the assessment is to begin, can nominate the person who is to do the assessment, and practitioners should be advised that this is really the best way of proceeding since it would be acutely problematic if the person so nominated subsequently refused – it is suggested therefore that prior consent from the person conducting the assessment is sought – and finally the order can have effect for such period not exceeding 7 days beginning with the date specified in the order.

It should be noted that the general principles governing the making of decisions by the court concerning the upbringing or welfare of children also apply to the making of child assessment orders. Thus, the court's primary consideration has to be the welfare of the child, although again, the courts are not required to have regard to the welfare checklist provided under s.1(3) CA 1989, Art. 3(3) C(NI)O and s.16(3) C(S)A 1995 as these have been held not to be applicable to child assessment orders. In addition, again it should be pointed out that no court should make an order under the Acts unless it considers that doing so would be better for the child than making no order at all – the 'positive advantage' principle referred to above (see s.1(5) CA 1989, Art. 3(5) C(NI)O 1995 and s.16(3) C(S)A 1995).

Concerns about children in other situations

It should, of course, be pointed out that where suspicions of abuse arise in certain other situations, the local authority may have the power to simply remove the child rather than being required to go to court to obtain an order to do so. This would be the case where the child is being 'accommodated' pursuant to s.20 CA 1989 or pursuant to a care order made under s.31 CA 1989 and concerns about the child have developed as a result of the child's care in a particular children's home or other residential placement or where the child is being cared for by foster parents (see also s.25 and s.52 C(S)A 1995, and Art. 21 and Art. 50 C(NI)O 1995).

Section 37 directions in other family proceedings

As was pointed out earlier, suspicions about a child suffering significant harm may also surface in the course of any family proceedings brought in the magistrates Family Proceedings Court, the County Court or the High Court in England, Wales and Northern Ireland and in the Sheriff's Court or Court of Session in Scotland. In such family proceedings, a Family Court Welfare Officer (or their equivalent, e.g. the Principal Reporter in Scotland) may have been requested to investigate the child's circumstances and has returned to court indicating that there is a degree of concern about the possibility of a child having suffered or being likely to suffer significant harm. The results of such an enquiry will generally have been in response to the requirement in s.1(3)(e) CA 1989 and Art. 3(3)(e) C(NI)O 1995 that in producing a report to the court the officer is required to identify any harm the child has suffered or may be at risk of suffering. Where the possibility of such harm has been identified, as was seen above in the case of *Re H* [1993] 2 FLR 541, then, in such circumstances, s.37 CA 1989 provides the court with the power to direct a local authority to undertake an investigation of the child's circumstances where it appears to the court that it may be appropriate for a care or supervision order to be made. (See also Art. 56 C(NI)O 1995 and s.56 C(S)A 1995, although note here that it is the Principal Reporter who should undertake the investigation.)

As has been noted above, where the court gives a direction under this section, the local authority is required when undertaking the investigation, to consider whether it should apply for a care order or supervision order with respect to the child (s.37(2) and Art. 56(2)). If the local authority decides that there are grounds for the institution of care or supervision order proceedings those proceedings may be commenced in the same level of court as the original family proceedings.

A further note on the jurisdiction of the courts

It should be noted that whilst all family proceedings courts, including the court for summary jurisdiction in Northern Ireland and the sheriff's courts are of equal standing, the county courts' jurisdiction in England, Wales and Northern Ireland have been classified according to the nature of the case being brought. Thus, county courts have been classified into Divorce County Courts, Family Hearing Centres and Care Centres by the Children (Allocation of Proceedings) Order 1991, Art. 2 for England and Wales. In Northern Ireland the situation is governed by the Children (Allocation of Proceedings) Order 1996, whereas in Scotland jurisdiction in relation to matters of jurisdiction is given to the children's hearings, with some powers also being granted to the sheriff with further provision to appeal to the sheriff principal (see s.51 C (S) A 1995). In England and Wales, the judges who can hear the proceedings in designated trial centres and the types of proceedings to which they are restricted, are provided in the Family Proceedings (Allocation to Judiciary) Directions 1991 and 1993 and as further amended. Where an application for a care or supervision order, or any associated orders, arises from a direction to conduct an investigation made by the High Court or County Court under s.37 CA 1989, then, provided that the court is a County Court Care Centre, the application can be made there or in such a Care Centre as the court which directed the investigation may order. Where a s.37 direction is made by the High Court, it has jurisdiction to proceed to hear the application for the care or supervision order made by the local authority.

Applications for care or supervision orders

Where concern over actual or potential significant harm to a child has not escalated suddenly with the need for resulting emergency protection orders, consideration should be given instead to initiating care or supervision order proceedings by way of issuing an application for such an order in the family proceedings court, or by way of an application for a children's hearing in Scotland. Such action may also be taken following on from an emergency protection order, the exercise of police powers of protection, the result of a s.37 investigation or the obtaining of evidence pursuant to an assessment done under the provisions of a child assessment order and in each case where social services have then determined that these initial orders must be followed up by longer-term protective orders such as care or supervision orders in England, Wales and Northern Ireland or to what are termed 'compulsory measures of supervision' with regard to children in Scotland (see s.52 C(S)A 1995).

Processing the application for care or supervision orders

Practitioners should note that an application for a care or supervision order will not at the first time of application result in the making of one or the other orders. It is most unlikely that a court at the first hearing would ever be able to be satisfied of the various threshold criteria laid down in s.31 and then of the demands in s.1(5) CA 1989 as to be able, immediately, to make a care or supervision order. This is why, of course, the Acts in England, Wales and Northern Ireland provide for the making of interim care or interim supervision orders (see s.38 CA 1989 and Art. 57 C (NI) O 1995). It must be stressed, however, that where social services make an application for an interim care or interim supervision order as their first application in proceedings for care and supervision orders, these will not be the only orders available to the court because s.38(3) CA 1989 also provides that the court may make a residence order although if it does so it must also make an interim supervision order with respect to the child unless satisfied that the child's welfare will be satisfactorily safeguarded without an interim order being made (see Art. 57(3) C(NI)O 1995). As the DOH (1991*c*, para. 3.35) Guidance states: 'the two main objectives of these powers are to enable the child to be suitably protected whilst proceedings are progressing where this is required, and to see that interim measures operate only for so long as necessary'. It should also be noted that interim care or supervision orders may be made either following a s.37 direction by the court to a local authority to investigate the child's circumstances, or indeed at any stage where it is felt that further investigation or assessment of the child is needed to be done by the local authority and that more time is there-fore required to do so. It is provided in the Act that an interim order made on the date of first application for a care or supervision order shall cease to have effect on the expiry of the period of 8 weeks beginning with the date on which the order is made and then if second or subsequent interim orders have to be made in order to allow for further investigation on behalf of any of the parties then such second and subsequent orders can only last for periods of up to 4 weeks at a time. At the expiry of each of the relevant dates a further application for a new interim care or interim supervision order has to be made and the courts again have to contin ue to be satisfied of the threshold criteria laid down in s.31(2) CA 1989 (see Art. 57(2) with reference to Art. 50(2) C(NI)O 1995). The threshold criteria that have to be satisfied before the court can make interim care or interim supervision orders are the same as those required for the making of a full care or supervision order under the provisions of s.31(1) (Art. 50(1) C(NI)O 1995). The only differ-ence is that where the court is looking to make an interim care or interim super-vision order it cannot do so 'unless it is satisfied that there are *reasonable grounds* for believing that the circumstances with respect to the child are as men-tioned in s.31(2)' (see s.38(2) CA 1989 and Art. 57(2) C(NI)O 1995). In addition it should be remembered that the requirements of both s.1(3) and s.1(5) CA 1989 must be observed in relation to the making of such orders and thus the courts must have regard to the welfare checklists and also to the fact that making an order must be better for the child than not making an order at all. The fact that both these requirements in s.1 have to be observed, in addition to the welfare paramountcy principle in s.1(1) CA 1989, is laid down in s.1(4), as the making of an interim care or interim supervision order is an order under Part IV Children Act 1989 and is thus incorporated as being 'the circumstances' mentioned in sub-section (4) in the opening words of s.1(3) CA 1989. (See for the comparable Northern Ireland provisions Art. 3(1), The Paramountcy Principle; Art. 3(3), The Welfare Checklist; Art. 3(5), The Positive Advantage Principle.) Interim care and interim supervision orders therefore are similar to full care or supervision orders in that the welfare checklist does apply to such orders, whereas as was noted ear-lier, the welfare checklist does not apply to any applications being made to the court for emergency or other protection orders such as child assessment orders.

The 'threshold criteria'

It must be remembered that before the court can make an interim care or super-vision order, it has to be satisfied that there are reasonable grounds for believing that the circumstances with respect to the child are as mentioned in s.31(2) (see also Art. 57(2) C(NI)O 1995). In addition, of course, a court can only make a care order or supervision order under the provisions of s.31(1) CA 1989 if it is satisfied of the so-called 'threshold criteria'. Providing practitioners keep in mind that under the requirements for interim care or supervision orders one simply has to establish that there are 'reasonable grounds for believing that the circumstances with respect to the child are as mentioned in s.31(2)' then there should be no dif-ficulty in obtaining an interim order if one so satisfies the court. To establish what exactly is required it is necessary to look at the terms of s.31(2) CA 1989 (Art. 50(2) C(NI)O 1995). S.31(2) provides that 'a court may only make a care order or supervision order if it is satisfied:

(a)   that the child concerned is suffering, or is likely to suffer significant harm; and

(b)   that the harm, or the likelihood of harm is attributable to –
     (i)   the care given to the child, or likely to be given to him if the order were not made, not being what it would be reasonable to expect a parent to give to him; or
     (ii) the child's being beyond parental control'.

There are therefore a number of different constituent elements contained within the so called 'threshold criteria'. The first element of this (which has already been discussed – see above at page 207) is that the child at the centre of the proceedings 'is suffering, or is likely to suffer significant harm' (see also Art. 50(2)(a) C(NI)O 1995). The issue of the standard of proof required has also been discussed (see above) and it was noted there that care proceedings are civil proceedings and therefore the standard of proof required was proof on the balance of probabilities with stronger evidence being required in respect of more serious allegations (see p. 206 in relation to the debate on *Re H and R*). It has to be remembered of course that in applications for interim care or supervision orders all that has to be proved at this stage as contrasted with that which must be proved at the final hearing of the application for the care or supervision order is that the person making the application for the interim orders has 'reasonable grounds' for believing that the circumstances with respect to the child are as mentioned in s.31(2), s.38(2) and see Art. 57(2) C(NI)O 1995.

Having therefore established that the applicant has reasonable grounds for believing that the child is suffering, or is likely to suffer, significant harm, then one must go on to establish that the harm or likelihood of harm is attributable to: the care given to the child or likely to be given to the child if the order were not made, not being what it would be reasonable to expect a parent to give to the child; or that the child is beyond parental control. In looking at the issue of the care being given to the child many academics have always argued that this first alternative of the second limb has always posited a standard of care rather than that it was the care in every case to be given to the child by a parent. In other words one was talking about an objective standard of parental type care which one would expect a parent to ensure that the child received, rather than that the limb was focusing on care which could only be given by a parent or parents. Others, however, had argued that this first alternative in the second limb of the threshold criteria was focusing exclusively on the fact that the care given to the child was not that which would be reasonably expected to be given by the child's parents themselves. This issue came up for consideration by the Court of Appeal in *Re B and W* [1999] 2 FLR 833. In this particular case a 7-month-old baby had suffered serious shaking injuries, caused by at least two violent shaking incidents. When the injuries had been inflicted the child was being cared for by a childminder during the day and by her parents for the rest of the time. The local authority applied for care orders in respect of both the baby and the childminder's own 10-month-old child. At the full care hearing, the first instance judge was unable to make any finding as to whether the injuries the baby had suffered occurred while she was in the care of her parents or in the care of the childminder. With reluctance, therefore, the judge dismissed both applications on the basis that, because he could not attribute the harm which the child had suffered to the care or absence of care given to the child by any one of the possible adults, the threshold criteria in s.31(2)(b)(i) had not been met. Instead, he made an order under the Children Act 1989, s.40 placing both children in care pending an appeal by the local authority and the guardian *ad litem*. In the Court of Appeal the local authority's appeal against the refusal to make a full care order in relation to the baby of the parents was allowed but the judge's refusal to make a full care order in respect of the childminder's child was dismissed. Thus the Court of Appeal found that the threshold conditions in relation to the 7-month-old baby who had suffered the serious shaking injuries had been met specifically under s.31(2)(b)(i), although whether a care order should be made was a matter to go back to the judge for a rehearing. The Court of Appeal determined this on the basis that where harm had actually been suffered by a child, there was no need to prove that 'the harm was attributable to a failure by one or more identified individuals before making a care order'. The court stated that to meet the threshold criteria, the harm suffered by, or anticipated to, the child had to be attributable to an absence of proper care, to the objective standard laid down in s.32(2)(b)(i) CA 1989. 'Attributable' denoted, said the Court of Appeal, a cause or connection of some kind, but not necessarily a strong connection. However, the degree to which an individual was responsible or culpable for the harm was not relevant. The court said that the task of caring for children was often shared between parents who were living apart, grandparents and other relatives and official and unofficial childminders. Where the task was shared in that way and a child suffered serious harm through lack of proper care, that child, said the Court of Appeal, should not be left at risk simply because it was not possible for the court to be sure which part of the care network had failed. On the other hand, said the Court of Appeal in the case of the childminder's child, the threshold condition being considered was the risk of future harm, and because it had not been proved that the childminder had caused the 7-month-old baby's injuries, it could not be said that a risk of future harm to the childminder's child had been established. The judge had therefore been right at first instance not to have made a care order in respect of this child.

The case of *Re B and W* reported in 1999 was given leave to appeal to the House of Lords and was heard by their Lordships on 30 and 31 January 2000 but, under the name *Lancashire CC v B* [2000] 1 FKR 583. The House of Lords dismissed the appeal by the child's parents against the making of the care order and ruled that the phrase 'care given to the child' referred primarily to the care given by a parent or parents or other primary care givers, but where, as in this case, care was shared, the phrase could be taken to include the care given by any of the care givers. Their lordships found that this interpretation was necessary to allow the court to intervene to protect a child who was clearly at risk, even thought it was not possible to identify the source of the risk. Their Lordships emphasised that it by no means followed that because the threshold conditions had been satisfied, the court would go on to make a care order, and when considering cases of this type, judges should keep firmly in mind, in the exercise of their discretionary powers, that the parents had not been shown to be responsible for the child's injuries. The steps taken in this case had been those reasonably necessary to pursue the legitimate aim of protecting the child from further injury, which was an exception to the guarantee for respect for family life contained within Article 8(1) European Convention, as provided for in Article 8(2).

The second alternative to the second limb of the threshold criteria is that the harm or risk to the child is attributable to the 'the child's being beyond parental control' (see s.31(2)(b)(ii)). Again, there have been remarkably few reported cases on this particular alternative. Nevertheless in *M v Birmingham City Council* [1994] 2 FLR 141, a 'wayward, uncontrollable, disturbed and periodically violent' teenager who had originally been accommodated by the local authority under s.20 was made the subject of a care order by the court, despite her mother's evidence that she could in reality control the child. On the evidence of the teenager's own behaviour the court was unable to agree with the mother and found that the child was beyond the parents' control and therefore not likely to receive the requisite degree of care necessary to prevent her having suffered, continuing to suffer and being likely to suffer significant harm. Stuart-White J. indicated that s.31(2)(b)(ii) might apply to a state of affairs which may be in the past, present or future. In *M* the teenager concerned was in local authority accommodation but the courts nevertheless held that the child was beyond the parental control of both mother and partner and thus it has been argued that the reference to 'parental' control is wide enough to include non-parents caring for a child at least where they have parental responsibility.

It should also be said that it is possible although certainly not necessary for both the alternatives of the second limb to be satisfied at the same time. In the case of *Re O* [1992] 2 FLR 7 (and see above) Ewbank J. indicated that the situation of the child not attending school in the circumstances of that case established *either* a lack of reasonable parental care *or* the child being beyond parental control, as required for each of the alternative limbs to be satisfied.

In addition to satisfying the court that there are reasonable grounds to believe that the threshold criteria laid down in s.31(2) of CA 1989 are satisfied, the applicant for an interim care or supervision order is further required to satisfy the court that making an order is better for the child than making no order at all – the 'positive advantage principle' provided by s.1(5) and that the court has had regard to the welfare checklist laid down in s.1(3).

In addition to satisfying all the requirements of s.31(2) and s.38(1)(2)(3), social workers applying for interim supervision orders would be well advised to read the further conditions laid down in the remaining provisions of s.38. It has already been stated that the first interim care or supervision order can last for a period of anything up to 8 weeks but then second or subsequent orders can only last for a period of 4 weeks at a time. Where the court makes an interim care order or supervision order, however, it is also able to give such directions (if any) as it considers appropriate with regard to the medical or psychiatric examination or other assessment of the child; but the legislation further provides that if the child is of sufficient understanding to make an informed decision they may refuse to submit to the examination or other assessment (see also Art. 57(6) C(NI)O 1995). It has already been noted that a similar provision is included within the provisions on emergency protection orders by virtue of s.44(6) and (7). The provision in these sections giving the child the right to refuse any such examination or assessment is referred to as a so-called *Gillick* provision. In debates upon the Bill and in the light of the sometimes quite awful experiences of children in the Cleveland controversy, it was argued that children should have the right to refuse medical examination and/or assessment. However, in the first case on this point under the section where an interim care order had been made, and a 15-year-old girl had refused to comply with the direction as to psychiatric assessment made upon her, and indeed refused to emerge from the bedroom in which she had barricaded herself for several months, the local authority instead resorted to the inherent jurisdiction of the High Court under s.100 CA 1989. Douglas Brown J. in *South Glamorgan County Council* v *W and B* [1993] 1 FLR 574 ruled that the High Court under its inherent jurisdiction has the power to override the child's right to object granted by Parliament in the statute and contained in the provisions of s.38(6). This is, of course, the point at which children's rights to their own autonomy collide with children's interests in being protected (see Lyon 1994). From the point of view therefore of the social work practitioner, if one has obtained such a direction either in an emergency protection order (see s.44(6) and (7)) or in a child assessment order (see s.43(7) and (8) or in s.38(6))) then if the practitioner believes that the child's greater protection demands their wishes being overruled, resort will have to be made to the High Court under the provisions of s.100 CA 1989 in order to enable the Court's inherent jurisdiction to be invoked and the child's wishes overruled.

It should be noted also that in relation to interim care and supervision orders the court can also include a direction that there is to be no medical or psychiatric examination or assessment, or that there should be no such examination or assessment unless the court directs otherwise. These provisions are clearly intended to enable the court to retain control of the situation and to ensure that no unauthorised medical examinations or assessments are performed on a child without the protection conferred by the provisions of s.38.

There has been quite a considerable amount of case law on various issues associated with interim care or supervision orders. In relation to the issue of the basic threshold criteria and the applicant having to prove to the court and the court having to be satisfied that it has reasonable grounds for believing that the s.31 thresholds are satisfied, Douglas Brown J. in *Re B* [1993] 1 FLR 815 held that where there was evidence before the court to satisfy the test that a girl was likely to suffer significant harm arising from allegations of serious sexual abuse, and that difficulties had arisen over the attribution of that harm, he stated that it was enough that he had had reasonable grounds for believing that the s.31 threshold criteria would be satisfied. As he put it, 'I have not got to be satisfied that they exist in fact before making an interim order'. In that case, an assessment of the child was critical in being able to attribute blame and to correctly make final orders and therefore an interim care order was made which ensured that the local authority could properly carry out its investigative and assessment process.

As Waite L. J. in *Re G* [1993] 2 FLR 839 at 845 observed:

the regime of interim care lay down by s.38 is designed to leave the court with the ability to maintain strict control of any steps taken or proposed to be taken by a local authority in the exercise of powers that are by their nature temporary and subject to continual review. The making of an interim care order is an essentially impartial step, favouring now the one side or the other, and affording no-one, least of all the local authority in whose favour it is made, an opportunity for tactical or adventitious advantage.

Further as Cazalet J. observed in *Hampshire County Council* v *F* [1993] Fam. 158–165;

justices should bear in mind that they are not, at an interim hearing, required to make a final conclusion; indeed it is because they are unable to reach a final conclusion that they are empowered to make an interim order. An interim order or decision will usually be required so as to establish a holding position, after weighing all the relevant risks, pending the final hearing. Nevertheless, justices must always ensure that the substantive issue is tried and determined at the earliest possible date. Any delay in determining the question before the court is likely to prejudice the welfare of the child [see s.1(2) of the Act].

It would appear to be the case that the courts have been fairly insistent that interim orders, instead of final care orders, should always be used if important evidence remains outstanding or unresolved; for example, where assessments are still being made and their outcome is awaited, most especially where such assessment will assist the court in reaching its final decision. The court's power to order assessments under the provisions of s.38(6) is thus clearly important. In the case of *Re C* [1997] AC 489, the House of Lords was considering a case in which the child had suffered unexplained injuries whilst in the care of parents and an expert had opined that the injuries were non-accidental. The local authority social workers themselves recommended an in-depth assessment involving both parents and child being placed at a residential unit. In this they were supported by the guardian *ad litem* for the child and the clinical psychologist whom they had consulted. The local authority initially indicated their resistance to the recommendation because of the costs and then latterly because of the lack of explanation for the injuries by the parents and because of their unstable relationship. By the time of the appeal, the local authority indicated that rehabilitation could expose the children to an unacceptable level of risk and therefore they were not prepared to pay the sum of between £18 000 and £24 000 for the specialist residential placement, which in any event, in their view, had little chance of success. The question before the House of Lords was whether the local authority could be ordered to carry out the assessment and the House of Lords ruled that both s.38(6) and s.38(7) (which empower the courts variously to direct that there should be any or no such examinations or assessments) must be broadly construed to confer jurisdiction on the court to order or prohibit any assessment which involves the participation of the child and which is directed to providing the court with material which is necessary to enable it to reach a proper decision at the final hearing. The House of Lords rejected the argument that the word 'assessment' had to be construed to be of the same type as medical or psychiatric examinations or assessments and they further rejected the argument that powers conferred by s.38 were confined to assessments 'of the child' and not of the parents in relation to the child. Lord Brown-Wilkinson pointed out that it was impossible to assess a young child divorced from either their environment or their parents. Their Lordships further rejected the argument that the local authority was better qualified than the court to decide whether assessment on such a scale is a sensible allocation of their limited resources. Lord Brown-Wilkinson pointed out that such an argument could not be made in respect of directed medical or psychiatric treatment under s.38(6), so why could it be made for other assessments. He stated that in any event to hold otherwise would be tantamount to allowing

the local authority to decide what evidence is to go before the court at the final hearing – to allow the local authority by administrative decision to pre-empt the court's judicial decision'.

His Lordship went on to state that, in his view, the 1989 Act

should be construed purposively so as to give effect to the underlying intentions of parliament. As I have sought to demonstrate, the dividing line between the functions of the court on the one hand and the local authority on the other is that a child in interim care is subject to the control of the local authority, the court having no power to interfere with the local authority decisions save in specified cases. The cases where, despite that overall control, the court is to have power to intervene are set out, inter alia, in s.38(6) and (7). The purpose of s.38(6) is to enable the court to obtain the information necessary for its own decision, notwithstanding the control over the child which in all other respects rests with the local authority. I therefore approach the subsection on the basis that the court is to have such powers to override the views of the local authority as are necessary to enable the court to discharge properly its function of deciding whether or not to accede to the local authority's application to take the child away from its parents by obtaining a care order.

It is submitted that nothing could be clearer than the House of Lords' ruling in this case that where the court deems that any assessment whether medical, psychiatric or otherwise is necessary to enable it to reach a final decision, then the local authority will have to comply with the orders and directions issued by the court.

The additional powers which social workers might seek in relation to the addition of exclusion requirements in interim care or supervision orders has already been discussed above (see above at page 199).

Preliminary hearings or other issues to be determined at the first interim care or supervision order hearing

Before the issuing of an interim order, or the hearing of such, the court may, pursuant to s.32 CA 1989, hold a preliminary hearing to determine the correct forum for the case (i.e which court would be best to hear the case), who are to be made parties, and the appointment of a guardian *ad litem* (under s.41). Legal Aid is automatically available for the child who will be represented by their own solicitor as well as by a guardian *ad litem*, and for the child's parents or the person having the care of the child at the time of the initiation of the proceedings. The arrangements concerning the provision of guardians *ad litem* are at the time of writing this manuscript under review and a new Children And Family Courts Advisory and Support Service (CAFCASS) is expected to be operational by April 2001. The new service is to be formed by the amalgamation of the Family Court Welfare Service, formerly under the supervisory control of the Home Office, the Guardian *ad litem* Service, formerly under the control of the Department of Health, and certain elements of the Official Solicitor's Office, formerly under the supervisory control of the Lord Chancellor's Department. Henceforward, guardians *ad litem* will come from the new CAFCASS, although at the time of writing it is anticipated that solicitors representing children will still be drawn from the Children's Panel, a specialist panel instituted by the Law Society comprising solicitors who are deemed to be properly qualified to represent children in care proceedings.

In addition to the solicitor and guardian *ad litem* acting on behalf of the child, it is possible that the solicitor will instruct Counsel, more particularly if proceedings are in the higher courts, thus there will be potentially solicitors and counsel for the child, and the parents and solicitors and counsel for the local authority. The position of the guardian *ad litem* acting on behalf of the child is one which was introduced following the *Maria Colwell Inquiry Report* in 1976, by the Children Act 1975. The guardian *ad litem's* duty is to put before the court what is in the best interests of the child, and in the first instance the guardian's duty is also to put before the court whether a solicitor should also be appointed for the child although the actual decision as to this is made by the court (s.41). The unique system of the dual representation of the child in care or supervision order proceedings, by a solicitor representing what the child wants (where they are capable of giving such instructions) and of the guardian *ad litem* representing what is in the child's best interests, was considerably strengthened by the provisions in the CA 1989 and the relevant rules of court made thereunder. (Similar provisions exist in the Northern Ireland legislation, see Art. 60 C(NI)O 1995 and children's hearing systems within the Scottish system have both the provision of the child safeguarded and the child's separate legal representative, see s.62 C(S)A 1995.)

As was stated above, the appointment of the guardian *ad litem* may well be made at the interim care order stage on first application or at a preliminary hearing or, indeed, it should be pointed out that a guardian *ad litem* may be appointed by the court when it makes an emergency protection order. In some situations, however, the court may be a little reluctant to do this if it feels that at the expiry of the emergency protection order it may well be that the local authority decides not to pursue care or supervision order proceedings.

The hearing for a final care or supervision order

It had been hoped that with the passing of the Children Act 1989 in England and Wales delay in civil child protection proceedings would be a thing of the past. As the years have gone on, however, delay has become an ever more serious problem with public law cases on average taking at least as long as they used to pre-implementation of the Children Act and in some cases longer. In her report 'Avoiding Delay in Children Act Cases', Dame Margaret Booth (1996) visited 29 of the 51 care centres in England and Wales and the remainder returned answers to detailed questionnaires which covered a range of aspects of children's cases. The report was an attempt to respond to the serious charge that delay in Children Act cases, particularly in public law proceedings, was seriously deleterious to the children concerned and that care cases could take between 6 and 23 months to reach a conclusion. The report was concerned only with the part in the care proceedings process played by the court, its administrative and support staff and the judges and lawyers. It identified many different reasons for the delays which occur at all stages in a child protection case including: lack of adequate resources; poor administration; lack of procedures for transferring cases from the Family Proceedings Court; lack of proper court control in the preparation of a case; difficulties arising with certain procedures including joinder of parties, the instruction of experts, discovery and assessments; listing problems; and lengthy hearings. Dame Margaret Booth put forward various proposals to try to ameliorate all of these problems and many steps forward have been made since the submission of her report in July 1996. It is still a problem, however, most particularly for the children concerned in such cases, that child protection proceedings can inevitably be drawn out particularly where there is a dispute over the main issues. It seems unlikely given the demands of the European Convention that much can be done to improve this particular problem since the Convention urges, in Article 6, the right to a fair trial in matters affecting the citizens' civil rights and obligations, and to proceed with undue speed may unduly prejudice the protection of that right under the Convention.

Once all the investigation, medical, psychiatric or other assessments have been completed and the guardian *ad litem* has completed their report in respect of the child, the court will be ready to proceed to the final hearing of the application for a care or supervision order.

The standard of proof required at the final hearing goes beyond that which has been required thus far for the issuing of child assessment orders, emergency protection orders or interim care or supervision orders. By s.31(2) the court may only make a care order or supervision order if it is satisfied on the balance of probabilities that the child concerned is suffering, or is likely to suffer significant harm; and that the harm, or likelihood of harm, is attributable to:

(i)   the care given to the child, or likely to be given to him if the order were not made, not being what it would be reasonable to expect a parent to give to him; or

(ii) the child being beyond parental control.

The requisite standard of proof has already been discussed in relation to the various limbs of s.31(2), as has the issue of the comparison of a child's health or development with that which can reasonably be expected of a similar child (see above). Once the court is satisfied that the relevant limbs of s.31(2) have been established, the court must then go on to consider which order, if any, it should make. Thus, once the threshold criteria have been established there is yet another stage for the court, sometimes described as 'the welfare stage', which requires the court to determine which order it should make based on what is in the best interests of the child. Thus, it is only where the constituent elements of s.31(2) have been proved, that the court will be unable to consider whether or not a care or supervision order is the most appropriate course of action or whether indeed it should support the making of other private law orders such as a residence order.

In order to assist the court in determining whether and which order to make, various parts of s.1 CA 1989 are held to be relevant to the court's determinations. Thus s.1(1) CA 1989 provides that when a court determines any question with respect to the upbringing of a child then the child's welfare shall be the court's paramount consideration. S.1(4) provides that where the court is considering whether to make care or supervision orders then it must apply the provisions of s.1(3), the welfare checklist. Finally, where the court is considering whether or not to make one or more orders under the Act with respect to a child, then s.1(5) applies which provides that the court shall not make the order, or any of the orders, unless it considers that doing so would be better for the child then making no order at all (the positive advantage principle) (comparable provisions exist in the C(NI)O 1995, Art. 3(1–5).

As well as being bound by these various principles of s.1 CA 1989, the court will also have before it the report of the guardian *ad litem* reviewing the history of the child's case and making certain recommendations to the court based on the guardian *ad litem's* investigation and interview with all the parties concerned including the child, where the child is old enough to put forward any views. Consideration of the guardian's report will enable the court to make a better informed choice as to which order, if any, it should consider making but in addition it should also have before it the local authority's care plan. In the case of *Manchester City Council* v *F* [1993] 1 FLR 419, Eastham J. emphasised that the care plans put before the court by local authorities should comply, as far as is reasonably practicable, with the Guidance (DOH 1991*a*) issued pursuant to the CA 1989. That Guidance advises (at para. 2.62) that although there is no set format for a care plan, it should be in writing and should set out the child's and the family's social history. It should go on to identify other key elements which should be included in the plan, such as identifying the child's needs and how these will be met, the nature of the proposed placement, arrangements for contact and rehabilitation, the duration of the placement and what is to happen if it should break down, as well as arrangements for the child's health care and education.

The importance of the care plan is that without having one before it, both the court and the guardian *ad litem* are unable to make any sort of judgement as to which of the potential orders or courses of action might be the most appropriate. This was emphasised by Wall J. in the case of *Re J* [1994] 1 FLR 253. The care plan put forward by the local authority should obviously be supported by the necessary evidence as was found in *Re H* [1998] 1 FLR 193. In the case of *Re CH* [1998] 1 FLR 402, the Court of Appeal quashed a final care order which had been made even though there had been outstanding expert evidence to bring before the court which would have enabled the court to scrutinise the care plan properly and to resolve differences of view between the guardian *ad litem* and the local authority. On the other hand, in *Re R* [1998] Fam. Law. 454, the Court of Appeal held on the evidence that there had been no realistic alternative to the making of an immediate full care order and that the judge at first instance had been mistaken in adjourning the hearing for 3 months to enable the local authority to reconsider its care plan.

In its Final Report in 1997, the Children Act Advisory Committee drew attention to the problems faced by some local authorities in drawing up care plans where the satisfaction of the threshold criteria depended on proof of specific facts, such as 'had a child been sexually abused or non-accidentally injured and, if so, by whom?' As has been pointed out, there might have been no prior history of inadequate parenting or social services involvement but until those questions could be answered, a care plan could not sensibly be made and that might lead to unacceptable delays in the proceedings. The solutions suggested by the Committee, and approved by Bracewell J. in *Re S* [1996] 2 FLR 773 is that there should be a 'split hearing': the first hearing should be held to determine whether the threshold criteria are met by proof of the relevant facts and once the criteria had been proved there could be a second hearing to consider the care plan and the relevant various reports and to decide what order, if any, should be made. The Committee advised that in order to avoid delay, it was essential that a decision to have a split trial should be made as early as possible in the proceedings, and that the case should then be timetabled as quickly and tightly as possible. In the case of *Re CD and MD* [1998] 1 FLR 825 the court criticised the local authority for its delay in seeking a care order and for not applying at a much earlier stage for a split hearing in relation to the issues.

At this second 'welfare stage' therefore, once the court has had an opportunity to read the guardian *ad litem's* report, and any other expert report which might be before the court, it must then determine whether or not the making of an order is better for the child than making no order at all (see so called 'positive advantage' principle). (For a detailed consideration of the two-stage process including the issue as to the benefits to the child of the making of an order, see the judgement of Booth J. in *Humberside County Council* v *B* [1993] 1 FLR 257.)

The court may be of the opinion, perhaps as a result of the guardian *ad litem's* report, or consideration of the care plan, that the making of a care or even a supervision order, would actually be the wrong order to make. The provision of s.1(4) CA 1989 enables the court to decide whether to make one of a range of orders which are available under the CA 1989, including the making, where relevant, of any of the s.8 orders which could be made in conjunction with a supervision order. (The s.8 orders available under the CA 1989, as they are under the Northern Ireland legislation, include a residence order, a contact order, a specific issues order and a prohibited steps order. The provision of s.8 should be consulted for the precise scope of these orders as space considerations do not permit detailed consideration herein.)

Any of the s.8 orders can be made, however, in conjunction with a supervision order. Thus, the local authority may have applied for a care order in respect of a child, and the guardian *ad litem's* report may recommend the making of a residence order in favour of grandparents or other relatives and the making of other s.8 orders in respect of the parents, such as a contact order in favour of the mother and a prohibited steps order in respect of the father, where residence has been given to the grandparents. Where the local authority or the court considers that contact should be supervised in any way, potentially this can be achieved by the making of a s.16 Family Assistance Order (see the comments of Booth J. in *Leeds City Council* v *C* [1993] 1 FLR 269). In order to determine that any order which the court makes is in the paramount interests of the child (see s.1(1) CA 1989, Art. 3(1) C(NI)O 1995), the court is required to consider the terms of the welfare check list set out in s.1(3) CA 1989, and Art. 3(3) C(NI)O 1995. These provisions set out for the court a very extensive checklist relating both to the background and circumstances of the individual child, as well as to the capability of any persons who might be seeking orders in respect of the child or in relation to whom the court is considering making any one of the orders available under the Acts. Where the court is proposing to make a care order, the local authority should, under the provisions of s.34(11) CA 1989 and Art. 53(11) C(NI)O 1995, further submit to the court the arrangements which are being proposed for the child to have contact with members of their family. Where the court is proposing that there should be no contact, or the family or child do not agree with the arrangements being proposed, an application will have to be made to the court to determine issues of contact under the provision of s.34 CA 1989 or Art. 53 C(NI)O 1995 (see further Lyon & de Cruz 2001).

S.34(1) CA 1989 and Art. 53 C(NI)O 1995 broke new ground by creating for the first time a presumption of reasonable contact with a child in care. This was emphasised in the case of *Re B* [1993] Fam. 301 at 311 where Butler-Sloss L.J. stated that

the presumption of contact, which has to be for the benefit of the child, has always to be balanced against the long-term welfare of the child and particularly, where he will live in the future. Contact must not be allowed to destabilise or endanger the arrangements for the child as in many cases the plans for the child would be decisive of the contact application ... The proposals of the local authority, based on their appreciation of the best interests of the child, must command the greatest respect and consideration from the court but Parliament has given to the court and not to the local authority the duty to decide upon contact between the child and those named in s.34(1) consequently the court may have the task of requiring the local authority to justify their long term plans to the extent only that those plans exclude contact between the parents and the child.

In agreement with this analysis, Simon Brown L.J. stated in the subsequent decision of *Re E* [1994] 1 FLR 146 that

if on a s.34(4) application the judge concludes that the benefits of contact outweigh the disadvantages of disrupting any of the local authority's long-term plans which are inconsistent with such contact, then, slow and reluctant though no doubt the judge would be to reach that conclusion, he must give effect to it by refusing the local authority's application to terminate the contact. That is not to arrogate to himself the task of monitoring or scrutinising the local authority's plan. That would be impermissible. Rather it is simply to discharge the duty which Parliament by s.34(4) has laid upon the judge.

In *Berkshire County Council* v *B* [1997] 1 FLR 171 the court again emphasised that since the child's welfare was paramount, contact should be ordered if it is in the child's interest, notwithstanding that the long-term plan of the local authority envisaged termination of parental contact. Simon Brown L.J. further observed in *Re T* [1997] 1 All ER 65 that contact should not be refused under s.34(4) whilst there remains any realistic possibility of rehabilitation of the child with the person in question. For comparable provisions see Art. 53(4) C(NI)O 1995.

Where, in a final hearing for a care or supervision order, the court has determined that one or the other order should be made despite the availability of other orders under s.8, then the provisions of s.31–33, s.35 and Sched. 3 would have to be consulted in detail. These provide respectively for the effects of the making of a care order or a supervision order and in the provisions of Sched. 3 the additional conditions which may be attached to a supervision order (for comparable provisions in Northern Ireland see Articles 52–54 and Sched. 3 C(NI)O 1995).

Additional protection available through the courts

Whereas in most situations the making of a care or supervision order will be sufficient to guarantee the long-term protection of the child who has suffered, or is at risk of suffering, significant harm, there may be situations in which the local authority will need additional protection for the child, or specific guidance in relation to some aspects of the care of the child. Where this is necessary, and where it is not possible by any other means (including the use of the provisions of CA 1989 or C(NI)O 1995) to acquire such protection, the local authority may have to seek to invoke the inherent jurisdiction of the High Court to obtain the relevant orders (see s.100 CA 1989 and s.173 C(NI)O 1995).

A local authority, which has a child in its care pursuant to a care order under s.31, is unable to use or benefit from the provisions of s.8 providing for the issuing of a prohibited steps order or a specific issues order (see s.9(1) CA 1989 and Art. 9(1) C(NI)O 1995). So instead, the local authority would have to apply to the High Court to be given leave to make an application for an order providing relevant protection under s.100 CA 1989 (Art. 173 C(NI)O 1995). The High Court in each jurisdiction may only grant leave where it is satisfied that the result the authority wishes to achieve could not be achieved through the making of any other order under the provisions of the CA 1989 or the C(NI)O 1995 and there is reasonable cause to believe that if the court's inherent jurisdiction is not exercised with respect to the child, the child is likely to suffer significant harm (s.100(4) CA 1989 and Art. 173(3) C(NI)O 1995). The situations in which the High Court's inherent jurisdiction may be invoked by the local authority include those situations where an injunction is required to prevent an abusing parent or child from going near or having contact with the child who has been made the subject of a care order and is in need of protection, as was the case in *Re S* [1994] 1 FLR 623 or, where some operative procedure is required in respect of the child, the child's parents are refusing to give consent and the relevant health authority or trust is concerned about accepting the consent to operative treatment provided by the local authority holding the care order who, nevertheless, are legitimately able to give it by virtue of the fact that making the care order has conferred parental responsibility on them by virtue of s.33(3) CA 1989 and Art. 52(3) C(NI)O 1995 (see further on this in Lyon & de Cruz 2001).

Appeals

Appeals in care and contact order proceedings against the magistrates' decision to make or refuse to make any order by the child, or by the parent, or by any other persons who have been made parties to the proceedings goes from the magistrates' court to the Family Division of the High Court in England and Wales (s.94(1) CA 1989), whereas in Northern Ireland it will go from the magistrates' court to the county court. There is, however, no right of appeal in the following situations:

1. Appeals against the making or refusal to make an emergency protection order, the granting of an extension of or refusal to extend the effective period of an emergency protection order, the discharge of or refusal to discharge the emergency protection order, or the giving or refusal to give any directions in connection with the order (s.45(10) as substituted by the Courts and Legal Services Act 1990, s.116 and Sched. 16, para. 19 for England and Wales; and Art. 64(9) C(NI)O 1995).
2. Cases where the magistrates' court has exercised its powers to decline jurisdiction because it considers that the case can be more conveniently dealt with by another court (s.94(2) CA 1989, Art. 166(5) C(NI)O 1995).
3. Appeals against decisions taken by courts and questions arising in connection with the transfer or proposed transfer of proceedings except as provided by orders made by the Lord Chancellor (under s.94(10) and (11) CA 1989 and Art. 166(14) and (15) C(NI)O 1995).

On hearing the appeal, the High Court, Family Division can make such orders as may be necessary (s.94(4) CA 1989 and Art. 166(8) C(NI)O 1995) including such incidental, consequential provision as appears to be just (s.94(5) CA 1989 and Art. 166(9) C(NI)O 1995) in order to give effect to its determination of the appeals. Any order of the High Court made on appeal, other than one directing a re-hearing by the magistrates, shall, for the purposes of the enforcement, variation, revival or discharge of the order be treated as if it were an order of the magistrates' court from which the appeal was brought and not an order of the High Court (see s.94(9) CA 1989, Art. 166(13) C(NI)O 1995). The role and powers of the appellate court and the court structures generally are considered in much greater detail in Lyon & de Cruz (2001), Chapters 3 and 6.

An appeal from a decision of a judge in a county court Care Centre or in the High Court is made direct to the Court of Appeal and there are no special rules relating to such appeals.

Protecting children in care

In order to cater for a large number of difficult situations with regard to the standard of care exercise in respect of children being looked after by a local authority, the CA 1989 and the C(NI)O 1995 provide for a system of reviews of cases to enable the child complainants' voice to be heard (see s.26(1)(2) CA 1989 and Art. 45(1) and (2) C(NI)O 1995). Where a child is complaining about harm occurring in either a residential home provided by the local authority, a home provided by a voluntary organisation or a foster home, then *Working Together to Safeguard Children* (para. 6.13–6.22) advises that social services must take such complaints seriously and investigate in the same way that they would for abuse occurring within the family setting.

Working Together to Safeguard Children (DOH 1999c) states that 'experiences show that children can be subjected to abuse by those who work with them in any and every setting'. It goes on to point out that 'all allegations of abuse of children by a professional, staff member, foster carer or volunteer (from ACPC member agencies) should therefore be taken seriously and treated in accordance with local child protection procedures ... It is essential that all allegations are examined objectively by staff who are independent of the service, organisation or institution concerned' (para. 6.13).

Both the system of reviews and the new representations procedure (established by local authorities under s.26(3) CA 1989 and Art. 45(3) C(NI)O 1995) were intended to ensure that children's complaints could properly be brought to the surface, particularly in the wake of residential child care scandals such as Leicestershire, Ty Mawr, Castle Hill, St Charles, Melanie Klein and Kincora. Those scandals had surfaced prior to the implementation of the Children Act 1989 in England and Wales in October 1991 but unfortunately further residential child care scandals have broken even since the implementation of the supposed protective procedures. The most recent publication, the Waterhouse Report entitled *Lost in Care* (Waterhouse 2000) has revealed that even where children attempted to complain and to use relevant procedures their complaints were not listened to and indeed it took a great deal even to persuade the then Conservative Government to appoint the Waterhouse inquiry in the summer of 1996. Had it not been for the independent report provided by John Jillings, which was taken up by the *Independent* newspaper it is doubtful whether the Government would ever have been persuaded to constitute this impressive and wide-ranging inquiry.

Unfortunately, the North Wales Tribunal of Inquiry, as it became known, revealed a catalogue of appalling physical and sexual abuse experienced by children in children's homes in North Wales. It is hoped that Utting's 1998 Safeguards Review in England and Wales and the 1997 Kent Report in Scotland will ensure that such appalling occurrences as those in North Wales cannot ever be repeated and further that the recommendations of the Waterhouse Report (Waterhouse 2000) are fully implemented in order to protect children being looked after by local authorities. The Government has put a great deal of money into the *Quality Protects* programme, making money available for local authorities to spend in achieving greater access for children to complaints procedures and such other sources of support as Children's Rights Officers but it remains to be seen whether enough has been done to ensure that children feel safe when making complaints about the system. Paradoxically, the Care Standards Act 2000 provides for a Children's Commission for Wales to be an independeent office to whom children can refer their complaints (see section 72), but no comparable provision has been made for any of the other jurisdictions. It has to be remembered that a child living within the system, be it one of residential care or in foster care, is not easily able to access relevant information about the complaints or representations procedure, and much more has to be done to guarantee such access. Once a child is possessed of the relevant information with regard to the complaints procedure there is then a two-stage process to be engaged in by the local authority which should involve independent members, and greater consideration has to be paid to the issue of children having access to an independent advocate to represent them in such difficult processes. There is such an imbalance of power between the child seeking to make any sort of representation and the panel sitting to hear such representations that it is at least questionable whether such procedures really do guarantee the further safety and protection of children or indeed comply with the provisions of Article 6 on fair trial under the European Convention. What should not happen is that we have any sort of knee jerk responses to the Waterhouse Report. To suggest, as some politicians have done, that more children should be placed in foster homes or that they should be more quickly adopted is potentially to jump from one frying pan into another fire. Foster or adoptive care is not necessarily the safest or even the best solution for some children and finding the right foster or adoptive home may not be easy (see Prime Minister's Review of Adoption 2000).

Important issues concerning liability in the tort of negligence

A chapter on the legal issues surrounding child protection would not be complete as we move into the new millennium without a consideration of very recent cases which have dramatically affected the potential liability of local authorities for the actions of their workers in the tort of negligence for failing to undertake child protection inquiries or for doing so incompetently. This will be even more particularly the case once the relevant articles of the European Convention on the Protection of Fundamental Human Rights and Freedoms comes into force through the implementation of the Human Rights Act 1998 in England and Wales on 2 October 2000. In the case of *X* v *Bedfordshire County Council* and Others [1995] 2 FLR 276 the local authority had received many complaints from relatives, neighbours, the NSPCC, the family's GP, neighbours, health visitors and social workers that children aged 5 and under were being severely neglected in their home, which was filthy, soaked with urine and spread with faeces. The children had been described as dishevelled, hungry and smelly and were apparently frequently locked out of the home. A child protection conference was finally held after a period of 4 years but it was decided not to place the children's names on the Child Protection Register and not to take any court proceedings. Finally, following repeat requests from the parents, all the children were placed in foster care and subsequently brought action for negligence which the local authority applied to have struck out. The court at first instance granted the local authority's application which was upheld by the Court of Appeal and confirmed by the House of Lords. The European Court, however, has issued a preliminary view that the facts of this case disclose *prima facie* breaches of Articles 3, 5 and 8 of the children's rights under the European Convention for the Proection of Human Rights and Fundamental Freedoms. In another case, *M v Newham L.B.C. and Others* [1995] 2 FLR 276 the local authority had arranged for a $4\frac{1}{2}$-year-old, whose name was already on the Child Protection Register, to be interviewed by a child psychiatrist with a view to establishing whether the girl had been sexually abused. The child had given a first name and the psychiatrist and/or the social worker had then concluded that the child had been abused by the mother's boyfriend. The child was made a ward of court and removed from her home and about a year later the mother saw a transcript of the interview and the local authority accepted that her boyfriend was no longer a suspect and the child was returned home. Both the mother and the child sought compensation from the local authority, the child psychiatrist and her employer. The claims of the mother and child were struck out by the court at first instance, this decision was upheld by the majority in the Court of Appeal and confirmed by the House of Lords.

In both these cases, although the local authorities could foresee damage to the children if they carried out their statutory duties negligently and it was demonstrated that the relationship between the children and the local authority was sufficiently proximate, the various courts held that it was not 'just and reasonable' to impose upon the local authorities a common law duty of care towards the children. The courts argued that it would be unjust and unreasonable since such a duty would split the whole inter-agency child protection system. It would be extremely unfair to hold liable merely one agency within any multi-disciplinary group and it was suggested that imposing liability on all participant organisations within the multi-disciplinary group would lead to impossible problems in determining the extent to which any one of them was negligent. It was also stated that the imposition of liability might make local authorities unwilling to take risks and encourage further, defensive investigations which would delay response and reduce the resources available for other social services activities. It was also stated that the nature of child protection work would mean that there would be a very great risk to local authorities of having to respond to many vexatious claims. It was also stated that the development of the tort of negligence to cover the administration of a statutory welfare scheme did not automatically follow on from any existing category of negligence. Additionally, in the *M v Newham* case, the court stated that psychiatrists and social workers did not owe duties to the mother and child for which their employers could be held vicariously liable. It was stated that these professionals were retained by the local authority and their duty was to the local authority alone. In this case, the House of Lords also held, overturning the Court of Appeal, that the psychiatrist had immunity because her examination had an immediate link with possible proceedings and the administration of justice required witness immunity for both civil and criminal proceedings relating to child abuse.

It has been stated by the Official Solicitor that the children in the X case undoubtedly suffered greatly from the alleged failure of the Child Protection Services and accordingly he has taken their case to Europe, since the European Convention was not then in force in England and Wales. He is arguing on behalf of the children that the lack of a remedy for this interference in their family life is in conflict with the children's rights under Articles 3, 5, 8 and 13 of the European Convention on Human Rights. The European court has accepted the reference and will go on to hear the case, which is known as *Z and Others* v *The UK*.

Nevertheless, despite this inauspicious start to attempts being made by children to sue the local authority, two other cases have revealed chinks in the armoury of the protection previously offered by the courts to local authorities in administering a statutory scheme of welfare. In *W* v *Essex County Council* [1997] 2 FLR 535 foster parents issued claims based in negligence for damages for sexual abuse of their own children by a 15-year-old foster child placed with them by the local authority. Despite their having sought assurances from social workers that a child who was a sexual abuser would not be placed with them and their three young daughters, such a child was placed with the foster parents. Hooper J., applying the 'just and reasonable' or 'public policy' test to the present case argued that the court had to bear in mind that the public policy consideration which had first claimed to the loyalty of the law was that wrongs should be remedied, and that if the allegations in the statement of claim were correct, the plaintiff's children and possibly the parents had suffered a grievous wrong and further, that the imposition of a duty on the local authority to provide the foster parents with all the information needed to enable them to care for the child, which information was required under the Foster Placement (Children) Regulations 1991 but had been denied to the plaintiffs, could not lead to conflict between the inter-disciplinary bodies involved, nor could it be against public policy. Hooper J. therefore ruled that the social worker placing a child with foster parents had a duty of care to provide the foster parents with such information as a reasonable social worker would provide and that the local authority was vicariously liable for the conduct of the social worker in that respect. Parts of the statement of claim relying on that duty and for corresponding reasons the foster parents' claim based on negligent mis-statement would not be struck out. Hooper J. went on to rule out the claim for misfeasance of public duty and also a claim for breach of contract specifically but the critical point was that he had allowed the imposition of a duty of care on social services and was prepared to hold that the local authority was liable for the conduct of its social worker in that respect.

In the even more recent case of *Barrett* v *Enfield London Borough Council* [1999] 2 FLR 416, the House of Lords held that a young man aged 24, who had been in the care of the local authority from the age of 10 months until he was 18, could make a claim for damages at common law for breach of statutory duty by the local authority and its employees. He had alleged failure to arrange for his adoption, inappropriate placements with foster parents and community homes, lack of proper supervision, and failure to obtain psychiatric treatment. He claimed that these contributed to deep-seated psychological and psychiatric problems leading to the failure of his marriage, alcoholism, criminal activities and the inability to find work. Both the judge at first instance and the Court of Appeal struck out the plaintiff's claim but the House of Lords held that it would be wrong to strike out his claim in the light of *W* v *Essex County Council* and also with reference to consideration based on the forthcoming implementation of the European Convention. The House of Lords therefore directed that the case should go back for hearing before a judge at first instance and it remains to be seen whether Mr Barrett is successful in his second attempt.

These cases and the possibilities opened up by the implementation of the Human Rights Act 1998 should sound warning bells in the ears of social workers, but more particularly in the ears of senior management within local authority social services departments. The resourcing of legal actions to defend potential claims which may be made in the future by children who argue that their lives have been damaged by social services is likely to be a problem and the more residential child care scandals are revealed pursuant to the North Wales Tribunal of Inquiry and its attendance at police investigations in over 30 other police force areas, the more likely it is that such claims will increase. It is certainly right that children who have been the subject of abuse such as that experienced in North Wales should be able to recover compensatory damages for the appalling neglect to which they had been subjected by those who were supposed to be providing care for them and there is no doubt that the principles of the cases referred to above will be opened up for further extension after 2 October 2000.

Conclusion

What has been provided here is only the briefest sketch of the provisions available to protect children under Parts IV and V of the Children Act 1989, the Children (Northern Ireland) Order 1995 and the Children (Scotland) Act 1995. As was indicated in the Introduction, the provisions in Parts VI–XII of the CA 1989, Parts VII–XI C(NI)O 1995 and Part II, Chapter 2, ss.31–38 C(S)A 1995, also seek to extend protection to children in whatever environments they are being looked after, but in many situations, if there are concerns about the child suffering significant harm, resort will have to be made to the relevant orders contained in Parts IV and V, CA 1989, Parts IV and V C(NI)O 1995 and Part II, Chapters 2 and 3 C(S)A 1995.

To many working with children and families, resort to the courts will be seen as a failure of all the agencies and systems designed to prevent children suffering harm. Whilst to a certain extent this may be true, it must also be acknowledged that there are situations in which resources, however plentiful, will simply make no difference or where serious and sudden outbursts of violence towards children can neither be predicted nor, in many cases, prevented.

Much does, however, remain to be done in the field of educating children so that they might develop their own preventive strategies, and little effort has been put into this area either by central or local government and particularly not in schools. Slogans such as 'information is power' and 'forewarned is forearmed' spring readily to mind when considering the plight of many youngsters who have to act in ignorance of what could be achieved if only they had been taught appropriate strategies. Of course, this raises the concern that discussing strategies and raising the profile of the issue of child abuse may encourage a proliferation of unfounded allegations, but the evidence now being provided by research into the incidence of child abuse and the testimony of adult survivors must make it all the more certain that we should work towards the notion that prevention is always, but always, better than cure.

In respect of the implementation of the Children Act 1989 in England and Wales, of the Children (Northern Ireland) Order 1995 in Northern Ireland and of the Children (Scotland) Act 1995 in Scotland, one has to ask whether the Government can really state affirmatively, in response to questions as to whether we have implemented the United Nations Convention on the Rights of the Child, that it has, in accordance with Article 19(1) taken all:

Appropriate legislative, administrative, social and *educational* measures to protect the child from all forms of physical, or mental violence, injury or abuse, neglect or negligent treatment, maltreatment or exploitation, including sexual abuse, while in the care of parents, legal guardians, or any other person who has the care of the child. (emphasis added)

Art. 19(2) goes on to provide that:

Such protective measures should, as appropriate, include effective procedures for the establishment of social programmes to provide necessary support for the child and those who have the care of the child, as well as for *other forms of prevention* and for identification, reporting, referral, investigation, treatment and follow-up of instances of child maltreatment and as appropriate for judicial involvement. (emphasis added)

In respect of both these provisions of Art. 19, it must be admitted that both the law and the practice, as thus far implemented by the relevant acts, within the UK jurisdictions fail to accord the necessary protection and support for the child and for those who might have the care of the child.

Acknowledgement

I am extremely grateful to Professor Kenneth McK. Norrie for setting me right with regard to several of the interpretations to be given to the Scottish legislation and in particular with regard to the impact of the relevant provisions of the Scotland Act 1998 on the issue of Human Rights.

References

Adcock M, White R (eds) 1998 Significant harm: it's management and outcome. Significant Publications, London,

Aldgate J, Tunstill J 1995 Making offence of Section 17 – implementing services for children in need within the 1989 Children Act. HMSO, London

Bainham A 1993 Care after 1991: a reply. 3 JCL 99 at p. 103.

Bedingfield D 1998 The child in need – children, the State and the law. Family Law, Bristol

Booth, Dame M E 1996 Avoiding delay in Children Act cases. Lord Chancellor's Department, London

Butler-Sloss, Lady Justice E 1988 Report of the inquiry into child abuse in Cleveland in 1987. Cmnd 412. HMSO, London

Dale P, Davies M, Morrison T, Waters J 1986 Dangerous families: assessment and treatment of child abuse. Tavistock, London

Department for Education and Employment (DfEE) 1995 Protecting children from abuse: the role of the education service. Circular 10/95. DfEE, London

Department of Health (DOH) 1989 The care of children: principles and practice in regulations and guidance. HMSO, London

Department of Health (DOH) 1991a Guidance and Regulations, Children Act 1989, Vol. II, Family support, daycare and educational provision for young children. HMSO, London

Department of Health (DOH) 1991b Guidance and regulations, Children Act 1989, Vol. 1, Court orders. HMSO, London

Department of Health (DOH) 1993 Children Act Report 1992. HMSO, London

Department of Health (DOH) 1994 Children Act Report 1993. HMSO, London

Department of Health (DOH) 1995a Child protection: messages from research. HMSO, London

Department of Health (DOH) 1995b Children Act Report 1994. HMSO, London

Department of Health (DOH) 1996 Children Act Report 1995. HMSO, London

Department of Health (DOH) 1999a Local Authority Circular (1999) 33, Health Services Circular HSC 1999\237, DfEE Circular 18/99: TV Quality Protects Programme: Transforming Children's Services 2000 to 2001. Department of Health, London

Department of Health (DOH) 1999b Convention on the rights of the child: second report to the UN Committee on the Rights of the Child by the United Kingdom 1999. The Stationery Office, London

Department of Health (DOH) 1999c Working together to safeguard children. The Stationery Office, London

Department of Health (DOH) 2000 Protecting children, supporting parents: a consultation document on the physical punishment of children. Department of Health, London

Department of Health and Social Services for Northern Ireland 1999 Children Order Report 1999.

Department of Health and Social Services for Northern Ireland 1996 The Children (NI) Order 1995: Regulations and Guidance, Vol. 6, Co-operating to protect children.

Farmer E, Owen M 1995 Child protection practice: private risk and public remedies, decision-making, intervention and outcome in child protection work. HMSO, London

Fox-Harding L 1991 Perspectives in childcare policy. Longman, London

Freeman M D A 1992 Children, their families and the law. Macmillan, London

Freeman M D A 1997 Childrens' rights and cultural pluralisms in the moral status of children. Martinus Nijhoff, Holland

Gelsthorpe L, Morris A 1999 Much ado about nothing: a critical comment on key provisions relating to children in the Crime and Disorder Act 1998.

Hansard, House of Lords 1989 Debates in House of Lords, Official Report, Vol. 503, col. 354 and 355.

Home Office, Department of Health, Department of Education and Science, Welsh Office 1999 Working together to safeguard children – a guide to inter-agency working to safeguard and promote the welfare of children, Quality Protects. The Stationery Office, London

Human Rights Act, para. 81 – Core Guidance for Public Authorities: A New Era of Rights and Responsibilities. Website ref: http://www.homeoffice.gov.uk/hrasection/hregpa.htm

Kent R 1997 The children's safeguards review. The Stationery Office, London

Lau A 1991 Cultural and ethnic perspectives on significant harm: its assessment and treatment. In: Adcock M, White R, Hollows A (eds) Significant harm. Significant Publications, Croydon

Lyon C M 1994 Whatever happened to the child's right to refuse. JCL 346.

Lyon C M 2000 Loving smack – lawful assault. A contradiction in human rights and law. Institute of Public Policy Research, London

Lyon C M, de Cruz S P 1993 Child abuse, 2nd edn. Family Law, Bristol

Lyon C M, de Cruz S P 2001 Child abuse, 3rd edn. Family Law, Bristol

MacKay, Lord Chancellor 1990 The Joseph Jackson Memorial Lecture, 139 NLJ 505 at 508.

Norrie K McK 1995 Current Law Statute Annotated 1995. Sweet & Maxwell, London

Parton N 1991 Governing the family: childcare, child protection and the State. Macmillan, London

Parton N, Thorpe D, Wattam 1997 Child protection, risk and the moral order. Macmillan, London

Prime Minister's Review of Adoption 2000 Performance and Innovation Unit. The Stationery Office, London

Scottish Office 1998 Protecting children: a shared responsibility. The Stationery Office, London

Scottish Executive Justice Department 2000 The physical punishment of children in Scotland: a consultation. Scottish Executive Justice Department, Edinburgh

Social Services Inspectorate (SSI) 1992 Court orders study: a study of local authority decision-making about public law court applications. Department of Health, London

Utting W 1998 People like us: the report of the review of the safeguards for children living away from home. The Stationery Office, London

Wall N 1999 Concurrent planning: a judicial perspective. 11 CFLQ p. 97–108 at p.98.

Waterhouse R 2000 Lost in care: the Report of the Tribunal of Inquiry into the abuse of children in care in the former county council areas of Gwynedd and Clwyd since 1974. Department of Health. The Stationery Office, London

Welsh Office 1995 Protecting children from abuse: the role of the education service, Circular 52/95. Welsh Office Education Department, Cardiff

Making enquiries under Section 47 of the Children Act 1989

Corinne Wattam

> It is never enough simply to comply with the letter of the state of procedures ... There is always an overriding professional duty to exercise skill, judgement and care. (Kimberly Carlile inquiry, DOH 1991b)

INTRODUC-TION

The process of making enquiries is directed by local procedures, all of which cover the requirements stated in *Working Together*.[1] Such procedures can only offer a broad outline; they cannot convey every aspect of the enquiry. Like all rules they have to be applied. The recipe for application – skill, judgement and care – is a good one. However, these attributes are something of a moving feast. How do practitioners know when they get it right? The standards by which they are judged appear to veer from interventionist to non-interventionist, doing too much or doing too little. Practitioners involved in the social aspects of welfare, and particularly child protection, must daily confront these difficulties. Is it better for the child to remain with their natural parents in a potentially dangerous situation, or to remove them and risk the longer-term effects that family separations can cause? What constitutes a dangerous, or 'at risk' situation, and what emphasis should be placed on strengths?

Crucial decisions are made early on in the process of intervention upon which the quality of a child's life might depend. This chapter aims to review some of the research which might inform decision-making. It also considers the official guidance which must be attended to, and some of the practice implications which result.

Review of recent research and literature

Where do referrals come from?

It can be seen from Table 11.1, which summarises the results from recent studies,[2] that the child is generally not the referrer, although some authorities appear to be better at attracting self-referrals than others. This places practitioners in a difficult position from the start. Unlike ChildLine, for example, where the child is phoning for help and advice, the subject of local authority enquiries has generally not volunteered themselves. The onus is therefore on professionals to establish what, if anything, has happened and on what basis help will be needed. Thus, from the beginning there is a particular emphasis. Parents, who on average

[1] The version of *Working Together to Safeguard Children* quoted in this chapter is the September 1999 draft.
[2] Studies reported in Table 11.1 are based on recent research commissioned by Local Authorities with Dr David Thorpe at Lancaster University, with the exception of CAPCAE which was commissioned by the EC.

Table 11.1 *Soures of referrals*

	CAPCAE	Northern LA	Midland LA	London LA
Date	1997	1998	1998	1998
Subject child	3	0	5	2
Other child	0	1	2	n/a
Maltreater	0	n/a	2	0
Parent/guardian	9	15	11	14
Relatives	2	8	4	1
Friends/neighbours	2	2	5	3
Medical practitioner	2	1	0	2
Hospital	7	4	6	5
Other health	7	5	4	6
Mental health	3	2	1	0
Social work	18	6	1	5
School	19	9	15	32
Day care	0	1	2	3
Police	19	10	12	10
NGO	1	1	n/a	2
Anonymous	4	29	20	0
Other	3	7	5	7
Not stated	1	n/a	0	4
Number	316	245	205	212

CAPCAE (Concerted Action on the Prevention of Child Abuse in Europe): final report submitted to the EC in December 1998

refer 12% of cases, may see the enquiry as intrusive, the child might not be willing to talk further or cooperate with enquiries. Information must be obtained from a range of relevant but indirect sources and, from the point of reporting, the right to protection must be carefully balanced against the rights of privacy and self-determination. At the same time the enquiry must address the wider needs of the child (DOH para 2.26).

Schools are a major source of referral revealing the importance of awareness training, which also covers issues of reporting. Health professionals are also a key referral source and are likely to see more children who have experienced maltreatment than they actually refer. The professional sharing of information about children for whom there are concerns has been a long standing problem in child protection (DOH 1991, MacLeod 1996). The Data Protection Act gives clear guidance on the sharing of personal information. Consideration should be given to how much personal information needs to be shared and what to do when consent is not given or cannot be sought. Briefly, disclosure of confidential information can be made for the purposes of the prevention or detection of crime. All forms of cruelty, neglect, physical and sexual assault can be designated as crimes so in that sense, confidentiality can legally be broken in relation to the reporting of any of these acts. It remains the case, however, that some children will wish to maintain confidence (Wattam 1999). This might prejudice the detection of crime and may well prejudice its prosecution and thus, although debatable, its prevention. One study which interviewed teachers who had been involved with cases of children who had, or may have been abused, found that teachers generally reported their concerns. However, the length of time taken to do so varied. A key factor in taking the matter further was the 'confidentiality trap' (Wattam 1989). The interaction required to break a confidence was complex, and not a matter easily addressed by procedures. Teachers found the experience difficult and three methods of getting out of the trap were identified: attempting to get the child to tell someone else, attempting to get the child's permission to tell someone else and asserting the right to tell others by telling children it would be in their best interests. Whilst these methods were ultimately successful, the time between the child's first account and the report varied from immediate referral to a wait of 1 year. Teachers and other professionals can now discuss concerns with the designated member of staff for child welfare or child protection, but the issue of confidentiality remains one which must be approached with care, respect and sensitivity on a case by case basis.

A varying percentage of referrals are anonymous or from the general public. There is a suggestion that anonymous referrals need careful screening on the basis that they are more likely to be unsubstantiated (Besharov 1988). The range of anonymous referrals in the studies reported in Table 11.1 suggests that some authorities may be better than others at clarifying the information source; however, the anonymity of referees should be respected (Carlile inquiry, 1987).

Joint working

There is a very clear mandate that the police and social services should work together in the investigation of child abuse (DOH 1999). *Working Together* requires local authorities and police forces to develop inter-agency protocols on information sharing:

Each ACPC should have in place a protocol agreed between social services departments and the police, to guide both agencies in deciding how s.47 enquiries and associated police investigations should be conducted, and in particular, in what circumstances joint enquiries are necessary and/or appropriate. (para. 5.31)

The forum for deciding how joint working should be undertaken in individual cases is the 'Strategy Meeting'. Strategy meetings should be held in all cases where there is the suspicion that a crime has been committed. This usually means cases of sexual abuse and serious physical abuse and neglect.

The benefits of combining the roles of child protection and criminal justice in the investigation are, on the surface at least, quite evident. If both needs can be met from one investigation this saves resources and reduces the level of intervention which should mean an improvement for children and families. However, there is no research supporting the view that the outcome for children and families is better under a joint working approach. Conversely, there is some concern that joint working has actually made the process more intrusive. If the police and social workers are involved at the very early stages of investigating a report it immediately highlights the potentially criminal nature of the allegation.

Messages From Research (DOH 1995) pointed out that one of the key deficiencies of the child protection system was the lack of inter-agency coordination at all stages of the child protection process. *Working Together* has reiterated the importance of practitioners in all relevant agencies being aware of the signs of abuse and of information sharing between agencies. However, it is not always easy or comfortable for professionals who base their approach on openness and trust with parents to initiate or become involved in the enquiry process. The Doreen Aston inquiry, for example noted:

... some conflict in philosophy and expectation of the health visitor, on the one hand facilitating and supporting individuals and families requiring an open, honest and direct relationship with parents whilst ensuring other professionals were kept fully informed. On the other hand, because a health visitor is usually afforded easy access to the home there is a social policing role in relation to early identification of abuse with a view to protecting the child. This can lead to loss of parental confidence and trust. A balance must therefore be maintained between these two approaches.

This is a difficult balance to strike, and one faced by social workers who must work within the principles of partnership with parents and parental responsibility.

Partnership

A great deal has been written about partnership with both parents and children. This is a key principle underpinning the making of enquiries under s.47, yet, like confidentiality, it presents a number of dilemmas. Views from children and families show that their expectations of the enquiry process are high. Practitioners must obtain trust through demonstration of their competence (PAIN *et al.* 1997). In addition, those about whom enquiries are made valued honesty and respect, demonstrated in terms of recognising rights and individual needs and including these in decision-making. Practical applications would be keeping to plans, scheduling meetings to take account of need, respecting wishes in allocating workers (particularly in relation to ethnicity and gender) and ensuring that everyone feels they have been listened to. Fairness was also important and is demonstrated through enquiries being conducted in a just and open manner. Information is central: children and families require clear, comprehensive information at a level which reflects their knowledge and understanding. Shemmings & Shemmings (1996) identify four key conditions for building partnership which summarise these principles:

- openess and honesty
- answerability
- even-handedness (avoiding rigidity combined with fairness)
- sensitivity.

Each of these principles is relevant to the making of enquiries, as they are to all child welfare practices.

Some children and families will want advocacy during the enquiry process. Advocacy in child protection is a relatively new area led from the ground by advocacy projects, some of which represent families, others only children and young people (Boylan & Wattam 1997, Boylan & Wyllie 1999). Professionals or members of the community not connected with the case can act as advocates for children.

Assessing the likelihood of significant harm

Initial and core assessments will need to be done according to the *Framework of Assessment*, which replaces the now out of date *Orange Book*. The philosophy behind the *Framework* is that the child's needs, including the need for protection, should be assessed in the context of the parents' capacity to respond and the wider circumstances of the family. If referrals have not come directly from the family, and the principles of partnership and supporting families take priority, then the assessment of the likelihood of significant harm having occurred, or occurring in the future, must take place within this context.

Traditionally, this area of work has been framed as 'risk assessment'. The search for the grail of answers, the method that will detect which child will be harmed and which will not, has resulted in nothing substantial. Whilst some factors will alert professionals to potential danger, these are not necessarily the factors that have been focused on in the more orthodox risk assessment literature, and all methods will produce false-positives and false-negatives (Dingwall 1989). The *Framework of Assessment* does not address risk assessment, per se. A focus on risk will narrow the assessment and will ignore the wider issues which may be more important for the child's longer-term welfare.

Practitioners must have some knowledge of risk factors in order to carry out the investigation. Research shows that 'gut feeling' or professional judgement are not very effective tools for assessing risk – and practitioners tend to be distracted by such factors as the status of the referrer and the degree of cooperation being shown by parents (Cleaver & Freeman 1995). Research has shown that certain factors may predispose a situation to be harmful or injurious to a child. Analysis of this research and repeated studies have also revealed that such factors do not necessarily mean that a child will be abused. Many of these attributes have been derived from studies of reported and/or registered abuse. Caution should be expressed for two reasons. First, it is generally accepted that there is a level of under-reporting, and we therefore know very little about the characteristics of unreported abuse and perpetrators. Secondly, correlation is not a cause. The nature of child abuse is complex, and it can have many causes (see Corby 1993 for a review). It may be that some of the more salient predictors of potential abuse have not yet been identified. Whatever the case, at the enquiry stage practitioners can only obtain basic information. This will be about the carers and their capacity to care, family and environmental factors, the child's current state and developmental needs (DOH 1999).

Factors concerning carers and their capacity to care are such things as their emotional, physical or mental health status (Falkov 1996, Stevenson 1998), their current involvement in domestic violence (either as a victim or perpetrator) (Hester *et al.* 1999) and their level of awareness of the child's needs and willingness or ability to meet them (Stevenson 1998). Family and environmental factors have to do with identifying external sources of stress, particularly recent changes in family circumstances, the degree of social integration or isolation, and also sources of extra-familial support. Practitioners are directed to assess the child's needs using the framework offered by the LAC materials (Ward 1995). These include the child's health, education, emotional and behavioural development, identity, family and social relationships, social presentation and self-care skills. Lessons from inquiries and other research suggest two further issues for assessment: the visibility of the child and opportunities given to the child to talk freely and be taken seriously (DOH 1991, Wattam & Woodward 1996). If a child about whom there are concerns has been 'missing' from school, day care, or the neighbourhood for what appears to be an unusual length of time or for which there is questionable reason this should alert practitioners to ensure that the child is seen, interviewed and listened to. Care must be taken not to prejudice future evidence in such interviews but the child's safety is the paramount concern.

Assessment, even at the early stages of making enquiries, should take into account the dynamics of the situation rather than focusing on factors alone. For example, a parent may be abusing drugs but this in itself is not the danger to the child. The danger could arise from the parents leaving needles on the floor, being 'high' when they are looking after young children, and so forth. Risk factors such as 'parent is a substance abuser' (or Schedule 1 offender, or teenage mother etc.) are only indicators of potential danger to the child and need to be explored further.

Decision-making

Many studies have shown that a considerable amount of filtering goes on during the investigation stage, which results in many cases dropping out of the system (Besharov 1986, Gibbons *et al.* 1995, Thorpe 1996, Parton *et al.* 1997). The criteria identified by research which underpin the decision to take no further action may not always be accurate. Cleaver *et al.* (1998), in a review of the

Authority	Child Concern (s.17)%	Child Protection (s. 47)%
Northern	78	22
Midlands	65	35
London Borough	75	25
Home County	69	30

Table 11.2 *Distribution of child care referrals* (Thorpe 1999)

research literature, found certain features of decision-making which can lead to mistaken conclusions about the safety of a child. These included:

- not enough weight being given to information from family, friends and neighbours
- not enough attention paid to what children say, how they look and how they behave
- attention being focused on the most visible or pressing problems which means that other warning signs are not appreciated
- pressures from high status referrers or the press, with fears that a child may die, leading to over-precipitate action
- assuming that when a professional has explained something as clearly as they can, the other person will have understood it
- assumptions and pre-judgements about families leading to observations being ignored or misinterpreted
- parents' behaviour, whether cooperative or uncooperative, is often misinterpreted
- when faced with an aggressive or frightening family, professionals are reluctant to discuss fears for their own safety and ask for help.

All of these need to be taken into account during the initial assessment.

Rather than filtering cases out with no further action, the emphasis in all local authorities is now towards ensuring that children in need are also attended to and that families receive supportive services. The question enquiries must direct themselves towards is whether the child is suffering, or likely to suffer significant harm, and/or whether they are a child in need. One recent research approach has examined the distribution of referrals in four authorities. It reveals a remarkable consistency for the percentage which fall into the s.47 category and, though using the different terminology of child concern, the percentage for children in need.

The data in Table 11.2 suggest that between one-fifth and one-third of all referrals will be cases which require s.47 enquiries. Working on the basis of approximately 160 000 referrals each year (DOH 1995) this amounts to between 35 000 and 56 000 cases.

Analysis of policy issues

There are six essential areas of policy which are relevant to the investigative process: the Children Act 1989, *Working Together under the Children Act 1989*, the *Framework for Assessment*, the Youth Justice and Criminal Evidence Act 1999, the *Memorandum of Good Practice on Interviewing Children*, and the UN Convention on Children's Rights.

Working together to safeguard children

The Children Act 1989 provides framework for care and protection. Under s.47 of the Act, local authorities have a duty to make enquiries to enable them to decide what action should be taken to safeguard and promote the child's welfare.

Section 17 gives the local authority the general duty to promote the welfare of 'children in need'.

Working Together combines the relevant sections and principles of the Act with guidance on inter-agency cooperation, management of child protection and the enquiry and assessment processes. The new version of *Working Together* is designed to address the deficiencies of the previous system which were identified in *Child Protection: Messages from Research*, and to take into account changes in practice in the last decade. All Area Child Protection Committee (ACPC) child protection procedures should conform to the guidance in *Working Together*. ACPCs are now required to supplement the information to provide more detailed guidance and inter-agency protocols for local use. All practitioners involved in child protection should be familiar with *Working Together* and the advice it contains.

Working Together divides the enquiry into two processes, the initial assessment and the s.47 enquiry. It also makes provision for emergency action in those situations which warrant immediate protection for children.

The initial assessment

Working Together says the initial assessment should:

- be completed within a maximum of 7 working days of the date of referral
- be carried out using the framework set out in *A Framework for Assessing Children in Need and their Families*
- address the questions:
    - what are the needs of the child?
    - are the parents able to respond to the child's needs? Is the child being adequately safeguarded from significant harm, and are the parents able to promote the child's health and development?
    - is action required to safeguard and promote the child's welfare?
- involve: seeing and speaking to the child (according to age and understanding) and family members as appropriate; drawing together and analysing available information from a range of sources (including existing records); and obtaining relevant information from professionals and others in contact with the child and family
- seek parent's permission before discussing a referral about them with other agencies, unless such a delay or discussion may place a child at risk of significant harm
- ask:
    - is this a child in need? (s.17 of the Children Act 1989)
    - is there reasonable cause to suspect that this child is suffering, or is likely to suffer, significant harm? (s.47 of the Children Act 1989).

The outcome of the initial assessment determines what action will be taken next. If the assessment results in a suspicion of actual or likely significant harm, then a s.47 enquiry will be instituted. The objective of local authority enquiries conducted under s.47 is to determine whether action is needed to promote and safeguard the welfare of the child or children who are the subject of the enquiries.

Section 47 enquiries should be initiated by a strategy discussion which plans the intervention and decides whether a single-agency or joint enquiry should be undertaken. The enquiry should conclude that the original concerns either have been substantiated or not, and should lead to appropriate action to ensure the child's needs are met where necessary.

The court has powers to concern itself with assessment at emergency or interim stages and with the child's contact with parents. There are a range of orders

An *Emergency Protection Order* can be granted if the court is satisfied 'that there is reasonable cause to believe the child is likely to suffer significant harm or the authority is investigating under Section 47 (i.e. reasonable cause to suspect significant harm) and access is frustrated' (DOH 1991*a*, para. 5.7, p. 26). The court can specify how long it will have effect, up to a maximum of 8 days (extendible in certain cases).

A *Child Assessment Order* can be applied for after investigation under s.47, where an emergency situation is not identified but the parents are not cooperating. It has to be shown that 'all reasonable efforts were made to persuade those caring for the child to cooperate and that these efforts were resisted'. The Order can last for a maximum 7 days. Assessment should be designed to secure enough information to decide what further action if any is necessary. The child may refuse to consent to assessment.

A *Recovery Order* can be made to assist the recovery of a child who is in care, under an Emergency Protection Order or in police protection, where there is reason to believe that the child has been unlawfully taken away, or is missing for some other reason.

which can be brought into the s.47 enquiry process to enforce social work intervention. Three orders were created by the Children Act 1989, in relation to the investigative process: an Emergency Protection Order, a Child Assessment Order, and a Recovery Order (*Working Together* provides details of these). In addition, the police have powers to take children at risk into police protection, and to obtain warrants to search premises.

Most cases do not go to court. If they do, before the case is heard there can be an initial hearing called a directions appointment. This will give directions to everyone concerned about how the case should proceed and can include: agreement on a timetable for the case, appointment of a guardian *ad litem*, decisions about whether the case should be transferred, consideration of attendance of the child and other directions as appropriate, for example, contact or assessment.

The Youth Justice and Criminal Evidence Act 1999 and the Memorandum of Good Practice

The Youth Justice and Criminal Evidence (YJCE) Act 1999 builds on the reforms originally introduced by the 1988 and 1991 Criminal Justice Acts. There has been a concerted policy shift towards making the process of giving evidence easier for children and young people.

In 1987 a working group issued a report, generally referred to as the Pigot report, which commented on extending provisions for child witnesses. Recommendations made by the group included:

- abolishing the competency requirement
- child witnesses should be interviewed as soon as possible after the event and that the interview be video taped
- cross-examination of children should take place in chambers
- full committal proceedings should be abolished.

These recommendations were intended to make the process easier for children and to reduce the need for children to have to give their testimony in open court.

The Criminal Justice Act 1991 abolished the competency requirement, allowed for committal proceedings to be by-passed under certain circumstances, and permitted video recorded evidence to be admitted, but only for evidence in chief. The YJCE Act 1999 introduced special measures which effectively provide for implementation of the Pigot recommendations if these measures are applied for and agreed. Thus children may be heard in private and may be aided by the use of interpreters. These changes, combined with an increase in awareness of child sexual abuse cases and the desire to prosecute them, has served to intensify the focus on the child victim as a potential witness. Whilst the giving of evidence in court will come later in the child protection process, its influence begins at the initial assessment stage. This is because evidence gained at the early stages, including interviews with the child, will be relevant later on and must be gathered with prospective use in mind.

Justice Pigot recommended a Code of Practice for practitioners to ensure that evidence would not be prejudiced during the initial assessment of cases. As a consequence, the Home Office published the *Memorandum of Good Practice* (Home Office & Department of Health 1992). This document provides advice on video recorded interviews with child witnesses for criminal proceedings. The *Memorandum* builds on the '*Working Together* approach', in particular the need for the police and social services to jointly investigate cases of child abuse to combine 'the interests of the child and justice.'[3]

The offences which apply to the making of video recorded interviews cover physical abuse, cruelty, neglect and sexual abuse. The interview should equate with a witness statement of the first detailed account given to the police and should be conducted as soon as is practicable. There are three reasons for this. First, there has been much controversy over the possible contamination of evidence by practitioners and parents prior to the initial interview. Secondly, it is considered better to get as recent an account as possible from the child in the light of research on memory and recall. Thirdly, a recent complaint has more validity in law. As a consequence, video interviews have now become an important consideration early on in the enquiry process and must be discussed, where relevant, at the strategy meeting.

Planning and assessment of the child's development, circumstances, background, competence and availability for cross-examination is emphasised prior to the interview. It is advised that the child's agreement to video should be sought, and if they are too young to understand, the views of parents or carers should be listened to. Written consent is not necessary.

The interview itself should go at the child's pace, but as a 'rule of thumb' should last for less than an hour. It will be phased, as follows:

Rapport – this stage helps the child to relax and supplements the 'base line' knowledge obtained in planning. Crucially, it allows the interviewer to explain the ground rules for discussion, such as: the need to tell the truth, and the acceptability of saying 'I don't know' or 'I don't understand'.

Free narrative – The child is asked to recall everything they can remember about the alleged offence in their own words. Prompts can be made about information mentioned by the child, for example: 'Did anything else happen?'

Questioning – This stage begins with open-ended questions and progresses to specific, non-leading questions, closed questions and, as a last resort, leading questions. The aim is to ask as few questions as possible, to elicit as much free

---

[3] The Home Office issued an updated version of the *Memorandum* in 2000. The new version, like *Working Together*, emphasises the wider needs of the child, and brings the *Memorandum* into line with the new legislation.

narrative as possible, and to avoid leading questions which are likely to be edited out and invalidate the interview.

Closure – It is essential to make sure that the child is not in distress at the end of the interview. Neutral topics can be returned to, the child should be asked if they have any questions, and a contact name and telephone number given.

The *Memorandum* emphasises that these are not therapeutic interviews, and that once they have been completed, it should be possible for 'appropriate counselling and therapy' to take place. The Crown Prosecution Service should be informed about this. The legal constraints to conducting the interview are clearly outlined, and practitioners are advised to abide by the basic rules of evidence. These include: avoidance of questions which assume disputed facts or suggest an answer (leading questions), steering away from talk about previous statements or what others have said (hearsay) and avoiding reference to the character of the accused.

There are a number of administrative and organisational issues relevant to recording, access, storage, copying and handling of tapes outlined in Part 4 of the *Memorandum*. In principle, copying should be avoided, access restricted and storage and handling carefully monitored.

UN Convention on Children's Rights

This Convention was ratified by the British Government in 1991. It is relevant to the investigative process in at least two ways. First, it sets out basic rights that pertain to all children. These are broadly covered by the Children Act and include:

- All actions concerning the child should take full account of their best interests.
- The rights and responsibilities of parents are respected.
- Child's right to express an opinion and to have that opinion taken into account in any matter or procedure affecting the child.
- Right to obtain and make known information and express views unless they violate the rights of others.
- The right to protection from interference with privacy, family, home and correspondence, and from libel/slander.
- The State's obligation to protect children from all forms of maltreatment perpetrated by parents or others responsible for their care.

Secondly, a number of investigations may concern the assessment of behaviour which is alleged to be bad for the child. In this context it should be noted that the following rights apply:

- The child's right to freedom of thought, conscience and religion, subject to appropriate parental guidance and national law.
- Child's right to meet with others and to join or set up associations, unless the fact of doing so violates the rights of others.

Practice implications of research and policy

Competing interests

There are competing interests in the enquiry process, to do with rights, responsibilities, need, protection, prosecution and justice. All of these must be balanced with optimum outcomes for children in mind.

Research on the referral process shows that it is selective in ways which may have been inappropriate: with an over-emphasis on protection and a lack of attention to need. All current policy directs practitioners to redress the balance. This is controversial because research on the child protection process reveals it has selective concerns, and thus need is selectively defined. First, research clearly indicates that a large amount of significant harm to children is not reported (Besharov 1988, La Fontaine 1990, Wattam & Woodward 1996, Booker *et al.* 2000). Thus, advice and policy is based only on knowledge from a system which has been ineffective for child protection. Secondly, families referred for child protection reasons may not contain children in need but rather they may be referred by mistake (false-positives). In such circumstances it is unlikely that the enquiry process will lead to the uptake of family support services. Thirdly, the extent of children in need in the UK is generally acknowledged to be greater than the 160 000 annual referral rate (consider, for example, the numbers of children living with domestic violence, severe poverty and homelessness). Thus the initial assessment of need will be limited to those that are referred. Fourthly, there is an indication that children of black and ethnic minority families remain marginalised in research and whilst guidance and policy must take account of ethnicity and need practice appears to reflect some ignorance and racism (Dutt & Phillips 1996). Fifthly, research suggests that disabled children are more vulnerable to abuse yet there is considerably more that needs to be done to ensure their access to equitable initial assessments becomes a reality (Westcott 1999). Finally, there is a gender bias in child protection which is not addressed (Otway 1996), despite clear gender issues being identified in various research studies: the high proportion of men who appear to be child sexual offenders, the higher proportion of girls who appear to be their victims (Finkelhor & Dzuiba-Leatherman 1994), the high proportion of single female parents referred for child protection concerns (Thorpe 1996) and the focus on mothers and mothering in the enquiry and assessment process (Farmer & Owen 1995, Parton *et al.* 1997, Kitzinger 1999) (see Featherstone's chapter in the *Handbook* for a further discussion of gender issues in child protection). All of these selective concerns are legitimated by the need to protect children from abuse or otherwise support children in need. The implications for practitioners, simply stated but still difficult to put into practice, amount to the need for application of clear anti-discriminatory practice principles (Thompson 1997).

Individual workers will have to come to judgements in each particular case, and within different working arrangements. Much hinges on the relationship in the field between social workers and the police when trying to balance protection, prosecution and welfare. In addition a great deal depends on the moral and cultural framework within which individual practitioners operate, particularly in relation to children's rights, parental competence and participation.

The implications for practice are twofold. Firstly, that decision-making should be guided by the needs of the child, and not the balance of power in social and working relationships. Secondly, that practitioners need opportunities to review and be more objective about their decision-making criteria, to learn how these might affect enquiries and their outcome.

A shift from treating children's accounts forensically

Since Cleveland, there has been an increasing emphasis on obtaining evidence for both criminal and care proceedings, and the impetus in such cases has been to establish the validity of an allegation and identify who was responsible. This has meant that children's contributions to the enquiry process have been either as victims who may be potential witnesses, or more generally as objects of evidence. The shift in policy and implementation of the UN Convention heralds a change towards more participatory, information sharing approaches with children and young people. The enquiry process must actively involve children and seek information not for validity, but to engage them in the process of assessing need.

Confidentiality

Child protection requires a close working relationship between agencies at individual and joint agency and management policy level. Practitioners from other agencies are not only carrying out their own agency functions, they are also helping the local authority to discharge its child protection duty. In terms of sharing information, there is often concern about confidentiality. *Working Together* stresses the importance of agencies sharing information in any situation in which a crime is suspected. Professional confidentiality, e.g. that between an adult psychiatrist and a patient, should be breached when there is a reasonable suspicion that a child has been significantly harmed.

On the other hand, information given to a professional in confidence should not be disclosed to another professional without the consent of the service user. *Working Together* lists the professional codes of practice for doctors and nurses, and also the Data Protection Registrar's checklist for setting up information sharing arrangements. The implications of the advice is that information should be disclosed only with the user's consent unless maintaining confidentiality is likely to lead to significant harm of a child. In that case only the relevant information should be disclosed, and, wherever possible, the user should be informed of the breach of confidentiality.

Disclosures by children should be treated in the same way. It is important to discuss carefully with the child the implications of sharing information with others and the need for doing so. These discussions should take into account the child's age and understanding. It is far better to obtain the child's approval to sharing information. Failure to do so may well result in the child retracting the allegation or otherwise undermining the investigation.

Interviewing the child

It should never be assumed that something has happened to a child. Important decisions have to be made at the strategy stage to weigh up whether or not it is necessary to conduct an interview under the *Memorandum on Good Practice*. Practice experience shows that this is not always in the child's interests, particularly if the child:

- does not consent
- is exhibiting life-threatening behaviour and needs immediate therapeutic support
- is not yet ready to discuss details of the alleged offence.

The style of interview will depend on the age and characteristics of the child and the nature of the allegation. For those who have suffered long-term abuse and who are traumatised by events that have occurred, a more sensitive and gradual approach may be required. Decisions must be made and be justifiable in terms of the child's welfare.

Some key issues

Recording

Records must be accurate and clear, reflect all the work which is being done and all information known regarding the family:

> they should contain clear details of the investigation, assessments, the decisions agreed, the basis on which they were made and the plan on which work is based.
>
> (DOH 1991*a*, p. 26)

Records are accountable. They may be used by the court, they can be accessed by clients, and they may be scrutinised under case review procedures. Distinctions must therefore be made between fact, opinion and hearsay, and confidentiality of source information should be respected.

The medical examination

Definitive physical signs and symptoms of sexual assault are rare (Royal College of Physicians 1991). Although it is possible that medical findings are present in fewer than half the cases where children have been sexually assaulted (Glaser & Frosh 1988), it is difficult to state categorically that these signs can be conclusive evidence of abuse. Cases of physical assault and chronic neglect or failure to thrive are more likely to have medical evidence. However, in some cases the sign or symptom may appear to be quite minor, such as small finger tip bruising on the face or back. The social and historical context of the injury is therefore essential and should be obtained before the medical is conducted.

Medical evidence is important for three reasons: to reassure the child and family that there is nothing physically wrong, to ensure that the child receives appropriate treatment wherever necessary, and to obtain forensic evidence for use in court proceedings.

Once again the general principle of obtaining the informed consent of the child and family applies. This means that the medical examination should be carefully explained to the child, in an age-appropriate way. Where the parents do not consent, but the child does, the 'Gillick' principle[4] applies. Gender of examiner is important and children should be given a choice. There has been some concern that the medical examination can contribute to a feeling of 'secondary abuse' for the child, however sensitively the practitioner may handle it, particularly in cases of sexual assault. When consent is refused an Emergency Protection Order or Child Assessment Order can be applied for. However, grounds for carrying out a medical need to be very clear in such cases.

The distinction between forensic and medical evidence is important because cases may fail to proceed on the basis that there is no medical evidence, and forensic evidence tends not to be sought. In cases of child assault, evidence is narrowly defined in terms of the alleged actions on the body. However, other forensic evidence which might corroborate a child's account can sometimes be present, such as fibres on clothing, bedding and so forth. The child's sense of what happened to them needs to be fully explored, and not dismissed if the adult interpretation does not give a medical sign consistent with it.

---

[4] The Gillick decision affirmed the right of a competent child to take decisions about their own medical treatment.

Conclusion

This chapter has presented a review of research, policy and practice in relation to making enquiries under s.47 of the Children Act 1989. The enquiry process is essentially an information gathering and an information sharing exercise. It is process requiring the skill of judgement in order to assess and balance the immediate and long-term interests of the child, the need for prosecution and justice, and the need for intervention and respect for individual privacy and freedom. A key component of the process is the ability to justify actions in these terms, and to carefully record all information. The initial contact with the child and family set the tone for the rest of the process. It is therefore vitally important that the practitioner is able to engage with the child and the carers in a way that deals with the strong feelings of anger, denial and fear that the process can generate.

Further reading

Hagel A 1998 Dangerous care: reviewing the risks to children from their carers. The Bridge Child Care Development Service/PSI, London

Lyon C, Parton N 1995 Children's rights and the Children Act 1989. In: Franklin B (ed) The handbook of children's rights: comparative policy and practice. Routledge, London

Platt D, Shemmings D 1996 Making enquiries into alleged child abuse and neglect: partnership with families. Pavillion, Brighton

Westcott H, Jones J 1997 Perspectives on the Memorandum: policy, practice and research in investigative interviewing. Arena, Aldershot

References

Besharov D J 1988 The need to narrow the grounds for state intervention. In: Besharov D J (ed) Protecting children from abuse and neglect: policy and practice. C C Thomas, Springfield, Illinois

Boylan J, Wattam C 1997 Advocacy and child protection: a literature review. Report for the Children's Society.

Boylan J, Wyllie J 1999 Advocacy. In: Parton N, Wattam C (eds) Child sexual abuse: responding to the experiences of children. Wiley, Chichester

CAPCAE 1998 Moving towards effective prevention strategies for child maltreatment in Europe; a report to the EC. Available from the Coordinator, Faculty of Health, University of Central Lancashire

Cawson P, Wattam C, Brooker S, Kelly G 2000 Child maltreatment in the United Kingdom: a study of the prevalence of child abuse and neglect. NSPCC, London

Cleaver H, Freeman P 1995 Parental perspectives in cases of suspected child abuse. HMSO, London

Cleaver H, Cawson P, Wattam C 1998 Risk assessment in child protection. NSPCC, London

Cleaver H, Wattam C, Cawson P 1998 Assessing risk in child protection. NSPCC, London

Corby B 1996 Risk assessment in child protection work. In: Kemshall H, Pritchard J (eds) Good practice in risk assessment and risk management. Jessica Kingsley, London

Department of Health (DOH) 1991 Child abuse: a study of inquiry reports 1980–1989. HMSO, London

Department of Health (DOH) 1995 Child protection: messages from research. HMSO, London

Department of Health (DOH) 1999 Framework for the assessment of children in need and their families: consultation draft. The Stationery Office, London

Dingwall R 1989 Some problems about predicting child abuse and neglect. In: Stevenson O (ed) Child abuse: public policy and professional practice. Harvester Wheatsheaf, Hemel Hempstead

Dutt R, Phillips M 1996 Race, culture and the prevention of child abuse. In: National Commission of Inquiry into the Prevention of Child Abuse. Childhood Matters, Vol. 2, Background Papers. HMSO, London

Falkov A 1996 Study of Working Together 'Part 8' Reports: fatal child abuse and parental psychiatric disorder. ACPC Series 1996, Report No. I. Department of Health, London

Farmer E, Owen M 1995 Child Protection practice: private risks and public remedies – decision-making, intervention and outcome in child protection work. HMSO, London

Finkelhor D, Dzuiba-Leatherman J 1994 Victimisation of children. American Psychologist, 49 (3): 173–183

Glaser D, Frosh S 1988 Child sexual abuse. Macmillan, Basingstoke

Hester M, Pearson C, Harwin N 1999 Making an impact: children and domestic violence. Jessica Kingsley, London

Home Office, Department of Health 1992 Memorandum of good practice on video recorded interviews with child witnesses for criminal proceedings. HMSO, London

Kitzinger J 1999 Who are you kidding? Children, power and the struggle against sexual abuse. In: James A, Prout A (eds) Constructing and reconstructing childhood, 2nd edn. Falmer Press, London

La Fontaine J 1990 Child sexual abuse. Polity Press, Cambridge

Lewisham Social Services Department 1989 The Doreen Aston Report. Lewisham Social Services, Lewisham

London Borough of Greenwich 1987 A child in mind: protection of children in a responsible society. The Report of the Commission of Inquiry into the Circumstances Surrounding the Death of Kimberley Carlile. London Borough of Greenwich, London

MacLeod M 1996 Talking with children about child abuse. ChildLine, London

Otway O 1996 Social work with children and families: from child welfare to child protection. In: Parton N (ed) Social theory, social change and social work.

PAIN, NISW, NSPCC 1997 Enquiries into alleged child abuse: promoting partnership with families. A policy and practice guide for elected members, senior managers, first line managers and practitioners. NSPCC, London

Parton N, Thorpe D, Wattam C 1997 Child protection: risk and the moral order. Macmillan, Basingstoke

Royal College of Physicians 1991 Physical signs of sexual abuse in children: a report of the Royal College of Physicians. Royal College of Physicians, London

Shemmings D, Shemmings Y 1996 Building trust with families when making enquiries. In: Platt D, Shemmings D (eds) Making enquiries into alleged child abuse and neglect: partnership with families. Pavillion, Brighton

Stevenson O 1998 Neglected children: issues and dilemmas. Blackwell Science, Oxford

Thompson N 1997 Anti-discriminatory practice, 2nd edn. Macmillan, Basingstoke

Thorpe D 1996 Evaluating child protection. Open University Press, Buckingham

Thorpe D 1999 Individual local authority research reports (Restricted Circulation). Department of Applied Social Science, Lancaster University, Lancaster

Ward H 1995 Looking after children: research into practice. HMSO, London

Wattam C 1989 Teachers' experiences with children who have been or may have been sexually abused. Occasional Paper No. 5. NSPCC, London

Wattam C 1999 Confidentiality. In: Parton N, Wattam C (eds) Child sexual abuse: responding to the experiences of children. Wiley, Chichester

Wattam C, Woodward C 1996 And do I abuse my children … NO! In: National Commission of Inquiry into the Prevention of Child Abuse, Childhood Matters, Vol. 2, Background Papers. HMSO, London

Westcott H 1999 Communication. In: Parton N, Wattam C (eds) Child sexual abuse: responding to the experiences of children. Wiley, Chichester

Assessment

Margaret Adcock

INTRODUC-TION

It is an accepted principle that good assessment is the foundation of sound child care protection work and planning (Department of Health (DoH) 1989). The research over the last 10 years suggests, however, that it is questionable whether agreement exists as to what constitutes good assessment at various stages in the child protection process, whether it actually happens in practice and whether assessment is subsequently linked with effective intervention.

The Department of Health published a *Guide to Comprehensive Assessment* in 1988 but this was not intended to be a guide to initial investigations. Its purpose was to assist long-term planning after completion of the initial investigation. In a study of child protection in four areas of Wales, Giller *et al.* (1992) found that over 75% of children dropped out of the child protection system at a point between referral and the decision of a case conference to register the child or not. The researchers claimed that there were no qualitative differences between the cases which dropped out and those which were ultimately registered. Decisions on registration were not guided by policy documentation or research findings. The researchers asserted that 'In the absence of clear guidelines to document acceptable and unacceptable levels of risk, subjective evaluations emerge'. Moral judgements were made by staff on such issues as normal chastisement and parental respectability, which influenced the likelihood of the child's name being placed on the register.

Registration itself did not guarantee thorough assessment and planning. There seemed to be no Social Services Department guidance or formats for assessments. There was no discussion in any of the documentation on different models of assessment, or any possibility of linking the type and depth of assessment to the severity of the cases. As a result, staff were left to formulate their own views on the purpose and methods of assessment.

Other research on assessment pointed to different approaches in short-term assessment and decision-making, depending on whether the case was physical or sexual abuse (Corby 1993). Assessment in cases of physical abuse tended not to be based on research findings and resulted in decisions favouring non-removal of children.

In assessment of the long-term outlook for the child and the kind of intervention needed, both Dale et al. (1986) working with physical abuse and Bentovim *et al.* (1988) working with sexual abuse claimed some success with their methods of assessment and intervention in difficult cases. They emphasised the need to focus on the assessment of the carer's capacity to acknowledge the abuse. Corby took the view that statutory agencies could not replicate the highly skilled and detailed assessment and intervention practice described by these authors. He suggested that the issue for the policy-makers, if these kind of approaches were desirable, was who should implement them and how they should be resourced.

In 1995 the Department of Health published *Child Protection: Messages from Research* which summarised the key findings from 20 research studies commissioned by the Department. Some of the key findings were:

- Over half the children who were the subject of s.47 (section 47 of the Children Act 1989) enquiries received no services as a result of professionals' interest in their lives. Too often, enquiries were too narrowly conducted as investigations into whether abuse or neglect had occurred, without considering the wider needs of the child and family.

- Enquires into suspicions of child abuse could have traumatic effects on families. Professionals could still do more to work in partnership with children and families.
- Discussions at child protection conferences tended to focus too heavily on decisions about registration and removal, rather than focusing on future plans to safeguard the child and support the family in the months after the conference.
- While inter-agency work was often relatively good at the early stages of enquiries, its effectiveness tended to decline once the child protection plans had been made, with social services left with sole responsibility for implementing the plans.

In 1998 a Social Services Inspectorate (SSI) study investigated the process of assessment by social workers in a range of contexts – selected social services departments, voluntary organisations and health settings. One aim of the study was to inform the development by the DOH of the new *Framework for Assessing Children and Families*. The study suggested that confident and effective practice depended on workers being able to distinguish between the values which they and their agency supported, the theoretical framework set by their agency and/or their professional background and the demands of legislation and guidance. Where practitioners were specific, three main perspectives were said to underpin their practice: an ecological approach which allowed for a holistic assessment of individuals in their environment, a developmental approach which set an assessment of the child in normal child development and a systems approach which focused on the whole family and interactions within it.

The SSI concluded that:

- Clarity and system in the application of theory to practice was important in every case, even where an eclectic approach was important. Data could not be analysed without a theoretical framework.
- Where assessment was a starting point for establishing a treatment plan, understanding the basis on which judgements were being made was important; where assessment in some way incorporated treatment, it was crucial.
- Where assessments involved work with very troubled families, a clear known framework based on theory elaborated by experience and review was fundamental to good practice.

Working Together to Safeguard Children (DOH 2000*a*) and *Framework for the Assessment of Children in Need and their Families* (DOH 2000*b*) attempts to deal with the issues raised by the research discussed above. The aim of this chapter is to describe the investigation and assessment model recommended in the statutory guidance, to consider some of the practice issues involved in the process, and to link these to relevant research findings.

Legal, policy and practice issues – the Children Act 1989

The Children Act 1989 is more specific than previous legislation as to when a local authority must investigate or may assess a child's circumstances. The duties of investigation and assessment are set out in Part V of the Children Act and include the requirement for a court direction in respect of medical and other assessments where there is an emergency protection or an interim care order. They should be considered in conjunction with the guidance in *Working Together* (DOH 2000*a*).

All work where significant harm to a child is suspected or confirmed requires an assessment to be made, both of the health and development of the child and of the child's needs. *Working Together* states 'sometimes a single traumatic event may constitute significant harm'. More often significant harm is a compilation of significant events both acute and longstanding, which interrupt, change or damage the child's physical or psychological development. Some children live in family and social circumstances where their health and development are neglected. For them it is the corrosiveness of long-term emotional, physical or sexual abuse that causes impairment of health and development to the extent of constituting significant harm. In each case it is necessary to consider any ill treatment alongside the family's strengths and supports.

Differing values

It is important for practitioners to be aware that the research suggests that, although there is agreement between the different professions and with the general public about what constitutes child maltreatment, there is often disagreement about the relative seriousness of it as a criteria for intervention. Boehm (1962) found that social workers, doctors, clergy, nurses and teachers were more likely to perceive the need for intervention than lawyers and businessmen. She suggests that the explanation may be that the latter are more likely to value individual freedom, legal rights and minimal intervention.

Giovannoni & Bercerra (1979) found that amongst the general public there were marked ethnic and social class differences in the perceptions of the relative seriousness of different kinds of maltreatment. For example, black mothers rated matters pertaining to supervision and basic child care as more serious than other respondents. Hispanic mothers were more concerned about sexual abuse and sexual mores. Amongst white respondents, lower education and lower income were related to ratings of greater seriousness. They state that the notion that the labelling of maltreatment by white middle class professionals as simply an imposition of their values on lower class people and those who are not white is clearly over-simplistic.

The definition of assessment

All professionals who become involved in child protection work are engaged in assessment of some kind in their daily work. It is highly likely, however, that their definitions of assessment and the purposes for which it is used will differ. Trowell (1993) suggested that there is often failure when professionals come together in multidisciplinary work in child protection to share and clarify definitions. Misleading assumptions are then made about other colleagues' meanings and activities. This can lead to confusion, antagonism and lack of cooperation. As a consequence, children and families may not receive the protection and help they need.

The following examples of different professional assessment activities and aims were shared in a group, which was looking at working together in multidisciplinary assessments.

Midwife

- Assessment of the well-being of the unborn baby and health of the mother.
- Purpose to ensure live healthy mother/child and safe environment.

Health visitor

- Assessment of family functioning and any areas of stress, either ante- or post-natally.
- Purpose to assess needs and mobilise any necessary resources.

Family centre worker

- Assessment of family functioning and parenting skills.
- Purpose to prevent family breakdown and assess whether child(ren) can stay at home.

Social worker

- Assessment of family problems and any deficits in the care of the child(ren).
- Purpose to identify any unmet needs of the child and any risk of harm, and to offer appropriate services.
- Assessment of parent's ability to protect the child.
- Purpose to contribute to statutory investigation of significant harm and subsequent decisions about need and child protection.

Speech therapist

- Assessment of feeding and communication skills in relation to child development and functioning in the family.
- Purpose to identify and address any communication problems.

Health therapist

- Assessment of ongoing health and development of children.
- Purpose to assess any cause for concern.

All these activities contribute to the promotion of the welfare of children and their protection from significant harm. All are part of the new *Framework for Assessment of Children in Need and their Families* (DOH 2000*b*). Most of these assessments will not, however, be undertaken with the primary aim of contributing to social services child protection investigations and assessments, although they may all contain information which could at some stage be highly relevant. All professions therefore need to understand the new assessment framework (DOH 2000*b*). They also need to understand each other's roles and functions and what their particular assessment could contribute to safeguarding and promoting children through the new assessment framework.

Working with families in partnership

Before looking at the detail of the process of assessment, consideration needs to be given to the context in which it should take place. Under the Children Act, working in partnership is an integral part of all work with children and families. It must form the basis of all assessment work. *Working Together* para. 7.2 (DOH 2000*a*) states that, 'Family members have a unique role and importance in the lives of children, and children attach great value to their family relationships. Family members know more about their family than any professional could possibly know, and well-founded decisions about a child should draw on this knowledge and understanding. Family members should normally have a right to know what is being said about them, and to contribute to important decisions about their lives and those of their children'.

'Where there are concerns about significant harm to a child, social services departments have a statutory duty to make enquiries and, if necessary, statutory powers to intervene to safeguard the child and promote their welfare. Where there is compulsory intervention in family life in this way, parents should be helped and encouraged to play as large a part as possible in decision-making and planning processes' (DOH 2000*a*, para. 7.3).

'Partnerships do *not* mean always agreeing with parents or other adult family members, or always seeking a way forward which is acceptable to them. The aim of child protection processes is to ensure the safety and welfare of a child, and the child's interests should always be paramount. Some parents may feel hurt and angry and refuse to cooperate with professionals. Not all parents may be able to safeguard their children, even with help and support. Especially in child sexual abuse, some may be vulnerable to manipulation by a perpetrator of abuse. A minority of parents are actively dangerous to their children, other family members, or professionals, and/or unable to change' (DOH 2000*a*, para. 7.5).

'Those working together to safeguard children should agree a common understanding in each case, and at each stage of work, of how children and families will be involved in child protection processes and what information should be shared with them. There should be a presumption of openness, joint decision-making and willingness to listen to families and capitalise on their strengths, but the guiding principle should always be what is in the best interests of the child' (DOH 2000*a*, para 7.6).

'Agencies should be honest and explicit with children and families about professional roles, responsibilities, powers and expectations, and what is and is not negotiable' (DOH 2000*a*, para. 7.7).

'Working relationships with families should develop according to individual circumstances. From the outset, professionals should assess if, when and how the involvement of different family members – both children and adults – can contribute to safeguarding and promoting the welfare of a particular child or group of children. This assessment may change over time as more information becomes available or as families feel supported by professionals' (DOH 2000a, para. 7.8).

In a discussion about partnership, the Family Rights Group (1992) commented that respect for statutory rights and the attitudes of professionals were perceived by families as all important. These rights need to be incorporated into all assessment work.

Under the Act, parents are entitled to:

- information/consultation about procedures, planning and decision-making
- involvement in child protection conferences
- access to complaints procedures
- exercise parental responsibility, subject to the limitations of s.47, 37 and 31
- withdraw children from accommodation.

Attitudes should reflect the following principles:

Respect for persons

This is possible even in difficult situations. Salter (1988) describes this in relation to sex offenders. She says 'the critically important factor is the simultaneous capacity of the worker to extend respect to people as human beings, to empathise with their pain, and to believe in their capacity to do better in the future while not colluding with their sexual abuse a single inch.'

Willingness to allow and encourage the expression of anger

Anger is almost inevitably present when restrictions are placed on an individual parent's freedom of action. The worker needs to express empathy and then to explain which areas are non-negotiable and which are the areas where the client still has free choice. (Rooney 1988).

A sense of fairness and natural justice

Morrison (1990) describes this as comprising the opportunity of advance warning, of prior consultation, of being heard to object, of representation, of knowing the full circumstances of the decision and of appeal.

Honesty, directness and openness combined with empathy and support

Crittenden (1991) points out the similarities between parental failure to care for and protect the child and the failure of society to protect its weaker and more vulnerable members from poverty, victimisation and discrimination.

The nature and process of assessment under the children act

Working Together to Safeguard Children (DOH 2000*a*) and the *Framework for the Assessment of Children in Need and their Families* (DOH 2000*b*) replaces *Protecting Children: A Guide for Social Workers Undertaking a Comprehensive Assessment* (DOH 1998). Much of the thinking of *Protecting Children* about children's development and carers' capacity to respond to children's needs has been incorporated in the new *Framework for Assessment*.

The *Framework* is based on the requirement to gain a thorough understanding of:

- the developmental needs of the child
- the capacity of the parents and caregivers to respond appropriately to those needs
- the impact of wider family and environmental factors on parenting capacity and the child.

These are described as three inter-related systems or domains, each of which has a number of critical dimensions. The interaction or the influence of these dimensions on each other requires careful exploration during assessment, with the ultimate aim being to understand how they affect the child(ren) in the family. This analysis of the child's situation will inform planning and action to secure the best outcomes for the child. All assessment activity and subsequent planning and provision of services must focus on ensuring the child's welfare is safeguarded and promoted.

The *Framework* emphasises the need to treat assessment as a process rather than an event. In evaluating the results of the assessment and planning a response, practitioners will be expected to consider the totality of the child's development and any unmet needs rather than focusing too narrowly on a need for protection.

Working Together (DOH 2000*a*) identifies the following stages of work in individual child protection cases:

- Referral and recognition
- Initial assessment
- Next steps – no suspected actual or likely harm
- Next steps – suspected actual or likely significant harm
- Immediate protection
- Strategy discussion
- S.47 enquiries and core assessment
- The outcome of s.47 enquiries – decisions about further action
- Initial Child Protection Conference
    (i)   to review information obtained about the child's health, development and functioning and the parents/carers capacity to ensure the child's safety and promote the child's health and development
    (ii)   to make judgements about the likelihood of the child suffering significant harm in the future
    (iii) to decide what future action is needed to safeguard the child and promote his or her welfare, how that action will be taken forward and with what intended outcomes
- Completion, within 42 days of beginning the initial assessment
- Child Protection Review Conference
- De-registration.

Risk assessments

Risk assessment is a term that is frequently used without practitioners being clear exactly what is meant or when it should take place. The initial investigation has often been described as a risk assessment. A risk assessment should be defined as the systematic collection of information to determine the degree to which a child is likely to be abused or neglected at some future point in time (Doueck *et al.* 1992). It should be linked to the question of whether the child is safe in the current living situation. It could be argued that this assessment of risk should be taking place throughout the child protection process.

It is important to remember, however, that a 'risk assessment' will provide only one part, albeit an important one, of the core assessment required by *Working Together*. It should enable practitioners to decide whether the parents have the capacity to keep the child safe from harm. The other two important aspects are the child's developmental needs and the parental capacity to meet those needs.

There are various models of risk assessment. Workers often are presented with checklists of so-called risk factors and an additive approach is adopted, whereby the more worrying factors there are, the more risky the case is thought to be. Doueck *et al.* (1992) describe and evaluate three models which are widely used in the USA. All modes include risk factors which relate to the child, the caregivers and the maltreatment. All three models stress that there are connections between treatment planning and identified risk factors, and the assessment of risk should be based on competently trained staff and not on a single risk factor. It should be noted that all three models also claim that they promote comprehensive assessments. Doueck and colleagues conclude that there should be caution about the overall utility of risk assessment systems. First, questions remain about the reliability and validity of most models. Second, research indicates that there are problems about the adequate implementation of the models. Third, these models cannot replace competently trained staff. All the models Doueck reviewed required a staff trained and knowledgeable in human growth and development, parenting practices, the causes and effects of mistreatment and family dynamics.

Nevertheless, Jones *et al.* (1993) make the important point that one of the major advantages of risk assessment systemisation may lie less in the content than in the process which is involved in applying it.

When they (the workers) have to apply some sort of matrix to the problem they are faced with, the problem itself is broken down into more manageable bits. The process allows the worker to consider different elements of the situation, rather than being overwhelmed by one striking component of a child abuse case. I would argue that the all-important process of maintaining neutrality can be enhanced by such a process of analysis and consideration of the different elements of risk.

In a later publication, Jones (1998) sets out a series of stages which the practitioner can consider and apply to the individual case. He says that this process has been described as one of risk assessment though 'in many respects risk assessment is merely the description of good methodical practice to risky situations.' The stages are:

- Gather all relevant information from all domains, including positive and negative features.
- Weigh all factors, in order to define the current risk.
- Identify those future circumstances which might increase or decrease risk (considering all domains of risk and proposed treatment strategies).
- Assess the likelihood of successful intervention.
- Make a prognosis, based on the primary stages, identifying the likelihood of particular outcomes occurring (risk prediction).
- Risk management plan (who will notice changes and what will they do).
- When will the next review occur?

These stages are very compatible with those set out in *Working Together*.

Undertaking the assessment

The process of assessment

Assessment has several phases which overlap and lead into planning, action and review. The *Framework* defines the process as:

- acquisition of information
- exploring facts and feelings
- putting meaning to the situation, distinguishing the child and family's perceptions from those of professionals
- reaching an understanding, with the family, wherever possible, of what is happening, problems, strengths and difficulties, and the impact on the child
- drawing up an analysis of the needs of the child and parenting capacity as a basis for formulating a plan.

Initial assessment

After a referral has been received, indicating concerns about a child's welfare, an initial assessment must be completed within 7 working days. Using the dimensions from the *Framework for Assessment of Children in Need and Their Families* (DOH 2000*b*) the following questions should be addressed

- What are the needs of the child?
- Are the parents able to respond appropriately to the child's needs?
- Is the child being adequately safeguarded from significant harm, and are the parents able to promote the child's health and development?
- Is action required to safeguard and promote the child's welfare?

The process of initial assessment should involve seeing and speaking to the child (according to age and understanding) and family members as appropriate; drawing together and analysing available information from a range of sources (including existing records); and obtaining relevant information from professionals and others in contact with the child and family. All relevant information should be taken into account.

In the course of this assessment the social services department should ask:

- Is the child in need?
- Is there reasonable cause to suspect that this child is suffering or is likely to suffer significant harm?

The focus of the initial assessment should be the welfare of the child. It is important to remember that even if the reason for a referral was a concern about abuse or neglect which is not subsequently substantiated, a family may still benefit from support and practical help to promote a child's health and development (DOH 2000*a*), paras 5.13–5.16.

Sometimes there will be a need for an investigative interview with a view to gathering evidence for criminal proceedings. The *Memorandum of Good Practice* (Home Office & DOH 1992) should be followed as recognised good practice for all videoed investigative interviews with children.

It is emphasised in *Working Together* that enquiries should always be carried out in such a way as to mimimise distress to the child and to ensure that families are treated sensitively and with respect. As far as possible, enquiries should be conducted in a way that allows for future working relationships with families. The way in which a case is handled initially can affect the entire subsequent process (DOH 2000*a*, para. 5.44).

Core assessments

A core assessment replaces the former comprehensive assessment. A core assessment is deemed to have commenced at the point the initial assessment ended, or a strategy discussion decided to initiate enquiries under s.47 of the Children Act 1989 or new information on an open case indicated a core assessment should be undertaken. A core assessment must be completed in respect of every child who has been placed on the Child Protection Register.

A core assessment is defined in the *Framework* as an in-depth assessment which addresses the central or most important aspects of the needs of the child and the capacity of the parents or caregivers to respond appropriately to these needs within the wider family and community context. While this assessment is led by social services it is likely to involve other disciplines, either providing information they hold about the child or parents, contributing specialist knowledge or advice to social services or undertaking specialist assessments.

The core assessment should provide professionals with an opportunity to try and engage with a family in a dynamic process which would give them all an opportunity of gaining more understanding of the causes of the concern about the child, of what changes would be needed to resolve these and the potential for change. The assessment should offer parents and children an opportunity for reflection and consideration of their family functioning and the degree to which the children's needs are being met.

It is stated that specialist assessments may need to be commissioned by outside specialists, particularly if there are issues related to adult learning difficulties, mental illness, substance addiction, or dangerousness. The need for the assessment to be undertaken on a multidisciplinary basis is stressed throughout.

Those undertaking an assessment are required to make reference to relevant research findings and have a clear theoretical base for their work.

It is essential that practitioners and their managers ensure that practice and supervision are grounded in the most up to date knowledge. Practice is expected to be evidence based. Practitioners should use knowledge critically from research and practice about the needs of children and their families and the outcomes of services and interventions to inform their assessment and planning and learn from the experience of users of services – children and families. The combination of practice grounded in knowledge and evidence bases with the use of finely balanced professional judgement is the foundation of effective social services practice with children and families. (DOH 2000 *b* para. 1.57–1.59)

Assessment is firmly linked to analysis and subsequent intervention. It is stated that

The conclusion of an assessment should result in:

■   an analysis of the needs of the child and the parental capacity to respond appropriately to those needs;
■   identification of where intervention will be required to secure the wellbeing of the child or young person;
■   a realistic plan of action (including services to be provided), detailing who has responsibility for action, a timetable and process for review. (DOH 200b, para 4.1)

Managing the process of a core assessment

Planning the assessment

Before the core assessment begins, consideration needs to be given as to who should be involved in an assessment and how the work will be planned and managed. The more care that is taken and the more preparation that is done at this stage, the less there are likely to be irretrievable difficulties in the work with the family.

The core assessment is likely to take place in situations of existing or likely significant harm, where there are concerns about the impairment of health and development of the child and about parental capacity to meet the child's needs. The gravity of the situation for the child and their future development needs to be recognised. The information already available about the child and the parents, together with any environmental pressure and the family's response to professional intervention, needs to form the basis of the planning. The planning team needs to think about how best to establish an appropriate context for the work, to enable the workers to engage with the family and to process the work appropriately.

First, as far as possible the child(ren) need to be safe. A preoccupation with a high level of continuing harm or likely harm makes it very difficult for everyone to focus on developing understanding and explanations about what is going on in the family.

Second, the context for assessment must be created. As Morrison (1991) says, 'families are often defensive and reluctant to look at the real issues. The motivation for change is often greater in the agencies than in the family. Assisting families with deeply entrenched patterns of dysfunctional behaviour to make a serious commitment to change requires considerable skill, patience and effort.' Motivation to change comes from an interplay of internal and external factors. Families therefore, need a clear message from the social services department about the concern for the child and the need for an assessment.

Race, gender and the circumstances of the case clearly need consideration. It may be that different workers should work with different family members. Situations in which there has been very distressing harm or trauma may need more than one worker to mimimise the stress for the child. If the family is likely to have continuing crises throughout the assessment or feels extremely angry about initial investigation, it may be better for one worker to hold the case responsibility and for another to undertake only the responsibility for the assessment.

Involving families

The experience of workers who have undertaken assessments is that the initial negotiations with families to involve them and obtain their agreement to participate are crucial. Difficulties are likely to arise during the process if an assessment is started without the family understanding what the assessment is, why it is needed and how they might benefit from the outcome.

Thought needs to be given as to what the family might gain from the assessment and to discuss this with them. This will vary according to the circumstances. For some families, help with their child's behaviour difficulties is very important. Others may want the child's name removed from the Register. It must always be made clear that participation in the assessment does not guarantee the desired outcome but this will be attempted.

The assessment is usually undertaken by involving the family individually and in combinations in a series of activities and questions that seem appropriate for their circumstances and abilities, e.g. the use of Genograms, eco maps and homework between sessions. All these activities may lead to some change, as family members are encouraged to interact or behave or talk in different ways. The worker needs to be alert to recognise the moment when change is happening and to make constructive use of it.

Components of the assessment

The components of the core assessment are set out in the *Framework* (DOH 2000*b*, Chapter 8). All these components are important, although space only permits discussion here of three elements.

Causes for concern

It is important in most cases to start by exploring with the family what they think are the causes for concern about the child and their upbringing. The parents may have a different view from the professionals, and their concerns may be very relevant. They may not understand what the professionals' worries are. Giving parents an opportunity to discuss their own concerns may enable the professionals to help parents realise why other people are concerned.

An example of this was a 3-year-old girl called Sharon, who was thought by the paediatrician and health visitor to be developmentally delayed and not making progress because her mother did not stimulate her or exercise appropriate controls. The mother was seen as hysterical and unhelpful. The social services department became involved after Sharon's father beat her severely for her defiant behaviour. During the assessment, the mother revealed that she had thought there was something wrong with Sharon from the time of her very difficult labour and forceps delivery. Sharon had been a very difficult baby to care for, she was very unresponsive to her mother and then, when she finally became mobile, was restless and lacking in concentration. The mother had no support because her own parents were in Ireland. The next baby, born 2 years later, had no problems and this confirmed the mother's fears about Sharon. After the mother had discussed her perceptions, these were shared with the paediatrician. The latter agreed that Sharon might have some minor residual damage as a result of her birth but then reassured the mother that with help Sharon could now make good progress. This enabled the mother then to look at what she and her husband could now do differently to help Sharon.

It may be necessary for the worker both to provide factual information, to correct any misapprehensions, and to explain fully the concerns of other professionals. The parents may sometimes be quite ignorant of the significance of various forms of harm or importance of health and development. Hooper (1992) suggests, for example, that mothers in her research sometimes did not realise that certain sexual behaviours were abusive. The social worker may need to discuss the significance of a particular condition for a child with other professionals before they talk with a parent. They may also want the other professional to talk to the parent at some stage.

Discussions about the causes for concern will enable the professional to begin to make an assessment of two factors, which will need to be explored further in the discussions with the parents/carers about the child's perceptions, and about the parents/carers as individuals and the adult family relationships. The first is the non-abusing parent's willingness and ability to protect the child in the future. This is a key part of any assessment, particularly in cases involving sexual abuse or violence. Account needs to be taken of how recently the non-abusing parent has learnt about the abuse, what supports have been provided, and what have been the consequences of the disclosure, e.g. the abuser has left the home. Attention should be given to the parent's relationship with the abuser, e.g. there is a high likelihood of future violence to the non-abusing parent or, alternatively, there is some degree of collusion between the parents. The second factor is what responsibility the parents/carers take for the harm that has occurred, or is likely occur, and whether they are willing to work with the professionals to resolve the consequences and to see that the child is protected in the future. It is unlikely that many parents/carers will take complete responsibility for what has happened or may happen for some considerable time. Indeed, one of the main aims of treatment is to help them to do this. It is important to see, at the outset, however, whether any responsibility is taken, even in terms of agreeing that parents have a responsibility to try and ensure that their children do not come to harm.

The causes for concern about the child or their development, i.e. what is happening or is likely to happen to the child, the parents' perceptions of the child and child's perceptions of what has happened (if the child is old enough) should then provide a continuing point of reference for the assessment. The social worker should make use of these discussions in order to explore and develop with the parents an explanation of why it is that harm was/is occurring or is likely to occur or how the child is coping. Talking with the parents about the early history of the child, the circumstances of the pregnancy and birth, the child's development, personality and behaviour will help some parents in this process, particularly if attachment difficulties are the major cause of concern. For some parents it may be their first opportunity to think in some depth about the child and their needs, or to share with someone else the difficulties they have had in caring for the child.

An example of this was Darren, aged 9, who frequently had unexplained bruises, seemed to be scapegoated within the family, and whose behaviour was uncontrollable at school and at home. In looking at his history, it became clear that the pregnancy had been unplanned, that he had been born at a time when the mother was looking after the maternal grandfather, who was dying, and that his sister had been born 10 months later. The parents realised that they had never really had an opportunity to bond with Darren and that they had resented his demands. Father had, as a child, been expected to be quiet and obedient and had been severely chastised for any naughtiness and he had continued the same pattern with Darren. The parents were then able to use the social worker's help to promote the development of attachments and to modify Darren's behaviour.

The child

Assessment of what is happening to a child requires that each aspect of a child's developmental progress is examined, in the context of the child's age and stage of development. Account must be taken of any particular vulnerability, such as learning disabilities or a physical disabling condition and the impact they may be having on progress in any of the developmental dimensions. There must be a clear understanding of what the particular child needs to achieve successfully at each stage of development, in order to ensure that the child has the opportunity to achieve their potential.

The child's perceptions, wishes and feelings

The child's statements about their situation and what has happened are a very important source of information both for the assessment and its outcome. When shared with the parent(s), they can be a powerful lever for creating change within the family or a source of evidence that change is unlikely.

Wishes and feelings can be ascertained though observation and play, through talking with older children, and by gathering reports from those closely involved with the child, e.g. teachers and current carers.

Child development and attachments

It is very important to assess the child's attachments and developmental progress. The importance of a secure attachment for a young child cannot be overemphasised. It provides the child with a secure base from which to explore the world and to which the child can return when anxious and distressed. Fahlberg (1991) states that attachment helps the child to:

- Attain their full intellectual potential
- Sort out what they perceive
- Think logically
- Develop a conscience

- Become self-reliant
- Cope with stress and frustration
- Handle fear and worry
- Develop future relationships
- Handle jealousy.

Children who experience moves and separations may have defective or disordered attachments, which will affect their behaviour and development. It is important, therefore, to chart moves and to find out whom the child feels close to, as well as the quality of the attachment. Children may be ambivalent about a particular carer, or they may show considerable affection for an abuser, or they may feel they have to look after a brother or sister. These feelings need to be taken into account, together with the need to provide the child with secure attachment when plans are made for placement and contact.

Professionals need to understand the process and the stages of child development. Bentovim (1998) says 'current views on development emphasise that what matters for development is that the various systems – biological and physical – should be well integrated'. Development is about progression, change and reorganisation throughout life. Significant harm occurs because of a disruption of the tasks to be achieved at particular ages and stages of development. Each critical task of development interrelates and influences the other.

Bentovim describes the key tasks of development as:

- The regulation of feelings
- The development of attachments
- The development of a sense of self
- The establishment of adequate peer relationships
- Adaptation to school
- Long-term physical and mental health.

The effects of harm and/or the impairment of health and development

These are likely to be reflected in the child's behaviour, development, play and communication with other children and adults. Close observation and the provision of opportunities for the child to play and talk may be necessary in order to ascertain how the child is. Terr (1990), writing about post-traumatic stress, suggests that there is often a tendency for adults to concentrate on a child's apparent recovery, e.g. 'she doesn't talk about it' and to ignore signs of continuing distress.

Assessments of children should be undertaken by a professional who is experienced in observing and communicating with children and who has, or can gain access to, knowledge about the possible effects of the particular harm the child has suffered or is likely to suffer. If the assessment is likely to take several sessions, consideration will need to be given to the relationship that develops between the worker and the child, and what the child is encouraged to express. An abrupt withdrawal of a new, important relationship in which the child has exposed a lot of hurt, anger and grief may reinforce previous experiences of abuse and loss.

The possibility of change

The child's healing is most likely to be achieved by the provision of 'good enough' parenting. Changes in the parent(s) or a move to a different placement will help to secure this. However, some children may also need additional individual help to enable them to make progress. These are likely to be children with attachment problems, severe health or development or educational problems, or an experience of sexual abuse or other violence, or post-traumatic stress. This needs to be considered during the assessment.

The individual adult and the couple relationship

In working with the parents to compile these profiles, there are a number of areas at which it is important to look. Practitioners doing the assessment will wish to see how the parent(s) perceive themselves, whether this matches up to how others see them, and what value and self-esteem are displayed. It is very important to identify positive attributes and coping abilities as well as exploring difficulties both in order to obtain an overall picture and because these qualities are likely to be the basis for future changes. The process of acquiring the information will require meeting with the whole family, with the child, and with parent(s)/carers together and individually.

An overall picture

It is suggested in the *Framework* (DOH 2000*b*) that information should be obtained about parents in respect of:

- their understanding of the child's needs and development and what they are doing which is relevant to the child's developmental needs
- their comprehension of their parenting tasks and the importance attached to them
- the parent(s)/caregiver(s) response to a child and the child's behaviour or circumstances
- the effect this child has on them and the meaning the child has for them
- the extent to which they are responding appropriately to the child's needs and the areas where they are experiencing difficulties in meeting needs or failing to do so
- the impact of difficulties they may be experiencing themselves on their ability to carry our parental tasks and responsibilities (distinguishing realisation from aspiration)
- their ability to face and accept their difficulties
- their ability to use support and accept help
- their capacity for adaptation and change in their parenting response.

Observation of interactions is as critically important as the way they are described by the adults involved. The parenting tasks undertaken by fathers or father figures should be addressed alongside those of mothers or mother figures. A distinction has to be made clearly between the contribution of each parent or caregiver to a child's well being and development. Where a child has suffered significant harm, it is particularly important to distinguish between the capabilities of the abusing parent and the potentially protective parent. This information can also contribute to an understanding of the impact the parents' relationship with each other may have on their respective capacities to respond appropriately to their child's needs. In some families, a single parent may be performing most or all of the parenting skills. In others, there may be a number of important caregivers in a child's life, each playing a different part, which may have positive or negative consequences.

Killen Heap (1991) has developed categories and criteria for investigating and evaluating parental functioning and potential. These are similar to those in the Department of Health Guide. They include stress factors in the parents' childhood, adolescence and early adulthood, stress factors related to pregnancy and birth, socio-economic factors, social networks and relationship factors, immaturity, which encompasses dependent and demanding behaviour, lack of impulse control and lack of ability to postpone satisfaction of needs, to think in time perspectives, to observe the connection between actions and consequences, and lack of empathy. Unresolved problems which were considered to affect the parent–child interaction negatively were marital conflict, conflict from an earlier divorce, current separation or divorce conflict, life stage/role crisis, unwanted pregnancy, anxiety/aggression problem, unmet dependency need, and alcohol or drug problem. Seven central parental capacities were identified:

- capacity to perceive the child realistically
- capacity for realistic expectations as to the needs a child may satisfy
- capacity for realistic expectation as to the child's coping and achievement
- capacity for empathy with the child
- capacity for involvement with the child
- capacity to give priority to the child's developmental needs
- capacity to restrain aggressive behaviour towards the child.

Killen Heap (1991) analysed a group of abused and neglected children and their parents using these categories and followed them up 5–6 years later. She found that immaturity was of greater importance for parental dysfunctioning than emotional problems such as anxiety or depressive states or uncontrollable anger. The mothers who scored highest on immaturity also had the highest number of stress factors in childhood, adolescence and early adulthood. She concluded, 'the high covariation between stress factors in childhood, adolescence and early adult life is of note. The findings underline the need for a thorough investigation of the interaction in the family, the child's role in it, the parents background, their level of maturity, emotional problems, and their central parental capacity' (Killen Heap 1991, p. 56).

Not all parents, however, who were themselves abused and neglected go on to maltreat their own children. Egeland (1988) says, 'Our findings indicate that about one-third of parents who were abused as children are at risk for abusing their own children ... The most compelling findings were in the areas of relationships, where we found that mothers who broke the cycle of abuse were as children most likely to have an emotionally supportive relationship with another adult and were as adults more likely to have an emotionally supportive husband or boyfriend' (Egeland 1988, p. 97).

The possibility of change

Difficulties in any of the areas included in the assessment may contribute to the maltreatment of a child. Most practitioners now subscribe to a multidimensional causal model of child ill-treatment. However, it is important to consider the nature of the harm or likely harm to the child, and what this may indicate about the parents and the possibility of successful intervention. Geller(1992), who has written and researched widely on family violence, has stated, 'our research clearly indicates that there is not a "continuum of abuse" with severe abuse occurring because of increased stress and disadvantage. Instead there seem to be distinct categories of maltreatment. Thus parents who inflict sever injuries on their children or kill them, are categorically different from those parents whose maltreatment does not involved life-threatening harm'. He suggests that in such cases, 'child protection and child advocacy needs to replace family reunification as the guiding policy of child welfare agencies'.

The research suggests that a number of characteristics in the parent, in the parent–child interaction, in the child, in the nature of the abuse, in the social setting and in the professional help offered are associated with a more positive or a more negative prognosis (Jones 1998).

Negative factors include: continuing parental denial of abuse or impairment; parents who refuse help or do not cooperate with professional help; severe parental personality problems – antisocial, aggressive or inadequate; parental mental handicap with accompanying mental illness; persistent parental psychosis with delusions involving the child; abuse in childhood not recognised as a problem; severe physical abuse, burns, scalds, failure to thrive, mixed abuse; pervasive lack of empathy for the child; severe sexual abuse, involving penetration, and of long duration; sadistic abuse or that which includes slow premeditated infliction of pain and suffering; certain types of abuse cases, e.g. Munchausens by proxy, deliberate poisoning, scalding and burns.

Positive factors include: a non-abusive partner, acceptance of the problem and taking of responsibility; compliance, a normal attachment; parental empathy for the child; less severe forms of abuse; a good corrective relationship for the child; professional outreach to the family and partnership; more local child care facilities and volunteer networks.

The various factors in a case will need to be weighed relative to one another and a prognosis estimated in the light of the research findings and the likely ability of the parents to work with professionals and make use of any intervention. Most experts in the field would be likely to advocate the use of court orders to protect the child in cases with a poorer prognosis.

Completing the assessment

At the conclusion of an assessment there should be an analysis of the findings which provides an understanding of the child's situation and informs planning, case objectives and the nature of service provision.

It is suggested in the *Framework* (DOH 2000*b*) that the following questions will need to be answered:

- The precise nature of the child's needs
- The reason for them
- The priority for action and/or resources
- The potential for change in the child and family
- The best options to be pursued
- The child and family's response to the intervention
- How well the child is doing.

The analysis of the child's needs should provide evidence on which to base judgements and plans on how best to safeguard a child, promote their welfare and support the parents in promoting the child's welfare. In respect of those children on the Child Protection Register, this analysis of the child's needs should underpin the child protection plan (DOH 2000*a*, para. 5.87).

If practitioners have been able to involve the family fully in the assessment, the parents will have an understanding of the answers to these questions and they will be aware that they need to decide whether they wish to pursue any further changes that have been recommended and to continue working with professionals. Whilst the assessment is in process, family members should be given feedback and invited to comment on their understanding of what has been happening and to share responsibility for any blocks or lack of progress. Sometimes a parent, if invited to give an opinion on what an outsider or a court would consider to be their strengths and difficulties, will give a view that very much accords with that of the professionals. No change and understanding, despite repeated efforts to engage family members, will provide evidence of the difficulty in preventing future harm if the child remains within the family.

The evaluation of an assessment and the resulting decisions should, wherever possible, be made by a group of professionals which should include those who participated in the assessment as well as some with experience in the work but no direct involvement in the case. The longer and the more closely involved a professional has been with a family, the harder it is likely to be for them to have necessary detachment to make an objective assessment.

Further reading

Adcock M 2000 The process of assessment – how to synthesize information and make judgements. In the child's world – assessing children in need. NSPCC & The University of Sheffield, London

Adcock M, White R 1998 Significant harm: its management and outcome. Significant, Croydon

Hull M 1999 Effective ways of working with children and their families. Jessica Kingsley, London

References

Adcock M 1991 In: Adcock M, White R, Hollows A (eds) Child protection: a training and resource guide to the Children Act 1989. National Children's Bureau, London

Adcock M 1993 Investigation and assessment in child protection. In: Adcock M, Hollows A, White R (eds) Child protection update. National Children's Bureau, London

Adcock M, White R, Hollows A 1998 Significant harm: its management and outcome. Significant, Croydon

Bentovim A 1998 Significant harm in context. In: Adcock M, White R, Hollows A (eds) Significant harm: its management and outcome. Significant, Croydon

Bentovim A, Elton A, Hildebrand J, Tranter M, Vizard E 1998 Child sexual abuse within the family. John Wright, London

Boehm B 1962 An assessment of family adequacy in protective cases. Child Welfare 41: 10–16

Corby B 1993 Child abuse: towards a knowledge base. Open University Press, Milton Keynes

Crittenden P 1991 Treatment of child abuse and neglect. Journal of Human Systems 2: 3–4

Dale P, Davies M, Morrison T, Walters J 1986 Dangerous families: assessment and treatment of child abuse Tavistock, London

Department of Health (DOH) 1988 Protecting children. A guide for social workers undertaking comprehensive assessment. HMSO, London

Department of Health (DOH) 1992 The Children Act. Report 1991. HMSO, London

Department of Health (DOH) 1993 The care of children: principles and practice in regulations and guidance. HMSO, London

Department of Health (DOH) 1995 Child protection: messages from research. Assessment in child protection and family support. Report of an SSI study. HMSO, London

Department of Health (DOH) 1999 Working together: a guide to inter-agency cooperation for the protection of children from abuse. The Stationery Office, London

Department of Health (DOH) 2000a Working together to safeguard children. The Stationery Office, London

Department of Health (DOH) 2000b Framework for the assessment of children in need and their families. The Stationery Office, London

Doueck H J, Bronson D E, Levin M 1992 Evaluating risk assessment implementation in child protection. Child Abuse and Neglect 16: 637–646

Egeland B 1988 Breaking the cycle of abuse; implications for prediction and intervention. In: Browne K, Davies C, Stratton P (eds) Early prediction and prevention of child abuse. John Wiley, Chichester

Fahlberg V 1991 A child's journey through placement. Perspective Press, Indianapolis, Indiana

Geller R 1992 Family re-unification versus child protection. Update. National Center for Child Prosecution 5 (8):

Giller H *et al.* 1992 An evaluation of child protection procedures in four Welsh ACPC areas. Social Information Systems,

Giovannoni J, Bercerra R 1979 Defining child abuse. Free Press, New York

Hooper A 1992 Mothers surviving child sexual abuse. Routledge, London Jones D P H 1998 The effectiveness of intervention. In: Adcock M, White R, Hollows A (eds) Significant harm: its management and outcome. Significant, Croydon

Jones D P H, Hopkins C, Godfrey M, Glaser D 1993 The investigative process. In: Investigative interviewing with children. The Open University Press, Milton Keynes

Killen Heap K 1991 A predictive and follow-up study of abusive and neglectful families by case analysis. Child Abuse and Neglect 15 (3): 261–273

Morrison T 1991 Change, control and the legal framework. In: Adcock M, White R, Hollows A (eds) Significant harm: its management and outcome. Significant, Croydon

Prosser D 1992 Child abuse investigations: the families' perspective. PAIN, London

Rooney R 1900 Socialistation strategies for involuntary clients. Social casework. Journal of Contemporary Social Work

Salter A 1988 Treating child sex offenders and victims. Sage, London

Social Services Inspectorate (SSI) 1993 Evaluating performance in child protection. HMSO, London

Terr L 1990 Too scared to cry. Basic Books, New York

Trowell J 1993 International Society for the Prevention of Child Abuse and Neglect. Unpublished paper, Chicago

White R 1994 Investigation and assessment. In: Adcock M, White R, Hollows A (eds) Child protection: a training resource and guide to child protection under the Children Act 1989, 2nd edn. National Children's Bureau, London

13

Inter-professional cooperation and inter-agency coordination

Brian Corby

Brian Corby

INTRODUC-TION

The way in which various health, welfare and police agencies work together both at the individual and organisational level has been seen as *the* crucial factor in child protection work in England and Wales in recent decades. Almost all the public inquiries published since 1973 have highlighted failures of systems to act coordinately and failures of individuals to cooperate and communicate effectively in events leading up to children's deaths. This chapter charts in detail the way in which this emphasis on inter-agency coordination and inter-professional cooperation has developed during this period. It then considers the merits and demerits of current inter-agency arrangements and ways in which those professionals engaged in child protection work can best cooperate within these arrangements. First, however, attention will be paid to research into, and theorising about, inter-agency coordination in a range of fields, including child protection work.

Review of recent literature and research

There is an extensive collection of literature on collaboration between different professionals and agencies in the subject areas of management studies, organisation theory, and public and welfare policy. This has been excellently summarised by Hallett & Birchall (1992) from whose work much of the material in this section is drawn. They point out that there are three terms that are used almost synonymously – *coordination, collaboration* and *cooperation*. All three activities are characterised by arrangements between two or more agencies or institutions to work together to achieve common goals. The differentiating factor between the three terms is the degree of formalisation involved in the arrangements. Thus, coordination is seen as the most formalised, involving agreement between organisations at the highest level and the use of specifically allocated coordinative machinery; collaborative arrangements are characterised by looser, lower level agreements; and cooperation is the least formalised arrangement of the three.

The attraction of coordinative activity for managers and policy-makers is that it has the potential for achieving more than merely the sum of the collaborating parts operating independently. It can create an extra dimension and, therefore, an increased pay-off. This, the most commonly held view about coordination, is termed by some writers as 'the optimistic tradition' (Challis *et al.* 1988). Adherents of this viewpoint can see little fault in collaborative activities. They are considered worthwhile in terms of both outcome and process. There is, on the other hand, a 'doubter/sceptic' view, that which sees coordinating activity as having the potential to stifle individual creativity and initiative and impose unnecessary constraints (Weiss 1981). From this point of view, the assumption that coordination is inevitably the best way to achieve goals is questionable. Indeed, there is a distinct possibility that coordinative action can be misused as a substitute for shortage of resources.

There has been a good deal of research into those factors which enhance or inhibit coordinative activities in the field of public policy. Hallett & Birchall (1992) in their review of this research stress the importance of the following factors. First, the external environment has to be supportive of such moves and a perceived crisis is often needed to act as a catalyst. Second, there has to be a good degree of consensus between the collaborating agencies about the solution to the targeted problem. Third, there is a need for committed individuals to push ahead with collaboration. Fourth, coordination is assisted by the fact of different agencies having coterminous administrative boundaries, and fifth, there need to be financial incentives. Inhibitors include the reverse of the above conditions and other factors such as lack of trust between professionals, status and resource differentials, fear of loss of autonomy, and different agency priorities and working schedules.

Hallett & Birchall point out that most of the literature on the effectiveness of collaborative approaches emphasises the benefits. They refer to several studies of inter-agency approaches to child protection work which point to positive outcomes of coordination (Newberger *et al.* 1973, Wallen *et al.* 1977, Hochstadt & Hardwicke 1985, Mouzakitis & Goldstein 1985, Cohn & Daro 1987, Gilgun 1988). However, the usefulness of these studies is limited for a variety of reasons. First, they are all North American and not directly comparable with the systems we use in the UK. Second, most of the projects being evaluated are small-scale and time-limited. Third, the studies rely heavily on the views of professionals, who are often more concerned with process than outcome, and do not take into account user's views. Finally, they concentrate on collaboration at the interpersonal level without consideration of structural and organisational factors. There are a smaller number of North American studies which point to negative outcomes of coordinating activities, such as over-reliance on group processes for decision-making, diffusion of responsibility and overuse of routinised responses (Bourne & Newberger 1980, Byles 1985).

There have been only a small number of British research projects specifically examining the impact of multi-professional and inter-agency cooperation and coordination on child protection interventions (Hallett & Stevenson 1980, Dale *et al.* 1986, Birchall & Hallett 1995). There have been several more general studies of child protection work, which have placed some emphasis on coordination issues (Dingwall *et al.* 1983, Dale *et al.* 1986, Corby 1987, 1998, Farmer & Owen 1995, Thoburn *et al.* 1995, Moran-Ellis & Fielding 1996, Sharland *et al.* 1996), and there have been some studies looking at particular inter-agency arrangements, most notably those between police and social workers (Metropolitan Police & London Borough of Bexley 1987, Fielding & Conroy 1992). Most of the earlier studies have emphasised the difficulties and dysfunctions of cooperative practice. The studies in the 1990s, by contrast, have tended to paint a somewhat more positive picture. Other sources of information are public inquiry reports (Department of Health and Social Security (DHSS) 1982, Department of Health (DOH) 1991a) (although these inevitably highlight errors and failures in communication) and Social Services Inspectorate (SSI) reports, which tend to concern themselves mainly with the formal nature of inter-professional arrangements. It should be noted, however, that there are no studies that directly evaluate the effectiveness of inter-professional cooperation in terms of outcomes.

An analysis of policy issues

The need for better inter-agency coordination in child care work was recognised as early as 1945 when the inquiry into the death of Dennis O'Neill reported (Home Office 1945). In that case, two young children had been hurriedly placed by one local authority, in an unapproved foster home situated in the area of another local authority without proper agreement between the employees of either about their respective duties and responsibilities. Six months after the placement had been made, Dennis, aged 12, was beaten to death by his foster-father. Sir Walter Monckton, in his report, was critical both of the systems and of the individuals involved:

What is required is rather that the administrative machinery should be improved and informed by a more anxious and responsible spirit. (Home Office 1945, p. 18)

This need for better coordination between agencies was also reflected in a 1950 Home Office circular which recommended to Health, Education and Children's Departments that they set up coordinating committees to review their work with disadvantaged families with children (Home Office 1950).

The Maria Colwell inquiry

The comments on inter-professional coordination and cooperation in the Maria Colwell inquiry report in 1974 were crucial in determining the future of child protection policy over the next 20 years (DHSS 1974). Maria, aged 7, died as a result of neglect and beatings by her step-father. She was under a supervision order to one social services department, but living in an area serviced by another. She was attending school. Thus social workers, teachers and an education welfare officer were all involved with her in the last year of her life. So too were an inspector from the National Society for the Prevention of Cruelty to Children (NSPCC), a general practitioner (GP), housing officials and police officers, following allegations by neighbours of ill-treatment of Maria. While the report was critical of the work of individuals, most notably that of the social worker with responsibility for Maria's supervision order and that of the NSPCC inspector, its main conclusion was that 'The overall impression created by Maria's sad history is that while individuals made mistakes it was the "system", using the word in its widest sense, which failed her' (DHSS 1974, p. 86).

In fact, there was no formalised inter-agency system for dealing with child abuse in most parts of the country at this time, apart from the coordinating committees referred to earlier. Much was left to the initiative of individual workers. The child protection system, as we know it, was set up as a direct consequence of the Colwell report's findings. The structure that was established between 1974 and 1976 is essentially that which underpins today's child protection system. It consisted of three main components:

1. Area Review Committees (now termed Area Child Protection Committees) consisting of senior managers of all agencies with an involvement in child protection work: social services, police, health, education, housing and probation. The main function of these Committees was (and still is) to oversee the establishment of the child protection system, and to monitor its operation. In addition it was given responsibility for issuing procedural guidance to all practitioners and for identifying and meeting their training needs.

2. Non-accidental injuries registers (now termed child protection registers): These were instituted with the aim of highlighting for all agencies those children considered to have been abused or at risk of abuse.
3. Case conferences called to assess all allegations of child abuse unless they were considered of insufficient substance to warrant holding them. These conferences were to be attended by all agencies with an involvement with the family in question. A 1976 circular emphasised that the police should be present at all case conferences unless they felt that it was unnecessary to attend.

Thus, coordination between agencies was officially seen as the key to developing effective systems for dealing with the problem of child abuse. While in theory these mechanisms were joint and cooperative enterprises, in practice a great deal of emphasis was placed on the role of social services departments and to a lesser extent on the NSPCC. It should be stressed that there were no legal requirements imposed on professionals either to report abuse (as is the case in the USA) or to attend conferences. Social services departments, the NSPCC and the police were the only agencies with responsibilities laid down by law. Coordination between agencies with child protection functions was at this time an uneven and experimental activity that looked firmer on paper than in practice.

From Colwell to Beckford

Between the publication of the Colwell inquiry report and that relating to Jasmine Beckford in 1985 (London Borough of Brent 1985), there were 29 further inquiries into the deaths of children as a result of abuse (Corby *et al.* 1998). Most of the cases inquired into were dealt with under the new arrangements for child protection. Inevitably, therefore, in seeking an explanation for what happened in these cases, greater emphasis was placed on the individuals operating the systems. Failures by professionals to share information and to work together collaboratively were identified by a DHSS summary of inquiry reports published in 1982 as key factors contributing to the failure to provide children at risk with sufficient protection:

1. 'Cases usually involve several professions and two or more agencies, but effective work is hampered by ignorance or misunderstanding of respective functions'
2. 'All workers need arrangements for exchanging information and, where there is an overlap of function or activity, a clear and common understanding of the extent and purpose of each individual's involvement in the case'
3. 'Case conferences offer an important means of co-ordinating action, but they need to be called at appropriate junctures, to involve everyone with a contribution to make, and to be specific about who is doing what to what end' (DHSS 1982, p. 68).

Hallett & Stevenson (1980) outlined some of the reasons why this lack of cooperation was persisting. First, they pointed out that professionals, in their training and practice, developed separate identities and ways of working. They were often not trained to work in conjunction with other professionals on an equal basis. Second, they had different social statuses, levels of education and pay which served to reinforce divisions. This was particularly obvious in the case of doctors.

Third, there were major differences of perspective on child protection issues – at the time this was most evident in the contrasting views held by police and social workers. Fourth, there was no regular meeting point for ground level professionals to air issues other than in the heat of the case conference. Hallett & Stevenson went on to stress that one of the ways in which professional workers coped with these differences and difficulties was by resorting to stereotyping. However, this was a major barrier to the type of communication and good collaboration that child protection work required.

The Beckford inquiry 1985

Despite these continuing difficulties, the early 1980s saw few major developments in the working of the child protection system. The main ones were a broadening of the concept of child abuse to include neglect and low standards of care of children (see Chapter 1, in this volume), and the increasing dominance of the system by social services department personnel.

However, the inquiry report into the death of Jasmine Beckford (London Borough of Brent 1985) shook the system out of any complacency into which it might have fallen. This report was unequivocal in its view that the various statutory agencies should bear responsibility for what had happened:

> On any conceivable version of the events under inquiry the death of Jasmine Beckford on 5 July 1984 was a predictable and preventible homicide ... The blame must be shared by all these services (health, education, social services and magistrate's court) in proportion to their various statutory duties, and to the degree of actual and continuing involvement with the Beckford family. (p. 287)

Jasmine and her sister had both been seriously abused by Morris Beckford in August 1981. They had been made the subject of care orders and were returned to live with him and their mother in April 1982 after being in a foster home.

The report questioned both the wisdom of the decision to return these children home and the way it was reached – i.e. at a case conference attended only by social services personnel and chaired by a line manager. It felt that a health visitor should have been present and that the consultant paediatrician who had been involved at the time when Jasmine and her sister had been hospitalised should have been invited to attend.

It went on to criticise the ongoing monitoring arrangements, particularly the lack of involvement of health professionals. During the first 6 months of Jasmine's 'home-on-trial' period, there was no contact between the health visitor and the social worker. There were also no checks on her and her sister's health and development at the local health clinic. Neither the health visitor nor the GP was able to attend the case conference at which Jasmine and her sister were de-registered. In January 1983, Jasmine was placed in nursery school. No mention was made to the head teacher of the school that Jasmine had been abused or that she was still on a care order. The social worker felt that there was no need for the school to be involved in monitoring Jasmine's health and welfare. Consequently, when Jasmine's attendance at the school deteriorated, as soon it did, the head teacher did not consider this particular cause for concern. From the summer of 1983 until Jasmine's death in July 1984, she was seen only once by her social worker and not at all by the health visitor, despite many calls to the home. There was no liaison at all between these two workers.

There is little sign of good coordination of services in this case. The report paints a picture of social services personnel going it alone and not sufficiently involving other agencies. On this evidence, the communication problem that had evidenced itself in the Maria Colwell case had not been much improved by the child protection system it had generated.

The main responses of the DHSS to the Beckford inquiry report were eventually incorporated into the 1988 *Working Together* guidelines (DHSS 1988). These guidelines re-emphasised the importance of concentrating on protecting children in serious cases, using the term 'child protection' for the first time. They tightened procedures by placing greater responsibility on specialist child protection managers to operate the system and by stressing the need for all involved professionals, particularly health workers and teachers, to play more active roles in the child protection process. Finally, they tried to encourage broader responsibility for policy and training at Area Review Committee level by greater involvement of health authorities.

The Cleveland inquiry 1988

Before the shockwaves of the Beckford report had died down, the Cleveland affair broke (Butler-Sloss L.J. 1988). Child sexual abuse had been a cause for concern for a small number of doctors and social workers (mainly female) in Britain since the early 1980s. By 1986 there were nearly 6000 children registered on the grounds of sexual abuse. Pediatricians in Leeds had been particularly active in detecting signs of anal abuse of young children (Hobbs & Wynne 1986). A Mori Poll survey (Baker & Duncan 1985) had reported much higher rates of sexual abuse than previously imagined.

In this climate, two paediatricians in Cleveland, using the techniques pioneered by Hobbs & Wynne, diagnosed large numbers of children as having been sexually abused. They were fully supported in what they were trying to achieve by the child protection coordinator in Cleveland Social Services Department who had also developed a particular interest in the issue of child sexual abuse. Other agencies, however, most notably the police and police surgeons, were more sceptical about the new thinking on sexual abuse and thus a major split in the inter-professional network was created. Pediatricians diagnosed abuse and the social services department social workers, heavily influenced by post-Beckford developments, speedily removed children to places of safety. Meanwhile the police and police surgeons dissociated themselves from what was happening. The following extract from the Cleveland report emphasises the full extent of the breakdown of inter-professional cooperation:

A week later social workers referred another family of 3 as a result of the comments of the eldest child of 10 at school and the concern of her headmistress. Dr Higgs examined the first child with the consent of her mother, and found signs she felt were consistent with sexual abuse. Before she could examine the second child, the father arrived on the ward and removed the 3 children. He took them to a secret address. He was at the time required to report daily to the police who were unable to persuade him to divulge the whereabouts of the children. However, he agreed to the examination of the children by a police surgeon, and Dr Beeby was taken to the secret address. He examined the children in an upstairs room and found no abnormality. They were then returned home by their father; removed on a place of safety order obtained by Social Services and taken back to hospital. This time Dr Higgs examined all 3 children and diagnosed sexual abuse in respect of all 3. The following day Dr Irvine (police surgeon) examined the 3 children and agreed with the conclusions of Dr Beeby. Two weeks later, Dr McCowen, paediatrician from Northallerton, considered the signs suspicious and, later in June, Dr Roberts (police surgeon) and Dr Paul considered there was no abnormality. (p. 16)

The conflict was not confined to the actions of the professionals on the ground. The Cleveland report closely examined the working of the Joint Child Abuse Committee (the new name for the Area Review Committee adopted in line with the recommendations of the Beckford report). It concluded that this body had been entirely ineffective in sorting out the chaos which reigned in the spring and early summer of 1987 and that the reason for this was that it was not sufficiently recognised by senior managers in the different agencies as having any authority to do so. When the chips were down, agencies disowned the collaborative mechanism and pursued their own interests.

The Cleveland report (Butler-Sloss L.J. 1988, pp. 248–250) had much to say about inter-professional coordination. It stated that 'no single agency – Health, Social Services, Police or voluntary organisation has the pre-eminent responsibility in the assessment of child abuse generally and child sexual abuse specifically' (p. 248).

It went on to outline the need to set up Specialist Assessment Teams comprising primarily police, social workers and doctors to deal with problematic referrals of child sexual abuse. While this particular recommendation has been largely ignored, there can be little doubt that the Cleveland report had a massive impact on inter-professional cooperation, perhaps more than any inquiry report since that relating to Maria Colwell. It placed child protection work firmly back in the court of *all* agencies and emphasised the need for more attention to be paid to careful inter-professional planning of intervention into suspected cases of child abuse. In particular, it recommended that police and social services department workers should conduct joint interviews of children alleged to or suspected of having been sexually abused. It also affirmed the need for inter-professional training for child protection work: 'For example police officers and social workers designated to interview children should have joint training in their approach to this task' (p. 251).

In addition to these recommendations on inter-professional coordination, the Cleveland report made recommendations about the treatment of children and parents that have had significant effects on inter-agency practices. The most influential of these has been the requirement that they be more closely involved at every stage in the investigative procedure, including attendance at child protection conferences, an activity that had been considered unwise by the Beckford inquiry (London Borough of Brent 1985, p. 249).

From Cleveland to the present

The Cleveland inquiry report had a major impact on the final outcome of the Children Act 1989 and on the 1991 *Working Together* guidelines (DOH 1991*b*) which, at the time of writing are still in operation, but are currently being revised in the light of developments in the last 5 years (draft guidelines were issued to local authorities for comment in August 1999 – DOH 1999). Since Cleveland, there have been several key developments that have had an impact on arrangements for inter-professional coordination. The early 1990s saw new child protection concerns coming on the scene-Satanist ritual abuse, organised abuse and institutional abuse (see Chapter 1 in this volume). Concerns about the former have largely been dismissed now (see La Fontaine 1998), but events at Orkney (Clyde 1992), in particular the extensive interviewing of children by social workers, confirmed the need for more controlled arrangements for gathering evidence from children. The subsequent *Memorandum of Good Practice on Video Recorded Interviews with Child Witnesses for Criminal Proceeding* (Home

Office & Department of Health 1992) established accepted procedures for doing this and confirmed the need for joint police and social work investigations of serious allegations of child abuse. Special arrangements involving more top-led strategic planning are set out in the *Working Together* (DOH 1991*b*, DOH 1999) guidelines for dealing with organised abuse, which is by and large seen as a much more widespread and worrying form of abuse than Satanist ritual abuse (see Bibby 1996). Institutional abuse has been seen to be even more widespread, resulting in at least ten public inquiries in the 1990s (Corby *et al.* 1998) and extensive police investigations (Webster 1998). There has also been growing concern about how to respond to young sexual offenders and child prostitution.

In contrast to these developments, there has been a considerable shift in thinking about child abuse within the family. In response to the concerns about professional intervention practices at Cleveland, the Department of Health sponsored a series of major research projects into child protection practices. The findings of most of these projects were published by 1995 and summarised in a Department of Health publication, *Child Protection: Messages from Research* (DOH 1995). The main argument in this document was that there was too much concern being placed by professionals on incidents of abuse and insufficient emphasis on the more general quality of life experienced by children in many of the families referred for child protection reasons. More attention needed to be given to working with families 'low on warmth and high on criticism' than had previously been the case, because children in many of these families frequently suffered more long-term negative psychological consequences than those subjected to one or two acts of violence in families where the general emotional climate was less harsh.

The second half of the 1990s therefore has seen greater encouragement for professionals to work together with a view to providing more supportive (as well as protective) intervention in working with children and families in the community. This shift in emphasis is evident in the following excerpt from the new draft guidelines (DOH 1999):

Only in exceptional circumstances should there be compulsory intervention into family life: for example, where this is necessary to safeguard a child from significant harm. Such intervention should – provided this is consistent with the safety and welfare of the child – support families in making their own plans for the welfare and protection of their children. (para. 1.5, p. 11)

Implications for practice

In this section, focus will first be placed on the current state of inter-agency co-ordination in child protection work and then consideration will be given to ways in which professionals can make best use of the systems within which they work.

The current functioning of the child protection system

As has been seen, the mechanisms and systems for developing inter-professional coordination became far more sophisticated from 1975 to 2000. They also became considerably more complex and demanding, particularly following the added dimension identified in the *Messages from Research* document (DOH 1995).

The administrative/managerial functions of the child protection system still rest with what are now called Area Child Protection Committees (having been re-titled yet again in the 1988 guidelines). These bodies have a crucial function in ensuring that cooperation and collaboration between all the agencies involved in child protection work is effective. The current *Working Together* guidelines (DOH 1991*b*) stress the need for all agencies to be represented at these committees by people of sufficient weight to commit them to agreed courses of action. All agencies are also required to contribute to the financial costs incurred by their work. While this requirement represents a major improvement, nevertheless these committees still do not have full managerial authority over the child protection work carried out by constituent member agencies and this is seen as a continuing weakness by several commentators (Stevenson 1989, Walton 1993). It should be noted that the new draft *Working Together* guidelines (DOH 1999) do not provide a remedy to this problem.

The reporting of concerns about children at risk either to social services departments or to the police is still not legally required of other agencies but in reality, particularly as a result of Department of Health guidelines and circulars, such activity has become less and less subject to the discretion of individual workers. Once a child has been identified as being at risk it is now the duty of local authority housing and education departments and of health authorities to assist in any ensuing inquiry (see section 47(9) of the Children Act 1989). Some professionals, such as health visitors and GPs, have retained a degree of discretion about when to refer and what to refer, but they are now much more aware of child protection issues and much more involved in the child protection system than was the case even as late as the mid-1980s.

Since 1995 there has been more consideration given to the process of dealing with child protection referrals. The picture is not yet clear, but some authorities are trying to be more discriminating about which families need more general family support and which more urgent and authoritative child protection interventions. The former are more likely to be supported under section 17 of the Children Act 1989 and less likely to be processed further through the child protection system. Local authority departments are now required to develop coordinated policies to provide for all children, including specifically children in need, in the form of Children's Services Plans. At present, it is not clear what impact these developments are having but they could well provide a more structured, interdisciplinary base for coordinating services to families identified as in need through the child protection system.

Child protection conferences are generally more focused and formalised than has been the case in the past. This is partly due to the fact that, following the recommendations of the Jasmine Beckford report (London Borough of Brent 1985), they are mostly chaired by specialist child protection coordinators, usually social workers who have developed a good deal of expertise as child protection workers. As stressed earlier, another important factor in this respect has been the involvement of parents and children in conferences. This has forced professionals to consider more carefully the format of the procedures and to be more explicit about aims and objectives (Thoburn 1992). There have been further developments in the post-*Messages from Research* period in this respect, with the introduction in some areas of Family Group Conferences (Marsh & Crow 1998). These conferences, drawing on a model derived from New Zealand (Connolly 1994), are designed to be more family-centred than child protection conferences and at the same time to place more responsibility on the family to come up with solutions to the problems they face (with the help of the attendant professionals). Such arrangements are very much in their infancy and may have less to offer in situations where serious abuse is being considered. In families where the concerns are more general, however, the ideas behind Family Group Conferences seem to offer good (and challenging) opportunities for professionals to work together with each other in working with families.

In the post-case conference period there is now a clear expectation that the key worker will involve other important professionals, parents and, in some cases, children in constructing the details of a child protection plan and implementing it. The core group is the mechanism whereby this is to be achieved. This comprises those professionals with an ongoing role to play with the family concerned (often social workers, health visitors and teachers) and the family members themselves. This group is intended to work to the protection plan established at the conference and to report back to the conference for review and de-registration purposes. There has so far been little research into these groups (see, however, Christie & Mittler 1999). Clearly, like Family Group Conferences, they have the potential for positive inter-professional practice with families. Such work is, however, time-consuming and has resource implications. According to *Messages from Research*, continuing inter-professional work of this kind is relatively rare:

... the evidence from Hallett and Birchall would suggest that while there is good inter-agency co-operation at the point of assessing risk to a child, when it comes to delivering services there is less sharing and a poor allocation of roles; in many cases social services are left to shoulder the responsibility.

(DOH 1995, p. 36)

Despite these reservations, in many more ways than before and at several different stages, inter-agency coordination and inter-professional cooperation has become the accepted way of working in child protection cases. Referring back to the levels of coordination discussed by Hallett & Birchall (1992) at the start of this chapter, it is clear that by any set of criteria the child protection system, while not subject to legal regulations, is now at a relatively high level of formalisation. Communication and cooperation are now seen as essential requirements of child protection work, not merely forms of practice preferred by professional workers.

Inter-professional cooperation now

It is probably safe to say that the standard of inter-professional cooperation is now at its highest level since 1974. Nevertheless, one should not get carried away. Although Birchall & Hallett (1995) found in their survey of 339 professionals (social workers, police, GPs, teachers, paediatricians and health visitors) that 'most respondents assert that the coordinating system works fairly well and the majority report that others in the network are fairly easy to collaborate with', they also point out that 'significant numbers ... report substantial difficulties in particular facets of the machinery or in particular inter-professional relationships', and go on to conclude that the 'professional network is not a "team" that can give emotional support to the practitioners' (p. 241). The state of inter-professional cooperation identified by these researchers was one where there was agreement about a common procedural framework and the development of close working relationships between some of the professionals involved.

In the following review, current expectations of all the main professions involved in child protection work will be considered along with a commentary on the way in which they are carrying out their responsibilities.

The importance of the role of GPs is heavily emphasised in the 1991 DOH *Working Together* guidelines (and in the 1999 draft guidelines), as is the need for them to receive child protection training. Since 1987 there has been clear guidance for GPs from the General Medical Council stressing that they have a professional duty to disclose information when they consider a child is being physically or sexually abused. Prior to this there had been a good deal of uncertainty on their part about the ethics of breaking confidentiality in these circumstances. On the debit side, GPs are still not regular attenders at case conferences and most have remained on the sidelines of child protection training and ongoing collaborative work (see Birchall & Hallett 1995).

Health visitors have now also clarified their position over the issue of confidentiality (Smart 1992). The 1991 *Working Together* guidelines (DOH 1991*b*) recommend that each health authority should identify a senior health worker (health visitor, community nurse or clinical medical officer) to oversee child protection issues and improve inter-professional communication and collaboration. Despite the views of the Beckford report (London Borough of Brent 1985) and some commentators (Dingwall *et al.* 1983) that health visitors should play a more central role in child protection work, particularly with regard to the under 5-year-olds the profession has remained marginal (relative to social workers), influenced to some degree by the need to preserve good relationships with families which it feels to be essential to the provision of community health care and advice. It may well be that health visitors will be more comfortable with the developments towards a more family supportive approach (see Corby 1999). One of their frustrations in the past has been that they have felt unable to persuade social workers to work in a more preventive capacity, and this may now be remedied.

Paediatricians have over the years been less equivocal over the issue of confidentiality than other members of the medical and health professions. They played a lead administrative, as well as medical, role in the early stages of the rediscovery of child physical abuse and, as has been seen, they were in the forefront of important developments in the field of sexual abuse detection as well. However, the Cleveland affair threw into doubt their credibility as expert witnesses in such cases. Paediatricians are still key figures in child protection work, although their role has consequently diminished to some degree (see Chapter 1 in this volume). Their expertise in serious physical child abuse, including Munchausen's syndrome by proxy (Meadow 1985) remains an important, though at times controversial (Thomas 1996), contribution to the field.

The role of the police in child protection work has changed dramatically in the last few years. Before the rediscovery of sexual abuse in the mid-1980s, police officers had only become directly involved with families in those cases of physical abuse and neglect which were considered to be serious enough to warrant prosecution, and such cases were very much in the minority. Their other main function was (and still is) to furnish child protection conferences with details of relevant offences committed by adults suspected of abuse. They have developed a more central role in child protection work since the Cleveland affair and the publication of the *Memorandum of Good Practice* (Home Office & Department of Health 1992). They tend to take a lead role in joint interviewing (Fielding & Conroy 1992) and have been particularly prominent in the investigation of institutional abuse. Their work has been aided considerably by the development of specialist child protection and family teams. It is notable (Birchall & Hallett 1995) that police and social workers have developed much closer working relationships than before. Some commentators have been sceptical about the benefits of this closeness and consider that social services departments' central role and approach is being threatened by the more crime-focused emphasis adopted by the police (Kelly & Regan 1990). Others have argued that these new developments have contributed to a more consistent service being offered to children and families (Wattam 1990).

The role of schoolteachers and education welfare officers (see Peake, Chapter 16, in this volume) has not changed greatly over the past few years. As a result of the Beckford inquiry report, all schools are now recommended to have a child protection liaison officer and in general there is greater awareness of the issues, particularly with regard to sexual abuse, thanks to media publicity and inter-disciplinary training. Many schools have developed sex and safety education programmes. School personnel are much more closely involved in child protection plans than before.

Social services department social workers, while subject to high levels of criticism throughout the whole period in which child abuse has been a prominent public issue, have nevertheless retained the key central role in the system. The 1991 *Working Together* guidelines (DOH 1991*b*) guidelines recommended the employment of specialist child protection coordinators to oversee child protection systems, and this is now the norm. Social services department managers are seen as key figures in the administration of Area Child Protection Committees. Only social workers can assume the role of key workers and it is their responsibility to manage the child protection plan agreed upon at the case conference. Social workers have key statutory responsibilities and resources in relation both to abused children and all other children in need. The greater emphasis placed on the need to support families more fully since the publication of *Messages from Research* in 1995, will in all likelihood result in social workers retaining that lead role but with a broader more flexible perspective.

The NSPCC still retains its long-established statutory powers in the area of child abuse detection and investigation. In practice, it is moving away from work in this area and focusing more on therapeutic work with families in which children have been abused.

The probation service retains its responsibility to notify social services departments about discharged prisoners convicted of child abuse and to supervise offenders in the community. Probation officers have become increasingly involved in child sexual abuse work in relation to sexual offenders and have developed treatment programmes both for those in prisons and those on probation orders in the community.

The new draft guidelines (DOH 1999) incorporate a wider range of professionals than before, including mental health specialists (adults and children), housing officers, day services staff, guardians *ad litem* and the wider community. These additions reflect the broadening of concerns about child welfare highlighted in *Messages from Research* (DOH 1995).

Suggestions for improving inter-professional cooperation

It should be evident by now that good inter-professional liaison depends on the quality of systems, the quality of those working within them, and the interplay between the two. It has been argued that there has been a concentrated effort since the Beckford and Cleveland reports to improve the standard of child protection procedures, and that involved professionals as a whole are working together better than ever before. As long as we retain our present system for dealing with child abuse, with its reliance on agencies to work together in a voluntary way, it is crucial that the relevant professionals continue to develop open and trusting relationships in order to maximise their effectiveness. This has several implications for practice.

First, inter-professional training in child protection work should be obligatory at all stages of professional development – during training for qualification, and at in-service and post-qualification courses. (Clearly there needs to be some distinction between the sort of training required for specialist child protection workers and for those for whom involvement in child protection work forms only a small part of their overall responsibilities.)

Second, practitioners need to maintain an awareness of the multidisciplinary dimension of child protection work by ensuring that they have a clear understanding of the organisational requirements and duties placed on professionals from other agencies.

Third, there is need for regular dialogue between different professionals about what forms of behaviour they consider abusive (or seriously abusive) and why. Giovannoni & Becerra (1979) have demonstrated how occupational concerns and requirements can lead to widely differing definitions of abuse between different professional groups. Birchall & Hallett (1995) have confirmed that such discrepancies still exist particularly in relation to emotional abuse and neglect.

Fourth, there is a need to avoid stereotyping other professionals which, as Hallett & Stevenson (1980) have pointed out, serves only to create and strengthen separation and distrust, and fifth, there is a need to be clear about who has responsibility for what in carrying out a protection plan and the need to check it out if in doubt.

All these issues can (and should) be addressed in training. Some can be aided by systemic changes, such as the clear delineation of responsibilities and expectations at child protection conferences. However, there is still a need for all individual workers to take professional responsibility in these matters *over and above* the stated requirements of the system. In addition, those in consultative or supervisory capacities over professional workers should be particularly attuned to the need for good inter-professional relationships as an essential ingredient of child protection work and ensure that it is high on their agendas.

Conclusion

While there have been considerable strides forward in the past few years in improving inter-professional cooperation within the child protection system, there are still many outstanding broader issues to be addressed about this type of coordinative activity. We still know very little about the effectiveness of our current system, and little attention has been paid to alternative ways of organising child protection work such as the development of specialist inter-professional teams which was recommended for consideration by both the Cleveland report (see above) and the Kimberley Carlile report (London Borough of Greenwich 1987).

As Hallett & Birchall (1992) point out, in our determination to make our system work, we run the risk of seeing only the positive aspects of inter-professional work and thereby of ignoring the possible dysfunctions. For instance, some commentators have argued that the bureaucratic arrangements needed to ensure inter-professional cooperation have led to more defensive decision-making (Harris 1987, Howe 1992) and the elimination of the use of professional discretion and judgement on the part of individual workers (Finkelhor & Zellman 1991).

There are also factors such as costs and resources that have to be taken into account. The formalisation of the inter-professional system, particularly since 1985, has seen a major increase in the number of conferences held. These conferences are costly in themselves because of the amount of professional time that they consume and because the more comprehensive decisions being made at them entail the provision of more resources. The American system, which has experienced similar developments to our own, is seen by some to be so overloaded that it cannot achieve what it sets out to do (Krugman 1991).

These dysfunctions of the child protection system are currently being addressed within the Department of Health. The *Messages from Research* (DOH 1995) recommendations, to adopt a more family-supportive approach to referrals coming through the system, are intended to have the effect of reducing bureaucratic costs at the same time as providing a more effective and protective service to children and their families. Whether this can be achieved has yet to be seen. Some commentators believe that the shift will increase demand under section 17 of the Children Act 1989 which local authorities will not be able to meet without a considerable increase in resources (Tunstill 1997).

If the resource issue can be properly addressed, there can be little doubt that the shift in focus put forward by the *Messages from Research* document is to be welcomed because of the likelihood of a more flexible and positive response to families where children are considered to be at risk of maltreatment or poor standards of care. The challenge for professionals, and therefore for inter-professional work, is how to operate more flexibly and with greater discretion. We have spent 20 or more years developing a tighter and more carefully managed approach to child protection work in which, as has been seen, professionals have gradually developed greater trust with each other and more certainty about each others' roles and functions. Welcome though the new developments are, they nevertheless present a major challenge to some of these certainties and therefore to inter-professional cooperation in the future.

References

Baker A, Duncan S 1985 Child sexual abuse: a study of prevalence in Great Britain. Child Abuse and Neglect 9: 457–467

Bibby P (ed) 1996 Organised abuse: the current debate. Ashgate, Aldershot

Birchall E, Hallett C 1995 Working together in child protection: report of phase two, a survey of the experience and perceptions of the six key professions. HMSO, London

Bourne J, Newberger E 1980 Interdisciplinary group process in the hospital management of child abuse and neglect. Child Abuse and Neglect 4: 137–144

Butler-Sloss Lady Justice E 1988 Report of the inquiry into child abuse in Cleveland 1987. Cmnd. 412. HMSO, London

Byles J 1985 Problems in inter-agency collaboration: lessons from a project that failed. Child Abuse and Neglect 9: 549–554

Challis L, Fuller S, Henwood M *et al.* 1988 Joint approaches to social policy: rationality and practice. Cambridge University Press, Cambridge

Christie A, Mittler H 1999 Partnership and core groups in the risk society. Child and Family Social Work 4 (3): 241–248

Clyde, Lord 1992 Report of the inquiry into the removal of children from Orkney in February 1991. HC 195. HMSO, London

Cohn A, Daro D 1987 Is treatment too late? What ten years of evaluative research tell us. Child Abuse and Neglect 11: 433–442

Connolly M 1994 An Act of empowerment: the Children, Young Persons and their Families Act 1989. British Journal of Social Work 24 (1): 87–100

Corby B 1987 Working with child abuse. Open University Press, Milton Keynes

Corby B 1998 Managing child sexual abuse cases. Jessica Kingsley, London

Corby B 1999 The child at risk: working with families and the child protection system. In: Booth K, Luker K (eds) A practical handbook for community health nurses: working with children and their parents. Blackwell, Oxford

Corby B, Doig A, Roberts V 1998 Inquiries into child abuse. The Journal of Social Welfare and Family Law 20 (4): 377–395

Dale P, Waters J, Davies M *et al.* 1986 Dangerous families: assessment and treatment of child abuse. Tavistock, London

Department of Health (DOH) 1991*a* Child abuse: a study of inquiry reports 1980–1989. HMSO, London

Department of Health (DOH) 1991*b* Working together under the Children Act 1989: a guide to arrangements for inter-agency cooperation for the protection of children against abuse. HMSO, London

Department of Health (DOH) 1995 Child protection: messages from research. HMSO, London

Department of Health (DOH) 1998 Children and young persons on Child Protection Registers. Year ending 31 March 1998 – England. Department of Health, London

Department of Health (DOH) 1999 Working together to support children and families. Draft Guidance. Department of Health, London

Department of Health and Social Security (DHSS) 1974 Report of the committee of inquiry into the care and supervision provided in relation to Maria Colwell. HMSO, London

Department of Health and Social Security (DHSS) 1982 Child abuse: a study of inquiry reports 1973–1981. HMSO, London

Department of Health and Social Security (DHSS) 1988 Working together: a guide to inter-agency cooperation for the protection of children against abuse. HMSO, London

Dingwall R, Eekelaar J, Murray T 1983 The protection of children: State intervention and family life. Blackwell, Oxford

Farmer E, Owen M 1995 Child protection practice: private risks and public remedies: decision-making, intervention and outcome in child protection work. HMSO, London

Fielding N, Conroy S 1992 Interviewing child victims: police and social work investigations of child sexual abuse. Sociology 26 (1): 103–124

Finkelhor D, Zellman G 1991 Flexible reporting options for skilled child abuse professionals. Child Abuse and Neglect 15: 335–341

Gilgun J 1988 Decision-making in interdisciplinary treatment teams. Child Abuse and Neglect 12: 231–239

Giovannoni J, Becerra R 1979 Defining child abuse. Free Press, New York

Hallett C, Birchall E 1992 Coordination and child protection: a review of the literature. HMSO, London

Hallett C, Stevenson O 1980 Child abuse: aspects of interprofessional cooperation. Allen & Unwin, London

Harris N 1987 Defensive social work. British Journal of Social Work 17: 61–69

Hobbs C, Wynne J 1986 Buggery in childhood – a common syndrome of child abuse. Lancet 4 October: 792–796

Hochstadt N, Hardwicke N 1985 How effective is the inter-disciplinary approach? A follow-up study. Child Abuse and Neglect 9: 365–372

Home Office 1945 Report by Sir Walter Monckton on the circumstances which led to the boarding-out of Dennis and Terence O'Neill at Bank Farm, Minsterley and the steps taken to supervise their welfare. Cmnd 6636. HMSO, London

Home Office 1950 Children neglected or ill-treated in their own home. Joint Circular with the Ministry of Health and the Ministry of Education. HMSO, London

Home Office, Department of Health 1992 Memorandum of good practice on video recorded interviews with child witnesses for criminal proceedings. HMSO, London

Howe D 1992 Child abuse and the bureaucratisation of social work. Sociological Review 40 (3): 491–508

Kelly L, Regan L 1990 Flawed protection. Social Work Today 21.32: 13–15

Krugman R 1991 Child abuse and neglect: critical first steps in response to a national emergency. American Journal of Diseases in Childhood 145: 513–515

La Fontaine J 1998 Speak of the devil: tales of satanic abuse in contemporary England. Cambridge University Press, Cambridge

London Borough of Brent 1985 A child in trust: the report of the panel of inquiry into the circumstances surrounding the death of Jasmine Beckford. London Borough of Brent, London

London Borough of Greenwich 1987 A child in mind: protection of children in a responsible society. The report of the commission of inquiry into the circumstances surrounding the death of Kimberley Carlile. London Borough of Greenwich, London

Marsh P, Crow G 1998 Family Group Conferences in child welfare. Blackwell, Oxford

Meadow R 1985 Management of Munchausen's syndrome by proxy. Archives of Disease in Childhood 60: 385–393

Metropolitan Police, London Borough of Bexley 1987 Child sexual abuse: joint investigative programme: Bexley experiment: final report. HMSO, London

Moran-Ellis J, Fielding N 1996 A national survey of the investigation of child sexual abuse. British Journal of Sociology 26 (3): 337–356

Mouzakitis C, Goldstein S 1985 A multi-disciplinary approach to treating child neglect. Social Casework 66 (4): 218–224

Newberger E, Hagenbuch J, Ebeling N, *et al.* 1973 Reducing the literal and human cost of child abuse: impact of a new hospital management system. Paediatrics 51 (5): 840–848

Sharland E, Seal H, Croucher M, *et al.* 1996 Professional involvement in child sexual abuse. HMSO, London

Smart M 1992 Professional ethics and participation: nurses, health visitors and midwives. In: Thoburn J (ed) Participation in practice: involving families in child protection. University of East Anglia, Norwich

Stevenson O 1989 Multidisciplinary work in child protection. In: Stevenson O (ed) Child abuse: public policy and professional practice. Harvester Wheatsheaf, Hemel Hempstead

Thoburn J (ed) 1992 Participation in practice: involving families in child protection. University of East Anglia, Norwich

Thoburn J, Lewis A, Shemmings D 1995 Paternalism or partnership? Family involvement in the child protection process. HMSO, London

Thomas T 1996 Covert video surveillance: an assessment of the Staffordshire protocol. Journal of Medical Ethics 22: 22–25

Tunstill J 1997 Implementing the family support clauses of the Children Act 1989: legislative, professional and organisational obstacles. In: Parton N (ed) Child protection and family support: tensions, contradictions and possibilities. Routledge, London

Wallen G, Pierce S, Koch M, Venters H 1977 the interdisciplinary team approach to child abuse services: strengths and limitations. Child Abuse and Neglect 1: 3559–3564

Walton M 1993 Regulation in child protection: policy failure? British Journal of Social Work 23: 139–156

Wattam C 1990 Working together. Social Work Today 22 (3): 222–223

Webster R 1998 The great children's home panic. Orwell Press, Oxford

Weiss J 1981 Substance vs. symbol in administrative reform: the case of human services coordination. Policy Analysis 7 (1): 21–45

14

Case conferences in child protection

Margaret Bell

INTRODUC-TION

Case conferences are crucial tools in the management of children in need of protection. Indeed, despite criticisms of their unhelpful focus on risk assessment and the recent policy shifts toward a more overtly welfare-based child protection service, the most recent guidance under the Children Act 1989 (Department of Health (DOH) 2000*a*) has confirmed the pivotal role of the initial child protection conference within the system. It remains an inter-agency meeting, held after section 47 enquiries have established that a child may suffer, or be at risk of suffering, significant harm, where:

those family members, the child where appropriate, and those professionals most involved with the child and the family, meet to ... analyze in a multi-disciplinary setting ... all relevant information, to make judgements about the likelihood of a child suffering significant harm in future and to ... plan how to safeguard the child and promote his or her welfare.

(DOH 1999, p. 69)

At the same time, the guidance recommends much greater use of other inter-agency meetings, such as family support meetings, in cases where children's safety can be assured. Such developments are to be welcomed as part of the broader based framework for meeting children's welfare needs. However, many of the complex issues in the management of conferences and other meetings in child protection – so helpfully identified by Stevenson (1995) in the first edition of this *Handbook* – remain. This chapter will, therefore, describe the background to the current situation and explore some of the main areas of continuing debate in relation to the purpose and scope of these conferences – including pre- and post-registration practice, assessments of risk and need, professional roles and responsibilities and the experiences of the participants. It will draw, in particular, upon the research of Farmer & Owen (1995), Thoburn *et al.* (1995), a research study undertaken in 1992 by Bell of 83 initial child protection conferences in a northern city (Bell 1999), and another reporting 27 children's experiences of child protection investigations (Bell 2000*b*).

Background

Case conferences to register children at risk of abuse were set up following the publication of the Maria Colwell inquiry report in 1974. However, their central role within the child protection system, the status of the Child Protection Register and its purposes remained ambiguous until 1988 when *Working Together* made it clear that the primary function of the initial child protection conference was to provide 'a forum for the exchange of information between professionals'. Following the Children Act 1989, *Working Together* (DOH *et al* 1991) confirmed that the initial conference was an essential component in protecting children. Inviting parents and children to take part in the meeting was advocated, and more detailed guidance on how to involve families was provided to Area Child Protection Committees by the Challenge of Partnership (DOH 1995*a*). Also in 1995 a number of research studies on the workings of the child protection system were published (DOH 1995*b*) and these have profoundly influenced the development of policy and practice.

On the positive side, the research studies confirmed the successful role of the initial conference in protecting from further harm children who were registered. In examining 120 conferences in two authorities, Farmer & Owen (1995) found that, 20 months after registration, 70% of the children were considered to be protected and in 68% of cases the child's welfare needs were met. At the same time, however, the research raised grave concerns at the shortcomings of the system. The work of Gibbons *et al.* (1995) demonstrated that large numbers of children were filtered out of the child protection process at different stages without their needs being addressed. They concluded that since only one-quarter of abuse enquiries reached conference and, of those, approximately one-third were not registered, more flexible responses to child abuse referrals should be developed so that appropriate help could be provided. Other research studies clearly demonstrated that, as far as the families were concerned, the experience of the investigation overall and of being present in the meeting was often traumatic. Thoburn *et al.* (1995), Cleaver & Freeman (1995) and Bell (1999) concluded that more constructive ways of involving families in the conference needed to be established and that, wherever possible, other means of protecting children and of meeting their wider welfare needs should be found. Added to concerns raised by the research, Social Service Inspectors found variable practice, poor management of family involvement, poor quality of assessments and unclear child protection plans (Social Services Inspectorate (SSI) 1997). The most recent guidance, *Working Together to Safeguard Children* (DOH 2000*a*) thus attempts to respond to the strengths and shortcomings of the existing system by confirming the centrality of the initial conference while also defining the situations in which other routes for meeting children's needs might be used both prior to and after the initial conference.

The present situation

Where there are child protection concerns, a number of case conferences are likely to take place. Whenever there is reasonable cause to suspect that a child is suffering, or is likely to suffer, significant harm, the professionals and sometimes the family members should first have 'a strategy discussion' to decide on the need for emergency action, further enquiries and the provision of interim services and support. In cases where the child's safety can be assured – for example, where the perpetrator has left the household – interventions other than proceeding to an initial child protection conference are encouraged. Family group conferences or family support meetings are currently the most common alternatives. However, where concerns are substantiated an initial child protection conference should be held. The initial conference has a twofold purpose: to consider whether the child is at risk of significant harm and, if so, whether safeguarding the child requires inter-agency help and intervention delivered through a formal child protection plan. If both of these criteria are satisfied, the child's name should be placed on the Child Protection Register under the category(ies) physical, emotional, or sexual abuse and/or neglect. Each area covered by a social services department should keep a register – 'to make agencies and professionals aware of those children who are judged to be at risk of significant harm and in need of active safeguarding' (DOH 2000*a*, p. 61). Additionally, the conference should make recommendations to 'the core group' as to how agencies, professionals and the family should work together to ensure the child's safety, including agreeing timescales, an outline child protection plan and identifying a key worker. The core group meeting, comprising the key professionals and family members, should be held within 10 working days of the initial conference to develop and operationalise the child protection plan. Here written agreements should be made and a comprehensive assessment consistent with guidance in the *Framework for Assessing Children in Need and their Families* (DOH 2000*b*) must be undertaken. In the spirit of partnership, family group conferences are viewed as a positive option at this stage. Within 6 months a review conference should be held to consider the child's developmental progress, against the intended outcomes, and de-registration is encouraged as soon as the child protection issues are resolved.

This framework for child protection decision-making thus represents a clear response to the concerns identified in *Messages from Research* (DOH 1995*b*), that the sharp focus on risk assessment which the conferences have traditionally assumed should be balanced with attention to the welfare needs of all family members. Whether the framework of the existing system supports this shift in focus is a matter of debate. Arguably, conferences have too much to do, too little time to do it in and many of the tasks and functions conflict. Parton (1996) has advocated a wholesale dismantling of the system with the most serious cases of abuse being passed to the police for investigation and the therapeutic work to the voluntary and not-for-profit sector. I, and others such as Corby *et al.* (1996) and Littlechild (1998), have suggested that the conflicts and ambiguities agencies and practitioners face in this difficult and sensitive area of work are embedded in the system and that its central components require radical change. Further, as Armstrong (1997) has suggested, the requirement to merge child protection into the wider canvas of services for children has, at local level, produced confusion and a blurring of boundaries. In responding to a mass of other government initiatives – not all of which run in tandem – some authorities have neither the commitment nor funding to resource the development of pre- and post-registration services. The worry is that children diverted from the conference will remain unprotected.

To explore some of these issues in more detail I shall address the following core dimensions of the initial conference, and the related issues for other conferences in child protection:

- purpose – collecting and analysing information and making judgements of significant harm
- the social work role
- the experiences of parents and children
- the child protection plan and subsequent core group meetings and family group conferences.

Purpose

The objectives of conferences in child protection are to share and analyse the information presented, to make judgements about the likelihood of a child suffering significant harm and to decide, with the parents, family members and the child, the most appropriate future action. The initial conference has the additional task of deciding whether or not to place the child's name on the Child Protection Register. Each of these objectives is intrinsically problematic – in particular for the initial conference. Some arise from difficulties external to the conferences themselves, others from the complexity of the group process. First, I will discuss issues concerning the collection of information before the conference, then explore some factors affecting the presentation and analysis of information within the conference.

Information collecting

It hardly needs saying that the quality of the decisions made by the conference is determined by the quality of the information made available to it. As reported above, there are concerns about the level of skill and expertise of the social workers undertaking assessments and the quality of information presented (SSI 1997). The Department of Health addresses this by the more detailed guidance in the *Framework for Assessment* (DOH 2000b), and by the introduction in 2000 of a new post-qualifying child care award. The fact remains that the task of collecting and processing information for an assessment is immensely difficult. One of the difficulties identified is in accessing family members. Bell (1999) interviewed 22 social workers about their initial assessments and found only three believed they had seen most of the child's primary attachment figures and only six had seen the child alone before the conference. Farmer & Owen (1995) reported a similar pattern. The social workers explained that this was because some of the adults were violent, some had mental health problems, some were not cooperative and sometimes language was a barrier. Calder & Howarth (1999) suggest that collecting information can be particularly difficult from families from ethnic minorities, who construct barriers of secrecy because of their fear of racially motivated interventions. Equally, workers may avoid talking to children because the emotions triggered are painful and overwhelming, or because they lack the skill.

Although there may be practical constraints, it seems likely that avoidance and denial are among the strategies for managing the anxiety provoked by these transactions. There is increasing awareness that the emotional impact of the work affects who is seen and what information is processed (Bell 2000a). Gibbons et al. (1995) reported the presence of domestic violence in 27% of their sample of approximately 2000 child protection referrals. Farmer & Owen (1995) report higher rates. In analysing inquiry reports, Munro (1998) found social workers 'lost' key bits of information and failed to make connections between the abuse of mothers and risk to children. Milner & Humphreys (1996) found that social workers often failed to record the existence of violence in case notes or to report it to conferences, concluding that professional responses could be driven by the fear of intimidation and harassment, sometimes of a sexual nature. The emotional response of the worker should, of course, be addressed in supervision so that its significance in the overall assessment can be considered. However, reports suggest that lack of managerial support is common and that the quality and quantity of supervision is often inadequate (SSI 1997).

There is also evidence that social workers lack confidence in selecting information which is key to the conference. The research commonly describes how the focus of enquiry was on the incident of abuse, with less attention paid to family background or environmental factors which could provide explanations. In cases where families were already known to social services (41% in Bell's study, two-thirds in that of Thoburn et al.) the social workers relied on information on file. However, Thoburn et al. (1995) found that social work files were unreliable sources of information on family circumstances in the year prior to referral – for example, a serious loss by death or divorce was not recorded.

A number of factors, therefore, affect what information is collected, as well as the ways in which it is recorded, prioritised and presented. Other professionals, equally, may miss important bits of information, neglect to present them to the conference or fail to attend. The sparse attendance of general practitioners (GPs) at conferences, for example, has long been a source of concern (Stevenson 1995). Professional perspectives also influence expressions of concern and the ways in which these are prioritised (Cleaver & Freeman 1995). For example, in constructing a diagnosis of neglect professionals from different agencies may apply different indicators of vulnerability. In such cases, health visitors are more likely to prioritise hygiene, whereas doctors look at bruises, teachers at learning difficulties and social workers at parenting skills.

Sharing information

Problems about quality coexist with matters of process and interpretation, some of which arise from the difficulties of inter-agency communication, some from poor training and support and some from the presence of family members. There now exists a substantial body of literature exploring the ways in which inter-professional communications are affected by issues of status and power. Hallett (1995) described how professionals, such as teachers who may only attend one conference in their career, do not feel part of the 'inner core' and hence believe their contribution is unimportant, or feel inhibited in speaking. This creates confusion because while these attenders feel they lack the knowledge and experience necessary, their contribution is perceived by others – particularly the children – to be very important. Other professionals, such as health visitors and school nurses who play a key part in the safety of younger children, struggle to be assertive in the conference which they experience as being dominated by social services. It has been suggested (Parton 1996) that the price to be paid for closer working between police and social services through joint interviewing is some loss of confidence from health personnel. In some cases criminal proceedings are being pursued and this alters the dynamics of the conference. In an attempt to decrease the dominance of social services, some authorities have employed chairpersons who are independent of line management. In any event, it is the chairperson's responsibility to integrate all the professionals round the table, and failure to do so means a vital element in the system is missing.

It is generally accepted (see Bell 1999, Thoburn *et al.* 1995) that the presence of family members in the conference improves the quality of information available. Family members add to it and clarify key details, while the professionals are more rigorous and accurate in what they say. However, these benefits have to be balanced against some of the difficulties which have been identified. Some of the professionals in Bell's (1996) study found it difficult to express negative views about the family in front of them, fearing this might alienate parents and endanger their capacity to protect the child. From a health visitor:

I feel other information may have been presented and considered regarding the child's home situation especially mother's lack of protective skills, if she had not been there.

At the same time, parents objected to information about their family background being shared in the conference, as well as to the professional interpretation of some events or behaviours as abusive. This was also inhibiting. In some conferences, the families' presence was found to be distracting when they became upset, and there were logistic problems in managing conferences where, for example, the parents were separated and had secrets from one another or in situations of domestic violence. The role of the chairperson in managing these situations is key, but, again, they are dependent upon the quality of information made available before the conference to judge how these situations might best be managed, including whether anyone should be excluded. The new guidance recommends that family members should only be excluded if there is risk of violence or intimidation. However, as we know from previous inquiries (for example, Jasmine Beckford, London Borough of Brent 1985), no-one can be relied upon to act rationally when feeling frightened or intimidated.

Analysing information

While professionals are becoming more experienced and skilled in presenting information which the family may not like to hear, they seem less confident about interpreting and analysing it in front of family members. Howe (1999) has pointed out that collecting pieces of the puzzle is not enough: 'pieces have to be in place for pictures and patterns to be seen ... and then move on to the analysis' (p. 195). There is continuing concern about the poor analysis of information and the absence of theoretical application. As described above, the focus is on describing incidents of abuse or neglect, with concerns accumulating, but with little evidence that the dynamics of the family situation and the social context have been analysed in relation either to causation, or to the making of a protection plan. In considering why social workers are more interested in what has happened than why, Stevenson's (1995) conjecture that social workers deny the significance of socio-economic forces is supported by the research. Farmer & Owen (1995) and Gibbons *et al.* (1995) found little reference to material factors relevant to the family situation. In the conferences in Bell's (1999) study, observation suggested that the social workers became uncomfortable when families described appalling social conditions which they could do nothing about. At the same time, Stevenson suggests, social workers who may be more willing to explore the dynamics of family functioning have lost confidence in, or understanding of, theories which might facilitate this. The move toward case management may increase uncertainty in this area because it requires less involvement in assessment of and direct work with families. Stevenson concludes that situations in which neither material circumstances nor family dynamics are adequately explored 'is the worst of both worlds and that the conference is operating with little or no explicit content and with little discussion of causation, of whatever kind' (p. 230).

Inter-agency processes also contribute to the lack of debate in the conference about aetiology. I have already identified some of the ways in which disagreement in the conference were suppressed. The professionals said they thought it important to present a united front to the parents and in some cases suppressed disagreement or diluted the negatives. The investigating social workers reported that decisions about registration were made beforehand and only rarely changed as a result of information heard in the conference. Hallett (1995) also noted an absence of dissent and conflict between the different professionals, concluding that there was a tacit agreement to avoid deeper differences in the way situations were perceived. Corby *et al.* (1996) provide evidence that parents are also inhibited from disagreeing with the professionals. The imbalance of power makes it difficult for them to speak and they fear making a bad impression. They conclude that the process of removing conflict from the conference, added to the parent's belief that the decision had already been made, is more likely to alienate parents and make them apathetic than to empower them. In the 110 conferences he studied, the chairperson had a key role in encouraging and supporting the expression of different views and in managing conflict constructively, but was not always successful in achieving this.

All this suggests that the conference's primary function – to share and analyse information – has become secondary to its instrumental function of managing professional anxiety in this highly charged area of risk. The idea of the conference offering mutual support in anxiety-provoking situations is not new. In 1980, Hallett & Stevenson accepted this as a valid part of the process. Farmer & Owen (1995) also suggest that the formality of the conference and the routinisation of the procedures services to distance the participants from the emotional impact of the distressing information which had emerged during the investigation. However, while managing anxiety may provide an important function the push to consensus makes it more likely that the chairperson effectively makes the registration decision. While many chairpersons are highly experienced and skilled operators, a possible consequence is that the conference decision may not be owned by members of the conference group. This will have implications for post-registration commitment. It will also influence the way in which the family – who are present but do not contribute to the registration decision – perceive the roles and responsibilities of the different professionals in subsequent meetings.

Judgements of significant harm

Clearly, a number of inter-connected and complex factors affect the collection, sharing and analysis of information that is presented to the conference. However, chairpersons report that, even where information is shared openly, many of the professionals present in the conference shrink from giving an opinion on registration. It is doubtful whether the new guidance detailing the process and content of 'Information for the Conference' will help. It emphasises the need to 'take care to distinguish between fact, observation, allegation and opinion', but does not suggest how this can be done. Some of the problems here are philosophical – how are 'facts' defined, and how can moral judgements be justified? Much has been written about the moral nature of the discourse in child protection work (Wattam 1992, Parton 1996, and see Parton, Chapter 1, in this volume). The overview in *Messages from Research* (DOH 1995) describes very clearly the ways in which thresholds for determining abuse differ historically and culturally, as we have seen they may also between practitioners in the conference. The rates of children on and added to registers, and the categories used, vary regionally (Gibbons *et al.* 1995) and over time. For example, in 1997 the number of children registered under the category of neglect and emotional abuse is significantly higher than in 1993, whereas there was a reduction in the categories of physical and sexual abuse. However, there is little evidence of change in the way the threshold criteria are being applied. Since 1993, the number of children registered annually – 32 400 – has remained steady (Barker 1997).

There are real problems in distinguishing between fact, observation, allegation and opinion as well as in determining when the threshold of significant harm has been reached – or, indeed, how 'significant' is to be defined. Judgements of significant harm also require that culpability and intent are addressed. In cases of physical abuse and sexual abuse the medical evidence may be unequivocal in so far as the injuries and incident and the identity of the abuser are concerned. By contrast, in situations of marital breakdown or domestic violence, the children may suffer emotional abuse which is not identified because it remains hidden and is not the result of a specific act directed at the children. In cases of neglect there are unique difficulties in agreeing on the benchmark and in determining cause and effect. It is difficult to substantiate – it happens over time, although the conference agenda is built around a snapshot of the present – and proving intentionality or culpability may be implausible in the context of the environmental disadvantage in which many of these families exist. The following quote from one of the mothers in Bell's (1999) study well illustrates the gap between what parents and professionals consider to be abusive.

I do smack my children, and I believe in smacking them. But I love them. I try to keep them clean, but it's impossible where we live. And how would you manage as a single parent with three boys under 5, no money and a stinking damp house?

Dingwell *et al.* (1983) suggested that intention should be one of the three types of evidence used to confirm child abuse – the others being the child's clinical condition and the nature of their social environment. The research has demonstrated, however, some of the ways in which information is presented as evidence and then used to construe responsibility or culpability for the abuse. Again, this raises issues about fitness for purpose. I have already suggested that the conference has an instrumental function which obscures its primary purpose. Here I am suggesting that the conference is fulfilling a quasi-judicial function which is potentially unjust. The family members can hear what is said and contribute but – unlike the local authority – they do not have legal representation and are not well positioned to dispute 'the facts' or question professional opinion. Additionally, my interviews revealed that they are unclear about the basis of the registration decision and that the nature of their subsequent cooperation is 'voluntary'. All this raises questions about justice as well as process and effectiveness, especially where working in partnership is one of the imperatives.

The social work role

I have already mentioned some of the sources of personal and professional stress for social workers and suggested contradictory demands are made on them in the conference. First, the social work role in relation to the family is complex. This role requires them, at different times, to act in different roles – as advocates, reporters, supporters, negotiators. Not all of these roles sit comfortably together. Additionally, there are conflicts of role in acting for different family members whose interests may diverge. Separated parents, for example, may hold entirely different views on good enough parenting; or the child's right to be protected may conflict with what the child wants, or what the parents want. The interests and rights of wider family members may differ, but also need to be addressed and presented to the conference. Further conflicts of interest may be created by the need to act as an advocate for the family in the conference while at the same time gatekeeping and case managing the Authority's scarce resources. Arguably, the imperative to work in partnership renders the task even more difficult – especially when the authority cannot provide the service the social worker believes the family needs.

Second, in pursuing section 47 enquiries, social workers walk a tightrope between the care and control functions of their work. In offering practitioners choices at each stage of the enquiry regarding which model of care planning best suits the family situation *Working Together* (DOH 2000*a*) clearly emphasises the care dimension of their role. Where parents can be relied upon to protect their children – including in cases where serious concerns have been substantiated – they should be supported in doing so without resort to the initial conference, or without registration. However, the critical decision as to how, when and by whom the threshold of entry into the child protection system is determined remains, and remains with the social worker. Deciding not to hold an initial conference may well place additional high risk demands on practitioners already under stress and over-burdened. Alternatively, in pursuing registration, social workers may be perceived by parents to be taking up adversarial positions in which they are accorded control, while not having access to the resources the families want (Bairstow & Hetherington 1998).

Family participation

The participation of families in the conference has, for some time, been regarded as a key component of partnership practice. Even before the Children Act, some authorities had been including parents. Following the unequivocal guidance in *Working Together* (DOH 1991a), all authorities introduced family participation. Some favoured partial exclusion, believing the consideration of risk and registration decision could be compromised by the parents' presence; others (Farmer & Owen 1995, Thoburn *et al.* 1995) thought this the worst of both worlds from the parents' point of view. Early concerns about the impact of parents' presence on the decisions made, generally, have been allayed. In Bell's (1999) study, conferences with parents present were not less frequent, less well attended and did not lead to different registration outcomes. Professionals believed that most conferences were better with parents attending than without; the quality of information was better, and the parental perspective better appreciated. Parents who attended were, in general, glad that they were able to be present and believed that it was right that they should be present. However, one-third of the conferences in this study were rated as having particular difficulties linked to the presence of parents, such as those where the parents were denying the abuse. Parents are now routinely invited to the conference, and there are attempts also to include the wider family. In 1996, 75% of parents attended conferences (SSI 1997). Of course not all parents want to attend and much depends upon the way in which they are prepared (Longstaff 1998). A particular concern raised by the research is that the mother is the target of much of the work pre-, during and post conference. In Bell's (1999) study, 94% of the mothers were invited to the conference, as opposed to 44% of the fathers; 70% of the mothers attended and 24% of the fathers. Farmer & Owen (1995) found, further, that children were more likely to be registered if the mother was seen as responsible for the abuse or neglect. Such practices are potentially oppressive to men, women and children: while men are excluded, women are seen as carrying responsibility for protection of the child, and feel guilty when they fail. Equally, the child's key attachment may be to another adult altogether. While who gets invited to the conference should be a focus for the initial assessment, the evidence suggests that the net is not cast sufficiently wide and the spotlight is on the mother.

There are other thorny and important issues. All the research undertaken on parental participation has shown that, although many parents were glad to have attended, the conference was often experienced as intensely painful and humiliating. From one of the parents in Bell's study:

I don't think parents should go because it's too upsetting ... loads of people going through the same problem. If they'd understood how awful it was they'd have supported us. It felt like a trial with the police there.

Many of these parents questioned the relevance of the information presented which related to their family background or lifestyle, rather than the incident. They found the meetings too big and disliked the presence of police and of other professionals not directly involved. While three-quarters felt they had been listened to and fairly treated, most felt they had not influenced the decision of the conference.

There is still little research specifically on the experiences of black families. In tracking 120 conferences, Owen & Farmer (1996) found it difficult to locate cases where black children had been registered. Families were wary about participating, and women were discouraged by their male partners. Like their white counterparts, the black families reported distress and a sense of intrusion at being referred. None had asked for help and they had no understanding of what registration meant. Nevertheless, in 70% of these cases the family was engaged, and successful outcomes were enhanced when social workers were matched on the dimensions of race, gender and culture. In Bell's (1999) study more cases from ethnic minorities were described as difficult. It seemed the professionals lacked confidence in making judgements about child care practice, while the families lacked confidence in the system. As Korbin (1981) suggested, cross-cultural differences can produce, on the one hand, an unhelpful cultural relativism and, on the other, cultural blindness or superiority. Language also presented difficulty; some words necessary, for example, to describe sexual abuse do not exist in other languages. Working with interpreters brought additional difficulty, especially when they – as they often did – belonged to the same community as the family. There were particular problems in some families where the women did not speak English, or were not expected by their male partner to take part in discussions. In others, the values of the parents and the child diverged – as in where they held differing opinions about acceptable sexual and marital partners, or family rites of passage.

The extent to which parents participate in the conference is thus questionable. Farmer & Owen (1995) estimated that parents contributed to the conference discussion in 44 of the 71 conferences they attended; in 15 cases their contribution was extremely limited and in only 11 cases did they participate in an exploration of the relevant issues. Thoburn *et al.* (1995) found that only 8% of the parents attending could be described as participating in the assessment of risk, and only 2% about registration. Farmer & Owen argue for greater use of parent advocacy but, as Stevenson (1995) points out, this carries the dangers (notably when the advocate is a lawyer) that the conference becomes an adversarial encounter which makes establishing partnership difficult. The focus on risk assessment, implying a disregard of wider welfare needs, also makes it less likely that the conference will be experienced as positive by parents.

Corby *et al.* (1996) suggest that the process of removing conflict from the conference, added to the parents' belief that the decision had already been made, is more likely to alienate parents and make them apathetic than to empower than. Perhaps it makes more sense, on the basis of the research evidence above, to talk about enablement rather than empowerment. For the parents in Bell's (1999) study who had participated, the strong sense of having been fairly treated seemed to lessen feelings of anger, to encourage a more rational response and to allow for a more positive social work relationship to develop. Their involvement in the process did seem to lay a firmer base from which to proceed in cases where they were not in denial. However, the extent to which such relationships can be described as partnerships is debatable.

Children's participation

While great strides have been made in enabling parents to participate in the conference, consequently less attention has been paid to the participation of children. Nobody questions the child's right to participate. Local authorities have a duty under section 22 of the Children Act 1989 to ascertain the wishes and feelings of the child, and the child's right to influence decisions is a legal one. However, opinion is divided on how that participation is best effected so that the child's voice is heard without damaging the child in the process. Questions arise about how the views of the child are to be ascertained in relation to age, maturity, capacity and so on. Browne *et al.* (1992) have suggested that for children, abuse is a process, not an event. Taking a chronological approach to a process which is an important way of ordering experience for adults may not, therefore, be appropriate with children. Many children, particularly very young children, children with communication difficulties or children for whom English is not their first language, have great difficulty expressing their views. Adolescent children may be traumatised, silenced or confused about what they feel. Mars (1989) found that black female children were less likely to disclose for fear of a racist response. The impact of the child protection system itself will create fear and uncertainty. In interviews with children about their experience of child protection investigations, one of the mothers in Bell's (2000*b*) study vividly described the impact on the family:

When they heard my child had an injury it was madness with police and social workers turning up and all the neighbours watching. It was so embarrassing. I felt all that was unnecessary.

There is evidence that social workers find it difficult to engage with traumatised children. Bell (1999) found that only 27% of the social workers she interviewed saw the child before the conference and the level of immediate post-conference activity – including talking to the child – was low. Although the child was more frequently seen in Thoburn *et al.*'s (1995) study this was not always with the parents' agreement, in which case it had a negative impact on future relationships. Many social workers lack the training and confidence to engage with the child's feelings. In investigating qualifying training for childcare, Central Council for Education and Training in Social Work (CCETSW 1999) found wide variability in the teaching and testing of basic child care skills of observation and communication. At present, 'direct work' with children is more commonly located in post-qualifying and specialist play therapy training. There are, therefore, a number of factors which contribute to social workers' reluctance to engage with children.

   Children are rarely present at the initial conference. Some authorities occasionally include adolescent children, and there have been projects (see Scutt 1998) using child advocates. The more recent research on childrens' views on being involved in child protection investigations has built on earlier work which concentrated on interviews with children looked after outside the home (Stein & Carey 1986). Barford (1993) talked to 11 children from four different families. He found that the social workers' initial contact was often surrounded in uncertainty, with some children wanting to speak but unable to, and others finding themselves expected to talk but unsure what to say. Shepherd (1994) found that younger children had very little understanding of the process. Shemmings (1996) interviewed 34 children about their experiences of attending an initial conference and reported a range of views, with children saying they needed preparation and independent representation, and that their view had not generally been sought. Bell's (2000*b*) more recent study of 27 children aged 8–16 suggests that they are given information, but their understanding of what is happening is poor and their desire to engage, including attending the conference, was variable. A few who had not been invited wished to have been there; others were happy for their views to be presented by their social worker; yet others were uninterested or feared going. From a 16-year-old girl:

They asked me if I wanted to go ... I didn't want to – nothing would have persuaded me – I didn't know what to say – I used to get all confused. My Mam used to go and talk about school – I just didn't want to hear it – couldn't be doing with it – it got me mad because I'd done nothing wrong – it was the family's fault.

The research is therefore common in finding variation. Clearly, different children want different things with regard to participation, and age is not the main criteria in determining attitude. Many of the children interviewed by Bell were troubled about confiding in a public meeting what was happening at home, fearing that adults would react in ways they did not want and that they would lose control of their lives. What mattered to them was that there was someone there for them who listened and took seriously what they said, and who they could trust. So, while it is possible, as Butler & Williamson (1994) suggest, that the essence of engaging children is communication, Bell's study implies that factors other than a trusting relationship and good communication influence children's views about participation in meetings.

It seems that children, like their parents, need a lot of help to enable them to exercise choice in relation to how they participate in the decision-making process. Essential prerequisites are a relationship of trust within which the trauma of the process can be contained, skills in communicating with children and time and space within which information about what has happened and what will happen can be shared and digested. Real choices about the different ways in which the child's view can be heard need to be offered, and these include the use of an advocate, written messages, drawings and audio-tapes – as well as, in some cases, the child's attendance. Clearly the conference agenda must specify at which point the child's voice will be heard and the ensuing core group should always consider the child's wishes and feelings, and the ongoing need for children to be kept informed and seen alone. As with their parents, attention needs to be given to the gender and race of the social worker, and whether a change of worker after the initial conference would be appropriate. This should all be recorded in the minutes and written into the protection plan.

The child protection plan

The difficulties the initial conference faces in constructing a detailed child protection plan after dealing with the registration issues have been well documented. Farmer & Owen (1995) and Bell (1999) found that risk assessment had so dominated the majority of conferences that there was little time left to consider the second crucial element, the child protection plan. In Farmer & Owen's study, on average, only 9 minutes were devoted to the protection plan. Bell noted that the presence of parents increased the length of the meeting by 20 minutes, with the result that some professionals had to leave before important discussions on registration and planning took place. Further, as *Messages from Inspections* (SSI 1997) confirms, there is great variation in the quality of the plans made at the conference. Farmer & Owen (1995) noted variation from broad general statements to detailed specifications, and in over a third of the cases studied, important aspects were overlooked.

Even where conferences had constructed an embryonic plan the research has also identified poor post-registration practice. In exploring the practice of 22 social workers after the conference, Bell (1999) found that only six had visited the family in the week following the conference and inter-agency work was negligible. Hallett (1995) also described inter-agency collaboration as being 'much more highly developed up to and including the initial conference than it was thereafter' (p. 275). Calder & Howarth (1999) found that key workers felt over burdened by their responsibilities and that other agencies were reluctant to share the tasks. *Working Together* (DOH 2000a), therefore, reaffirms that the agencies involved should work together to cooperate in the post-registration work and lays out in much greater detail the subsequent actions. These include the management of core groups, written agreements and family group conferences, as well as the relationship between their responsibilities and those of the initial conference.

Core group meetings

Although *Working Together* 1991, had identified core group meetings as being the appropriate place where planning could be progressed and operationalised, there were no guidelines on who should chair them, whether parents should be present and whether they were making decisions which were properly the responsibility of the initial conference. The commitment of all members of the core group was not always high and procedures were not always adhered to. Calder & Howarth (1999) identified other issues for both practitioners and families in the core group, such as that family participation was reactive rather than proactive and that recording and written plans were poor.

In an attempt to address the lack of clarity and status of the core group as the focus for the post-registration work, the new guidance clarifies the respective roles of the conference and the core group in relation to the child protection plan. The conference should produce an outline child protection plan identifying risks, short- and long-term objectives and who should do what, when; the core group has responsibility for developing and operationalising the plan 'as a working tool'. Membership comprises all professionals who have direct contact with the family and key family members, including the child, if appropriate. It should meet within 10 working days of the conference, and record agreed action. However, while the inter-agency component of the core group is reinforced, the role of the key worker remains complex and extensive: 'to lead the core group, to maintain responsibility for managing the multi agency plan, complete the core assessment of the child and family, to co-ordinate the contribution of family members and other agencies, to put the child protection plan into effect and review progress' (DOH 1999, p. 76).

While this clarification of responsibility is long overdue – and the new framework and tools for conducting comprehensive assessments provide a much improved child centred, ecological framework – the tasks above remain complex and burdensome. The role of key workers as managers is emphasised, but the question of whether they (or others) should carry out the work with the family remains unclear. Also unclear is the question of who should chair the core group. Some authorities have, for some time, used conference chairpersons to chair this meeting in acknowledgement that social workers lack the necessary status, experience and skills. What is essential is that other professionals are kept on board, and that the families' responsibility for their children's care is actively maintained.

Family group conferences

One of the mechanisms for establishing the responsibility of the family – as opposed to that of the professionals – is the family group conference. Originating in New Zealand (Wilcox *et al.* 1991), family group conferences are meetings where all members of the wider family, including the child, meet together, and propose to the professionals the best ways for them of safeguarding and meeting the child's needs. Initially it was hoped that family group conferences might replace child protection conferences. However, in evaluating attempts in six authorities to introduce family group conferences, Marsh & Crow (1998) found the social workers' reluctance to engage with them a major factor in the decision not to use family group conferences to replace the initial conference. It seems that, despite the rhetoric of refocusing, social workers found it difficult to relinquish the policing aspect of their role. So, while the function of family group conferences in care planning was confirmed by the research, the difficulties encountered in using them suggested that their use in the UK is more limited than was originally hoped. *Working Together* (DOH 2000a), concludes that 'Family Group Conferences do not replace, or remove the need for child protection conferences – but may be valuable for children in need where a plan is required for the child's welfare' (p. 78).

Authorities will presumably make their own decisions as to the respective roles these two important planning groups occupy in the child welfare system – and that is as it should be. However, there still remain uncertainties about the role of the core group vis-a-vis the conference. In addition, the circumstance in which a family group conference might be used instead of, or alongside, the core group, are not addressed, although the descriptors of its function and purpose sound almost identical. If professionals are confused, families will be more so.

Family support meetings

Turning to pre-registration practice, other models of meeting are being developed to enable families to be helped without resort to conference. One authority in the north of England is piloting a twin track approach by which cases where there are 'moderate to serious child protection issues', but the family are acknowledging the reality of the situation and the need for help, are routed to a 'family support meeting' instead of to conference (I Bond, personal communication). The family support meeting, chaired by the principal social worker, involves all agencies and an action plan is identified. It is early days, but the results are generally positive. To date, half of the potential conference cases – mainly cases of general neglect – have been successfully re-routed. The principal social workers report that the families feel involved and that some professionals remain more committed to the ongoing intervention. However, others have been less convinced of the benefits; the police do not play a large part in the meetings, and paediatricians fear a minimisation of child protection concerns. Some of the difficulties identified in the development of family group conferences may also appertain here. The capacity to provide appropriate services is patchy, although the success of the project requires that they are available. Most importantly, the success of the project relies upon committed managers and project leaders providing encouragement and leadership to sometimes reluctant social workers, and social workers being convinced that management will share responsibility for the decisions made. Whether management can provide this support is questionable, particularly in the light of *Messages from Inspections* (SSI 1997) which reported that management systems had weaknesses, inaccuracy and variations.

So, while other types of meeting do give social workers a wider repertoire to bring into play and provide them with real opportunities to develop the care aspect of their role in some cases, some key issues remain. Many years ago, Dingwall *et al.* (1983) cautioned against the rule of optimism, and social workers who have learned the hard way will continue to be wary.

Conclusion

In the first edition of this *Handbook* (1995), Stevenson reviewed the knowledge base and research findings in relation to initial child protection conferences with reference to content and purpose, process, inter-professional cooperation and parent/child participation. This chapter looks again at those issues, re-examining some of the problems identified which still remain, while also exploring the ways in which progress has been made. The problems that still remain concern the ambiguous nature of the tasks and functions of the conference, the way in which the conference process mitigates against quality assessments of risk and need and the adversarial nature of the encounter which distresses parents and makes children's participation extremely difficult. Arguably the difficulties identified in these areas are embedded in the system, for the reasons discussed, and can only be addressed by a radical change in the decision-making process. Other models do exist which may be less adversarial and more likely to promote partnership. In comparing the experiences of English and French parents, Bairstow & Hetherington (1998) found that, while parents in both countries experienced similar problems, the English parents were more upset and less satisfied than their French counterparts. In France, as in Scotland, parents have direct access to the judge – or the panel – and experience the law as accessible and responsive to their needs. Most importantly, they felt the professionals were on their side. Although it seems ironic to propose that the ideology of rights which underpins our system mitigates against partnership, much of the evidence presented here in relation to the conference function and process leads to that conclusion. It does seem important, therefore, to acknowledge openly that the difficulties and conflicts identified do exist, and to consider more radical ways of engaging with them. A closer alliance with a more welfare-oriented court system may enable the conflicting welfare and policing roles that social workers currently occupy within the conference process to be more appropriately managed.

Turning to what is new, the development of frameworks for pre- and post-registration practice is encouraging if it reduces the need for more intrusive State intervention at all stages of the process. A welfare-based service is much more likely to promote opportunities for preventative and therapeutic work and to be experienced by families as supportive. Whether these developments will be adequately resourced remains to be seen. There are models of community development which lay the foundations for sound preventative work – such as Easterhouse in Glasgow, where lead staff help local people to establish services and activities which meet the needs of disadvantaged families, such as credit unions, community shops and after school clubs (Hearn 1995). However, such initiatives require continuing funding of the voluntary sector, close inter-agency collaboration and commitment from local and national government. Whether social workers feel comfortable doing this work also remains to be seen. The encouragement to shift, wherever possible, the focus of their work with children and families away from the heavy end of child protection to family support – an area traditionally staffed by unqualified workers – has left many social workers feeling confused and de-skilled. Finally, there is concern that, even where family support services exist, children who are at risk of harm may not be adequately protected without recourse to the initial conference. Littlechild (1998) cautions that, since the predictive factors in any case of abuse are often not clear, serious cases of abuse will be missed because an enquiry has not been fully pursued. Assessing risk is notoriously difficult and provokes much anxiety. If as is generally agreed, one of the functions of the conference is to manage professional anxiety, it is difficult to see where this containment will be held. Risk and need are two sides of the same coin – and the political shift toward family support is to be welcomed – but there are difficulties in doing this within the context of an inter-agency meeting set up to judge whether or not the incidents triggering the conference were abusive.

References

Armstrong H 1997 Refocusing children services conferences. Department of Health and London

Bairstow K, Hetherington R 1998 Parents' experience of child welfare interventions: an Anglo-French comparison. Children and Society 12: 113–124

Barford R 1993 Childrens' views of child protection social work. University of East Anglia Monograph, Norwich

Barker M (ed) 1997 Health and personal social services statistics for England. The Stationery Office, London

Bell M 1999 Child protection: families and the conference process. Ashgate, Andover

Bell M 2000a Social work responses to domestic violence within the context of child protection. In: McCluskey U, Hooper C A (eds) Psycho-dynamic perspectives on abuse: the cost of fear. Jessica Kingsley, London

Bell M 2000b Children speak out: the experiences of children and young people of child protection investigations. University of York, York

Browne K, Davies C, Stratton P 1992 Early prediction and prevention of child abuse. John Wiley, Chichester

Butler I, Williamson H 1994 Children speak: children, trauma and social work. Longman, London

Calder M, Howarth J 1999 Working for children on the Child Protection Register. Ashgate, Aldershot

Central Council for Education and Training in Social Work (CCETSW) 1999 Focused investigation into child care teaching on DipSW, Report Summary. CCETSW, London

Cleaver H, Freeman P 1995 Parental perspectives in cases of suspected child abuse: studies in child protection. HMSO, London

Corby B, Miller M, Young L 1996 Parental participation in child protection work: rethinking the rhetoric. British Journal of Social Work 26 (4): 99.475–493

Department of Health (DOH) 1995a The challenge of partnership in child protection: practice guide. HMSO, London

Department of Health (DOH) 1995b Child protection: messages from research. HMSO, London

Department of Health (DOH) 1999 Working together to safeguard children. Consultation document. The Stationery Office, London

Department of Health (DOH) 2000a Working together to safeguard and promote the welfare of children. The Stationery Office, London

Department of Health (DOH) 2000b Framework for the assessment of children in need and their families. Department of Health, London

Department of Health, Home Office, Department of Education and Science, Welsh Office 1991 Working together under the children Act 1989. A guide to arrangements for inter-agency cooperation for the protection of children from abuse. HMSO, London

Dingwall R, Eekelaar J, Murray T 1983 The protection of children: State intervention and family life. Blackwell, Oxford

Farmer E, Owen M 1995 Child protection practice: private risks and public remedies. HMSO, London

Gibbons J, Conroy S, Bell C 1995 Operating the child protection system. HMSO, London

Hallett C 1995 Inter-agency cooperation in child protection. HMSO, London

Hallett C, Stevenson O 1980 Child abuse: aspects of inter-professional cooperation. Allen & Unwin, London

Hearn B 1995 Child and family support and protection: a practical approach. National Children's Bureau Enterprises, London

Howe D 1999 Attachment theory for social work practice. Macmillan, Basingstoke

Korbin J (ed) 1981 Child abuse and neglect: cross-cultural perspectives. University of California Press, Berkeley, California

Littlechild B 1998 Does family support ensure protection of the child? Child Abuse Review 7: 116–128

Longstaff D 1998 Partnership: a social work perspective on preparing children and families for the initial child protection conference. MSW Thesis, University of York, York

Mars M 1989 Child sexual abuse and race issues. In: British Association for Adoption and Fostering (ed) After abuse papers: papers on caring and planning for a child who has been sexually abused. BAAF, London

Marsh P, Crow G 1998 Family group conferences in child welfare. Blackwell, Oxford

Milner J 1996 Men's resistance to social workers. In: Fawcett B, Featherstone B, Hearn J, Toft C (eds) Violence and gender relations: theories and interventions. Sage, London

Munro E 1998 Improving social workers' knowledge base in child protection work. British Journal of Social Work 28: 89–105

Owen M, Farmer E 1996 Child protection in a multi racial context. Policy and Politics 24 (3): 299–313

Parton N 1991 Governing the family: child care, child protection and the State. Routledge, London

Parton N 1996 (ed) Social theory, social change and social work. Routledge, London

Schofield G, Thoburn J 1996 Child protection: the voice of the child in decision-making. Institute of Social Policy Research, London

Scutt N 1998 Child advocacy. In: Cloke C, Davis M (eds) Participation and empowerment in child protection. Pitman, London

Shemmings D 1996 Involving children in child protection conferences. Social Work Monograph, University of East Anglia, Norwich

Shepherd A M 1994 Ensuring children's voices are heard in the child protection process and child care decision making: strategies for improving policy and practice. Advanced Practice Dissertation, University of East Anglia, Norwich

Social Services Inspectorate (SSI) 1997 Messages from inspections: responding to families in need: inspection of assessment, planning and decision-making in family support services. Department of Health, London

Stein M, Carey K 1986 Leaving care. Blackwell, London

Stevenson O 1995 Case conferences in child protection. In: Wilson K, James A (eds) The child protection handbook, 1st edn. Ballière Tindall, London

Thoburn J, Lewis A, Shemmings D 1995 Paternalism or partnership? Family involvement in child protection: studies in child protection. HMSO, London

Wattam C 1992 Making a case in child protection. Longman, Loughborough

Wilcox R 1991 Family decision-making: family group conferences: practitioners' views. Practitioners Publishing, Lower Hutt, New Zealand

Protecting children: the role of the health visitor

Sue Rouse

That there is a significant role for health visitors in the protection of children would appear to be without contention as evidenced by the inclusion of this chapter and the publication of much material over the years which addresses training in child protection specifically for health visitors (e.g. Stainton-Rogers & Iskander 1990, Armstrong 1994). There are also other works highlighting and addressing child protection issues which are specific to health visitors and nurses (Cloke & Naish 1992, Department of Health (DOH) 1992). However, the extent to which the role should focus on child protection issues and the way in which this fits into the broader public health and primary health care remit, can be the cause of some uncertainty on the part of both individual practitioners (Waters 1992) and on the part of those commissioning and managing the service. It would appear that, in caseloads where there is a high incidence of recognised child abuse, the role of the health visitor can become dominated by work in connection with child protection. This may well be appropriate in the light of the outcomes of local health needs assessment. However, child protection work must be set against the range of local health needs when commissioners of health visiting services determine public health priorities on behalf of their resident population. Indeed, health authorities are advised of the need to include child protection within their contracts for primary health care services (DOH 1991*b*). It must be remembered, however, that health visitors are the only members of primary health care teams whose role is aimed exclusively at improving the public's health through health promotion and ill-health prevention and this work entails addressing a wide range of competing priorities.

Health visitors, by the very nature of their work, are often involved in the primary prevention of child abuse and its recognition and referral and are regular participants in multidisciplinary interventions such as child protection case conferences and core groups. Their substantial role in child protection is recognised and endorsed by the arrangements for dedicated support and supervision mechanisms such as the appointment of specialist child protection advisors within health authorities and National Health Service (NHS) trusts. Their contribution and specialist expertise in the fields of child development and family health are acknowledged in publications such as *Working Together under the Children Act 1989* (DOH 1991*b*) and *Working Together to Safeguard Children* (DOH 1999*a*). However, in the greater scheme of things, child protection work forms a relatively small, if very important and anxiety-provoking, part of the role.

This chapter aims to examine the role of the health visitor in child protection in the light of the broader remit of public health nursing practice, the underlying principles of health visiting and some of the recent Government policy guidance on health and social priorities. This will be followed by a consideration of the nature and extent of the role at various stages in the child protection cycle with discussion of some of the difficulties and dilemmas involved. There will be some concomitant discussion of the skills, knowledge and support systems required in order for the role to be safely and appropriately performed. There is not scope within a short chapter such as this to address any issues in detail and the reader is directed to more in-depth texts on various aspects of the discussion throughout.

The principles of health visiting and the public health role

The principles of health visiting were published in 1977 (CETHV, 1977) and subjected to substantial review and ultimate endorsement in 1992 (Twinn & Cowley, 1992). The primary purpose of the role is founded in addressing issues of public health and health promotion. Indeed, this central focus is re-inforced by the role title within the new standards for community specialist practice in 'Public Health Nursing (Health Visiting)' (UKCC, 1992). The concept of public health indicates a population-based approach to care and poses the first of many potential dilemmas for health visitors in balancing community-based activities and group approaches with the individual home visiting which is central to their recognised role in child protection. However, there would appear to be some evidence that home health visiting helps in the prevention of child abuse (Gelles 1998).

The principles which form the foundation for health visiting practice are deliberately described in broad rather than specific terms so that they can be applied to the health needs of the moment and are not 'timed out' by changing health needs and priorities. They are:

- The search for health needs
- The stimulation of awareness of health needs
- The influence on policies affecting health
- The facilitation of health enhancing activities.

The principles can be applied to every client group within society and do not specify work with families with small children; a fact little recognised by those outside of the profession. However, this area of work continues to be central to the day-to-day workload of many health visitors and it is this 'routine' contact with young families that ultimately leads to health visitors' involvement in child protection work.

Using the broadly accepted definition of health which incorporates social, emotional and spiritual aspects as well as the more obvious physical and mental ones (World Health Organization (WHO) 1946), then the application of the principles within the field of child protection is clear. The search for health needs (or the need for a child to receive protection from actual or potential harm) relies on contact with large numbers of the population in order that both the potential for child harm and/or actual incidences can be identified. Stimulation of the awareness of health needs includes work within families which acknowledges potential or actual difficulties in the practical care and protection of children and encourages parents and other responsible adults to recognise and engage in their caring and protective roles. The facilitation of health-enhancing enhancing activities includes direct work with families on parenting and the provision of ongoing support as well as referral to other sources for help and advice. Finally, the influence on policies affecting health includes effective inter-agency working as well as the collection and analysis of data to inform future professional and service developments.

Following from the principles discussed above, the concepts of primary, secondary and tertiary prevention are often used to provide a framework for health visiting practice (Robertson 1991) with the emphasis lying in primary prevention and health promotion. A brief explanation of these levels of prevention as they relate to child protection is reproduced below:

- Primary prevention – prevention of occurrence of a child-abusing situation mainly through teaching or information-giving.
- Secondary prevention – prevention of the development of stress and tensions leading to child abuse mainly through surveillance and referral for support.
- Tertiary prevention – prevention of deterioration where child harm seems to have occurred, mainly through support.

This emphasis on prevention would indicate a clear contribution for health visitors in working with families where there has been no child harm but where the potential vulnerabilities can be detected and addressed so that child harm does not ensue. This part of the role is hugely important in terms of cost-effectiveness and the prevention of human suffering and yet is largely unrecognised as child protection work. In contrast, the secondary prevention role which manifests itself in the early recognition and referral of child harm and the tertiary role in providing continuing support and family based working following abuse as discussed in more detail by Browne (Chapter 3, in this volume), are widely recognised both within and outside of the profession. The tertiary prevention role for health visitors does not usually significantly involve them in therapeutic intervention but can be important following rehabilitation. This, in itself, presents a huge dilemma for those health visitors who have a large incidence of child harm within their caseload. In the first place, their broad remit which involves the provision of a public health service to the entire population, 'from the cradle to the grave' tends to become dominated by work with young families, and in the second, there is a propensity for this work to become dominated by secondary and tertiary level work rather than primary prevention. The potential for the underlying principles of practice to become lost in the face of such pressures looms large and can be re-inforced by the expectations of other professionals, often including social workers, whose role description sees the protection of children as the over-riding priority. None of this discussion seeks to undervalue the immense importance of child protection work, merely to place it in some perspective within the context of the total range of health visiting practice.

Policy and guidance

Various government policy and guidance documents refer to the role that health visitors play both in working with families and more specifically in child protection. Following the publication and enactment of the Children Act 1989, the Government's *Working Together* guidance (DOH 1991*b*) describes the contribution that health visitors may be expected to make in terms of preparing and supporting parents. This guidance has recently been subject to review and the new document emphasises the role of health professionals in the early identification and referral of children in need (DOH 1999*a*). This is clearly a role which arises out of a predominantly primary and secondary prevention approach as discussed above. The Home Office guidance on *Supporting Families* (Home Office 1998) re-inforces the view that work with the family as a client group remains central to the Government's perception of the role of the health visitor. Nevertheless, the publication of *Saving Lives: Our Healthier Nation* (DOH 1999) emphasises the centrality of coronary heart disease, stroke, cancer, accidents and mental health issues to the public health agenda of today as well as acknowledging the vital role that health visitors play in supporting parents and families. All of this serves only to emphasise some of the dilemmas of prioritising within health visiting (or public health nursing) practice and must impact upon the extent to which a significant role in child protection can be effectively combined with other important public health priorities.

Summary of current research

The role of health visitors or, more specifically, home visiting, in the prevention of child harm has been subject to some extensive research over the last 20 years. A systematic review of such studies, conducted in 1996 (Roberts *et al.* 1996), concluded that whilst it would appear that 'home visiting programmes have the potential to reduce significantly the rates of childhood injury *though* the relative effectiveness of professional versus non-professional home visits remains unanswered'. A subsequent systematic review of home-based social support for socially disadvantaged mothers (Hodnett & Roberts 1999) drew similar conclusions, stating that 'Postnatal home-based support programs appear to have no risks and may have benefits for socially disadvantaged mothers and their children, possibly including reduced rates of child injury'.

A review of the literature on the role of the health visitor in identifying and working with vulnerable families was conducted by Appleton in 1994 (Appleton 1994*a*). It was concluded that although health visitors were clearly involved in this work, there was little by way of empirically based research to describe this involvement. This review was followed up by Appleton's own study of health visitors' perceptions of vulnerability (Appleton 1994*b*), which concluded that health visitors tend to use their own professional judgement rather than official guidelines or checklists in assessing vulnerability, indicating that such checklists are inadequate measures of families' needs.

Most recently, a study carried out to examine the role of the Irish public health nurse (the Irish equivalent of the health visitor) in child protection (Hanafin 1998) resulted in the recommendation that, in view of the size and diversity of the role, they should focus on primary and secondary prevention and that the tertiary prevention role should, at best, be limited. This follows the work of Browne (1995), which concluded that greater support and training was required if health visitors are to be used to prevent child abuse and neglect.

It is clear, then, that the role of the health visitor in child protection is both acknowledged and of interest to researchers but that there is a need for further and more rigorous research into this area of health visiting practice, in order for it to be better understood and potentially, made more effective.

The nature of the health visitor/client relationship

The nature of the relationship between health visitors and their clients lends itself to the concept of working in partnership with parents as advocated by the Children Act 1989 and this has been the principal approach taken by health visitors for many years as acknowledged by Stainton-Rogers & Roche (1992). The educational and informative elements of primary prevention enable health visitors to work in an empowering and client-led way by encouraging informed parental decision-making in the light of information given, and by respecting parental autonomy in cases where choices which are adverse to positive health outcomes may be made. The exceptions to this approach occur almost exclusively in the event of concerns about child harm, when action may be taken without full parental agreement.

Health visiting is perhaps unique among the primary care professions in that the relationship with clients is not usually initiated in response to a clearly identified and acknowledged client need and as such is usually unsolicited in the first instance. There is, therefore, an element of early negotiation in gaining access to family homes and establishing a relationship of trust before the business of identifying and responding to health needs can begin. This rather tenuous basis for continuing contact with no statutory right of access to a family can often be at the root of difficulties in initiating child protection interventions. On the one hand, there may be early indicators of the need for intervention to protect a child from harm, but on the other hand, no substantial evidence to support a child protection referral. It is in circumstances such as these, where families may fail to recognise a (health) need, may turn away all offers of additional help and support and may threaten to refuse further access and cooperation, that a health visitor may feel most vulnerable and in need of support. Continuing the relationship with the family in question in order to monitor the situation and provide what support is acceptable may appear to be the only available option. Advice will usually be available in the form of both formal and informal supervision systems and access to colleagues from other agencies and this should be sought. However, the ability of other agencies to respond with the provision of preventative services is often limited by both availability of resources and acceptability to the family concerned. As a result, direct contact with the family and the day-to-day judgements which must be made often remain squarely on the shoulders of the individual practitioner. This type of situation often leads to concerns about 'social policing', where health visitors can fall into the trap of feeling that their role requires them to be on the scene if ever the family situation succumbs to pressures and child harm ensues. For example, in supervision a health visitor may describe their ongoing role with a family as 'just keeping an eye on things in case something happens' rather than being able to articulate a meaningful ongoing role within a family. In situations such as these, a balance must be sought between parental and professional responsibility and also between parental and child rights – a decision which is not easy or straightforward in many cases (Wattam 1992).

Having identified the risks in terms of all aspects of family health as well as the potential for child harm, as in all other cases, a plan of support and intervention must be negotiated and agreed with the family. For example, there may be an agreement for the health visitor to assist in addressing issues of behaviour management or to offer advice and information on improving family nutrition. In the absence of such an agreed plan, the health visitor is severely limited in their ability to take further action and must either adopt a more confrontational protective role, which is out of keeping with the usual preventive mode of intervention, or continue to monitor the situation and offer support, as before. The use of assertive communication skills can help to overcome this sort of dilemma, as indicated by Tattersall (1992). This potential dichotomy between the prevention and protection role which can appear to exist is discussed in more detail by Waters (1992).

The voluntary nature of the health visitor–client relationship requires scrupulous attention to issues such as trust and confidentiality. Families must be advised at an early stage in the developing relationship that, in some circumstances, confidentiality may be breached if it is felt necessary to do so in order to protect a child from harm or further harm. The timing and context for introducing this information can be extremely influential in determining whether a positive working relationship can be developed and subsequent work towards achieving positive family health outcomes can be agreed. It can sometimes be helpful to introduce this information in conjunction with a general discussion about the team approach to primary health care and the nature of information-sharing (with the client's consent) between different members of the team on a 'need to know' basis. For instance a mother will often be happy for the health visitor to discuss a health concern with the general practioner (GP) prior to a consultation.

A further aspect of the relationship between the health visitor and client families is the universal nature of first contacts with families following the birth of a new baby. This can be extremely effective in reducing any sense of stigma and facilitating the establishment of open and effective communication, and can often serve as an effective counterbalance to some of the tensions described above.

The primary prevention role – educating and supporting parenting

As indicated earlier, this is perhaps the most important role of the health visitor in the field of child protection. Universal contact with all families with young children, often in their own homes and with a purely health-promoting focus, is a unique feature of health visiting practice. There is an important educative role in assisting parents with the adjustment to their new roles and helping them to learn about their child's development and basic needs in order to enhance parenting skills. Health visitors can be influential in promoting positive parenting practices as advocated by Pound (1992). In addition, the provision of a listening ear in times of stress allows parents to talk through their problems and seek appropriate assistance or advice, thus helping to avoid a situation in which a child may become vulnerable to harm. Health visitors tend to work in partnership with parents seeking to empower and encourage personal responsibility for decision-making in connection with their own and their family's health needs. The need to work in a different and more assertive way when child harm is suspected can be a source of much uncertainty and stress and is discussed later in this chapter.

Perhaps an additional role within the field of primary prevention, and one which may not always seem so obvious, is the teaching of parents and potential parents about some of the factors which lead to child harm. This may help parents to recognise the need to seek help at an early stage. Similarly, knowledge of the philosophy of the Children Act 1989 and the aims of the child protection system may reduce fear of inappropriate intervention in the event of child harm. Gough (1995) concluded that such education programmes might do much to improve the effectiveness of interventions when they are needed.

Secondary prevention – early detection and referral

The nature of health visitor involvement with families leads to their role in the early detection of significant harm or the potential for significant harm to a child(ren). The search for health needs which may begin in the ante-natal period will encompass early identification of family stressors and/or other features which may predispose to child harm. The use of 'predictor checklists' in order to assist in this process has been subject to some criticism, as discussed by Reder *et al.* (1993) and Corby (1993), and is largely unformalised. However, information from statistical analyses of those factors which are often associated with child harm forms an essential element of the knowledge base used by health visitors for this purpose. Often, the most appropriate form of intervention at this time is referral for family support. This can take the form of interventions by voluntary organisations, self-help and support groups or assistance with access to services such as child care and benefits. Direct intervention in terms of providing a listening and/or counselling service can also be appropriate.

In circumstances where actual harm to a child is suspected, referral to investigating agencies as directed by local guidelines and procedures is the appropriate course of action. Research shows that 17% of referrrals to the child protection system come from health visitors and other health professionals (Gibbons *et al.* 1995). However, the referral is likely to be more effective if accompanied by as much supporting information as possible, particularly where there is no direct evidence or disclosure but only a collection of small indicators. In all but the most urgent cases, the collection of supporting information by consultation with colleagues such as the GP or the School Nurse can be extremely valuable. Thorough discussion of the cause for concern with the relevant family member before a referral is made is also indicated in the majority of cases. This helps to eliminate misunderstandings where there may be an acceptable alternative explanation for an injury or other sign/symptom and also facilitates the initial contact by the investigating agencies. Exceptional circumstances clearly exist where there is concern on the part of the referrer that such discussion may result in the child suffering further harm, or in the health visitor becoming vulnerable to harm as a result of such a discussion. There is, however, a need to take care in the collection of information to support a referral, in order to avoid encroaching upon and hindering the subsequent investigative inquiries. For instance, referral to a GP for physical examination should only be used where necessary to eliminate other potential explanations since there will almost certainly be a physical examination by specialists in child health and forensic medicine as part of the investigative procedure. However, Wattam (1992) discovered a tendency not to proceed to forensic medical examination in cases where the child had already been examined by a doctor.

However, the decision about whether to refer is often not straightforward and can be the cause of great anxiety. The potential effect upon both the family and the subsequent relationship with the health visitor in the case of a mistaken suspicion and referral is often central to the decision-making process. It is therefore essential that the support and advice of experienced colleagues is obtained where there is any doubt about the course of action to be taken.

Among those circumstances which can cause particular difficulty in deciding whether and when to make a referral are cases of failure to thrive or unexplained developmental delay, failure to gain access to a child and where there is domestic violence.

In the case of failure to thrive or unexplained developmental delay, referral should usually be made to the GP and, if necessary, to a paediatrician for further investigation before considering a child protection referral. The association between failure to thrive and emotional abuse or neglect was illustrated in the case of Jasmine Beckford as pointed out by Reder *et al.* (1993) and Corby (1993) and is now well recognised, though in the absence of other signs alternative possible causes should be eliminated before suspicion is aroused (Skuse 1989).

Accepting that the health visitor has no right of access to a house or a child, refusal by a parent or carer to allow or facilitate access is often a cause for concern. In many areas, local policy will advocate writing to parents/carers in these circumstances to ascertain that it is their intention to refuse the services of a health visitor or to offer alternative arrangements for service provision, if required. Such policies often advocate that both the GP and the Local Authority social services department are informed of the situation in writing in order that the health and well-being of the child can be monitored through other means if necessary. In the absence of other factors which give rise to concern, this is the only action which is reasonable. Attempts at imposing conditions in such circumstances serve only to reinforce concerns about a social policing role for health visitors. However, in cases where there are additional reasons for concern, there is provision under the Children Act 1989 for access to a child to be gained through a Child Assessment Order.

A case where there is domestic violence, even where there is no indication of the child(ren) being involved or even witnessing violence, should always be considered for potential referral. There is a growing body of evidence that children in situations of domestic violence are vulnerable to injury at least of an emotional nature and sometimes much worse, as in the case of Tyra Henry (London Borough of Lambeth 1987). A study by Gibbons *et al.* (1995) recorded domestic violence in one-quarter of cases of children on the Child Protection Register. Health visitors often work closely with mothers who live in situations of domestic violence, both supporting and encouraging them in choosing a more satisfactory way of dealing with the relationship and in monitoring the health and development of the children concerned. It would perhaps be impractical for all cases of domestic violence to be referred as cases of actual or potential child harm, though the health visitor must remain alert to the danger to children in these situations as well as alerting the mother to the risks. However, note must be taken of the findings of Farmer & Owen (1995) which would suggest that professionals tend to presume that mothers are responsible for the care of their children and too little attention is paid to domestic violence (DOH 1995).

Tertiary prevention – monitoring and support

In situations where child harm has been established and a child protection plan is in place, involvement by the health visitor takes the form of tertiary prevention, where the aim is to prevent further deterioration of the situation and to foster rehabilitation, where appropriate. For some health visitors, this aspect of child protection work can dominate the workload and must be managed carefully if the overall public health role is not to be severely compromised.

In situations where children are temporarily removed from the parental home, as well as continuing to monitor the health and development of the child(ren) there may be a role for the health visitor in providing continuing support for parents in preparation for a rehabilitation programme. Alternatively, or at the same time, there may be a role in advising foster carers on matters of the child(ren)'s health or development. Where the child(ren) remain(s) at home and there are detailed assessments being carried out under the guidance of the *Orange Book*, the health visitor may be able to contribute to this process by virtue of their knowledge of the family and its circumstances. However, whether there should be a specific and ongoing role for the health visitor in such a process is debatable. Membership of core groups for health visitors should be restricted to those circumstances in which there is a continuing preventative role which requires their specialist knowledge and expertise and is not appropriate in order merely to assist social workers with ongoing monitoring and assessment of the family situation. However, the work of health visitors and social workers often complements each other well, particularly where health visitors continue to offer support to children in need after child protection concerns have abated (DOH 1995).

Relationships with other disciplines and agencies

Collaborative work between various agencies is a cornerstone of public health practice and this is no less the case in child protection work. Numerous child death enquiry reports conclude that failure of good collaborative working and ineffective or inadequate inter-agency communication have contributed significantly to a child's death. Four key issues in connection with inter-disciplinary working are discussed below, though there are many others which could have been addressed.

First, there are those relationship difficulties which arise out of fundamental differences in terms of approaches to and the focus for practice. This is an issue discussed by Stevenson (1989). At least in part, the aim of this chapter has been to illustrate the nature of health visiting practice and the place of child protection work within it, for the benefit of workers from other agencies who may have very different roles and subscribe to very different principles underlying their work. It has been demonstrated in other contexts that increasing understanding of each other's roles enhances teamwork. Multi-agency management of child protection relies on a multidisciplinary team approach, particularly at child protection case conferences and within core groups. Therefore greater understanding of each other's roles in terms of underlying philosophies and priorities should enhance the overall approach to protecting children, although the findings of Wheeler (1992) would indicate that social workers and health visitors already have a good understanding of each other's roles.

One area of potential conflict and misunderstanding between health visitors and the investigative agencies of social services and the police occurs at the point of referral. As described earlier in this chapter, health visitors may feel the need for support in working with families about whom they have concerns but where concerns are insufficient to comprise the conditions for a child protection referral. However, they will often report that social worker colleagues have neither the resources nor the inclination to offer such support until a case of actual child harm is suspected or discovered. Social workers, in their turn, may feel that health visitors seek constantly to add to their workload by trying to offload cases for which they should be able and willing to accept responsibility. A difference of perception of what constitutes acceptable standards of care and parenting may possibly be attributed to the range of 'normal' encountered by health visitors and social workers respectively, in the course of their daily work. Such differences can often be overcome by the establishment of close working relationships with opportunities to discuss issues informally and perhaps arrange joint assessment visits in cases of doubt or disagreement.

In other cases, a police investigator may express frustration with a health visitor who has discussed with a family the intention to make a referral and thus allowed them the time and opportunity to collude on evidence to be given at investigation. A better appreciation of each other's position and day-to-day working priorities may help to resolve such potential conflicts.

A second issue in relationships with other agencies is the occasional perception on the part of other disciplines within health, and often colleagues within education, that the health visitor can be used as a 'half-way house' in cases of concern. Requests for health visitors to visit a family to 'check out' the home situation following concern on the part of a midwife, hospital nurse or teacher, can be interpreted as an attempt to pass on responsibility for a decision about whether or not there is a risk of harm to a child. In such cases there should always be further discussion between the professionals concerned before a decision about whether to, and who should, refer for further investigation is taken. However, the health visitor should maintain awareness of their own professional responsibility in the case of a failure to reach an agreement and may decide to refer independently.

The extent of the health visitor's duty of confidentiality becomes an issue when they have access to information which is held by a colleague, most notably a GP or hospital doctor. In circumstances where a health visitor becomes aware of information which has been given in confidence to another health professional but has been shared on a 'need to know' basis in accordance with good practice recommendations and this information gives rise to child protection concerns, there is a potential dilemma. The dilemma is easily resolved where the fellow health professional shares the concern and is prepared to make the appropriate referral and/or take the appropriate action. However, when this is not the case, there arises an important legal and ethical debate. The health visitor has a duty of care to the child as client, via their code of professional conduct, to take the necessary action to secure the child's protection but does not have ownership of the record required to substantiate the referral. In circumstances such as these, advice should be sought from the professional supervisor and a decision about the 'best' course of action in terms of what can best be professionally defended should be taken. The details of individual cases are likely to lead to different decisions in different circumstances. Decision-making will be based on an individual's interpretation and application of ethical principles and no general guidance can be given. It is important to note that, in terms of professional accountability, the decision must be taken by the practitioner themself and cannot be 'delegated' to the supervisor/advisor or employer.

A further area of potential conflict arises when a health visitor has concerns about a child within a family at the same time as a colleague is working with one of the adult family members as client. The health visitor may have concerns about the child's welfare which may or may not be connected with the adult's health problem. Potential conflict arises when the health visitor seeks to assess the need to take action to protect the child but can obtain neither support nor relevant information from their colleague on the grounds of client confidentiality. Such resistance may arise out of the desire to protect the adult client's right to confidentiality according to codes of professional conduct or an awareness of prejudices commonly held by others in cases such as mental illness or learning disability, for example. This would be in line with the findings of Finkelhor (1984). There may also be a lack of appreciation of the over-riding paramountcy of the welfare of the child in cases where child harm is suspected. Such situations can lead to conflict at case conference and can only be tackled through child protection awareness raising for health workers who do not normally work with children as suggested by post-Cleveland recommendations for training (Training Advisory Group on Sexual Abuse of Children 1988). In reality, these issues often remain unresolved in individual cases since the resolution lies in professional judgements and the interpretation of professional codes of conduct.

The multidisciplinary child protection system

Responsibility for the protection of children is recommended as one which should be shared between a range of both individuals and organisations (DOH 1999*b*). Social services departments of Local Authorities clearly have a central role but rely on the cooperation and support of all of the member agencies of the local child protection committees. Other than the administration of the local Child Protection Register, a central function of the multidisciplinary child protection system is achieved through the child protection case conference.

Health visitors are frequently called upon to attend and contribute to case conferences and are often able to make a significant contribution in terms of knowledge of the family concerned both prior to and during the period of concern. Their contribution is usually via a written report which will cover all aspects of child and family health along with any additional information relevant to the current cause(s) for concern. Good quality record-keeping is an essential requirement if accurate and reliable case conference reports are to be made. The current, almost universal, practice of making the parent the holder of the main child health record has many benefits in terms of encouraging parental responsibility and participation in matters of their child(ren)'s health. However, there may be difficulties when the health visitor requires access to the written records. In some cases this is overcome through the maintenance of separate and parallel records which are often kept by the health visitor in cases where there may be some cause for concern, though this may not always be so. In cases where there is no parallel record, the health visitor may need to gain access to the parent-held record in order to compile their report and this factor alone may pose a challenge to the partnership approach which has hitherto been central to the caring relationship. Parents will be aware of what has been recorded but may not be willing for this to be shared with others in difficult circumstances. However, the situation provides a good opportunity for sharing the proposed content of the case conference report and can be an effective way of beginning to prepare a parent for the meeting itself.

The actual case conference can be a stressful experience, especially for the inexperienced health visitor. Often, the relationship between health visitor and parent prior to the case conference will have been a collaborative one based on trust and perceived by the parent as largely supportive rather than challenging. It is also important to remember that any subsequent relationship will need to be re-established on a voluntary basis, and awareness of this can be the cause of some anxiety and uncertainty. This may be the first occasion during which a parent becomes aware of an inter-agency working relationship and they may feel that the meeting's focus upon the welfare of the child(ren) in question is to the detriment of their previous relationship with the health visitor. For this reason, it is important that information is presented in an objective and non-judgemental way and that concern for the child rather than judgements about the parents remains central to the content of the report. Parental attendance at case conferences also reinforces the need for information to be accurately compiled and based in factual observations so that discussion of the parents' interpretations of the situation and their positive participation in the case conference can be facilitated. This is an issue addressed in some detail by Peall (1992). This form of full participation in case conference discussions can serve to reinforce the perception of a partnership approach on the part of involved parents.

The multidisciplinary ownership of decision-making and recommendations is an aspect of the case conference which is often overlooked by staff from agencies other than the social services. It is important for health visitors to be aware that the case conference is not a vehicle for sharing information with social workers so that they, or the case conference chairperson, can make a decision about registration and recommendations to member agencies but that the whole process is intended to be multidisciplinary and multi-agency in its function. For this reason, it is important that the process is fully engaged in, and the health visitor needs to have a thorough understanding of the grounds for concern and the plans for dealing with the case in question. Any dissension should be stated and recorded within the minutes of the meeting. This is in order that the health visitor's participation in subsequent assessment and/or family work is fully informed and appropriate, especially if there is to be a court appearance.

Supervision and support

Although clinical supervision is recommended as good professional practice, it is still not universally established within health visiting. However, some form of supervision and support for child protection work is usually provided by employers. This is usually in the form of one or more practitioners who have extensive previous experience in the field and who are appointed as child protection advisors/specialists with an educational, practice development and support role. The question of whether those appointed to this role should also have a managerial relationship with the health visitors to be supervised is subject to debate. This is an issue covered in some detail by Parkinson (1992). There are clear managerial issues to be addressed during supervision such as monitoring of standards and identification of training needs. However, the provision of professional support and reassurance may best come from someone in a different role.

The amount and nature of support available is likely to vary from area to area and even from team to team, especially where primary care nursing teams are becoming more closely aligned with general practice and more independent of the employer's management and supervisory networks. However, given the stressful and uncertain nature of many aspects of child protection work, access to some form of peer or supervisory support is essential. Ideally, this would provide opportunities to discuss individual families within the caseload where there are concerns about harm to the children and would extend to those families not included on child protection registers but about whom there is concern. Sometimes there is a separate register or index of such families which forms the focus for supervision sessions. Whilst the expertise of the child protection advisor is undoubtedly of great benefit, an important aspect of supervision and support is the need for practitioners to understand that accountability for decisions made and actions taken remains with the individual and cannot be 'delegated' in any way to the supervisor. As well as the individual practitioner's need for support, the danger of the professional relationship becoming collusive and dangerous in the absence of objective supervision has been recognised and discussed elsewhere. Another important function of child protection supervision is to give assistance in the preparation of care plans, case conference reports and statements of evidence and to monitor the effectiveness and appropriateness of interventions against agreed objectives. This aspect of supervision helps to guard against the development of a social policing role as discussed earlier, and to focus on working towards the achievement of valid health outcomes for both the child(ren) and family.

Conclusion

This chapter has focused upon some of the dilemmas faced by health visitors in seeking to incorporate successfully the child protection role into the broader public health function. It has necessarily skimmed over the surface of many of the issues, and health visitors with child protection cases on their their caseload will need to refer to specialist advice, local guidelines and more detailed texts to help with their decision-making and skills development.

However, the chapter does aim to raise awareness of the nature of health visiting practice and the source of some of the dilemmas and difficulties faced in day-to-day practice among newly qualified health visitors and other professionals. It is hoped that, in this way, it will make a small contribution to inter-agency cooperation and collaborative working in the interests of those children who require the intervention of professionals to protect them from harm.

In terms of the future role of health visitors in child protection work, government policy would appear to support a strong role in working in partnership with parents in order to identify and meet the needs of children and families for prevention as well as protection.

Annotated further reading

Cloke C, Naish J (eds) 1992 Key issues in child protection for health visitors and nurses. Longman, Harlow
This book discusses a number of the issues touched upon within this chapter, including issues of race, culture and gender, which have not been addressed here. The format is easily readable and the contributors come from a variety of backgrounds and offer a number of perspectives. Reference is made to the relevant authors for further reading throughout this chapter.
Booth K, Luker K (eds) 1999 A practical handbook for community health nurses. Blackwell Science, London
This book contains a section of six chapters which deal with the child and family, and provides a valuable and practical overview of family and child-focused work. The book deals with issues which would traditionally be associated with the work of health visitors but acknowledges the growing role of other community-based nurses in working with families.
Violence Against Children Study Group 1999 Children, child abuse and child protection: placing children centrally. Wiley, Chichester
This book is another collection of writings by different authors and builds upon a previous publication by the same authors entitled: *Taking child abuse seriously*. It is written for a broad range of readers and addresses issues of theory, policy and practice, including a section on the role of various agencies within the child protection system.

References

Appleton J V 1994*a* The role of health visitors in identifying and working with vulnerable families in relation to child protection. Journal of Advanced Nursing 20 (1): 167–175
Appleton J V 1994*b* The concept of vulnerability in relation to child protection: health visitors' perceptions. Journal of Advanced Nursing 20 (6): 1132–1140
Armstrong H 1994 Child protection for health visitors: a training resource. HMSO, London
Booth K, Luker K (eds) 1999 A practical handbook for community health nurses. Blackwell Science, London
Browne K 1995 Preventing child maltreatment through community nursing. Journal of Advanced Nursing 21 (1): 57–63
CETHV 1977 An investigation into the principles of health visiting. CETHV, London
Cloke C, Naish J (eds) 1992 Key issues in child protection for health visitors and nurses. Longman, Harlow

Corby B 1993 Child abuse: towards a knowledge base. Open University Press, Milten Keynes

Corby B 1999 The child at risk: working with families and the child protection system. In: Booth K, Luker K (eds) A practical handbook for community health nurses. Blackwell Science, London

Department of Health (DOH) 1991*b* Working together under the Children Act 1989. A guide to inter-agency cooperation for the protection of children from abuse. HMSO, London

Department of Health (DOH) 1992 Child protection: guidance for senior nurses, health visitors and midwives. HMSO, London

Department of Health (DOH) 1995 Child protection: messages from research. HMSO, London

Department of Health (DOH) 1999*a* Working together to safeguard children: new government guidance on inter-agency cooperation. The Stationery Office, London

Department of Health (DOH) 1999*b* Framework for the assessment of children in need and their families: consultation draft. The Stationery Office, London

Farmer E, Owen M 1995 Child protection practice: private risks and public remedies, decision-making, intervention and outcome in child protection work. In: Department of Health (ed) Child protection: messages from research. HMSO, London

Finkelhor D 1984 Child sexual abuse: new theory and research. Free Press, New York

Gelles R 1998 Do child abuse prevention programmes work? The Brown University Child & Adolescent Behavior Letter, August 1998 at *www.psychlink.com*

Gibbons J, Gallagher B, Bell C, Gordon G 1995 Development after physical abuse in early childhood: a follow-up study of children on Child Protection Registers. In: Department of Health (ed) Child protection: messages from research. HMSO, London

Gough D 1995 Child abuse interventions: a review of the literature. In: Department of Health (ed) Child protection: messages from research. HMSO, London

Hanafin S 1998 Deconstructing the role of the public health nurse in child protection. Journal of Advanced Nursing 28 (10): 178–184

Hodnett E D, Roberts I 1999 Home-based social support for socially disadvantaged mothers (Cochrane Review). In: The Cochrane Library, Issue 2, 1999, Oxford, Update software

Home Office 1998 Supporting families: Green Paper. The Stationery Office, London

Parkinson J 1992 Supervision versus control: can managers provide both managerial and professional supervision? In: Cloke C, Naish J (eds) Key issues in child protection for health visitors and nurses. Longman, Harlow

Peall C 1992 Partnership and professional power. In: Cloke C, Naish J (eds) Key issues in child protection for health visitors and nurses. Longman, Harlow

Pound R 1992 Promoting positive parenting: new horizons for the prevention of child abuse? In: Cloke C, Naish J (eds) Key issues in child protection for health visitors and nurses. Longman, Harlow

Reder P, Duncan S, Gray M 1993 Beyond blame: child abuse tragedies revisited. Routledge, London

Roberts I, Kramer M, Suissa S 1996 Does home visiting prevent childhood injury? A systematic review of randomised controlled trials. British Medical Journal 312: 29–33

Robertson C 1991 Health visiting in practice. Churchill Livingstone, London

Skuse D H 1989 ABC of child abuse: emotional abuse and delay in growth. British Medical Journal 229 (6691): 113–115

Stainton-Rogers W, Iskander R 1990 You did everything possible: what if I got it wrong? Dilemmas in child protection for health visitors and school nurses. Department of Health and Health Visitors Association, London

Stainton-Rogers W, Roche J 1992 Putting it all together: the Children Act 1989. In: Cloke C, Naish J (eds) Key issues in child protection for health visitors and nurses. Longman, Harlow

Stevenson O 1989 Public policy and professional practice. Harvester Wheatsheaf, London

Tattersall P 1992 Communicating assertively to protect children in nursing practice. In: Cloke C, Naish J (eds) Key issues in child protection for health visitors and nurses. Longman, Harlow

Training Advisory Group on Sexual Abuse of Children (TAGOSAC) 1988 Post-Cleveland: the implications for training. TAGOSAC, London

Twinn S, Cowley S (eds) 1992 The principles of health visiting: a re-examination. Health Visitors Association and London

UKCC 1992 Standards for specialist practice. UKCC, London

Waters J 1992 'Protecting' children and 'preventing' child abuse: a consensus or conflict? In: Cloke C, Naish J (eds) Key issues in child protection for health visitors and nurses. Longman, Harlow

Wattam C 1992 Making a case in child protection. Longman, Harlow

Wheeler S 1992 Perceptions of child abuse. Health Visitor 65: 316–319

World Health Organization (WHO) 1946 Constitution. World Health Organization, Geneva

16 Enhancing the contribution of teachers to child protection

Anne Peake

INTRODUC-TION

The role of the teacher in situations where there are suspicions that a child is being abused may be pivotal. Teachers are the only professionals who are in regular daily contact with school-aged children, and they are in a unique position to monitor situations where there are concerns about a particular child. By dint of their training and the numbers of children in a particular age group with whom they have contact, teachers are also well equipped to identify those children whose behaviour, for whatever reason, falls outside the normal range. Yet there can be few problems faced by children that arouse teacher's anxiety quite like that of child abuse. The distress of the children, the complexity of the problem, the difficulties of investigation and the often unhelpful media coverage of the issue, all contribute to the very understandable levels of anxiety and sense of vulnerability which teachers feel.

This chapter addresses some of these concerns by setting out in detail ways in which teachers are uniquely placed to monitor children where there are suspicions of abuse, and by identifying frameworks within which children can be monitored by teachers in primary and secondary schools. It must be stressed at the outset, however, that although teachers can monitor children, the duty to investigate and take action always lies with the statutory child protection agencies. Once a child is known to be the victim of abuse, the provisions of the Children Act 1989 and the recently revised guidelines contained in *Working Together* (Department of Health (DOH) 1991) must be brought into play, together with the child protection procedures laid down by the local authority, which should be followed without delay.

Teachers therefore need to be aware of these and of the work of the statutory agencies, to liaise with them and adhere carefully to local child protection guidelines.

Schools should contribute to a co-ordinated approach to child protection by developing effective liaison with other agencies and support services.
(Department for Education and Employment 1995)

However, teachers have been left, and feel themselves to be, ill-equipped for their role in protecting children. The emphasis of initial teacher training is on teaching children knowledge and skills. There is no support from the Government that child protection training should be included in the initial training of teachers (Peake & Turner 1999). Yet the fact remains that teachers are dealing with children about whom there may be concerns, for at least 6 hours a day, 5 days a week, 40 weeks a year. Faced with a dearth of training, an awareness of anxiety-provoking concerns about a child(ren), and the need to work outside their professional group, it is no surprise that teachers feel uncertain.

One of the themes of this chapter is that teachers should not feel alone in the contribution they can make to protect children. Work done with a group of teachers who were all Special Educational Needs Coordinators (SENCOs) in Banbury, Oxfordshire produced a simple initial contact form for teachers to use. The form is designed to help teachers focus on what they know, organise their initial observations and have a basis on which to discuss their concerns with teaching colleagues and with other agencies. The form is useful in bringing some structure and consistency into the way teachers describe their concerns about children who may be being abused. It also can be used as a record of liaison with other agencies. While the main theme of this chapter is to consider the complexities of child sexual abuse, it is important to be clear that, sadly, children can be abused in many ways: physical injuries to the child, in situations where there is violence in the home, by being emotionally neglected or abused, when they are sexually assaulted or sexually assault other children/adults, and in cases of concern about persistent neglect. The form is reproduced here for other teachers to use (Fig. 16.1).

Fig. 16.1
Initial contact form for teachers

Initial Contact Form where there are Child Protection Concerns

Date........................ Type of contact..

Person/Agency Contacted...

Name of child .... **D.O.B.**..

Address ....

Parents' names ....

Other family members (if known)...

People visiting the house (if known)..

Child details

Age/developmental stage..

Race/culture/language..

Ability/Disability..

Temperamental factors...

Other features...

Current concerns (describe the problem)　　　| **Emotional** |

When first noticed..

(if relevant) Where do the problem behaviours occur?...

....

....

When do these occur?...

For how long do these behaviours continue?...

What usually has happened beforehand? ....

....

What usually happens afterwards?..

....

With what outcome?..

....

Fig. 16.1 (cont'd)
Initial contact form for teachers

School view of child

Appearance of the child

Physical:..

Dress:..

Attendance...

Attendance figures:..

Punctuality:...

Preparedness:...

Health

Known factors:...

Current concerns:..

Interaction with peers

Boys v girls: ....

Ages of preferred peers: ....

Structured v unstructured: ....

School experience of siblings:...

Interaction with adults

Preferred adult in school:...

School's interaction with parents:..

Home conditions (if known):...

....

Any additional comments:...

....

....

Action agreed following sharing the concerns: ....

....

....

Notes made by: ....

Distinctive features of child sexual abuse

Teachers have had a longer time to adjust to the procedures with regard to the physical abuse of children and their role within the procedures than is the case with child sexual abuse. Thus, although the main features of child sexual abuse are dealt with in detail in Section 1 of this book, the main issues are summarised here because it is important to be clear at the start about the ways in which child sexual abuse differs from the physical abuse of children. Child sexual abuse is an essentially different phenomenon from the non-accidental injury of children. The difference rests on five basic features.

1.   The incidence of child abuse is different from that of physical abuse. In child sexual abuse, the majority of the abusers are men (Finkelhor 1984).

A survey by Baker & Duncan (1985) has shown there to be no significant class or geographical differences, and the majority of the victims are girls. (This is discussed more fully in Section 1 by Creighton, Chapter 2 and Frosh, Chapter 4).

2.   The question of evidence sets sexual abuse apart from physical abuse. The nature of most sexual abuse is such that there is rarely, if ever, any evidence. Even in cases where there is evidence of abuse (Manchester 1979), it is often impossible to prove the identity of the abuser. If we have learned one lesson from Cleveland, it is that even when professionals are confident that there is evidence of sexual assaults on children, the evidence will be challenged and professional competence questioned. With the exception of brittle bone disease, there is rarely such a high level of controversy about the evidence in cases of the physical abuse of children.

3.   The issue of gender is central, not only in terms of the incidence of child sexual abuse, but also in terms of the intervention of professionals (Frosh 1987, see also Featherstone, Chapter 6, in this volume). Traditionally, professionals have given insufficient attention to the significance of the gender of the worker. However, from the child's point of view, the gender of the adult can determine how safe they feel. Additionally, girls need to see their same sex adult models in positions where sexual assault is seriously and effectively challenged. The issue of race needs consideration too, not least because of the position of women in some ethnic minority groups (see Phillips, Chapter 7, in this volume). Racism at both the individual and institutional levels of society places additional pressures on children from different ethnic/cultural groups which may affect their attitude to disclosure. The existence of positive adult models from their own communities who are active in child protection work may encourage children from ethnic minority groups to seek help.

4.   The problems of obtaining clear and reliable evidence have implications for the assessment of children. In the field of child sexual abuse, there is no equivalent to the regular medical examinations whereby a child's growth and physical well-being are checked after known instances of physical abuse. The professional dealing with suspected sexual abuse therefore has to face the problem of monitoring children without a specific baseline of checks that can be made. In addition, when someone who has been strongly implicated as an abuser, but has not been convicted, moves in with a family in which there are children, social services departments may be unclear as to the basis upon which they can judge whether the children in that household are safe or not, and how best to protect them.

5.   Child sexual abuse raises professional anxieties and divides workers more than other problems (Furniss 1983). It would be hard to imagine such an intense and long-lasting debate about whether children exaggerate, fantasise, or lie being conducted about other problems children present.

These features – the different incidence of sexual abuse, the question of evidence, the issue of gender, the difficulties of monitoring situations and the level of anxiety aroused – all combine to set child sexual abuse apart from physical abuse, and to make it a problem that saps the confidence of many workers. However, although the parameters of the problem are such that protecting children in such situations is not easy to resolve, particularly given the demands it makes for the coordination of different professional roles (see Corby, Chapter 13, in this volume, for a detailed discussion of issues of inter-professional cooperation), the protection of the child where sexual abuse is suspected is of paramount importance in view of the suffering and damage it can cause.

The role of the teacher in responding to suspicions of abuse

As a psychologist who has worked in both education and social services departments, I have frequently been approached by teachers seeking advice about the problem of suspected sexual abuse. Faced with this need for guidance, I began to think about detailing the ways in which teachers could make their own contribution to assessments concerning the child's safety. Not only are there particular features of the teacher's role which may make it very important but also, when abuse is suspected, the nature and sequence of professional involvement is critical. The following factors are of particular importance in informing any plans for intervention.

1. There is a need to collect evidence on which to base the plan for professional intervention to protect the child, or perhaps to make a case for the prosecution of the abuser, or to allay anxieties about possible abuse.
2. There is a need to avoid warning the abuser of the fact that there are suspicions. If an abuser becomes aware of such concerns before child protection agencies are in a position to act to protect the child, the abuser can be made more powerful. The abuser would be able to adjust their threats accordingly, and/or remove the child from the school setting, so that the capacity of professionals to act is diminished. They would also become more powerful in the eyes of the child because of their demonstrated capacity to resist efforts to intervene and to continue the abuse.
3. It is important that when professionals do intervene in the lives of children and families, they do so effectively. This involves not only collecting evidence and avoiding alerting the abuser, but also having a clear and coordinated programme of action, to which those professionals involved are committed. It is therefore important that the child protection network has time to plan intervention carefully where sexual abuse is suspected. There is nothing more dangerous than hasty and ill-prepared intervention. In the event of failure, this leaves the child even more isolated and powerless, whilst the power of the abuser in the eyes of the child is increased and the child's capacity to trust in the action of the professionals is severely damaged.

Given these considerations, the nursery worker, class or form teacher in daily contact with children can have an important part to play in collecting information for those agencies who have a statutory role in regard to child protection. Teachers are the *only* professionals who are in regular daily contact with children about whom there may be concerns about possible sexual abuse. They are in a unique position for monitoring suspicion for three main reasons.

1. Training for teachers, particularly for the infant/nursery sector, includes work on child development which is a helpful basis for considering children whose presenting behaviour is a focus for professional concern. This means that concerns about the behaviour of one child can be considered in the context of the normal development of children of a given age and ability.
2. Teachers are the only professional group in regular and almost daily contact with children about whom there may be concerns. So a teacher may make detailed observations of a child in a variety of situations involving a variety of interactions with peers and adults. Teachers can also have close and trusting relationships with some children which may make them feel safe enough to reveal some of their deeper anxieties.

3.   Most importantly, there is no professional group, other than teachers/nursery workers, who have regular daily contact with such large numbers of children of a given age group. They are, therefore, able to place their detailed observations of children about whom there are concerns, in the context of both knowledge of child development and regular experience of the normal range of children's behaviour. Teachers will constantly be comparing one child with approximately 25 other children of the same age on the basis of daily contact. The observation by a teacher that a child is different from their peers in specified ways can therefore be a powerful statement.

In my work advising teachers who are worried about what to do when there are suspicions of child sexual abuse, it became plain to me that there was a need for a locally agreed system of monitoring which enabled teachers to feel confident about their role in a field where professional anxieties are high. What was developed initially in conjunction with teachers was a standardised outline for monitoring children in school where particular situations or concerns suggested the need for further assessment. Two outlines have subsequently been developed, one for younger children and one for children in secondary schools. These have been agreed and accepted by one local social services department and provide a workable base for considering the role of the teacher in dealing with the suspicion of child sexual abuse. More generally, they may also provide the basis for developing whole-school policies for dealing with child protection in conjunction with local social services departments, which fit in with area child protection guidelines.

Monitoring children in school

By way of introduction, it is important to stress that teachers should be alert to overt signs of abuse. In the event of a child displaying any of the following overt signs of child sexual abuse, the teacher should inform the head teacher who should contact the nearest social services office:

- a child saying they have been touched sexually
- a third party saying a child has been touched sexually
- a child with injuries to the genital area
- a child giving clear evidence of an awareness of sexual behaviour, in drawings, play or talk
- a child who masturbates excessively.

In such cases, monitoring is not an option to be considered, since the involvement of the appropriate child protection agencies is clearly justified.

In suspected cases of child sexual abuse, however, systematic careful monitoring is essential. The following four points should be kept in mind when a programme of monitoring is undertaken.

1. Observation
2. Detailed recording
3. Open-ended activities
4. Safety of the child.

Observation

Careful attention needs to be paid to observing children in both structured and unstructured settings. Children may well show few, if any, warning signs in a structured busy classroom which may be fully occupying their thoughts, so that feelings, memories and insecurities are less likely to surface.

Additionally, for small children, the close presence of adults in structured situations may discourage them from acting out their inner feelings. The nature of child sexual abuse is such that there are enormous pressures on children not to reveal what is happening to them. Teachers' observations of children in unstructured settings such as playgrounds and playhouses in classrooms can also be very helpful, as can observations of behaviour during the usual classroom routines and activities.

Children, especially teenagers, who are socially aware and more able to control their feelings, may show few, if any, warning signs in structured busy classrooms. The demands of the timetable in terms of subjects, teachers and room changes may fully occupy their thoughts and time, and feelings, memories and insecurities are less likely to surface. The close presence of adults in structured situations may also discourage children from displaying their emotions. It is also the case for some abused children that school is the one place where they can feel safe and their wish to appear like other children provides them with a relief from the pressures at home. Older children can also be skilled in behaving in ways which meet the expectations of staff. For some children this is a relief they will not readily abandon. Also, with child sexual abuse there are enormous pressures on children not to tell what is happening, which for the teenager are particularly acute. Having kept the secret, quite possibly for some time, they feel implicated by their silence, and they are all too aware of society's condemnation of young people who have early sexual experiences, even the victims of child sexual assault. They are also more aware of the possible consequences of disclosure. Observations of children in different classroom settings (e.g. formal lessons, group work) and different responses to teachers of varying age and/or gender, should be compared with observations in more unstructured settings such as games or leisure periods, etc.

Detailed recording

It is important in recording any observations or comments about a child's behaviour that teachers also note the context in which it occurred. Context can be viewed in different ways, and therefore several examples are given.

1. The context could be the actual setting in which the behaviour was seen. Thus, for example with young children, the recording might note that the behaviour was observed 'during 10 minutes free play in the playhouse', or 'in a concealed corner of the playground not normally used by children playing at break', or 'when all the class were asked to write and draw about the weekend in their diaries' etc.

Context is particularly important in a secondary school setting, as children may move between several different situations in one timetabled day. The observations of differences in behaviour in different settings and with different adults can be extremely helpful, particularly if they are clearly recorded. Thus, for example with older children, the recording might note that the behaviour was observed 'during the time when children gather before registration'; or 'in a formal English lesson with a middle-aged male teacher'; or 'when all the class were asked to write about "the worst day I can remember"'; or 'in a concealed part of the playground by staff cars, where the children know they should not be' etc.

2. The context could also be provided by the behaviour of other adults or children. For example, the behaviour may be noted as a reaction when 'a teacher (male or female) touches the child's arm', or 'another child who tends to be clumsy pushed him/her', or the note might describe how the child responds to the

proximity of male adults. Attention must also be paid here to possible cultural differences in response, for example that of an Asian female child towards an adult male.

3.　The context can also be provided by the usual practices or routines in a given situation. For example, 'when children are asked to sit in a group close to each other', 'children always walk into assembly in this way', 'the PE teacher's routine for children changing for a lesson is', 'all children are told not to use the yard by the office', 'after school most children', 'if a child is late for school he/she is expected to', 'when letters are given out for parents' evenings', etc. Such contextual information should be followed by a description of the behaviour of the child being monitored.

It is, of course, important to be aware that many changes in behaviour which a teacher might notice may have nothing to do with sexual abuse and may be attributable to a wide range of other, less serious causes.

Open-ended activities

It is essential that any activities planned by teachers which may also be used for the purposes of monitoring should be balanced and open-ended. There should never be any room for the suggestion that a teacher might have led or biased a child's responses. For example, if children are asked to make a drawing depicting someone with sad/angry feelings, they should also be given the opportunity to depict glad/happy feelings with respect to the same person. Further examples are that if a class is asked to write a pen-picture of their fathers, they should also, at another time, be asked to write a pen-picture of their mothers, similarly, if they are asked to write about the 'worst day they remember', they should also be given the opportunity to write about 'the best day they remember'.

This approach has two advantages. First, it avoids leading children, which could have the effect of a child saying what they imagine will suit the teacher. Abused children are particularly sensitive to adult interest in their home life (maintaining a secret has made them thus). If an abused child feels an adult is taking too much interest, the child may withdraw and become even more guarded.

Secondly, this approach reflects the reality of children's worlds, which are that they often have ambivalent feelings about their situation, rather than feelings which are clearly positive or negative. They may well love their abuser and be reluctant to betray them. The child way well detest the sexual abuse but may have moved on to be sexually active in a way which they *do* enjoy, or which they feel might compromise any disclosure they might have to make about the initial sexual abuse.

Safety of the child

Child sexual abuse understandably arouses anxieties in adults concerned about children they suspect or they know are being abused. Unlike the physical abuse of children which can sometimes necessitate urgent action, child sexual abuse is rarely life-threatening, so with children suspected of being victims of child sexual abuse, it is better to begin a system of careful monitoring. This will enable professionals to clarify the basis for their concerns and, if necessary, to plan an effective form of intervention. However, child sexual abuse *might* become life-threatening if professionals intervene but fail to ensure the safety of the child, or if there is the threat of the child talking to an outside agency. Some children just run away in the face of possible attempts to help them disclose. This then places the child at even greater risk, and beyond the reach of much of the help that is available.

Monitoring children in primary school

The monitoring of young children about whom there is concern is best carried out by the child's teacher. Regardless of who does this, however, it is of over-riding importance that observations are objective, recorded systematically and without bias.

The headings outlined below constitute a range of parameters which teachers can use as a basis for monitoring children. Some ideas and explanations are given to help the teacher doing this for the first time. It may be best to record observations in a notebook which can be kept confidentially and in a secure place. Exercise books are probably best avoided for this purpose because of the obvious risk of confusion with other exercise books, resulting in the record falling into the wrong hands.

These headings can be put on separate pages, with examples of behaviours or incidents (including dates, times and the context) entered under the appropriate headings. The book will then contain a range of observations in chronological order organised under respective headings. This will provide a clear basis on which a teacher can give a structured report on a child to a social worker, police officer, or to a case conference. Systematic monitoring is a continuous process which can be time-consuming, since it may take weeks to establish a clear and detailed picture of a child's behaviour. Systematic and effective monitoring therefore requires both time and perseverance.

Once it is clear that a child is the victim of sexual abuse, the statutory child protection agencies are responsible for investigation and intervention, and the provisions of the Children Act 1989 and the revised guidelines contained in *Working Together* (DOH 1991) must be brought into play, together with the child protection procedures laid down by the local authority, which should be implemented without delay. In the early stages of concern, however, the very special contribution of the teacher to any subsequent multi-agency work can be in terms of the quality of the monitoring of children believed to be at risk. The following are suggested as parameters which will help to ensure the quality of that monitoring.

Attendance

Details of dates and times are all-important, since patterns of absence can often be very revealing: for example, absences on a particular day may coincide with the presence or absence of a particular parent and/or caretaker; children can be brought in late by one adult but on time by the other. It is possible that repeated reasons for absences given to the school may not be being brought to the attention of the family's doctor and this can be checked out by the school nurse, where there is one.

Mood changes

Children may show changes of mood during the day, perhaps becoming quiet and tense towards the end of the day when home time is anticipated. Children's behaviour may also change if the adult who collects them from school is different from the one who brought them.

Contact with parents

The school's contact with parents may also shed light on a child's situation. Although there may be obvious and common-sense explanations, such as domestic arrangements or a parent's work patterns, details of which parent comes to school and their responses to encouragement from the child's teacher to be involved in the child's education may be important. The interaction between parent(s) and the child's teacher can often be a lifeline for the non-abusing parent but a threat to an abuser. Teachers need to be aware of this two-edged effect.

Children's body language/behaviour

So often, and particularly with young children, body language can speak volumes. Observations can be made of children with their parent(s) and/or caretakers, and of any different responses of children to adults according to the gender of the adult. Children can also show signs of change in body language which vary with the time of the day or the day of the week. For example, a child may well show signs of tense, or apathetic, or otherwise unusual behaviour towards the end of a school day. This may be because the child is anticipating returning to an abusive situation at home. Similarly, a child might show changed body language/behavioural change before and/or after weekends, which may coincide with contact visits, staying with relatives, the presence of a baby-sitter in the home, etc.

Some children may display overt signs of distress such as marked changes in eating patterns (over-eating, refusing to eat, extreme faddiness) or a sudden onset of daytime, or reported night-time wetting and/or soiling. There may be a deterioration in a child's demeanour, with the child becoming increasingly unresponsive, aggressive, tense, etc., or children may display bruises, problems when walking and/or sitting on chairs or on the floor. Teachers noting such behavioural signs of distress should note the dates of these changes and any contemporaneous events in the life of the child being monitored.

Any sexualised behaviour is extremely significant and should be noted carefully, although it should be interpreted with caution. Children can only learn sexualised behaviour from others, either by being abused, by being present during adult sexual behaviour or by watching sexually explicit or pornographic videos/films. However, children below the age of 8 displaying sexualised behaviour are unlikely to learn such detailed behaviour from seeing adult sexual behaviour (they usually think the adults are cuddling or wrestling). They are also unlikely to learn sexualised behaviour from pornographic videos or films, since with younger children, their short concentration span coupled with their limited capacity to grasp the details and meaning of what they see, make it unlikely they will mirror what was on film in their play (although children aged 8 or over would certainly be able to concentrate and remember images and behaviour seen on video). In young children, therefore, the most likely explanation of sexualised behaviour is that they are or have been sexually abused.

Children's language

Young children are unlikely to verbalise what is happening to them in a clear way. This is because they may well not have the language for body parts and sexual behaviour, or they may well be too young to speak about what is happening to them. Even very young children will have deduced or been told, tricked or threatened that what is happening to them must be kept secret. Therefore, they may not feel they have permission to tell, and so they will often speak in analogous terms about snakes that spit at them, tickling they don't like, monsters that gobble them, etc.

This should be recorded carefully, noting the exact words used by the child rather than adult equivalents. Unless teachers have been specially trained for such work, however, and are acting after consultation and with the agreement of the statutory agencies, they should not actively explore any such comments with a child.

Children's play

Teachers are the best judges of normal age-appropriate play because of their training in child development and their expertise with large numbers of children in given age groups. So, for example, an observation by a reception class teacher that a particular child was the only child in the class to play with a toy in a given way may be significant, as the teacher will be comparing the child with approximately 25 other children. No other professional is in a position to make such observations.

Obviously, there are many aspects of children's play which could be detailed here, and it is worthwhile to stress again the need to consider more obvious and less worrying explanations. However, any aspects of play which seem to be out of the ordinary should also be considered in the light they could possibly shed on a child's safety. A child can often act out with a toy ways which may mirror an abusive situation – for example, play with a teddy bear having breakfast and going to school, and then a child saying 'Teddy doesn't want to go to bed'. For many children it is easier to talk about teddy's fears than to talk about their own. Dolls, glove puppets, soft toys, playhouse corners and telephones can be useful. Any such incidents should be noted carefully, but the teacher should avoid becoming directly involved in the child's play or any attempt to investigate further.

Children's drawing/writing

Whilst teachers also need to be extremely cautious in forming conclusions on the basis of children's drawings and/or written work, children often express a great deal of themselves in this way. No one drawing or type of drawing, in terms of figures drawn or colours used, is necessarily indicative that a child is being sexually abused, and an enormous range of self-expression through such media is to be expected. However, on occasions, children's drawings may be a useful index of their fears and feelings, and when children draw people with genitalia the possibility that this might be a cause for concern should be considered. Other kinds of drawings may also need careful consideration, such as children who draw themselves or small children in pictures where they are calling for help. Such evidence should be noted carefully and, if there are doubts about its possible significance, expert advice sought from an educational psychologist or from social services.

Many teachers make use of a weekly diary session for all the class. This can be a very useful way of monitoring a particular child. For example, a child's account of their weekend at home may reveal potentially important information about events and people which should be carefully recorded. If the class has a time for each child to write their own diary each week, it may well be useful to consider who in the family gets most mentioned and who does not, what are the times when different adults are alone with a given child, and does the child always write about being out of the house rather than in the house, etc.

Often a link can be made between drawing/painting and writing. For example, if a class is asked to draw and paint pictures of being happy/sad/angry in which work is done with the class on colours and lines in art, each child could then write about a time when they were happy/sad/angry, or the group of children can be helped to list words connected with being happy/sad/angry. The responses of the child being monitored could then be noted. The advantage of doing this as part of a class lesson is that the teacher is not singling one child out and suggesting *that* child is happy/sad/angry. Also, the responses of the child being monitored can be compared with those of a group of peers.

Medicals, physical education (PE)

A child who is being or has been sexually abused may well react differently from classmates when the time comes for PE/games lessons and/or before a school medical. Teachers are now aware that PE/games lessons, where children undress, provide a useful weekly point to check children known to be at risk of physical abuse for tell-tale signs of injury. Teachers monitoring children who may be sexually abused should consider the extent to which they might also use this weekly opportunity for observation. Signs such as torn clothing, blood stains on clothes, the smell of semen on a child's skin or clothes, an unusual reluctance to undress, or an apparent shamefulness about being undressed, or a disinhibition which is out of keeping with the norm of the age group of children may be of some significance.

However, there are obvious dangers in making such observations, not least the risk that the teacher might be accused of taking an inappropriate interest in the child, and such opportunities for observation could only be taken after careful consideration and prior discussion with a senior colleague. Physical examination by a teacher should not, of course, be contemplated under any circumstances.

Children who are being sexually abused may also often make veiled references to their plight in the guise of psychosomatic complaints. They may well present in school with headaches, stomach-aches and pains. A note should be kept of the frequency of such complaints, and the school nurse kept informed. An abusing parent/adult may well keep a child away from school when medicals are planned. If a child who is being monitored is away from school for a medical, this should be noted and followed up.

Monitoring children in secondary school

The following is a suggested outline for teachers to use for monitoring children in secondary schools who are either already known or are suspected to have been sexually abused by someone known to them. One major way in which secondary schools *differ* from primary schools is that the children have several different subject teachers each year. They could have between four and eight different teachers in any one day. This raises the obvious question about which teacher should coordinate the monitoring of a child about whom there are concerns. No one teacher in a secondary school will be in a position to shoulder the whole task of monitoring a child. A nominated teacher will therefore be needed to coordinate the contributions of all the teachers involved with that child, and there is no obvious answer as to who this should be. Options range from the form tutor, the year head, the teacher who sees most of the child, the teacher the child likes most, to the teacher with special responsibilities for special needs and/or child protection. In selecting the teacher to coordinate the monitoring, there are three particular issues to bear in mind.

1.   Although there are obvious advantages to this being a teacher who has regular contact with the child about whom there are concerns, this may not always be possible and will depend to some extent on the organisation of the school. What is more important is that the coordination of the monitoring should be well organised and effective, and this does not necessarily require a teacher who knows the child well. The coordinator must ensure that staff involved in

monitoring are clear about what behaviours/incidents to record and how to record them. What is important is that teachers actually making the observations are those who regularly interact with the child.

2. In addition to being suitable in other respects, the teacher who takes on the task should be willing to do so. As mentioned above, child sexual abuse can raise many anxieties about children and about the consequences of recognising abuse for the child, the family, the teachers and the school. For some, it also raises anxieties about their own attitudes to child sexual abuse, such as being able to accept that it does happen. Sadly, for some, it may also raise spectres from their own past, since some teachers are themselves survivors of child sexual abuse. This may make them more or less willing to undertake coordinating the monitoring of a child. So for a variety of reasons, it is important that the teachers selected to coordinate the monitoring in a secondary school should be willing to do so.

3. The coordinator needs to have ready access to information on child sexual abuse and the support of other professionals to perform this task. Much relevant information, together with references which may be followed up, is contained in other chapters in this handbook. Additional information and support could also be sought by contacting: the member of school staff with overall responsibility for child protection; the local social services Child Protection Training Officer; and specialist agencies such as the NSPCC, ChildLine, etc. In some authorities, there are also special services for consultation which teachers are encouraged to use (Peake 1991). The teacher who takes on this task also needs the personal and professional support of immediate colleagues.

This is intended as a basic outline which teachers can adapt in ways which suit the particular needs of the child about whom they are concerned and the features of the school situation in which they are working. Since secondary schools differ widely in their organisation, it will also be necessary to adapt the ideas according to the pastoral care system of the school.

Most children who are being sexually abused and attending secondary school have been abused for some time and have developed strategies for achieving a precarious balance between being a victim of abuse and 'surviving'. There is a sense of strength in doing this, and adults should not challenge this without clear and effective plans to guarantee a child's safety and an end to the abuse. Careful monitoring enables professionals to become clear about the basis of their concerns and to plan an effective form of intervention, involving the agencies which can protect children. Schools are not able to offer such protection.

The teacher selected to coordinate the monitoring needs to collect information/observations systematically from all the teachers who have contact with the child about whom there is concern. The following sequential plan may well be useful.

1. The support of the head teacher, or the special needs/child protection teacher, or the head of year is sought to determine a plan for monitoring the child.
2. A meeting is arranged for all those who teach the child about whom there is concern. They are all given an opportunity to hear and discuss the concerns.
3. All the subject teachers are given the headings from the monitoring outline and asked to make a written record of behaviour/incidents over a specified length of time. Teachers could be asked when recording their observation to do so using the following framework:
    - details of the incident/behaviour
    - where it took place
    - when it took place
    - with whom it took place

- the duration of the incident or the intensity of the behaviour
- the frequency of the behaviour
- the sequence of the behaviour (following what/before what did the behaviour occur).

4. At the end of the period of monitoring, the coordinating teacher collects the written records of the other teachers and assembles incidents/behaviours recorded by different teachers under the headings as listed. So, for example, for attendance there would be incidents/behaviours recorded by all the subject teachers under that heading.

5. The coordinating teacher may well see patterns emerging in the incidents/behaviours recorded by different teachers. The monitoring will then contain a range of observations in chronological order by different teachers organised under the respective headings. This will then be a clear basis upon which the coordinating teacher can give a structured report on a child to a social worker/police officer, or to a case conference.

It is worth emphasising that, as with younger children, systematic monitoring is a continuous process which can be time-consuming, since it may take weeks to establish a clear and detailed picture of a child's behaviour. Systematic and effective monitoring therefore requires both time and perseverance.

Once it is clear that a child is the victim of sexual abuse, the statutory child protection agencies are responsible for investigation and intervention, and the provisions of the Children Act 1989 and the revised guidelines contained in *Working Together* (DOH 1991) must be brought into play, together with the child protection procedures laid down by the local authority, which should be implemented without delay. Children who are sexually abused have a variety of needs – legal, medical, social, emotional and often educational – and so need the combined work of a variety of professionals.

In the early stages of concern, however, the very special contribution of the teacher to any subsequent multi-agency work can be in terms of the quality of their monitoring of children believed to be at risk. The following are suggested as parameters that will help to ensure the quality of that monitoring.

Attendance

Details of dates and time are all-important, since patterns of absence can often be very revealing. For example, absences on a particular day may coincide with the presence or absence of a particular parent and/or carer. It may be that notes written to explain absences are always written by one parent and not the other. Repeated reasons for absences given to the school may not be being brought to the attention of the family's doctor. This can be checked by the school nurse if there is one, whilst repeated complaints of headaches, stomach-aches or urinary tract infections should be followed up. Older children may well provide quite plausible explanations for absences or injuries, and often it is the frequency and/or pattern of absences that is revealing. A child may reveal anxieties by changes of moods within a school day or week, perhaps becoming tense and quiet towards the end of the day, when home time is anticipated. Such a child may well seek out opportunities to stay behind after school to delay going home.

Contact with parents

The contact between parents and secondary school teachers is less than that between primary school staff and parents, not least because secondary school children often travel unaccompanied to and from school. It is nevertheless important to be aware of the frequency and quality of the school's contact with parents and to consider the light this may shed on a child's situation. Although there may be obvious and common-sense explanations, such as domestic arrangements or a parent's work patterns, details of which parent comes to the school for parents' evenings and open days, and their responses to encouragement to participate in the child's education are important and should be monitored where practicable.

When letters are given out for children to take home to parents, the child's reactions/comments should be noted where possible. If the child and parent(s) are seen together in school, does the child's demeanour differ from what the teacher would expect, and in what ways does the child's demeanour alter? The interaction between parent(s) and the child's teacher can often be 'a lifeline' for the non-abusing parent, but a 'threat' to an abuser. An abused child will watch this interaction closely, since such children are sensitive to the moods and wishes of adults. Abused children need adults who are prepared to put children first and are seen to do so.

Children's body language/behaviour

Body language can communicate the existence of problems, but less so with older children than with younger children, since they often behave in a way which is designed to conceal the existence of sexual abuse. Observations can be made of a child with their parents(s)/carers, which may indicate different responses to adults according to the individual or the gender of the adult. For example, a child may shun proximity to men and/or be especially aggressive towards men. A child may show signs of tense, apathetic or other inappropriate behaviour which is most apparent on particular days. This may be because abuse is occurring at particular times of the week or it may coincide with the visits of relatives etc. Since children at risk are often the least able to express how they feel, or to seek out appropriate and effective help, frequently the only indication of their unhappiness is the existence of inappropriate behaviour.

The ethos of the school and the responses of school staff to children displaying inappropriate behaviour may influence the signals abused children use and the likelihood of their talking about any underlying unhappiness. Rudeness to a teacher may be dealt with as only attention- and confrontation-seeking and therefore as a disciplinary issue. If, however, the reasons for the rudeness are unhappiness stemming from abusive experiences, the child may find it more difficult to trust staff and to explain.

Helpful conditions for a child exist where school staff are visibly prepared to accept that children may have a variety of reasons why they misbehave, that the reason for the misbehaviour is sought from the child and discussed, and that staff are able to demonstrate that while some behaviours are clearly not acceptable, the children are accepted. Signals used by sexually abused children often include the following:

- suicide attempts/self-mutilation
- children who run away from home/school
- relationship problems with peers and adults
- changes in mood, both gradual and sudden
- children who hurt or assault other children/adults.

Suicide attempts/self-mutilation

Surveys of adult survivor organisations indicate that the vast majority of survivors of child sexual abuse seriously considered or attempted to end their lives as teenagers. Teenage years are a time of rapid upheaval, physically, socially and emotionally, for all children. Most teenagers experience mood changes and periods of poor self-confidence. However, very few contemplate, talk about and/or attempt to kill themselves. Those that do are saying very clearly that their lives are intolerable and that they see no way out other than to end their lives. No suicide talk/attempt or incident of self-mutilation should be ignored or dismissed. Adults should not use their own perspectives on the child's suicide talk to attempt to judge the seriousness of the child's intentions. Children who attempt suicide, if not in contact with their family doctor, should be referred to the educational psychologist/education social worker/local social services office/child psychiatrist so that the causes, including the possibility of sexual abuse, can be explored.

Children who run away from home/school

Children, even teenagers, are entirely dependent on adults for their well-being and safety. Adults provide children with shelter, food, love, attention and guidance. No child casually or deliberately puts themself at risk for no reason, and children who run away are giving a clear cry for help. Such children are likely to be dealt with by the social services department or the police, and this is not primarily an issue requiring action by teachers. Such an incident should not be viewed in isolation, however, since it may assume added significance if other behavioural anomalies have been observed in school.

Relationship problems with peers and adults

Adolescence is a time when children begin to distance themselves from adults and to gravitate to their peer group. Children who have been or are being sexually abused tend to be isolated, however. The pressures on such children not to to tell isolate them from other significant adults in their lives. A child may often want to tell a sympathetic teacher or school nurse, but the pressure to keep silent may be too great and militate against this. These pressures also isolate children from their peers. This is especially so for teenagers. If classmates are talking of first dates, how can a child who has been sexually abused for years want or be able to join in? The isolation goes still further, since the abuse may isolate children within their families, from their non-abusing parents and their siblings. It is this isolation that leads many abused children to believe that they are the only child to whom this has happened, and it underpins their problems in relating to both peers and adults.

A sexually abused teenager may well maintain a distance between themself and adults in school in a variety of ways, such as being very well-behaved, quiet and never in the forefront or available to adults; or by being so churlish and difficult that adults readily dismiss them as unworthy of any teacher's efforts; or by establishing contact with adults based on reasons which mask the child's real need for adult contact, such as excessive helpfulness or repeated health complaints.

Abused teenagers will often have few, if any, close or lasting peer friendships. Such friendships may well not be allowed by the child's abuser. There is a strength in children's closeness with each other which can be a challenge to the power of an abuser. So, friendships are often discouraged or forbidden. The child may well not want close friendships, fearing rejection should the secret become known. Often, abused children have such a poor sense of self-esteem and confidence that they do not believe they are worthy of friendships and do not attempt to make any, or the friendships they do make are with the more antisocial/disaffected groups where they feel they will be judged less harshly or where they can gain some status and positive regard.

Children do, of course, vary in this as in many other respects, and the exis-tence of such factors on their own will not necessarily signify the existence of abuse. They may, however, be significant as a small part of a much larger pattern of behaviour and may provide important supplementary or confirmatory evidence.

Changes in mood, both gradual and sudden

Many teenagers display changes of mood as a result of normal hormonal changes and, in any event, the usual secondary school situation makes it hard to monitor changes in mood in individual children. Subject, teacher or room changes affect the way children behave and feel during the school day. For any child, a double period of their least favourite subject, particularly on a Friday afternoon, may well account for a great deal!

However, careful monitoring may well reveal that all teachers who take a child at the end of the day find that the child is withdrawn and tense, perhaps indicat-ing a fearfulness about home time. As discussed earlier, a weekly pattern of act-ing-out or withdrawn behaviour may well coincide with events at home such as contact, weekends with grandparents, outings with an uncle etc. Gradual changes in children are even harder to notice, particularly if teachers have daily contact with a child over several years. Checking previous school reports/records may reveal that a child's attendance, work patterns and/or behaviour have deteriorated over time.

Children who hurt or assault other children/adults

Children who are confused, frightened, or being hurt do often build up defences to protect themselves from further perceived threats. Older children are able to do this more effectively than younger children. Their capacity to contain their own emotions and be aware of the demands of others and of situations are such that many teenagers mask the warning signs of their own abuse. Teachers should be alert to the possibility that children who hurt or assault other children and/or adults are losing control of themselves.

Such behaviour may reflect a variety of factors, including poor role models at home, or involvement in a delinquent or gang subculture. However, the question needs to be asked why a child is behaving thus, rather than assuming we know the answer. Children can also hit out at other people because they are under pres-sure. They may hit out at people who have done nothing to hurt or frighten them because they cannot hit out at the people who *have* hurt and frightened them. Socialisation processes can lead to gender differences in children's reactions so that sexually abused boys are more likely to hit out, acting out their anger and hurt. Details of any such assaults need to be carefully recorded, noting the date, time, age and gender of the victim, and the nature of the assault, including details of what was said and done.

Children's drawing/writing

Whilst teachers also need to be extremely cautions in forming conclusions on the basis of their students' drawings and/or written work, children often express a great deal of themselves in this way. No one drawing or type of drawing, in terms of figures drawn or colours used, is necessarily indicative that a child is being sex-ually abused, and an enormous range of self-expression through such media is to be expected. However, on occasions, children's drawings may be a useful index of their fears and feelings, and teenagers are particularly adept at using drawings in metaphorical ways. Drawings will seldom be explicitly about child sexual abuse, but they may provide a basis for the teacher to be concerned enough to seek expert advice (from the educational psychologist or from child protection workers) and to consider whether the child should be monitored more closely.

Older children will often respond to ideas for writing in very individual ways. It is helpful if programmes of work for helping children to express themselves include ideas or prompts which might be an opportunity for children to write about what is happening to them, although any such idea should obviously be used in some overall curriculum context for a whole group or class.

The advantages of monitoring an individual child's drawing/writing in the context of a piece of work for the group/class is twofold. Firstly, the one child about whom the teachers feels concern is not singled out in ways which would suggest the child is happy/sad/angry/at risk etc. So children who perhaps shun approaches by adults can be monitored as soon as there is any concern without unduly making a child feel threatened. Second, the responses of the child who is being monitored can be compared with those of a group of peers. Such comparisons are often very helpful in alerting teachers to a child's fears and feelings.

Health complaints, medicals, PE

For many secondary school students, complaining about an ache or a pain is a way of avoiding unpopular lessons or activities, or it may be a normal part of adolescence, such as the onset of menstruation in girls. It may, however, be a more 'respectable' way to bid for attention than to talk of being unhappy and needing help. Certainly, going to an adult with a health complaint provides a cover to keep inquisitive peers at a distance. Children may often present with repeated and/or trivial health complaints, such as headaches, stomach-aches, pains, feeling sick etc.

Whichever way children present with health complaints, they should be taken seriously, listened to, and offered advice and help. Some such complaints will be invented, but many will be related to real illnesses, and schools have a duty to be alert to the health of their pupils. Some real health complaints may well seem not to be founded on actual symptoms at all. Even if this is the case, the teacher and/or welfare assistant and/or school nurse if there is one, who listens carefully and is sympathetic, is showing a child that they take what the child has to say seriously and are prepared to listen. This may be a child's first step to approaching adults outside the family, and the response with which they are met may determine future approaches from the child.

Many adolescents go through a period of not wanting to participate in physical activities, and this is often associated with the physiological changes which they are experiencing. However, a child who is being sexually abused may well react differently from classmates when the time comes for PE/games lessons. Teachers are now well aware that PE/games lessons, where children undress, provide a useful weekly point to check children known to be at risk of physical abuse for tell-tale signs of injury, and those monitoring children who may be sexually abused should consider the extent to which they might also use this weekly opportunity for observation.

However, there are obvious dangers in making such observations, not least the risk that the teacher might be accused of taking an inappropriate interest in the child, and such opportunities for observation should only be taken after careful consideration and prior discussion with a senior colleague. Marks are perhaps less likely to be seen on older children, and since abused children are often aware of the consequences of disclosure they are also likely to provide plausible explanations for any marks. For these reasons, it is all the more important that any obvious marks are noted, concern expressed and the child's responses noted. However, physical examination by a teacher should not, of course, be contemplated under any circumstances.

Medicals are also an opportunity to talk to children about their well-being, and although teachers are not directly involved in these, visiting medical staff should be alerted to any concerns. A child may well feel more able to talk to someone with a medical background whom they do not see everyday. Notes on a child's absences and health complaints should also be shared and discussed with visiting medical staff, and if a child who is being monitored is away from school during a medical this should be noted and followed up.

Finally

As with the previous outline, the above is also intended to help in situations where teachers suspect a child is being sexually abused, and to provide some practical monitoring of a child. Teachers need always to remember, however, that they should never shoulder alone the concern about a child they suspect is being abused. The sexual abuse of children is a crime and needs to be reported to one of the agencies with statutory powers to deal with the problem, namely the social services, the NSPCC or the police. Where there is a suspicion that a child is being abused, advice might also be sought from the educational psychologist and/or education social worker, and social services should be informed.

It is also important that whenever a decision is made to undertake monitoring of a child in a school setting, a record is kept of the process of monitoring which includes details of timing, discussions with colleagues, follow-up action taken and dates set for further reviews. The notebook in which the notes relating to the monitoring of the child's behaviour are kept should contain a record of these.

Issues arising from using a system of monitoring

The monitoring guidelines outlined above have been welcomed by both education workers and social services workers. Several issues have arisen as a consequence of the outlines being used on a regular basis. The debate around these issues has served to define and clarify views both within the profession and between professionals about the role of the class teacher. The issues that have arisen are as follows.

Parental involvement

Most child protection procedures usually, and quite rightly, include the need for early discussion of concerns with parents. The Children Act 1989 lays great emphasis on partnership with parents (see Petrie & Corby, Chapter 20, in this volume), and there has obviously been much debate about the stage at which the practice of monitoring children in school should be discussed with parents. This clearly needs to be decided in consultation with senior colleagues and child protection workers.

As discussed earlier, if a discussion with parents is held too soon this may only serve to alert the abuser and make them more skilful. For example, to explain that sexual abuse is suspected because of a child's drawing of a man with genitalia is to provide the basis for future threats to that child, not only about telling, but also about what the child draws in school. This makes it possible for the abuser's threats to become more specific, but also for them to appear to have knowledge of what the child does in situations separate from them. This can make the abuser seem more powerful and can seem to the child to be a betrayal by other adults in their life. Such a precipitous warning to an abuser could result in that child never doing such a drawing again.

Obviously, the aim of the monitoring guidelines is not to undermine the right of parents. What is clear is that most arguments about the rights and civil liberties of parents/adults cut across the needs that some children have for protection, given the simple fact that the majority of children who are sexually assaulted are assaulted by adults who are in their families or known to their families beforehand. It is obvious, therefore, that some kind of balance needs to be struck.

Where there are specific grounds for suspecting abuse, it would seem in everyone's interest that those grounds are refined and made more specific, so that they can be discussed with parents by the appropriate authorities, while at the same time providing a basis for effective protective action if necessary. It needs to be remembered that these outlines for monitoring children in school are specifically designed to be useful in situations where there are suspicions of child sexual abuse which need to be substantiated or eliminated. It is in the interests of everyone that when such concerns are aired, there is clarity about the evidence on which they are based. These guidelines are one way of achieving this clarity.

Local authority open records

Many local authorities are now adopting the system of open records, to which parents have access. The advice to teachers in the monitoring outlines is that they record their observations in a notebook. It is quite clear that the matter is not one for the child's record at that stage. It is important that any record of discussions involved in planning the monitoring of a particular child should include specific decisions made about the nature of the record of the monitoring which is to be kept, and the stage at which the school's concern would be discussed with the child's parents, entered on the child's record and discussed with professionals from other agencies.

The timing of monitoring

It has become increasingly evident that there needs to be parameters to the timing of any arrangements for monitoring a child. It is clear, however, that when a teacher suspects that a child in their class is being sexually assaulted, these concerns should be discussed immediately with the head teacher and with a member of the local social services department, e.g. the duty officer at the local office, the allocated social worker if the family is already known to social services, or the child protection coordinator for that authority. If the suspicions are unclear, the discussions may well centre around the ways in which the outline for monitoring can be adapted to clarify the situation.

It is also important to remember that where the evidence is quite clear – for example, a child is displaying overtly sexualised behaviour in a way which is out of keeping with the normal range of behaviour for a child of that gender, age and ability – then the decision could well be that monitoring by school would not be an appropriate course of action on its own, and that an investigation of possible abuse should be initiated according to the local area child protection guidelines. So the decision to start monitoring needs to be made first and foremost on the basis of the level of concern about the risk to the child.

A second consideration in the decision to monitor a particular child must be to determine the period of time over which monitoring takes place. Monitoring must take place over a reasonable period of time, and it must be geared to the level of concern about the child and to any difficulties envisaged in establishing an effective and comprehensive system. Thus, where the level of suspicion is quite high, the decision with regard to monitoring may well be to monitor the child more intensively over a shorter period of time.

Any decision about the length of time over which the monitoring takes place should also include a decision about when the monitoring should be reviewed and by whom, and arrangements made accordingly. The central point is that monitoring needs to be a flexible system that, while providing a standard framework, remains sufficiently flexible to meet the needs of individual children and the level of professional concern about these children.

One issue that has arisen from the use of the outline by teachers has been the need to stress that monitoring is not an activity in itself that protects children. It is one means of aiding the work of other professionals to do just that. So there is no virtue in monitoring a child about whom there is concern if the results are not communicated to local child protection workers. There is also a danger that monitoring, which provides a specific and clear role for teachers, can be seen as an end in itself and used as a means to avoid the difficulties of implementing local procedures with regard to child protection. It is therefore always important to distinguish between situations where monitoring is sufficient and those where action is needed.

The important point is that monitoring should have a clear start and end. The duration of the monitoring should be geared to the level of concern about an individual child, and there should be consultation between professionals at all stages. Decisions made should be clearly recorded.

Professionals' use of the monitoring guidelines

Obviously, the above outlines for monitoring were written specifically for teachers, and in using them many have demonstrated their skills and expertise in ways which have contributed greatly to the protection of many children. Given a specified role in the collection of information, teachers are extremely skilful in the observations they make, and in their capacity to place those observations in the context of daily contact with children and also the range of normal behaviour of children.

The outlines have also been found to be useful by social workers or education social workers. It is often the case that the initial concerns about possible risk to a child do not arise in school, but rather arise in the context of family work done by social workers or education social workers. These professionals frequently need to obtain information about a child in different settings from those in which they see the child, and they will often approach the child's teacher to ask for additional information which may clarify their concerns. The outlines have been useful for them in clarifying what they can expect from, and the basis on which to approach, a teacher. This has led to a greater level of consistency within the authority that uses the outline in terms of what social workers and education social workers ask of teachers.

Teacher confidence

Currently, the confidence of teachers is at a very low ebb, partly because of their vulnerability to being accused of sexually abusing their own students, and because of the pressures involved in delivering the National Curriculum. Some reluctance to take on what might be seen as a social work role is therefore, perhaps, to be expected. The introduction of this system of monitoring has, however, resulted in an increased level of teacher confidence. The outline recognises the ambiguities of any situation where there is the suspicion of child sexual abuse and the levels of professional anxiety that this produces. In asking teachers to take on the specific role of monitoring children in school, it is helpful to be able to give them a standard outline which can then be modified to take account of their particular concerns, the particular situation within their school, and the child about whom there is concern. The fact that there is something specific for the teacher to do often helps to reduce their understandable reluctance to get involved.

Increased levels of teacher confidence have been particularly apparent in child protection conferences. Teachers who attend, having previously been given the outline for monitoring children in school, are usually quite clear about the information that has been collected. Often the information the teacher has been able to provide has encouraged discussion of the roles of other professionals and other basic information which has to be collected.

The outlines have also made clear where the contribution of the teacher ends and where the work of statutory child protection workers begins. However, a note of caution needs to be sounded. The introduction of a monitoring system for use by teachers brings with it the challenge of court work. Evidence from monitoring by teachers will increasingly be used in courts, and teachers are going to need training, reassurance and support to do this work. However, the signs are that when teachers do present the results of balanced and careful monitoring, the courts are more able to protect children.

Inter-agency conflict

Other chapters in this section of the *Handbook* address the issue of inter-professional relationships in some detail (see Corby, Chapter 13, in this volume). However, the introduction of a system of monitoring where child sexual abuse is suspected has helped to reduce inter-agency conflict. When teachers are clear about the role they can play in child protection work, their anxieties about children are less likely to lead to tensions between themselves and workers from other agencies. Those who have participated in case conferences know all too well the way in which such tensions can be generated by a lack of awareness of others' roles, responsibilities and authority. The outlines enable teachers to become a more integral part of the child protection process in which the emphasis is on multidisciplinary teamwork, based on clear and realistic expectations of the roles of all concerned.

Conclusion

The sexual assault of children by adults known to them is a difficult situation which arouses anxiety in all who care about the welfare of children. My message is that teachers have a key role in dealing with the suspicion of abuse, but that this role needs to be clarified. Given clear parameters for monitoring, teachers can make a powerful contribution to the assessment of risk. The essential point is that teachers can monitor the situation of a particular child, but the duty to evaluate their observations and take action always lies with the statutory child protection agencies. Teachers need to be aware of the work of these agencies, liaise with them and adhere to local child protection guidelines.

Annotated further reading

David T 1993 Child protection and early years teachers. Open University Press, Milton Keynes

This is an extremely useful book for teachers, covering the different forms of child abuse. It has a helpful first section on understanding child abuse which sets out clearly the historical, social and legal contexts to abuse. The book then goes on to look at how schools and teachers respond to child abuse both in terms of concerns about individual children and also in terms of developing a whole school approach to child protection. The book contains information, practical advice and some attention to the feelings this difficult work raises for teachers.

Peake A, Rouf K, Michaels M 1996 Working with sexually abused children. Brookes University, Oxford

This is a resource pack for professionals, parents and children. It contains nine practice papers for professionals on a range of areas in the field of child sexual abuse: suspicion, assessment, group work, one-to-one work and consultation. There is a very comprehensive set of INSET materials for teachers in schools who may wish to develop their knowledge and understanding of child sexual abuse. The pack has accompanying annotated bibliography of leaflets and books for parents and children which can be ordered separately.

Brown H, Craft A 1989 Thinking the unthinkable. Family Planning Association Education Unit, London

This is a collection of papers on the problems of child sexual abuse for people with learning difficulties. The papers cover a range of topics from the need for safeguards and keeping safe programmes, to issues to do with the law and sexual abuse of adults with learning difficulties. It is a helpful set of papers, seeking to begin to chart a very difficult area of work. The book is useful in that at the end of each paper there are a set of key questions for professionals wanting to make practice-based developments to protect children and adults with special needs.

Rouf K 1991 Into Pandora's box. Children's Society, London

It is important in our work in the field of child sexual abuse to listen to the voices of children. This is a collection of poems and drawings by a young Asian woman about what it means to be abused and to be black. The complex and conflicting emotions contained in the poems remind us all of the dilemmas for children who are abused by trusted adults. Without such brave reminders, our practice would be impoverished and irrelevant.

References

Baker A W, Duncan S P 1985 Child sexual abuse: a study of prevalence in Great Britain. Child Abuse and Neglect 9: 457–467

Department for Education and Employment (DfEE) 1995 Protecting children from abuse: the role of the education service. Circular No. 10.95. HMSO, London

Department of Health (DOH) 1991 Working together under the Children Act 1989. A guide to arrangements for inter-agency cooperation for the protection of children against abuse. HMSO, London

Finklehor D 1984 Child sexual abuse: new theory and research. Free Press, New York

Frosh S 1987 Issues for men working with sexually abused children. British Journal of Psychotherapy 3: 332–339

Furniss T 1983 Mutual influence and interlocking professional-family process in the treatment of child sexual abuse and incest. Journal of Child Abuse and Neglect 7: 207–223

Manchester A H 1979 The law of incest in England and Wales. Journal of Child Abuse and Neglect 3: 670–682

Peake A 1991 Consultation: a model for inter-agency cooperation in child sexual abuse. In: Ussher J (ed) Gender issues in clinical psychology. Routledge, London

Peake A, Turner J 1999 Helping teachers to help children. In: Calder M C, Horwath J (eds) Working for children on the Child Protection Register. Arena/Ashgate, Aldershot

17 Court proceedings and court craft

Mary Lane, Terry Walsh

INTRODUCTION

Many professionals believe that good child protection practice means avoiding courts as far as possible – a view in Department of Health (DOH) guidance following the implementation of the Children Act 1989. However, this legislation was influenced by the findings of major child abuse enquiries, especially that social workers failed to use their legal powers to protect children or abused families with those powers. It is unsurprising therefore that the Act took many decisions about children away from social workers and gave them to courts, to be determined with the objectivity of the 'due process' of law (see Parton, Chapter 1, in this volume). Consequently, it is vital that social workers, health professionals and carers who testify in court have the skills to do so competently. It should not be assumed that because the welfare of the child is paramount in care proceedings that the judiciary will always follow the professionals' view of what is best for children. This chapter gives practical and realistic guidance in preparing for, and giving evidence in, court.

Families often find courts 'frightening and daunting' (Murch & Hooper 1992); many professionals share that view and experience. The advice in this chapter is based upon the premise that knowing more about what happens in court and why, and how lawyers approach *their* tasks will better equip witnesses for successful court appearances. It is important, however, to be realistic about the way courts are, rather than as we might want them to be. Despite the pressure for family courts to be 'non-stigmatic responsive institutions employing conciliatory procedures' (Murch & Hooper 1992), courts hearing child protection matters are not 'user friendly', they are still formal and adversarial. Witnesses should therefore acknowledge the particular nature of legal proceedings and adapt behaviour and attitudes accordingly when in the court arena.

Much misunderstanding may be caused between the 'caring' professions and the legal profession because the latter is steeped in tradition and adapts slowly to modern life. Judges are predominantly white, middle class, middle-aged to elderly men, and most magistrates have conservative life experiences. The judiciary are therefore likely to regard all those who come before them in the light of the usual stereotypes. Women projecting unconventional images of motherhood or femininity may have their evidence devalued, and the discrimination experienced by members of ethnic minorities generally may be present for professionals in court. It is the authors' experience that the extensive training given the judiciary in recent years has caused them to bend over backwards to demonstrate rejection of outdated and stereotypical attitudes towards those from the ethnic minorities who appear before them, so that such professionals are often carefully given extra respect. Female professional witnesses giving evidence about children will have the advantage of more credibility, at least initially, than their male colleagues, and all witnesses with qualifications and experience will have enhanced status in court, whatever their gender or race, especially if they have the qualities consistent with those of credible professionals.

Success as a witness does not require unthinking collusion with values and methods discordant with those most cherished, but compliance with the procedures and etiquette peculiar to legal forums is necessary. Court is not the place for professionals to challenge such values or methods with hostile or dismissive behaviour and witnesses should remember that they are not in court on their behalf, but to achieve decisions which protect the child. It is important to acknowledge the particular nature of legal proceedings and adapt behaviour and attitudes accordingly when in the court arena. For example, some inexperienced professional witnesses seem to believe that if they dress casually for court, they can make the whole proceedings more relaxed. This simply does not work, however, and is more likely to make witnesses feel uncomfortable when surrounded by the formally dressed.

Two particular aspects of the legal system are now outlined to assist readers' understanding. Since both solicitors and barristers have rights of audience in family courts, the word 'advocate' is used for both, meaning the lawyer in court.

The adversarial method

A social work academic has written of courts as 'a context in which winning is more important than an exploration of all possibilities and options. Social workers seek to have their plans ratified on the basis of selected and selective evidence' (Ryburn 1992). However, the partisan approach this deplores is not a matter of choice when courts are asked to resolve disputes. Professionals may find it hard to accept that their 'non-judgemental' approach may have to give way to taking sides and that, on occasion, the partisan approach requires that they say things in court about others, in their presence, which compassion would leave unspoken. The conduct of the British court process has its foundation in the adversarial method whereby justice is arrived at through a verbal contest between two or more advocates, according to formal rules designed to achieve a fair hearing for all of them, with each challenging the other's version of events and presenting their own in the best light in order to persuade independent arbitrators to decide in their favour. Adversarial hearings are most ferocious in criminal courts and whilst some legal decisions and procedural methods have tempered the combatant nature of family court proceedings, e.g. relaxed rules of evidence, they have not destroyed it. The position at present is that whilst care proceedings are adversarial, efforts are usually made to conduct the hearings in a non-adversarial way.

There are, however, new developments ahead, stemming from the European Convention on Human Right and the Human Rights Act 1998 which may halt the erosion of the adversarial method in family proceedings, in order to protect the right to a fair trial for *all* parties (see Lyon, Chapter 10, in this volume). Once in court, witnesses may find their own experience less adversarial than anticipated, but it is still necessary to prepare, psychologically and evidentially, for combat, especially in relation to challenging cross-examination.

The power of oral evidence

In family courts, disclosure of each witness's evidence is required in advance of the hearing. Detailed knowledge of what will be said in court does not, however, make the outcome of hearings certain – the judiciary make their decision *after* witnesses have been seen and heard. Oral evidence can be more powerful than written, because the judiciary has much more than words on paper available to them. They can take into account witnesses' demeanour, appearance and attitudes in assessing the value and credibility of their evidence. For the same reason, oral evidence can weaken or even destroy a witness's case. In other words, convincing testimony is a matter of not only of the evidence given, but the way in which *it is given*.

Taking instructions

Solicitors accept their clients' instructions, but not uncritically – they should identify weaknesses in cases, give realistic appraisals of the likelihood of success, or suggest viable alternatives. In first meetings between solicitor and witness, the history of the case is discussed if not already known by the solicitor. Witnesses should give their solicitors as much detailed information as possible, including, where appropriate:

- *Family tree*, a diagram of the members of the family, their names, dates of birth, and relationship to each other;
- *Chronology* in date order, of significant events, including the beginning (and end) of the witnesses' involvement with the case. Solicitors will value witnesses' expertise about the emotional, or medical impact of events (e.g. repeated admissions to care, shaking a young baby, etc.) and may need help in linking facts to theory (e.g. the effects of abuse, known risk factors, etc.)
- *Names and addresses of other potential witnesses*, e.g. previous health visitors, or the colleague who witnesses a crucial incident, and if possible an opinion as to their likely attitude to giving evidence.

It is also the case that to be forewarned is to be forearmed. Sometimes errors, omissions etc. occur, even in the most professionally conducted cases. Since they may be used by opposing advocates to attack witnesses, it is vitally important that in the privacy of interviews with their own solicitors, witnesses raise these, so that they can be taken into account, and their potential to damage evidence be defused.

Preparing evidence

The adversarial method is the basis of the approach taken by lawyers to the preparation and presentation of evidence. A legal textbook has the story of a judge, exasperated by constant interruptions from advocates, asking, 'Am I never to hear the truth in this matter?' – the answer came back from one of them, 'No, my lord, you will hear the evidence'. Advocates must not lie or mislead the court but do select and shape the information provided by their clients into evidence, presenting the court with that which is persuasive in their favour, and dissembling what is not, rather than giving an all-inclusive exposition.

Turning information into evidence

Teachers of advocacy skills suggest that evidence is prepared by concentrating on six or seven of the strongest and most crucial points arising from the information – the 'pillars' on which the case is constructed – and discarding points which are weak or peripheral. The next exercise is to play 'devil's advocate', often with the help of the future witnesses, by trying to predict the points and arguments which might be advanced from the other side to demolish these pillars, what their pillars might be and how they can be demolished. Witnesses might puzzle at the omissions or the emphasis placed on particular aspects of evidence by the advocate but there comes a time, after all the thought and preparation before court, for witnesses to rely on advocates' skills and judgement.

Expert witnesses are those whom the court (judge or magistrates) decides are experts. Formal qualifications are not always necessary. For example, a person with lengthy experience of fostering can give expert evidence about foster care. All professional witnesses have some expertise, but in consultation with their solicitors should consider whether the effective presentation of a particular case in court requires support from those having more, e.g. sufficient practice experience to give valid evidence about the prospects of an adoptive placement of a boy of 9.

Witnesses should not be offended if their solicitor suggests an expert be brought in as witness and may know someone amongst specialist colleagues. If, for example, the other side is calling a consultant psychiatrist, consideration will have to be given to calling an equally weighty expert to counter that evidence. It is galling when experts reiterate what social workers already know, but the reality is that the evidence of doctors, especially consultants with strings of letters after their names, is accepted more readily than that of 'mere' social workers.

Advocates with experience in child protection litigation will build up their own lists of experts and know their abilities (or lack of them!). The trend towards 'court appointed' experts, usually via the guardian *ad litem* and agreed by all parties, is welcome but does not prevent the commissioning of further experts by one or more party if the court is persuaded of the need.

Leave of court for expert advice

The court must give permission for an expert to examine a child for the purposes of giving evidence. Without leave, the evidence may be excluded (Rule 18).

Research evidence

Research-based evidence backing up a witness's views will be welcome by advocates, but any research offering alternative views should also be mentioned. A witness intending to use research in evidence should be able to quote chapter and verse and to answer questions about it, as well as deal with contradictory research with which a cross-examiner might challenge the witness. A good advocate becomes an instant expert on any subject!

Evidence of what children have said

Social work witnesses giving evidence about what children have said may be challenged about their familiarity with the two documents (as far as lawyers are concerned) most relevant to interviewing children about abuse – the 'Cleveland' Report (Butler-Sloss, L.J. 1988) – even if the issue before the court is not *sexual* abuse – and the guidelines in the *Memorandum of Good Practice on Video Recorded Interviews with Child Witnesses for Criminal Proceedings* (DOH 1992). The latter is about children's evidence in criminal proceedings but is expected to be complied with whenever children are interviewed about alleged abuse (see Williams, Chapter 19, in this volume).

Witness statements

Rules of court require that written statements of the evidence to be given by all witnesses are prepared and submitted to court in advance of the hearing. Sometimes this does not happen but the intention is to ensure that as much evidence as possible can be agreed, that oral evidence is given on contentious matters only, and to enable each party to prepare their case in the knowledge of what they have to challenge or counter. Statements are either prepared by the solicitor or the witness, who should ask the solicitor to check them. The statement is signed by the witness after carefully ensuring, even though the wording may not quite be their own style, that the contents are true. The sanction of perjury applies to untruthful or misleading statements.

Witnesses should be aware of, and prepare their evidence in the light of where their evidence 'fits in' with the other evidence to be given. This can be ascertained from advocates and by reading other witness statements, e.g. are they the principal witness setting out the case for a care order, in a supporting role giving evidence about a crucial incident, or an expert witness on a particular point? This will be especially important if the witness is not in court throughout the hearing and therefore does not hear the evidence given before theirs. The DOH handbook *Reporting to Court under the Children Act 1989* (Flin & Spencer 1990) gives valuable and easily accessed guidance to writing statements.

New evidence

After witness statements are submitted to court, new evidence can only be given with the leave of the court. The solicitor should be informed immediately of any significant developments in the case after written evidence has been submitted, so that the other parties can be informed as soon as possible and are not 'ambushed' in court.

Using written evidence in court

Giving oral evidence is not a test of memory. In most court hearings, a bundle of all the documents filed in the proceedings will be available in the witness box, including the witnesses's statement. This bundle should be paginated so that when a particular statement is the subject of examination the witness is referred to it by the page number. At the same time as the witness turns to the document, so will the judge and advocates, so there is no need to panic looking for the right page.

Witnesses may be asked about dates or events which are not in their statement or anywhere in the bundle. This is usually a diversionary tactic by the cross-examiner, an attempt to weaken credibility by demonstrating that a witness cannot remember a certain date or the exact words used at a particular time. Whilst witnesses should always bring their files to court, they should not take them to the witness box because of the rule of evidence about 'memory-refreshing documents', i.e. if used *in the witness* box, files or other records must, at the request of opposing advocates, be submitted to their scrutiny. However, if the *judge or magistrates* regard the information requested by the cross-examiner as necessary, and if witnesses cannot give it without looking at their file, they may direct a brief adjournment so that a professional colleague of the witness in court, or the advocate for the witness, can extract it from the file. Copies of the relevant record must then be made available to all the advocates.

Directions hearings

These are relatively informal court hearings, in the weeks or months before the final hearing, to identify evidence which is agreed or remains in dispute as statements and reports become available, and to decide procedural matters. These include obtaining leave for expert evidence, and timetabling – establishing when all the evidence will be ready, all witnesses available – and setting a date for the final hearing. It is unusual for witnesses to give oral evidence at directions hearings, but the crucial parties should attend so that they can give instructions to their advocates on the directions being requested and check dates being suggested in their diaries.

Personal preparations for court

Do not underestimate the importance of dress and appearance – it should be smart and 'sober', the kind of clothes worn to an important interview. Dressing casually to try to lessen the ceremonious or intimidatory nature of court may be seen as disrespect. Formal clothes may also increase witnesses' confidence and sense of occasion. Keep makeup and jewellery toned down. Badges, whatever worthy causes they espouse, risk damage to witnesses' credibility, because of the possibility that the judiciary assessing the witness hold different views.

Witnesses should read over their evidence the night before court but not burn the midnight oil. They should also get to court in time – at least half an hour before the start of the hearing. Witnesses will need time to compose themselves and ensure they are comfortable. Witnesses who are unavoidably delayed on the morning of court should ensure their advocates are notified so that an adjournment can be requested. An advocate will not start a hearing with vital witnesses absent.

Viewing the courtroom

Another good reason to arrive early is the opportunity to have a look at the courtroom before the hearing starts. The object is to become familiar with the layout, e.g. where you will be sitting, where the witness box is, and the distance between the witness box and where the judiciary is sitting (important for adjusting the loudness of the voice). Ushers (black gown or badge and clipboard) will usually oblige by showing witnesses around whilst the courtroom is empty. Dealing with nerves is an occupational hazard of court witnesses but, up to a reasonable level, is conducive to good performance. Nerves are also a reassuring sign that the witness's physiology is normal – adrenalin is pumping around the body to produce alertness. Witnesses who are not nervous may perform badly because they are too blasé or overconfident. Take whatever stress-reducing measures are available, except alcohol and other mood changing substances. It may be reassuring to know that even the most experienced advocates are frequently anxious before court, but most have developed ways of concealing it in public.

It frequently happens, for a number of reasons, that on the morning the hearing is to start all is suddenly agreed at the court door, or there is an unexpected adjournment. Whilst this means a day or more of unpleasantness is avoided, it can leave witnesses feeling frustrated and disappointed. If this happens, take advantage of the opportunity of unexpected free time to do something relaxing and pleasant, to recharge batteries and come back down to earth.

Outside the courtroom

The time immediately before going into court is valuable for negotiations with the other parties by your advocate. Sometimes the reality of actually being at the court door focuses minds positively on compromises that might avoid or shorten the battle ahead and your advocate will need your instructions. If the advocates go into 'huddles', which exclude key professional witnesses and seem to be making 'deals', join in to ensure your views are part of the debate. But beware of being overheard – valuable clues to your strategy can be picked up this way.

The court hearing

In family courts, all witnesses will usually be allowed to remain in court throughout the proceedings, both before and after giving evidence.

Order of examination of witnesses

The applicant for the order, which is the substance of the court case, is the first to call witnesses to give their evidence and all the applicant's witnesses are examined at this stage. Each witness is examined 'in-chief', first by their own advocate, and then cross-examined by the advocate(s) for other parties. They are then re-examined by their own advocate. Those challenging the application call their witnesses next and all their witnesses are examined at this stage. Children's evidence is usually last to be heard – guardians *ad litem* and all their witnesses (and/or occasionally the children) are examined at this stage.

If witnesses have not finished giving their evidence when there is a break in the hearing – for example at lunch or the end of the day – they are forbidden by rules of evidence from speaking to their own advocates or other witnesses about any aspect of the evidence and may be asked questions when next in the witness box to check compliance with this rule.

Final speeches

When all the witnesses have been heard, advocates may give a summary and overview of their case to the judiciary.

Announcing the decision

The magistrates or judge may give their decision and their reasons at the end of the hearing, or 'retire', giving their decision an hour or two later. Judgement can also be reserved to another day.

Giving oral evidence

Witnesses can make a good start to their 'performance' by walking confidently and purposefully into the witness box. All eyes, including those of advocates for other parties, will be on the witness at that point and a lot can be revealed about them. The impression should be of a witness at ease with what they are about to do.

Taking the oath or affirmation

Every witness promises to speak the truth, by religious oath or non-religious affirmation. This is the judiciary's first encounter with the witness and first impressions count. The oath or affirmation should be un-rushed, pronounced with sincerity and solemnity, looking at the judiciary. Since affirming is still relatively unusual, the usher or clerk should be warned in advance of the witness going into the box so that the correct card is readily available, or better still, the witness should memorise the words so that the card is not needed. Credibility might be affected by jarring the smooth administration of the affirmation if the card has to be hunted for round the courtroom.

Christian oath

Taking the Bible/New Testament in the right hand:

I swear before Almighty God that the evidence I shall give shall be the truth, the whole truth and nothing but the truth.

Affirmation

This needs practice, as the phrasing is awkward:

I do solemnly and sincerely and truly declare and affirm that the evidence I shall give shall be the truth, the whole truth and nothing but the truth.

Non-Christian oath

If the witness's religion demands a non-Christian religious form of oath or other ceremony which the court is unlikely to know, the usher or clerk should be told before court starts so that the necessary book or equipment can be obtained – or witnesses could bring their own.

Sit or stand?

After the oath/affirmation, the judge or magistrates may invite the witness to sit – do not do so until invited. Thereafter, sitting or standing is for each witness to decide whichever feels right in that particular setting. Witnesses of small stature or having quiet voices should, when giving evidence in the high-sided witness boxes in some formal courts, stand so that they can be seen and heard and to maximise their 'presence' in the court! Whether sitting or standing, however, avoid slouching and be upright and alert.

Addressing the judiciary

Witnesses are giving evidence to magistrates or judges only – it is they who must be convinced by it. Witnesses may look at the advocates when listening to questions, but should look at the judiciary when giving the answers. This breaks the normal rules of conversation and seems alien at first, but witnesses should remember that although evidence is given to the court by way of questions and answers, it is not conversation – more about this later. Eye contact with the judiciary should be maximised, within reason, to increase credibility. The occasional smile – in an appropriate place – is a good way of establishing rapport. It is important to speak clearly and pace the reply to take account of the fact that most judges and magistrates make their own notes of the evidence – watch the pen or keyboard! Judges or magistrates should be addresses as follows:

The Family Proceedings (Magistrates) Court – 'Your Worships', 'Sir' or 'Ma'm'
County Court – 'Your Honour'
High Court – 'My Lord/Lady' or 'Your Lordship/Ladyship'.

There are times during oral evidence when witnesses may need to create a pause, or emphasise some particular aspect of their evidence, especially when a cross-examiner is making damaging inroads. The witness who looks the judiciary in the eyes and says, 'Your Worship (Honour etc.) I would like to say,' guarantees that for the next few minutes the questions stop, and the judiciary give the witness their full attention.

Qualifications and experiences

If a brief account of their present occupation, professional address, qualifications and experience is not in their statement, this is the first the court will hear about professional witnesses. These details should be stated briefly but clearly. Prepare a succinct CV in advance – every professional witness should know how many years they have been a social worker or health visitor without having to count them up in the witness box! Witnesses should also give the full name of their qualifications, not just the initials 'CWSQ' or 'RSN'. If employed in an unusual capacity or by an organisation with which the judiciary may not be familiar, the witness should give a short explanation (e.g. community link worker, family centre staff). Modesty about being a manager is out of place in court – the witness is aiming to impress the judiciary with their knowledge, experience and seniority.

Examination-in-chief

The first evidence witnesses give is via questioning by the advocate acting for them. The purpose of evidence-in-chief is to put before the judiciary the evidence in support of the case. In essence, evidence-in-chief is an oral repetition of a witness's statement and this stage is often dispensed with to save time.

However, giving some evidence-in-chief in full allows witnesses the opportunity to add power to the written word with colour and detail, e.g. the statement referring to concerns about domestic hygiene can be brought to life with graphic details! Also, in this earlier stage of giving evidence via a friendly advocate asking the questions, witnesses can show confidence and competence, thereby establishing credibility with the court and 'settle into' the role of giving evidence before coming under attack in cross-examination.

The technique of evidence-in-chief

Evidence-in-chief should be a relaxed exchange between witness and advocate, with the flow of questions and answers easy and rhythmic, like a long rally in tennis or the movement of a metronome, and *seem* like conversation. Advocates use their skills to ask questions in a way that allows the evidence to be brought out with convincing impact on the court, emphasising the facts and details which are essential to proving the case. Witnesses give answers to the judiciary, but occasional eye contact with the advocate will maintain the teamwork between advocate and witness.

Leading questions

A leading question only has one answer. For example, if a crucial piece of evidence were that a child told the witness they did not want to see their father again, a leading question would be, 'Did she tell you she did not want to see her father?' Rules of evidence prohibit the witness's own advocate asking leading questions during examination-in-chief. Hence the need for careful preparation, so that witnesses will know in which direction their advocates are going if questions sound obscure, or several questions are need to reach the same point that leading questions get to directly! The clue to the answer to a non-leading question may lie in key words, e.g. 'did she *say* anything to you about her *father?*' Although witness and advocate know the answer, no leading questions have been asked.

In family courts, the rule excluding leading questions in evidence-in-chief is often relaxed to the point of being ignored, but that will not become apparent until the actual hearing and the witness should be aware of it as part of their preparation for evidence-in-chief.

Leading questions can be asked in cross-examination and frequently *are* in order to try to put words into the witness's mouth.

Cross-examination

This is without doubt the aspect of giving evidence which causes greatest apprehension. Curiously, many 'helping' professionals seem to regard cross-examination as an experience which must be suffered passively, but there is no rule that witnesses must endure it without defending themselves and their evidence. Indeed, a witness on behalf of a child has a duty to defend their evidence under challenge in cross-examination, although at all times remaining polite and dignified.

Psychologist Rhona Flin argues that 'torturing' witnesses by cross-examination is not an effective way to ensure truth emerges (Flin & Spencer 1990), but cross-examination is a time-honoured and central element of the adversarial method. Cross-examination is verbal chess – it can be intellectually stimulating and even exciting but a few survival techniques can make it an experience in which the witness is victor, not victim.

The aim of cross-examination

Cross-examination is for advocates to destroy or weaken the evidence given 'in-chief' by attacking or undermining it, or the credibility of witnesses, and introducing evidence favourable to their case – usually in the form of alternative explanations or re-interpretations of what the witness has said.

In family courts, cross-examination is likely to be less ferocious than in criminal courts, and the bullying advocate who reduces the witness to tears risks alienating the judiciary and giving witnesses the 'sympathy vote'. However, if aggressive cross-examination is successfully denting the credibility of witness or evidence, a court may allow it to continue. Cross-examiners try to devalue or negate any aspect of witnesses or evidence, which include qualifications, experience, memory and attempts to demonstrate witness bias or misunderstanding. Cross-examiners may try to make witnesses muddled or lose confidence, or contradict themselves and although it may *feel* like a personal attack, it is not. Goading witnesses into losing emotional control, getting angry or upset, is part of an advocate's tactics. Seeing it as such, and maintaining professional dignity, will help witnesses rise above it.

Surviving cross-examination

Survival depends on preparation begun long before the court hearing. Witnesses who have done their work competently, and made adequate recordings, should have little to fear when faced with searching questions about their work. Having well-organised evidence, thoroughly prepared, with the potential weaknesses covered in work with the solicitor, with the main points of evidence in their statements will also help witnesses to avoid being muddled or thrown off balance. Witnesses who have mastered all the facts and know the main pillars of their cases will be hard to undermine. Giving evidence-in-chief with confidence and panache may assist survival in cross-examination because advocates watch witnesses during this stage and make their own assessments of their strengths and weaknesses. Witnesses who appear vulnerable may attract more challenge than strong ones. Body language should be just as calm and confident in the witness under cross-examination as during evidence-in-chief. Backing away in the farthest corner of the witness box or loosing eye contact with the judiciary will help the cross-examiner by signalling that the witness is feeling threatened.

In evidence-in-chief, the witness and advocate work together to establish an easy flow and rhythm to the questions and answers. In cross-examination, witnesses should try not to allow the advocate to set the pace or establish a rhythm, because the advocate thereby gains control of the encounter and is able to push and pull witnesses in dangerous directions. Interrupt the rhythm by giving long answers when short ones are expected (and vice versa), ask for questions to be repeated, or drink a glass of water.

Witnesses are not obliged to give the exact answers the cross-examination questions require. Again, it is not conversation. Anyone who has observed some politicians being quizzed by journalists could learn from their technique of giving answers *they* want, whatever the questions! If an advocate insists on a simple 'yes' or 'no' answer, the witness could give it, and then add elaboration or explanation, weakening the impact of the first answer, just as the cross-examiner is about to move on to the next question. Alternatively, witnesses, facing the judiciary, could say that in their opinion, a simple 'yes' or 'no' answer is inadequate and go on to give the appropriate answer. Witnesses should look at the judiciary to give their answers. In fact, *it is not necessary to look at the cross-examiner at all.* Witnesses feeling threatened by advocates can help themselves by not looking in their direction even during the questions. Not only does this prevent intimidation by cross-examiners' body language, but also it conveys an unspoken message to the judiciary that the cross-examiner is of no importance and can be ignored.

Whenever possible in answer to cross-examination questions, witnesses should take opportunities to restate to the court the main points of their evidence-in-chief, so that the court's attention is drawn back to that, not the cross-examiner's distortion of it.

Multiple cross-examination

In each court hearing, one advocate is on the witness's side, and will conduct the examination-in-chief and re-examination, and all the other advocates, representing other parties in the case are entitled to cross-examine that witness. This could mean three or more cross-examinations! This may not be the nightmare it seems at first because in reality, some of the advocates in a multi-party case, for example for the guardian *ad litem*, may be on the same side as the witness they cross-examine, sharing on behalf of their clients the witness's view about what the court's decision should be.

In preparing for court, witnesses should ascertain from their own advocates, and from reading witness statements, which of the other advocates is 'friend' or 'foe', or 'friend' on some issues and 'foe' on others. Witnesses can then take advantage of the rule permitting leading questions in cross-examination by allowing themself to be 'led' by the friendly advocate, in the knowledge that the interests of the cross-examiner and the witness coincide.

Re-examination

When cross-examination has finished, witnesses may be tempted to relax and let down their guard. They should, however, remain alert. The next questions are from their own advocates again in re-examination.

The purpose of re-examination is to repeat parts of the witness's evidence and/or repair damage to it sustained in cross-examination. For example, if during cross-examination witnesses became confused, or their credibility shaken, questions in re-examination will be directed at untangling the confusion, correcting misunderstandings and putting the evidence 'back on the rails'. Alternatively, advocates may want their witnesses to remind the judiciary of some important points so that the last words they hear are a restatement of the witness's evidence-in-chief before cross-examination dented it.

Leading questions cannot be asked in re-examination, so questions from one's own advocates may again be indirect, or long-winded. Witnesses should re-establish eye contact with their advocate to facilitate the communication and teamwork.

After giving evidence

Witnesses will usually be permitted to remain in court after giving their testimony but if they have other demands on their time, the judiciary should be asked by their advocates to 'release' them. This request is usually granted if all parties agree.

Witnesses remaining in court can assist their advocates by making notes of other witnesses' evidence when their own advocate is cross-examining and giving further instructions to their advocates as other evidence unfolds, by passing notes or whispering. This should not be done with such frequency that it causes irritation or distraction, or creates the impression that the advocates were poorly instructed in the first place. When listening to other evidence, witnesses should sit in an impassive but respectful manner, not agreeing or making disapproving noises or expressions of shock or amazement.

███

After the decision

When the magistrates or judge have given judgement, professional witnesses should take the news calmly and with dignity, whatever the outcome. Witnesses should expect to feel tired and sad after a court hearing, even if they get the decision they wanted. This is partly because of the adrenalin draining away – but mostly because child protection decisions inevitably involve loss to one party or more. This is the time to seek supportive debriefing from trusted colleagues.

Like most things which are worthwhile, developing skills and confidence as a witness in court takes practice and experience. A respect for, and acceptance of, the unique rules and procedures of the judicial process are a good beginning. Whilst social workers and health professionals have different training and often different values from lawyers, there is no reason teamwork cannot be achieved, with roles and skills being complementary, ensuring that the right decisions are made for children who need the protection of the courts.

References

Butler-Sloss, Lady Justice E 1988 Report of the enquiry into child abuse in Cleveland, Cmnd 412. HMSO, London

Department of Health (DOH) 1992 Memorandum of good practice on video recorded interviews with child witnesses for criminal proceedings. HMSO, London

Plotnikoff J, Woolfson R (eds) 1996 Reporting to court under the Children Act 1989. HMSO, London

Flin R, Spencer J R 1990 The evidence of children: the law and psychology. Blackstone Press, Oxford

Murch M, Hooper D 1992 The family justice system. Rule 18 (1) Family Proceedings Court (Children Act 1989) Rules 1991; Rule 4.18(1) Family Proceedings Rules 1991. Family Law, Bristol

Ryburn M 1992 Contested adoptions. Adoption and Fostering Journal 16 (4): 29–38

The work of the guardian *ad litem*

Ann Head

The decision of a social services department to institute care proceedings is clearly a very serious one, which may result in a child's compulsory, and even permanent, removal from their family. In addition to the procedures described in the preceding chapters, there is a further safeguard for the child in the court's appointment of a guardian *ad litem* (hereafter referred to as a GAL), a person independent of the local authority, whose prime duty is to safeguard the interests of the child. The appointment of GALs and their duties under the Children Act 1989 are matters dealt with under section 41 of the Act and in the Rules of Court. The assumption is that a GAL will be appointed in the great majority of public law cases.

For the purpose of any specified proceedings the court shall appoint a guardian *ad litem* for the child concerned unless satisfied that it is not necessary to do so in order to safeguard his interests.

(Children Act 1989, s. 41(1))

The concept of a GAL, in the sense of a person appointed by a court to safeguard the interests of a child in the course of legal proceedings, has been known in adoption proceedings since the Adoption Act 1958. The extension of the concept to the field of public law resulted from a need for the child in care proceedings to be represented by a voice independent of the local authority bringing proceedings and of the child's parents. This was highlighted by the Field Fisher inquiry into the death of Maria Colwell (Department of Health and Social Security (DHSS) 1974), a child who had been returned from foster care with relatives to her mother and step-father, and who subsequently died at the hands of her step-father. The inquiry report drew the conclusion that an independent social worker's views of Maria's best interests would have been helpful to the court in that case. A further pressure to secure an independent voice came from David Owen's Children Bill 1974, which directed attention to the need for independent legal representation for children.

in any proceedings relating to a minor in any court, separate representation should be considered and, if appropriate, the child should be made (if not already so) a party of the proceedings.

(Children Bill 1974, clause 42)

The Children Act 1975 reflected both these identified needs and the views of the Houghton Committee (1972) on adoption, in making provision for courts to appoint GALs in care proceedings. Full implementation of the provisions had to wait until 27 May 1984, when it became mandatory for local authorities to establish panels of GALs and reporting officers (ROs) who would be available to act in the full range of care and related proceedings, as well as in adoption and freeing for adoption cases. The task of the reporting officer is to interview parents who wish to consent to an adoption order, and to advise the court whether the consent is given freely and with the full understanding of its implications.

Early studies of the work of GALs drew attention to the wide variations in the number of appointments in care and related proceedings, consequent upon the degree of discretion allowed in the 1975 Act. Murch & Bader (1984), for example, commented as follows:

Diversity is a theme which runs throughout the scheme: diversity between local authorities of comparable size in the number of cases which came to court; diversity in courts' practice, concerning both the criteria used in order to separate representation in the first place, and the stage at which this is done, that is, on application after the initial hearing; diversity between courts with comparable workloads in the proportion of cases in which GALs are appointed.

The Children Act 1989 addressed this question of diversity and it extended the range of work to be encompassed by GALs. It also directed that the courts were to appoint a GAL, unless they were satisfied that it would not be in the child's interest to do so. The duties which now fall to the GAL, set out in the *Manual of Practice Guidance for Guardians* ad litem *and Reporting Officers* (Department of Health (DOH) 1992*a*), are to advise the court on the following matters:

1. Whether the child is of sufficient understanding for any purpose, including the child's refusal to submit to a medical or psychiatric examination, or other assessment that the court has power to require.
2. The wishes of the child in respect of any matter relevant to the proceedings, including the child's attendance at court.
3. The appropriate forum for the proceedings, basing the criteria for the transfer of cases on:
   i. exceptional complexity, importance or gravity; The quick brown fox jumps ove
   ii. the need to consolidate with other proceedings, for example, adoption and contact applications;
   iii. urgency.
4. The appropriate timetabling of the proceedings, or any part of them, always bearing in mind the dictates of the Children Act, s. 1(2) regarding the avoidance of delay.
5. The options available to the court in respect of the child and the suitability of each such option, including what order should be made in determining the application.
6. Any other matter on which the Justices' Clerk or the court seeks the guardian's advice, or concerning which the guardian considers that the Justices' Clerk or the court should be informed (DOH 1992*a*).

In practice, the GAL's duties will involve appointing a solicitor for the child (Family Proceedings Court Rules 1991, rule II (a)), identifying to the court any person whose party status in the proceedings would help to safeguard the child's interests (rule II (6)), accepting documents on behalf of the child (rule II (8)) and conducting a full investigation of all the circumstances of the case (rule II (9)) which will lead to the production of a written report (rule II (7)) making recommendations as to the course of action which will best promote the child's interests. The GAL is bound by the court's obligation to reduce delay and to have regard to the matters set out in the welfare checklist (see Chapters 8, 14 and 16, in this volume).

The duties of the GAL are many and varied. It is perhaps helpful to consider the type of tasks involved, which I suggest are as follows.

Practical

As laid out in the court rules: appointing a solicitor, aiding the swift and efficient conduct of the proceedings, advising on matters to be considered by the court. There has been an increasing stress on the 'case management' role of the GAL, who is required to attend all directions hearings (see Bell, Chapter 14, in this volume), with a view to advising the court of any matters which may affect the child and to avoid delay in the proceedings.

Investigative

Gaining a full picture of the case from documentation and from those professionally and privately involved with the child.

Analytical

Teasing out the issues from conflicting arguments and reaching reasoned conclusions, based on experience, research findings, expert advice and a detailed consideration of the facts of the case.

Representational

Promoting in court the child's best interest as perceived by the GAL and the child's wishes and feelings, and defending the GAL's conclusions in the face of challenges by other parties.

Explanatory

Interpreting the process of investigation in a sensitive manner to the child. An advancement of the child's understanding of their situation is a legitimate aim of the GAL's intervention; this point is well made by Schofield & Thoburn (1996).

Research

The role of the GAL in family proceedings is a new one, although comparable systems in Scotland (the curator *ad litem*) and in the USA pre-date the setting up of panels in the UK.

Early studies of panels of GALs and ROs focused on the wide variations there were between local authorities in the size of the panels, the personnel appointed and the use made of the service by the courts. Those acting as GALs, the overwhelming majority of whom are experienced social workers, are either freelance, fee-attracting, local authority employees offering a service to a neighbouring authority's panel on a reciprocal basis, or employees of another agency, usually a voluntary agency or a probation service. In Coyle's (1987) study of the work of GALs, of 130 GALs interviewed, 54% were employed full-time with a voluntary or statutory agency and 29% were self-employed; a further 14% were self-employed with voluntary or statutory agencies. The figures quoted in the Children Act 1989 Report for panel membership at 31 March 1992 show that the numbers of fee-attracting or self-employed GALs had risen to 56.6% – local authority employees accounted for 28.1%, and probation officers and members of voluntary organisations accounted for a further 15.2% (DOH 1992b).

It is clear from the change in the figures over 6 years and from the reduction in overall numbers of GALs (2366 in 1989–1990 to 1327 in 1992) that there has been a general trend away from large numbers of workers doing a small amount of work each, in favour of smaller, more work-intensive panels, composed primarily of self-employed GALs. There is some evidence of a North/South divide, with reciprocal panels composed of local authority social workers being more common in the north of the UK, and panels of mainly or solely fee-attracting GALs predominating in the south of the UK. In one or two places in the north of the UK, teams of dedicated GALs have been employed and this model may have attractions when new plans for court welfare services are developed.

Feedback from the courts has been generally enthusiastic about the work of GALS. Justices' Clerks interviewed in the course of Coyle's (1987) study commented favourably on the help given by GALs to the courts in resolving difficult cases, and on the quality and general acceptability of the reports produced. Many of the clerks were, however, concerned about the delay in concluding cases where a GAL had been appointed. There is no clear evidence, however, about whether GALs contribute significantly to delays and, if so, in what ways. As the Social Services Inspectorate (SSI) has argued, further research is needed before the causes and effects of delays in making decisions about the future of abused children become clearer (Socio-legal Centre for Family Studies & University of Bristol 1993).

Several studies have described the weight given to recommendations made by the GAL. As a recent SSI report comments, 'Courts put great weight on the GALs' contributions and followed their recommendations in over 90% of care and related proceedings in the sample' (SSI 1990). A case which went to appeal not long after the establishment of GAL panels, called for the following comment from Sir John Arnold, then president of the Family Division:

It is well established in relation to appeals from magistrates that if they fail to follow the advice which they receive – for example from a probation officer, without any justification for that failure, then the appeal will ordinarily be allowed. Exactly the same consideration must apply, in my judgement, to the views of the Guardian *ad litem*.

(Devon County Council v Clancy [1985])

There has been some research undertaken to elicit the views of children about the representation of their wishes and feelings by the GAL. Masson & Oakley (1999), for example, comment:

focusing on the child and looking at care proceedings from the standpoint of the children involved in them highlights parts of the process not previously examined in studies of guardians *ad litem*, solicitors and court proceedings. Despite Butler-Sloss L.J.'s often repeated statement that the child is a person, not an object of concern, 'children and their concerns have been omitted from much of what is written about court proceedings for children's protection. This study has tried to redress that balance'.

Appraisal of the work of GALs is a subject which has exercised the Department of Health and panel managers. Most panels have introduced appraisal systems, requiring GALs to be interviewed about their work and to produce examples of written reports, and advice about the GAL's competence is sought from courts and solicitors. More recently there has been an emphasis on obtaining feedback from children, parents, social workers and others involved in the court process. The moves towards formal appraisal of GALs and the increased gathering of feedback are important because of complaints that GALs were formerly subject to very little control or oversight, a situation which allowed some poor or 'maverick' practice to flourish unchecked.

Since the DOH's issue of guidelines to panel managers, there has been an expectation that panels will be organised on similar lines across the country, and that mechanisms for appointment, appraisal and dismissal of GALs will be in hand, guided by a panel advisory committee. It is acknowledged that panels will have different compositions, but there is some argument that a relatively small, well-occupied but flexible panel works best (DOH 1992*b*). Evidence also suggests that qualified and experienced social workers are most likely to have the knowledge necessary to be a GAL, and that GALs must keep abreast of research and practice developments by having access to high-quality training and adequate support.

Plans are in hand for the reorganisation of the GALRO service, as a result of the Government's stated intention to combine it with the Family Court Welfare Service (formerly part of the Probation Service) and that part of the Official Solicitor's Department which deals with children matters. It remains to be seen to what extent the present independent GALRO service will survive; the challenge remains as set out by the Bristol Report on Child Representation (Murch *et al.* 1990):

To design a management structure which preserves autonomy of decision-making and practitioner control over the management of individual cases but is able to monitor professional standards and evaluate both effectiveness and efficiency.

Independence

A key quality of the GAL system, as envisaged in the 1970s, was independence. It was seen as essential that the GAL should be independent of the social services department bringing proceedings, and of the child's parents or other relatives. Care has been taken from the inception of the role to ensure that the person appointed as GAL has no prior knowledge of the case, unless, of course, it is a reappointment for the same child in fresh proceedings. Thus, it has been seen by every study as a major flaw that the GAL service continues to be a responsibility of social services departments. As the joint ADSS/ACC/AMA* officers stated in their report, dated April 1986:

Almost all sources doubted whether true independence of GALs/ROs can be compatible with a local authority's responsibility to set up, administer, train and finance the panels.

(Quoted in Coyle 1987)

Similarly, Independent Representation for Children in Need (IRCHIN) commented:

If panel members are to work independently and are to be seen to be working independently, they must be free from outside pressures and constraints. This is extremely difficult unless they have an independent administrative structure from which to operate ... the difficulty with the present arrangement is that panels are funded and administered by the local authorities.

(IRCHIN 1985*a*)

Following the implementation of the Children Act 1989, attempts have been made to distance the administration of panels from the managerial structure of social services departments by the appointment of panel managers working with advisory committees which have independent representation, and by the setting up of complaints boards, again with independent representation.

These attempts to organise panels of GALs separately from the structure of social services departments, whose work it is the responsibility of GALs to appraise, are clearly to be welcomed. However, to most outside professionals and, more importantly, to many families involved in family proceedings as a result of

---

* Association of Directors of Social Services, Association of County Councils and Association of Metropolitan Authorities.

allegations of child abuse, such improvements do not detract from the fact that GALs are paid by social services departments. That the Government has allocated funds specifically for the administration of panels does not answer the widespread objections to the service being located within social services departments.

In November 1991, Cornwall GALs took the issue of budgetary independence to Judicial Review, following an attempt by the Director of Social Services to impose time limits on the amount of work that could be done by a GAL on a particular case (R v Cornwall County Council [1992]). The President of the Family Division, Sir Stephen Brown, found in favour of the GAL: 'This case underlined the importance of guardians *ad litem* being seen as officers of the court whose professional decisions should not be constrained by the administrative dictate of social services' (quoted in Murch & Hooper 1992).

The case did, however, illustrate the vulnerability of the GALs, who work very much as individuals and who, in the Cornwall case, had to request personal donations from other guardians across the country in order to cover their costs in bringing the action to Judicial Review.

The proposed reorganisation of existing services under the new Children and Family Court Advisory and Support Service (CAFCASS) will bring the GALRO service under the control of the Lord Chancellor's department, which should remove the longstanding concerns about independence whilst local authorities had the management of panels.

Resources

GALs have been criticised for making unrealistic recommendations about the plans which should be made for children, suggesting the use of resources that are not available and thereby causing dissatisfaction and disappointment to children and their families. It is not difficult to envisage the basis for such complaints, particularly given the aspirations of the Children Act to ensure the cooperation of all the authorities concerned with children and their families (section 27) and to provide a wide range of services to children in need (section 17).

Should the GAL be recommending an ideal or a realistic course of action for the child? Many other professionals concerned with children may have asked themselves what aspirations for children are reasonable. To take an example, should the GAL recommend that a mother and baby be kept together in a therapeutic and educational environment even though no such facility exists in the area, or should the discussion focus on what might be the next best solution – perhaps the placement of the baby in foster care with liberal contact for the mother? I take the view that it is the responsibility of the GAL to consider all the options, discussing the merits and disadvantages of each, and making it clear why certain options are unlikely to be viable. It is only by making clear statements about the absence of necessary resources that GALs will be able to build up a case to show the negative, and often ultimately costly, effects of lack of provisions.

A further argument about resources concerns the diversion of finances and skilled personnel away from hard-pressed social services departments into the GAL service. It is undeniable that social workers and front-line professionals like teachers and health visitors are under extreme pressure as a result of increasing demands for their services and cut-backs in local and central government funding. GAL panels have undoubtedly taken some experienced workers from actual or potential posts in social work teams. As the National Children's Bureau's submission to the House of Commons Social Services Committee states:

One further cost ... has been to deprive existing child care teams of senior members. It is important that ways are found to encourage such experienced personnel to return to local authority child care work after a period as guardians, bringing back with them the additional expertise gained from working as a guardian.

(National Children's Bureau 1988)

However, the issues involved in child abuse cases which come before the courts are extremely serious, and the GAL system does ensure that each case is looked at by an experienced social worker with specialist expertise, whose sole perspective is the welfare of the child. It is clearly important that the expertise of the GAL service is fed back into the work of social services departments in a constructive way. It may also be the case that a substantial number of freelance GALs have been attracted to the work specifically because it can be done flexibly and accommodated with other responsibilities, professional or personal. The SSI (1990) report made this point:

The growth in the number of freelance members has been marked. They were a previously untapped source of scarce, skilled labour, and have provided a flexible workforce useful in meeting the uneven demand for the service.

Financial constraints

There is likely to be continuing tension between GALs and local authority social workers in the area of finance. To social workers, it can appear that the GAL has no financial constraints and can do work the key social worker cannot do, either because of lack of time or because a directive from management forbids it. GALs do have a great deal of personal freedom to decide how much work to do on the child's behalf, and this freedom has received legal sanction in the Cornwall judgement mentioned earlier. It remains to be seen whether this will change in the context of the CAFCASS.

However, both social workers and GALs are committed to providing optimum services for children and their families at a time of reduced public finances, and there is a responsibility on panel managers to ensure that the resources of their members are used economically. GALs are gaining confidence in limiting their work, underlining good local authority practice where it is observed, restricting their work where a case is overwhelmingly made out and reserving major pieces of intervention for those cases where the issues are complex or very finely balanced, or where there appear to be major flaws in the local authority's or parents' cases.

It is incumbent upon the GAL to seek the views of all those who may have a contribution to make relevant to the child's future, and frequently the GAL is able to talk to important people whose views have not previously been heard. A class teacher at the child's school (or a playgroup or nursery worker for a younger child) may have a very particular account to give of the child's activities, behaviour or friendships. These workers may not have had a chance to attend a case conference. Equally, a relative living at a distance, or friends from a previous home area, may have important views to contribute but may not have been interviewed by the local authority social worker.

Sometimes workers from other disciplines and relatives and friends of the child are very relieved to be able to speak freely to the GAL, appreciating the GAL's position of independence, particularly if they have reservations about the local authority's case, or if they have had previous unfortunate experiences with a social services department. It is therefore essential that the GAL should be at liberty to research any views that may be pertinent to the child's future. Some critics have referred to the unfairness of a 'Rolls Royce' service being offered to some children and not to others, but the emphasis, particularly since the implementation of the 1989 Act, on bringing before the court only those cases that have been impossible to solve in any other way, perhaps indicates that these cases involve the children who deserve the most thorough examination of all the circumstances and options. As the IRCHIN *Training Notes* (1985*b*) state:

> Firstly – and most fundamentally – is (the point) summed up by Brenda Hoggett in her book *Parents and Children*, 'any child whose future has to be decided in litigation has already been deprived of his best interests.'
>
> (Hoggett 1985)

Another financial constraint on a service composed largely of self-employed individuals is the absence of back-up for essential resources needed by the GAL. GALs are responsible for their own office administration, training, library and professional support. There is a sense in which this is right and proper if they are to function as independent professionals, but the inevitable consequences are an unevenness in the resources at the disposal of individual GALs, and a reluctance amongst many to involve themselves in training and organisational events when these have to be paid for and when they represent a serious loss of earnings.

Plans for reorganisation, assuming that they include centralised office facilities, will benefit GALs and help provide a more consistent service.

Causes of delay

One of the early concerns about the appointment of GALs in care proceedings, as mentioned earlier, was that this would cause a delay in dealing with child care cases coming before the courts. Murch & Bader (1984), in their early survey, report the views of many Justices' Clerks: 'cases chosen for GAL reports now take much longer to complete, both in the preparatory stages, and in the trial itself'.

This is echoed in the SSI report published 6 years later: 'The demand for the service has increased and GALs and ROs have generally taken longer to complete cases than had been anticipated' (SSI 1990). There is a danger in assuming that all delay is harmful to the child. Clearly, there are some cases where an adjournment of the final hearing for a specific purpose, for example, to allow a piece of intensive work to be undertaken with the parents or to allow a child to build up a link with an absent relative, can be very beneficial to the child.

There is also a view that the potential increase in the number of parties, following the implementation of the Children Act 1989, has of itself added to delays. The GAL has a clear responsibility quickly to locate and interview anyone who may have a right to be appointed as a party, and to advise the court of the benefits or otherwise to the child. Recent case law suggests that party status is unlikely to be given to relatives whose case is very similar to that of another party (G v Kirklees M.C., 31 July 1992).

Delays in appointing a GAL to the proceedings continue to be a problem in some parts of the country. The Cleveland inquiry drew attention to the unwarranted delay caused by the need to appoint a GAL (DHSS 1988), and the more recent SSI report (1990) concedes that there is still cause for concern:

> Although there was some evidence of improvement in the time taken between request and appointment of GALs and ROs, long delays were still common. Undoubtedly this has been detrimental to the interests of many children because they have had to wait too long for major decisions about their lives to be made.

There are some indications that delays in appointment of GALs occur more frequently in those panels which rely heavily on GALs who are social workers for a neighbouring authority. Where panels employ a majority of freelance guardians, or those who work exclusively as GALs, delays are not apparent and an appointment can usually be made in time for the GAL to be present at the first interim hearing of the case, or at an emergency protection order hearing. A few panels now operate a duty system to ensure that even hearings held at very short notice can benefit from a GAL's attendance.

The trend towards long, drawn out hearings is a concern, but it is perhaps a consequence of a desire to hear the maximum amount of evidence in the most complex and bitterly contested cases. Justices' Clerks who complained that, 'sometimes more information merely serves to confuse the issue' (Coyle 1987) would surely not suggest that information should be withheld in child abuse cases merely to expedite the outcome. There is a responsibility for the GAL to make a clear summary of the issues and to indicate which particular matters are central and disputed. If these are clearly set out at a directions hearing, and a proper timetable for the filing of reports is made and adhered to, delays should be kept to a minimum. However, the GAL is, above all, the child's representative and should sanction or request delay where this is essential to ensure that the child's needs are met. As the *Manual of Practice Guidance for Guardians* ad litem *and Reporting Officers* states:

The purpose of their liaison and communication with the court is not to ease the passage of the case through the courts as an end in itself, but to secure the welfare of the child by so doing.

(DOH 1992*a*)

Guardians around the country report a rise in cases that 'settle', obviating the need for a costly, contested final hearing. There are clear benefits to a process of mediation and compromise which leads to an agreed order, but it can also be important to have evidence heard and tested in such a way that all parties can move forward.

Implications for practice

Understanding and interpreting the child's wishes and feelings

The United Nations Convention on the Rights of the Child 1989 has been influential in bringing the wishes and feelings of children into prominence. Articles 3 and 12 are particularly pertinent to children involved in court proceedings (see Butler, Chapter 9, in this volume).

Communicating effectively with children and interpreting their wishes and feelings is perhaps the central task of the GAL. It is far from being easy, given the time limits of the GAL's role and the number of people with whom the child may already have had to communicate prior to the guardian's arrival. As Masson & Shaw (1986) have commented:

The notion (central to the function of the guardian *ad litem*) of an independent person coming in to take a fresh look at a child's situation runs into difficulties in the face of the reluctance of most children to confide readily in unfamiliar adults.

Nevertheless, the GAL has a unique opportunity to spend time with the child playing, talking and observing, in order to put forward as comprehensive a view as possible of the child's wishes and feelings. Most GALs have developed a wide repertoire of games, stories and toys to engage younger children, and a variety of techniques to explore the feelings and views of older children. Some children, although young, can offer a sophisticated account of their history and family members as well as clear wishes of their own, whilst others can do little more than indicate where their feelings are very raw, or where they are strongly attracted to a particular person.

Often children's behaviour is a more powerful indicator of their feelings than what they actually say. For example, a child may insist that they definitely wish to return home, but on being told that this is not thought by the court to be in their best interests, may respond with relaxed and settled behaviour in their foster home and at school.

Some commentaries on the Children Act 1989 suggest that it puts undue emphasis on the child's wishes and feelings, at the expense of a proper consideration of the child's best interests. This is illustrated by a recently reported private law case in which a 12-year-old child who, having spent her whole life with her mother, was made the subject of a residence order in favour of her father after a brief court hearing during which she had expressed a preference to live with her father. An unidentified psychiatrist commented that:

> The Act completely misunderstands child psychology. In a case like this, the child's comments should obviously be taken very, very seriously. But, that's not the same as acting upon them without proper evaluation.
>
> (Phillips 1993)

In the even more complex arena of child abuse, it seems to be crucially important that the GAL, whilst listening carefully and sympathetically to the child's views, does not put more responsibility on the child than is appropriate.

Waite L.J. in Re T (child representation), put the issue very succinctly:

> Children should have attention paid to their views, but be spared the risk of making, through lack of insight, understanding or maturity, choices which accord with their wishes but are in conflict with their genuine interests.
>
> (Quoted in Wall 1998)

Legislation allows for the child to put their own views directly to the solicitor appointed, and for the solicitor to take instructions separately from the child if those instructions differ from the GAL's. To take instructions from the child alone, the solicitor must decide on the child's capacity so to do. The *Guide for Guardians* ad litem *in the Juvenile Court* (DHSS 1984) sets out the position clearly.

Court rules provide that the GAL gives instructions to the solicitor except where the solicitor considers, having taken into account the views of the guardian, that the child wishes to give instructions which conflict with those of the guardian and is able, having regard to his age and understanding, to give instructions on his own behalf. In these circumstances the solicitor has a clear duty to act on instructions from the child.

This is, in my experience, a rare occurrence, but even in these circumstances there is provision for the court to hear both about the child's wishes and feelings and an independent view as to their best interests.

Consulting widely on the child's best interests

As has been stated earlier, it is difficult to talk in terms of the child's best interests when their future has to be decided by a court. One is generally looking at the least detrimental alternative among possibilities that are much less than ideal.

The early DHSS guidance to GALs, which reflects the wording of the Court Rules to Magistrates 1970, stated that, 'The guardian *ad litem*'s first and paramount consideration must be the need to safeguard the child's best interests *until he achieves adulthood*' (DHSS 1984; italics added).

This was a high, perhaps impossible, expectation and the wording has not been included in subsequent legislation, although the *Code of Ethics* produced by the National Association of Guardians *ad litem* and Reporting Officers (NAGALRO 1991) has a similar aspiration. There are issues on which it is very difficult to determine the best long-term interests of the child. Disputes over contact for a child who is in the care of the local authority can be particularly difficult. It can be argued with equal force both that an abused child is distressed and unsettled by contact with the abusing parents, and that it is in the child's long-term interests to retain contact with their natural family. In such finely balanced decisions, it seems important to have a reasoned view expressed by an independent person who will be biased neither towards the understandable aspirations of the parents, nor towards the equally understandable views of substitute carers, but who is seeking to determine the best interests of the child.

Judith Timms of IRCHIN, sums up well the task of the GAL in reconciling different views as to the best interests of the child:

> Panel members can be presented with numerous different interpretations of the child's best interests, as viewed by the local authority, the social worker, the solicitor, other involved professionals, the natural family, the foster parents, and – most importantly – the child. It is in attempting to balance these differential interpretations that panel members will be confronted with the most onerous aspects of their role, while bearing in mind that 'best' interests can quickly become 'vested' interests in an adversarial situation.
>
> (Timms 1985)

Evaluating conflicting evidence

Following on from the last issue, the GAL, in completing the investigation may have to reconcile conflicting evidence from equally well-qualified professionals, or from apparently equally convinced private parties. GALs will inevitably have to take into account their own observations and attempt to test their hypotheses. Masson & Shaw (1986) offer an interesting comment on this issue:

> Perhaps the most marked difference of approach we noted is between those guardians who tend to take the 'facts' of the case as given, and those who adopt a more creative approach, testing and to some extent re-working the material to see if there is scope for changing the facts. For example, is a child's opposition to parental contact a fact to be respected or one to be explained and possibly modified? Is lapsed parental contact to be taken as given or should the guardian attempt to discover the reason for this lapse or perhaps propose a contract approach to restoring contact. (p. 38)

I would suggest that, faced with conflicting evidence on important issues, GALs have no choice but to make their own clear observations known, if necessary setting up situations in which hypotheses can be tested.

It is clear that the GAL's case will be very influential in court, particularly when other professional views are polarised. It is an important part of the role of the GAL to indicate the wide range of opinion there may be in relation to a particular case, before making clear the grounds for their own opinion. Other parties may omit or gloss over pieces of evidence that do not fit comfortably with their case, but the GAL has an obligation to put the whole picture before the court.

Promoting good practice

The preceding paragraphs make clear that the GAL needs to be particularly well-informed in the face of conflicting evidence and opposed views on the child's best interests. Sometimes a particular case will require an enormous amount of research, and in other cases knowledge of professional viewpoints and an ability to evaluate the merits of each will be required. The GAL has an advantage in having a constant workload of very different cases, and is likely to have had considerably more concentrated exposure than the social worker. This is particularly true of problems and syndromes that are on the increase or are newly recognised – for example, drug addiction, AIDS, Munchhausen's syndrome by proxy and sexual abuse.

There is a responsibility on GALs to seek to promote good practice in the care of children, by disseminating research findings, questioning poor practice and validating examples of good practice. The SSI (1990) report *In the Interests of Children* states that the GALs support the local authority's case in 84% of cases. This does not take account, however, of those instances where the GAL's involvement may cause the local authority to modify their application or their plans, or to withdraw unfounded applications completely. Research is awaited on the influence of GALs on local authority practice from the point of view of both parties.

It is the impression of the writer that the early influence of the GAL in court proceedings has somewhat waned, partly as a result of local authorities being more confident in advancing their own views and partly as a result of the rise in importance of the 'expert'. It is to be hoped that decisions about children will increasingly be made according to the quality of evidence given, from whichever source it comes.

It must be said that the GAL's viewpoint is restricted to a brief period of time, and the longer time perspective of the social worker and others should never be under-rated. However, a re-evaluation of a well-known situation by an independent person can sometimes identify a new way forward which merits consideration.

Summary and conclusions

Situations of child abuse that are brought to a court for consideration will involve the appointment of a GAL, an independent person who is almost always an experienced social worker. The appointed GAL will have the task of representing to the court the child's wishes and feelings, and recommending a course of action that will be most likely to promote the child's best interests. In order to fulfil this task, the GAL will need to get to know the child as well as possible in a defined period of time and conduct a thorough investigation of all the circumstances of the case, consulting widely and using their experience and knowledge to evaluate conflicting opinion and research evidence.

Court proceedings, when a family's problems and relationships are exposed to public scrutiny, can be traumatic and distressing, and it is an important responsibility of the GAL to ensure that the case is properly and expeditiously carried forward, and that the child's welfare is paramount. It is to be hoped that the involvement of exclusively child-centred workers will lead eventually to improvements in the legal system which will reflect the needs of children as well as adults and which will ensure that children who have been abused in their own families are not further abused by the court process.

Annotated further reading

Adcock M, White R (eds) 1985 Good enough parenting. British Agencies for Adoption and Fostering, London

This book contains useful chapters on the assessment of parenting (Margaret Adcock) and an invaluable discussion on 'good enough', borderline and 'bad enough' parenting (Christine Cooper).

Adcock M, White R, Hollows A 1991 Significant harm: its management and outcome. Significant Publications, Croydon

This collection of papers focuses on assessment of harm against the background of the Children Act 1989. The contribution of David P H Jones on the effectiveness of intervention is particularly helpful to GALs in deciding whether rehabilitation of an abused child to their family is likely to be viable, and there is also a useful chapter by Annie Lau on cultural and ethnic perspectives.

Aldgate J, Simmonds J (eds) 1988 Direct work with children. B T Batsford, London

Although this collection of papers is aimed primarily at social workers, its themes of listening to children and helping them to make sense of their past experiences, as well as planning for the future, are relevant to the work of GALs. Case examples are taken from the work of students on the Advanced Diploma in Social Work with Children and Families at Goldsmiths' College, and, in that the work of the students was strictly time-limited, it offers useful suggestions for the intervention of GALs.

Department of Health and Social Security (DHSS) 1985 Social work decisions in childcare. HMSO, London

A useful summary of research relevant to child care decision-making, based on nine research reports. (See DHSS 1991, for an update of this report.)

Department of Health and Social Security (DHSS) 1991 Patterns and outcomes in child placement. HMSO, London

This is an update of the DHSS (1985) report on similar focuses and messages from research, but against the background of the Children Act 1989.

Hetherington R, Cooper A, Smith P, Wilford G 1997 Protecting children: messages from Europe. The Stationery Office, London

A book which sets child protection issues in a European context and challenges assumptions by presenting alternative visions of how children can best be protected.

King P, Young I 1992 The child as client. Family Law, Bristol

This book was written specifically for solicitors who represent children, but it covers the principles that must govern the work of a GAL, and it deals in considerable detail with the partnership between the GAL and the solicitor. The book discusses the practical steps that are necessary in order to ensure that the child's case is properly put, and it also covers ethical issues and problems of communication and assessment.

Masson J, Oakley M W 1999 Out of hearing. Representing children in care proceedings. NSPCC and John Wiley, London

This comprehensive picture of representation for children is based on interviews with older children who were involved in court proceedings and on the views of professionals seeking to assist them.

Reder P, Lucey C (eds) 1995 Assessment of parenting: psychiatric and psychological contributions. Routledge, London

A useful compilation of contributions from experts in the field of parenting and risk assessment.

References

Coyle C 1987 The practitioner's view of the role and tasks of guardians *ad litem* and reporting officers. Barnardo's Research and Development Section, London

Department of Health (DOH) 1992*a* Manual of practice guidance for guardians *ad litem* and reporting officers. HMSO, London

Department of Health (DOH) 1992*b* Children Act Report 1991 HMSO, London

Department of Health and Social Security (DHSS) 1974 Report of the committee of inquiry into the care and supervision provided in relation to Maria Colwell. HMSO, London

Department of Health and Social Security (DHSS) 1984 Guide for guardians *ad litem* in the juvenile court. HMSO, London

Department of Health and Social Security (DHSS) 1988 Report of the inquiry into child abuse in Cleveland 1987. HMSO, London

Hoggett B 1987 Parents and children, 3rd edn. Sweet and Maxwell, London

Independent Representation for Children in Need (IRCHIN) 1985*a* Representing children. IRCHIN, Wirral, UK

Independent Representation for Children in Need (IRCHIN) 1985*b* Training notes for guardians *ad litem* and reporting officers. IRCHIN, Wirral, UK

Masson J, Oakley M W 1999 Out of hearing. Representing children in care proceedings. NSPCC and John Wiley, London

Masson J, Shaw M 1986 Guardians *ad litem* in care cases. University of Leicester, Centre for Law and Social Work Research, Leicester

Murch M, Bader K 1984 Separate representation for parents and children: an examination of the initial phase. Family Law, Bristol

Murch M, Hooper D 1992 The family justice system. Family Law, Bristol

Murch M, Hunt J, Macleod A 1990 Representation of the child in the civil courts – research report for the Department of Health. Summary of conclusions and recommendations. Socio-Legal Centre for Family Studies, University of Bristol

National Association of Guardians *ad litem* and Reporting Officers (NAGALRO) 1991 Code of ethics, code of practice for guardians *ad litem* and reporting officers. Statement of policy in regard to equal opportunities. NAGALRO

National Children's Bureau 1988 Review of progress on children in care. Submission to House of Commons Social Services Committee

Phillips M 1993 Ninety minutes to lose a daughter. *Guardian*, 13 February

Schofield G, Thoburn J 1996 Child protection. The voice of the child in decision-making. Institute for Public Policy Research, London

Social Services Inspectorate (SSI) 1990 In the interests of children, an inspection of the guardian *ad litem* and reporting officer service. HMSO, London

Socio-Legal Centre for Family Studies, University of Bristol 1993 Avoidable delay in care proceedings. Conference report. Department of Health, London

Timms J 1985 The task of the guardian *ad litem*. In: IRCHIN (ed) Training notes for guardians *ad litem* and reporting officers. IRCHIN, Wirral, UK

Wall J 1998 What about the children? Issues in public and private law relating to welfare and legal representation, Seen and Heard 8 (3):

19

Child protection and the criminal justice system

John Williams

John Williams

INTRODUC-TION

Children who have been the victims of abuse may be called upon to give evidence in criminal proceedings if it is decided that prosecution of the perpetrator is appropriate. Very often their evidence, and their demeanour when presenting it, will be crucial to the outcome of the proceedings. Children may also be called upon to give evidence as bystander witnesses, especially of abuse within a family. For most adults the potential trauma that a child may experience through reliving their experience is unimaginable. The formalities and the adult setting of a courtroom will further add to the child's experience.

Many areas of the civil law process have addressed the issues surrounding the appearance of children as witnesses. Although falling far short of perfection, child care proceedings endeavour to recognise the vulnerability of children and to make appropriate allowances. It is encouraging to note that significant improvements have been made to the way in which children are assisted in giving evidence in criminal proceedings, although there is always room for improvement. There is an increased awareness by those involved in the criminal justice system of the need to recognise the vulnerability of children.

However, in criminal proceedings, care also has to be taken to balance the welfare of the child with the rights of the accused. This will be of even greater importance now the Human Rights Act 1998 is in force. Until recently, very little was done to make the criminal courts less threatening to children giving evidence. The interest shown in this area illustrates the concern of professionals, parents and children regarding the potential for further abuse of children by exposing them to a system that fails to recognise their special status. This chapter considers the policy issues behind the law and explains the implications for the various professionals and individuals who have contact with child witnesses in the criminal courts.

Review of literature and research findings

The impact of the criminal justice process on vulnerable witnesses is a burgeoning area of research. Although initial interest was merely an offshoot of the increase in awareness of the plight of victims in general, it continues to develop into a discrete area of research. The early work of Hardin on the potential for the use of a guardian *ad litem* in America provided an impetus for research in this country (Hardin 1987, Spencer 1990). The study of child victims conducted by Morgan & Zedner (1992) provides a basis for exploring ways of enhancing the plight of child victims, revealing the shortcomings of the present *ad hoc* response to the needs of child victims.

Morgan & Williams (1992) made a number of suggestions as to how procedures could be improved. They point out that the reforms should not be seen as a panacea – children may still suffer avoidable trauma even with the changes accomplished by the Criminal Justice Act 1991 (Morgan & Williams 1992,

1993). Importantly, research findings dispel the myth that children are unreliable witnesses and compulsive liars, or are unable to distinguish fact from fantasy (Goodman & Helgeson 1985, Jones 1987). This has done much to remove the prejudice against child witnesses.

A number of research studies have been undertaken on the plight of the vulnerable witness and the working of the procedures in place to protect them. More recently, Davies & Westcott undertook a major review of the research literature on interviewing children. Their report, *Interviewing Child Witnesses under the Memorandum of Good Practice: A Research Review,* provides an excellent summary of the main research findings (Davies & Westcott 1999). A Home Office Interdepartmental Working Group also looked at vulnerable witnesses more generally. It made a number of important recommendations on the protection of vulnerable adults and children in the criminal justice system. Many of these recommendations were implemented by the Youth Justice and Criminal Evidence Act 1999 (Home Office 1998*a*).

Cassel & Bjorklund's (1995) work on questioning children during interviews also provides some useful guidance on repeated suggestive interviews. Similarly, Bull (1995) stresses the importance of the rapport stage of interview under the *Memorandum of Good Practice* (Home Office & Department of Health. 1992). The Scottish Office (1998*a*) guidance on 'appropriate adults', although not applicable to children, identifies a very valuable model for the introduction of a support person in England and Wales. It's emphasis on joint working and careful planning, plus a clear understanding of agency responsibility, is an excellent template for future developments. The research has clearly identified weaknesses in the system. The 1999 Act has gone some way towards addressing these, but only in the courtroom environment and that is only one part of the process.

An analysis of the policy issues

The question of children giving evidence in criminal proceedings highlights the tension between the legitimate objectives of the criminal justice system and the emphasis placed by the civil law process on the welfare of the child. This is inevitable as each is seeking to achieve an objective that may, although does not necessarily, conflict with the other. One important area of conflict between the two systems is that in general terms, the criminal justice system seeks to determine guilt or innocence. It also provides safeguards for the accused by, for example, placing the burden of proof on the prosecution, and by the laws of evidence. Civil law child protection proceedings are, however, designed to safeguard and promote the welfare of children (see s. 1 Children Act 1989). This tension does not mean that the needs of child witnesses cannot be accommodated within the criminal justice system, or that the rights of those suspected of abuse or neglect should be ignored in civil law care proceedings.

Each system must ensure that it does not fatally compromise its own principles to an unacceptable level. This is particularly important when considering the different standards of proof required by the criminal and civil systems. The criminal courts require proof beyond all reasonable doubt, whereas the civil courts operate on the basis of the balance of probabilities. The clear dividing line between the two is, in some instances, becoming blurred. The House of Lords in Re H (minors) (Sexual abuse; standard of proof) [1996] AC 563) held that the more serious the nature of the behaviour alleged in care proceedings, the stronger the evidence must be. Lord Nicholls said,

Built into the preponderance of probability standard is a serious degree of flexibility in respect of the seriousness of the allegation. Although the standard is much the same, this does not mean that where a serious allegation is in issue the standard of proof required is higher. It means only that the inherent probability of an event is itself a matter to be taken into account when weighing the probabilities and deciding whether, on balance, the event occurred.

Jane Fortin is quite rightly sceptical about the claim by Lord Nicholls that this approach does not mean that the standard of proof is higher. This argument, she claims, 'bears all the hallmarks of casuistry' (Fortin 1998, p. 384).

Clearly the criminal justice system must ensure that it protects the right of the accused to a fair trial. This has even greater significance with the implementation of the Human Rights Act 1998. This Act incorporates the rights and freedoms contained in the European Convention on Human Rights into the law of the UK. Under the Act, it is unlawful for a 'public authority' to act in a way that is incompatible with the Convention. Section 6 of the Act includes in the definition of public authority 'a court or tribunal' as well as any other body whose functions are 'functions of a public nature'. Article 6 of the Convention provides for the right to a fair trial. It states:

In the determination of his civil rights and obligations or of any criminal charge against him, everyone is entitled to a fair and public hearing within a reasonable time by an independent and impartial tribunal.

Article 6 does not make reference to any rights of witnesses and victims, especially those who may be vulnerable through age or disability. This does not mean that their rights are ignored under the Convention. The European Court has emphasised the importance of having regard to the interests of witnesses.

It is true that Article 6 does not explicitly require the interests of witnesses in general, and those of victims called upon to testify in particular, to be taken into consideration. However, their life, liberty or security of person may be at stake, as may interests coming generally within the ambit of Article 8 of the Convention ... Against this background, principles of fair trial also require that in appropriate cases the interests of the defence are balance against those of witnesses or victims called upon to testify.
(Doorson v Netherlands [1966] 22 EHRR 330, para. 70)

Similarly, in Baegen v Netherlands, the Commission was of the view that,

in criminal proceedings concerning sexual abuse certain measures may be taken for the purpose of protecting the victim, provided that such measures can be reconciled with an adequate and effective exercise of the rights of the defence.
(A/327-B [1995] para. 77)

The Court and the Commission provide little guidance on how the balance between the interests of the accused and witnesses is achieved. However, they do affirm the principle underlying the legal protection provided by domestic law, namely that witnesses do have recognised rights within the judicial system.

In spite of such tensions, the criminal justice and civil law systems can work together very effectively. This is illustrated by the procedures in place for the joint investigation by police and social services of child abuse. *Working Together to Safeguard Children* (Department of Health (DOH) 1999) emphasises the point that the police 'recognise the fundamental importance of inter-agency working, as illustrated by well-established arrangements for joint training involving police and social work colleagues' (para 3.48). The more general responsibility of the police towards the welfare of the child is recognised by the fact that the police should be informed of cases of suspected abuse even though further action by them is not envisaged (para 3.51). Morgan & Zedner (1992) found in their early study that a number of difficulties have arisen, mainly because of the different philosophies of the two agencies. However, despite their different cultures and statutory frameworks the two agencies have succeeded in developing a more integrated approach to interviewing children. The success of joint investigation is illustrated by the fact that it has been developed in the majority of police forces in England and Wales (Conroy *et al.* 1990).

It should not therefore be impossible to create a workable rapprochement between the civil and criminal processes. It is essential, however, that the differences between the two systems are recognised and not ignored. It is also necessary to ensure that children are prepared for these differences.

Implications for practice

Pre-trial

Courtrooms are not designed to accommodate the special needs of children and other vulnerable people. Evidence shows that children are particularly vulnerable when appearing as witnesses in criminal proceedings and are likely to be highly stressed (Spencer & Flin 1993). This is likely to affect the child's ability to give evidence in the courtroom (Goodman *et al.* 1992). According to Flin, 'The question of children's stress during the pre-trial period is extremely significant because prosecutors may decide whether to proceed with a case on the basis of the child's emotional fitness to testify' (Flin 1990). Anything that can be done to minimise the stress will improve the quality of the evidence given by the child. It will also help to reduce the 'secondary victimisation' which can result from a courtroom appearance (Sanders *et al.* 1997).

Pre-trial preparation for children is essential. However, it is important to recognise that there is a distinction between helping the child prior to appearance in court and coaching the child. Any attempt to coach the child as a means of preparing them would run the risk of the testimony being excluded. The *Child Witness Pack* (Home Office 1993), which has been replaced by the *Young Witness Pack* (National Society for the Prevention of Cruelty to Children (NSPCC) 1998), is designed to give children and young people an idea of what will happen when they appear in court. Part of the pack is a booklet for parents and carers and also a handbook for practitioners. In Scotland, the Lord Advocate's office has published *Going to Court as a Witness*, aimed at 5–12-year-olds and 12–16-year-olds (Scottish Office 1998*b*). The *Child Witness Pack* was evaluated in 1995 and the majority of respondents found that it was useful, although there was some concern over the style and suitability for target groups (Plotnikoff & Woolfson 1995). However, research indicates that these packs are only used for 25% of children (Annon. 1996).

Unfortunately, it is unclear which statutory agency has the duty to provide pre-trial support for child witnesses (Sanders *et al.* 1997). As is often the case where a number of different agencies are involved, there is a lack of clarity of responsibility. Any child about to face an appearance as a witness in criminal proceedings could come within the definition of a child in need under the Children Act 1989. Arguably the child's health or development could be significantly impaired without the provision of assistance (s.17(10)(b) Children Act 1989). However, difficulties may be encountered if the social services authority is taking a leading role in the prosecution process. A conflict of interest may arise which may be partly avoided by involving the voluntary sector in the provision of support, whilst the statutory agency retains responsibility for the investigative process. A number of other agencies will be involved, including health, education, the Court Service, the Crown Prosecution Service and the police (Victim support 1996). A Home Office Interdepartmental Working Group recommended that, 'Agreement would need to be reached on a local basis on who should be responsible for preparing the vulnerable or intimidated witness for court' (Home Office 1998*a*, para. 6.43).

Crown Courts have a Child Witness Officer (CWO) who is responsible for coordinating facilities for children and who also liaises with other agencies who have responsibility for child witnesses. A key part of the CWO's duties is to arrange for child witnesses to visit the court beforehand to familiarise themselves with the environment. The CWO also has responsibility for trying to ensure that such cases are dealt with speedily.

The lack of coordinated pre-trial support remains an area of concern. Morgan & Williams, writing in 1993, argued that,

At present preparation and support for child witnesses is carried out on an *ad hoc* basis in England and Wales. Advice and practice vary considerably around the country. Although the provision of support both before and during the trial has been advocated, no one inside the criminal justice system has a clear responsibility to provide information about the court process to child victims and their families; to liaise with others about the child's needs; to assist the child required to give evidence (for example, by arranging an advance visit to the court or by reading the child's statement); to support the child in court, or to explain the court's verdict.

Similarly, Morgan & Zedner's (1992) research shows that support, when offered, is often marred by lack of continuity or by the inexperience of those providing it. It is disturbing that more recent research indicates that this is still the case. Provision of pretrial support is uneven across the country and national standards are required (Plotnikoff & Woolfson 1995, Home Office 1999). Any revision of the *Memorandum of Good Practice* should contain guidance on the value of pre-trial preparation.

Welfare of the child

The welfare principle as found in the Children Act 1989 does not apply to the criminal justice system, although under s. 44 Children and Young Persons Act 1933, a criminal court when dealing with a child or young person 'brought before it as an offender or otherwise, shall have regard to the welfare of the child or young person'. Two points arise from this, first, the section does not just apply to offenders, it also applies to witnesses. Second, the court need only 'have regard' to the child's welfare; unlike the Children Act 1989 their welfare is not paramount. Another crucial difference between the two statutory duties is that under the Children Act 1989, the welfare principle is something that operates not only in the courtroom environment, but also in everyday social work practice. However, the duty in the 1933 Act only operates within the courtroom. The reasoning behind this is that only the court can balance the competing interests of the child's welfare and the rights of the accused to a fair trial (see R v Highbury Corner Magistrates, ex parte Deering [1997] 1 FLR 683 and R v Liverpool Magistrates Court, ex parte Pollock [1997] COD 344). The courts will be alert to the need to fulfil their duty to the defendant. Nevertheless, the court in R v X, Y and Z [1990] 91 Cr App Rep 36 emphasised that judges must ensure that the system operates fairly 'not only for the defendants but also to the prosecution and to the witnesses'. This is consistent with the thinking of the European Court outlined above.

What can be done to protect the welfare of child witnesses? Prior to the Youth Justice and Criminal Evidence Act 1999, there was some doubt as to what level of support a child witness could be given in court. There was some support for the view that a social worker could sit alongside the child to 'comfort them when necessary' (see Lord Lane C.J. in R v X, Y and Z), and the Pigot Report (1989) had recommended the use of an intermediary or communicator in court to assist the child, but this recommendation was not implemented in the Criminal Justice Act 1991. However, the 1999 Act introduces a number of special measures, which may be available to child witnesses in certain circumstances (see below). Under s.29, a special measures direction may provide for any examination of a child witness (however and wherever conducted) to be conducted in the presence of an interpreter or other person (an 'intermediary'). The role of the intermediary is to facilitate communication between the persons conducting the examination and the child. The intermediary will communicate to the child the questions asked and then communicate any answers given in reply to them. The intermediary can explain the questions or answers if it is necessary to enable them to be understood by the child or person asking the questions. An intermediary will be extremely useful for very young children – it is interesting to note that in Scotland a boy aged only 4 years was enabled to give evidence from behind a screen in a criminal trial (*Glasgow Herald* 10 August 1999) In addition, intermediaries will be invaluable for children with learning disabilities or communication difficulties, groups previously denied access to the criminal courts.

Helpful though the intermediary will be, it does not cover those situations where the child needs the more general support envisaged by Lord Lane. Somebody needs to have responsibility for ensuring that the child is not hungry, tired, or feeling too isolated, and that appropriate regard is had to the child's well-being. A social worker, or similar person, sitting beside the child whilst they are giving evidence, is one way of meeting such needs. However, great care has to be taken to ensure that such arrangements do not compromise the defendant's rights. In R v Smith [1994] Crim LR 458, a social worker sat beside a 12-year-old witness and talked quietly to her when she broke down in tears. Arising from this, the Court of Appeal gave guidance on the nature of assistance that could be given by a support person. The Court recognised the need to balance the interests of the child and those of the accused but held that if a support person is used then they should say as little as possible, and ideally nothing, to the child whilst they are giving evidence. Judges do have discretion to adjourn proceedings if the witness becomes too distressed to continue. In extreme cases the judge may declare that the examination of that person should proceed no further (R v Wyatt [1990] Crim LR 343). The Home Office Interdepartmental Working Group recommended that children should have the option of being accompanied by a support person when giving evidence in the TV link room (Home Office 1998*a*, para. 10.22).

A number of practical difficulties arise when a child is required to attend court to give evidence. The physical environment is unsuitable for children. Courts are unfriendly and often lack even the basic amenities for children and their carers. There is always the risk that they will bump into the alleged perpetrator or witnesses for the defence. Practical matters such as food and toilet facilities can often be overlooked as nobody has overall responsibility for such matters. Parents are often inappropriate for providing such support, as they may be involved in the proceedings. Social workers, teachers and health professionals may also have been involved in preparing the case. It has been suggested that the court ushers should perform this role. However, they have many other duties and are probably perceived of by the child as being part of the court and consequently part of the problem.

Morgan & Williams (1993) advocate the appointment of a support person for the child when at court. The appropriate adult scheme in Scotland provides an example of how such a person could be introduced in England and Wales. Although the scheme applies only to vulnerable adults, the general approach is adaptable for use with child witnesses. Unlike the scheme in England and Wales, an appropriate adult is available in Scotland for victims and witnesses navigating the criminal justice system. The appropriate adult would be with the vulnerable person throughout the interview and preparation for the trial, and also be present to support the witness when giving evidence. The scheme has much to commend itself to the treatment of child witnesses in England and Wales.

The conduct of any hearing involving child witnesses requires sensitive handling by the judge and the lawyers involved in the defence and prosecution. Not all judges will recognise the special needs of child witnesses. They may interpret enabling the child to present their testimony with minimum distress as unfairly adding to the weight and value of their evidence. However, to place a child witness, who in cases of child abuse is probably the most crucial witness, in a position which is disadvantageous solely because of their tender years, is tantamount to denying them the protection of the criminal law. A video produced by the NSPCC, *A Case of Balance*, is aimed at judges and lawyers and addresses the question of balance between the competing rights of witness and defendant.

The courtroom environment

Whereas wigs and gowns may add something to the majesty of the law, they do little to provide the supportive environment necessary to enable vulnerable child witnesses to give evidence. In practice, such quaint traditions will render the experience that much more traumatic. The practice has arisen of judges and lawyers removing their wigs and gowns when a child is giving evidence. Section 26 Youth Justice and Criminal Evidence Act 1999 enables a court making a special measures direction to provide for the wearing of wigs and gowns to be dispensed with during the giving of the witnesses' evidence. A special measures direction may also require the child to be provided with 'such device as the court considers appropriate with a view to enabling questions or answers to be communicated to or by the witness despite any disability or disorder or other impairment which the witness has or suffers from' (s.30). This includes not only microphones, but also special devices for children who have hearing impairments.

The Court of Appeal in R v Smellie [1919] 14 Cr App Rep 128 held that where there was a fear of a witness being intimidated, the witness could give evidence out of sight of the accused. The Court of Appeal supported this in R v X, Y and Z. The argument against such arrangements was that the accused has the right to face their accusers. The provision of screens is now covered by s.23 Youth Justice and Criminal Evidence Act 1999. As part of a special measures direction the court may provide for the child giving evidence, or being sworn in, to be prevented by means of a screen or other arrangement from being seen by the accused. However, the child must be capable of being seen by (and seeing) the judge and jury, the lawyers and anybody who may be acting as an interpreter or intermediary. Although the introduction of new technology, such as interactive and pre-recorded videos, may reduce the need for such measures, they will still be important for those cases where the technology is unavailable or the witness does not wish to take advantage of it.

Another important way of protecting the welfare of the child is to protect their anonymity during the criminal process. The court may, in cases concerning decency or morality, direct that the courtroom be cleared of members of the public when children or young people give evidence (s.37 Children and Young Persons Act 1933). This does not apply to *bona fide* members of the press. However, s.45 Youth Justice and Criminal Evidence Act 1999 enables the court to restrict the reporting and publication of information that would lead to the identification of a witness, complainant or defendant under the age of 18 years. Section 44 (when in force) will impose reporting restrictions from the beginning of a criminal investigation if a child under the age of 18 years is involved. They will also be enforceable throughout the UK. Applications can be made to the court to lift these restrictions. It is a criminal offence to breach such restrictions, but there are a number of defences. It is a defence if the person charged did not know at the time of the disclosure that the publication included something covered by a reporting restriction, or that they had no reason to expect that a criminal investigation had begun, or that the public interest demanded publication and that consequently the restriction was substantial and unreasonable. It is also a defence if the person charged had the written consent of the child's parent or guardian (other than when they are the accused) provided they are reminded of the need to consider the welfare of the child. A child aged 16 or 17 years can also give a valid consent. (See s.44–50 – these provision are not yet in force.)

Children giving evidence

Prior to the Youth Justice and Criminal Evidence Act 1999, children could, at the discretion of the court, give evidence-in-chief (see Lane & Walsh, Chapter 17, in this volume) by means of a pre-recorded video interview. The child could then be questioned during the actual trial by means of a live television link (see s.32 & 32A Criminal Justice Act 1988). These facilities were available to witnesses under the age of 14 years in cases of violence or cruelty, and under the age of 17 years in the case of sex offences. On the whole, these provisions work reasonably well, although Davis *et al.* (1995) reported that technical problems sometimes made it difficult for juries to assess the evidence of the child (Home Office 1999). The Home Office Interdepartmental Working Group made a number of recommendations for the reform of these provisions. It recommended that there should be only one age limit regardless of whether the offence was one of violence or a sexual offence. The proposed age limit was under 17 years (Home Office 1998a, Rec.65). This proposal was implemented in the 1999 Act (s.16(1)(b)). Witnesses under 17 years will always be eligible for help and in certain circumstances this can continue if they turn 17 years before the trial ends. The special measures available to eligible witnesses are outlined in Table 19.1.

Courts will not be able to award any of these special measures until the Secretary of State notifies it that those measures are available in its area (s.18(2)).

Section 21 makes further special provision for child witnesses. Three groups of child witnesses are created:

Provision	Section
Provision of screens so that the witness cannot see the defendant	(s.23)
Giving evidence by a live television link	(s.24)
Allowing evidence to be given in private	(s.25)
Removal of wigs and gowns	(s.26)
Allowing a pre-recorded video interview with the witness to be admitted as evidence-in-chief	(s.27)
Allowing a pre-recorded videoed cross-examination to be admitted in place of a live cross examination	(s.28)
Use of an approved intermediary	(s.29)
Use of communication aids	(s.30)

Table 19.1   *Special measures available to witnesses under the Youth Justice and Criminal Evidence Act 1999*

1. Children giving evidence in sexual offence cases
2. Children giving evidence in a case involving an offence of violence, abduction or neglect
3. Children giving evidence in other cases.

Children in groups 1 and 2 are, under the Act, in need of 'special protection'. Children in group 3 will have a video recording admitted as evidence-in-chief and will be cross-examined through a live video link at the trial. There will be a presumption to this effect unless giving evidence in this way would not improve the quality of the child's evidence. However, for children in need of special protection there is a stronger presumption in favour of a video recording being admitted as evidence-in-chief unless it would not be in the interests of justice to admit the video evidence (s.27(2)). Child witnesses in sexual offence cases will then be cross-examined at a pre-trial hearing, which will be recorded on video, unless they inform the court that they do not want to give evidence in this way. Those involved as witnesses in violent offence cases will give any further evidence through a live link at the trial.

The *Memorandum of Good Practice*

The experience of the use of pre-recorded videos in wardship cases is not a very happy one. A series of cases reported in 1987 1 FLR highlighted some of the problems involved for the legal process when considering pre-recorded video interviews with children. To overcome these problems the Home Office, in conjunction with the Department of Health, published the *Memorandum of Good Practice* (1992), although it's status is not that of a code, as was recommended by Pigot (1989). Instead, it is voluntary 'but should be followed whenever practicable to try to ensure that a video recording will be acceptable in a criminal court' (p. 1). A key theme in the *Memorandum of Good Practice* is the need to develop further inter-agency working (see Corby, Chapter 13, in this volume). A number of different agencies will be involved in investigating cases of child abuse; these include social services, education, police, health and the voluntary sector. Section 27 of the Children Act 1989 encourages an interdisciplinary approach to the provision of Part III services. As noted above, these may include provision for children giving evidence in criminal proceedings. In addition, s.47 places a duty on education, housing and health to help social services investigate cases of suspected abuse. Clearly an *interdisciplinary* rather than a *multidisciplinary* approach is desirable. Practitioners will need to prepare carefully 'in order to make the best use of the reforms, both in the interests of the child and of justice' (p. 2).

A revised version of *Working Together to Safeguard Children* was published in 1999 (DOH 1999). Inter-agency work is a key theme running through *Working Together*. The Policing and Crime Reducing Crime Unit of the Home Office examined the training needs of police officers involved in joint investigation of child abuse cases (Home Office 1998*b*). It made a number of recommendations and gave expression to a number of concerns at the application of the principles contained in the *Memorandum*. Police officers identified a number of areas where training needed to be improved. These were:

- aspects of child development (e.g. children's concept of time)
- interviewing suspects
- the tactics and behaviour of sex offenders.

The report also highlighted the need for trainers to have greater operational experience. *Working Together* picks up the training theme. Single agency training is essential. Home Office research, for example, found that police officers were given very little training or guidance on the legal principles underlying the procedures they were required to follow when investigating child abuse (Home Office 1999). However, joint training should be provided whenever possible. *Working Together* states that 'inter-agency training should complement the training available to staff in single agency or professional settings' (para. 9.2). The purposes of inter-agency training are identified as:

- A shared understanding of the task, processes, principles, roles and responsibilities and local arrangements for safeguarding children and promoting their welfare
- Coordinated services at both strategic and individual case level
- Improved communications between professionals including a common understanding of key terms, definitions and thresholds for action
- Effective working relationships based on respect and an understanding of the role and contribution of different disciplines
- Sound decision-making based on information sharing, thorough assessment, critical analysis and professional judgement (para. 9.7).

These training objectives precisely identify the joint working culture necessary to ensure that the child's passage through the criminal justice system is as user friendly as possible within the constraints of the law. *Working Together* requires that all investigative interviews with children should 'be conducted by those with specialist training and experience in interviewing children' (Home Office 1999, para. 5.38). The *Memorandum* should be followed as 'a recognised good practice guide for all investigative interviews with children' (para. 5.40).

Under the *Memorandum*, interviewers must have clear objectives that are consistent with the main purpose of the interview. It may be difficult, however, to identify with the necessary degree of clarity what the main purpose of the interview is. Davies & Westcott (1999) identified one possible tension that may arise. A video taped interview may serve as the initial step in a criminal investigation, an inquiry into whether the child is in need of protection and also the examination-in-chief at the trial (Home Office 1999). These tensions could lead to the evidence gathered being incomplete or inadmissible or of little probative value. That main purpose 'is to listen *with an open mind* to what the child has to say, if anything, about the alleged event'. Interviews are not to be referred to as therapeutic interviews, or as disclosure interviews (p. 3). Although the *Memorandum of Good Practice* states that counselling and therapy may take place after the interview, it also points out that the defence may wish to know what form it has taken, which unfortunately may be an inhibiting factor. Practitioners must familiarise themselves with the detail of the *Memorandum* in its entirety. The following account merely highlights some of the main issues.

A pre-recorded video interview is part of the evidence child witnesses present to the courts and as such it is subject, so far as is realistically possible, to the laws of evidence. The most common difficulty is how to avoid asking a leading question. These may be perfectly proper in other types of interview, but as evidence before the court they may attract, at best, adverse comment by the judge and, at worst, be excluded. Although courts may take a relatively sympathetic view of leading questions used when interviewing child witnesses, this is by no means certain and it is essential that their use is minimised or avoided altogether. Research has shown that adult and child witnesses are susceptible to repeated suggestive questioning, with children under 6 years being especially vulnerable (Cassel & Bjorklund 1995, Leichtman & Ceci 1995). For detailed guidance on leading questions, see Parts 3A and paras 3.51–3.55 3B of the *Memorandum*. Guidance is also offered on the use of previous statements (paras 3.56–3.60) and references to the character of the accused (paras 3.61–3.63).

Great care has to be taken in choosing the venue for the interviewing of child witnesses. Ideally, purpose-built facilities should be available, and special arrangements must be made for children with disabilities. Suspect interview rooms should not be used. Appropriate amenities should be provided (refreshments, toilets, waiting areas, etc.). In the case of younger children, toys should be available in the waiting area, although the *Memorandum* stresses that anatomically correct dolls are unsuitable. The use of dolls is an area of considerable controversy since there is no agreed design for such dolls, and there is no agreement on how they should be used during the interview (Davies & Westcott 1999). The Home Office review of research on the working of the *Memorandum* identified the need for more research on the use of dolls before recommendations could be made on their use in interviewing. Relying on the research of Bull (1995) and Lamb *et al.* (1996), the review concludes that when a child appears to demonstrate abuse with the aid of a doll, the interviewers should follow this up with verbal questioning to confirm that this is what the child intended to convey (Davies & Westcott 1999).

Although the *Memorandum* does not specify the type and quality of the equipment to be used, practitioners must bear in mind that faulty or inadequate equipment may render the video inadmissible. Technical guidance is to be found in Annex F of the *Memorandum*. Courts will require detailed information about the equipment and the venue. The *Memorandum* suggests that practitioners should strive to achieve the same quality as the live television link used in courts.

Part 2 of the *Memorandum* deals with procedure before the interview and exhorts the interviewers not to conduct an interview without adequate planning, even when the interview has to be conducted at short notice. One important feature of planning is to understand what information is required for the purposes of the alleged offence; Annex D provides guidance on these matters. The *Memorandum* lists a number of developmental factors, which the interview team should consider. These should cover assessing the child's development, use of language, social and sexual understanding, concepts of time, ideas about trust, the child's present state of mind, cultural background and any disabilities (see paras 2.3–2.10). On the question of language, it is essential that the interviewers use language that the child is capable of understanding. Bull (1995) argues that it is important to assess the child's linguistic abilities at the rapport stage of the interview, something that is not always done.

The length and duration of the interview is important and should, so far as is possible, be planned in advance. Davies & Westcott (1999) noted that although the *Memorandum* suggested a length of 1 hour as a 'rule of thumb', officers were criticised for going beyond that time. It appears that the majority of interviews last for less than 1 hour (Davies & Westcott 1999). It may be better to exceed 1 hour, however, rather than rush the pace of the interview, which may work to the disadvantage of the child. Davies felt that in 43% of cases the child had been rushed into the questioning phase (Davies *et al.* 1995). In exceptional circumstances it may be necessary to exceed 1 hour, as ideally only one interview should be conducted. However, there may be cases where a further interview may be needed. A supplementary interview should only be carried out if the investigation team is fully satisfied, following consultation with the Crown Prosecution Service, that it is needed. It should be video-recorded. Interviews should proceed at the child's pace and not that of the interviewers. Multiple interviews are not always bad, however. The review of research concluded that,

> It is important to distinguish between multiple interviews which are properly planned and sensitively conducted and repeated interviews, driven by adult priorities and assumptions, rather than the needs of the child. This latter form of repeat interviewing can lead to distorted testimony and have harmful effects upon the child.
>
> (Home Office 1999, p. 24)

Where there are breaks, these should be carefully noted as they will have to be accounted for when applying for leave. Reasons for any breaks, and their duration, will need to be recorded, and the court may want to be satisfied that child witnesses are not coached during the recess. Regard must always be had to the normal routine of children (e.g. their normal bedtime, see paras 2.17–2.21). On the question of who should be interviewers, the *Memorandum* suggests it should be a person who has, or is likely to be able to, establish rapport with the child, can communicate effectively with them and who has a proper grasp both of the rules of evidence and the elements of criminal offences (see para. 2.23).

Police officers and social workers should be flexible and willing to respond to particular situations. The presence of a second member of the interviewing team during the interview will be helpful, although it is desirable that only one member interviews during any single phase. Guidance is given on when somebody who is not part of an interviewing team can interview children (see paras 2.22–2.26). Part 3A recommends a four-phase approach to the interview (Table 19.2).

Regard must always be had to the special needs of those children who have communication problems or learning disability. This is especially important as the *Memorandum* emphasises the importance of free narrative account. When

Table 19.2 *Four-phase approach to child interviews*

Phase	Designation	Purpose
Phase 1	Rapport	To settle the child and relieve anxiety
Phase 2	Free narrative account	To enable the child to give account in their own words
Phase 3	Questioning	To find out more about the alleged offence
Phase 4	Closing the interview	To ensure that the child has understood the interview and is not distressed

interviewing such children there may be a need for greater flexibility. Davies recommends that this issue needs to be addressed in any new edition of the *Memorandum*.

Summary of key issues

The protection available for child witnesses has improved considerably as a result of legislation, the attitude of the judiciary and a greater awareness of the issues by practitioners. The recent changes to the law by the Youth Justice and Criminal Evidence Act 1999 continue this trend and place on a clearer statutory footing the range of protection that may be available. Pre-recorded video interviews still give some cause for concern. The *Memorandum of Good Practice* is still a very valuable guide to the way in which they should be conducted. However, it is essential that this is now revised, as research has identified a number of gaps and shortcomings.

Interdisciplinary working is as essential now as it was at the time of the first edition of *Working Together to Safeguard Children*. Although funding problems can sometimes be used as a reason for agencies to withdraw from joint working and concentrate on their core activities, this must be resisted. The problems facing children about to give evidence are so complex that no single agency or profession has the expertise or responsibility to cope. Involvement of the courts and the Crown Prosecution Service is essential. An important aspect of interdisciplinary work is joint training. This is given much greater emphasis in the revised *Working Together*. The *Memorandum* emphasises the importance of careful planning and getting the interview right first time. There is no going back to correct mistakes. Mistakes may result in the video being excluded.

One area where further action is required is that of providing a support person for children during the investigative process, courtroom appearance and after the trial is over. The Scottish 'appropriate adult' scheme has much to commend itself and would enable the child to have a single support person to help them navigate the entire process. Coordination between the various officials and agencies concerned is crucial. A properly appointed support person would be able to ensure that this takes place and that the child's passage through the criminal justice system is as smooth as possible.

With the implementation of the Human Rights Act 1998 the courts may be called upon to consider in greater detail the balance between the rights of the defendant and the rights of the child witness. The European Convention on Human Rights does envisage witnesses having rights in the system – whether the courts think that the current balance is appropriate remains to be seen.

Conclusion

For children, the giving of evidence in criminal proceedings in whatever form will be a traumatic and distressing experience. Although recent changes in the law and procedures have done something to minimise the trauma and distress it is essential that these are not seen as a panacea. It is still essential to listen to children and what they want. Do they want to use the new technology? Do they want to appear in open court and face the defendant? How do they feel about giving evidence? The danger with having procedures in place is that they become the norm, regardless of what an individual child actually wants. Only by listening to children can we properly prepare them for giving evidence by whichever method is decided upon.

References

Anonymous 1996 Victim support. *Times* 17 September

Bull R 1995 Good practice for video recorded interviews with child witnesses for use in criminal proceedings. In: Davies G, Lloyd-Bostock S, McMurran M, Wilson C (eds) Psychology, law and criminal justice: international developments in research and practice. de Gruyter, Berlin

Cassel W, Bjorklund D 1995 Developmental patterns of eyewitness responses to repeated and increasingly suggestive questions. Law and Human Behaviour 19: 507–531

Conroy S, Fielding N G, Tunstill J 1990 Investigating child sexual abuse: the study of a joint initiative. Police Foundation, London

Davies G M, Westcott H L 1999 Interviewing child witnesses under the *Memorandum of Good Practice*: a research review. Police Research Series, Paper 115. The Stationery Office, London

Davies G, Wilson C, Mitchell R, Milsom J 1995 Videotaping children's evidence: an evaluation. HMSO, London

Department of Health (DOH) 1999 Working together to safeguard children. The Stationery Office, London

Flin R 1990 Child witnesses in criminal courts. Children and Society 4(3): 264

Fortin J 1998 Children's rights and the developing law. Butterworths, London

Goodman G S, Helgeson V S 1985 Child sexual assualt: children's memories and th law. University of Miami Law Review 40: 181

Goodman G, Taub E, Jones D, *et al.* 1992 Testifying in criminal court: emotional effects on child sexual assault victims. Monographs of the Society for Research in Child Development 57 (5), serial no. 229

Hardin M 1987 Guardians *ad litem* for child victims in criminal proceeding (1986–1987). Journal of Family Law 25 (4): 687

Home Office 1993 Child witness pack. HMSO, London

Home Office 1998*a* Speaking up for justice. Report of the Interdepartmental Working Group on the treatment of vulnerable or intimidated witnesses in the criminal sustice system. The Stationery Office, London

Home Office 1998*b* Child abuse: training investigating officers. Police Research Series, Paper No 94. The Stationery Office, London

Home Office 1999 The admissibility and sufficiency of evidence in child abuse prosecutions. Home Office Research and Statistics Department, Research Findings No 100. The Stationery Office, London

Home Office, Department of Health 1992 Memorandum of good practice on video-recorded interviews with child victims in criminal proceedings. HMSO, London

Lamb M, Hershkowitz I, Sternberg K, *et al.* 1996 Investigative interviews of alleged sexual abuse victims with and without anatomical dolls. Child Abuse and Neglect 20: 1239–1247

Leichtman M, Ceci S 1995 The effects of stereotypes and suggestions on preschoolers' reports. Developmental Psychology 31: 568–578

Morgan J, Williams J 1992 Child witnesses and the legal process. Journal of Social Welfare and Family Law 14: 484–496

Morgan J, Williams J 1993 A role for a support person for child witnesses in criminal proceedings. British Journal of Social Work 23: 113–121

Morgan J, Zedner L 1992 Child victims: crime, impact and criminal justice. Clarendon Press, Oxford

National Society for the Prevention of Cruelty to Children (NSPCC) 1996 A case for balance. NSPCC, London

National Society for the Prevention of Cruelty to Children (NSPCC) 1998 Young witness pack. NSPCC, London

Pigot T 1989 Report of the advisory group on video evidence. HMSO, London

Plotnikoff J, Woolfson R 1995 Prosecuting child abuse: an evaluation of the Government's speedy progress policy. Blackstone Press, London

Sanders A, Creaton J, Bird S, Weber L 1997 Victims with learning disabilities: negotiating the criminal justice system. Occasional Paper No 17. Centre for Criminological Research, University of Oxford, Oxford

Scottish Office 1998*a* Interviewing people who are mentally disordered: 'Appropriate Adults' schemes. Scottish Office, Edinburgh

Scottish Office 1998*b* Going to court as a witness. Scottish Office, Edinburgh

Spencer J R (1990) Children's evidence in legal proceedings in England. In: Spencer J R, Nicholson G, Flin R, Bull R (eds) Children's evidence in legal proceedings: an international perspective. Spencer, Cambridge

Spencer J R, Flin R H 1993 The evidence of children: the law and the psychology. Blackstone, London.

3

INTERVENTION AND TRAINING ISSUES IN CHILD PROTECTION

The chapters in this third section of the *Handbook* focus, broadly speaking, on those aspects of the child protection process which follow comprehensive assessment and case conference decisions and recommendations: namely, the implementation of the child care plan in out-of-home care for the child, or the provision of a variety of helping services for victims of abuse, whether as children, adolescents or adults, and their families. The concluding chapter in the section discusses the training of professionals in relation to child protection. In the introduction to this section of the first edition of the *Handbook*, we drew attention to the fact that significant resources and a large proportion of multi-agency work focused on the early stages of the child protection process, and that relatively little attention or resources had been given to the later stages of the process. This imbalance had been criticised by a number of writers, including Hallett (1995) and Lynch (1992) who questioned the wisdom and morality of a system which devoted significant resources to case identification and the determination of case status without offering significant and effective help. There has since then been some attempt to remedy this, and Nigel Parton, in Chapter 1 of this edition, discusses the extent to which in the intervening period there has been a shift in policy and practice towards supporting and working with families who come into the child protection system.

Despite this, many of the concerns about the provision of therapeutic help and family support which we identified in the earlier edition remain. In practice, the role of the social worker has continued to be predominantly that of case manager, involving the dual role of assessor and enabler with the 'ability to make a proper assessment of need and to ensure that a range of services is available to meet that need' (James & Wilson 1991). There is therefore little evidence of any increased involvement on the part of workers in statutory settings in the undertaking of therapeutic work. Consequently, therapeutic help, such as that described in the ensuing chapters, is likely to be offered by health workers or social workers in settings such as family centres or family service units.

This has two important implications. First, the skills involved in undertaking assessments and in drawing up care plans that include therapeutic work need to be clarified. Second, the current haphazard pattern of providing services needs to be recognised and changed. There continues to be very little information concerning the effectiveness of different therapeutic approaches with different problems and at different stages in children's lives, and services within a locality usually seem to have developed piecemeal and are dependent on the individual interests and talents of the individual practitioner. There is a need for research which would both help develop a more systematic framework of provision and guide practitioners in referral decisions. In the absence of this, the material in the chapters in this section will assist the practitioner in developing plans for children.

The first two chapters address issues that relate to all aspects of the child protection process, i.e. issues of partnership and communicating with children, but are seen to have particular relevance to this part of the process. Steph Petrie and Brian Corby (Chapter 20) explore the nature and meaning of the concept of partnership with parents in the context of its history and other requirements for working in partnership (with children and with other agencies) which are embodied in the Children Act 1989. They suggest that definitions of partnership are elusive, but that there is a consensus that for true partnership to exist there must be an element of power-sharing: partnership is then most difficult to achieve in compulsory intervention. Nonetheless, the small amount of available research suggests that the absence of parents from decision-making is usually detrimental to children. In the context of a section that focuses on services provided under Part III of the Act (i.e. 'less compulsory' forms of intervention) but that includes a focus on out-of-home care, this finding is important, suggesting as it does the principles that should inform all such intervention.

The following chapters concern the provision of help to victims of abuse either as individuals or in the context of families or in groups, or through intervention which involves caring for children away from their birth families. The first chapter on individual work with children (Margaret Crompton, Chapter 21) considers a broad range of interventions that may be undertaken, exploring the professional principles that need to inform all communications with children, and a variety of means, such as life story books, music, drama and storytelling, to enhance these.

In Chapter 22, Virginia Ryan provides a detailed discussion of one particular approach to therapeutic work with children, that of non-directive play therapy. This approach will be familiar to many readers from the work of Axline, who adapted Rogerian client-centred therapy with adults to child therapy. However, its theoretical and practice base, described here, has recently been more rigorously developed. We selected this particular approach for inclusion in the *Handbook* from a range of possible child therapies because it offers a robust and relatively brief method of working with children, particularly in statutory settings. A limitation, perhaps, of this approach is that although practitioners will be familiar with the core Rogerian skills on which it is based (for example, the use of congruence, reflection, acceptance and non-directiveness) it does require further training to be used effectively.

Katy Cigno's chapter on behavioural work (Chapter 23) explores the different ways in which this approach may be used in work with troubled children and their families. She considers three applications of the approach, namely parent–child interaction, parent training and work with children who have failed to thrive, where research suggests this way of working may be particularly effective. This chapter may also be seen as an example of preventative work with children and families where there are concerns about the quality of care.

In Chapter 24, Arnon Bentovim discusses therapeutic work with abusive families, which he stresses needs to be undertaken in the context of a consultation process with social services and the courts. He explores the distinction between family therapy approaches and family approaches, before considering questions concerning indicators for and against involving the whole family in therapy, and practice issues at different phases of intervention, both in cases of child physical and child sexual abuse.

In the next chapter on therapeutic work, Anne Bannister (Chapter 25) describes the use of groups in child protection settings. She reviews issues in relation to planning and conducting groups for children and adolescents, giving detailed practice suggestions and a case example of a group with four children who had been severely abused. In a separate section, she considers particular problems and styles of working appropriate for groups of adults, both for adult perpetrators who may be mandated by the courts and for adult survivors of abuse.

The needs of this last group form the focus of the final chapter concerning approaches to helping (Chapter 26), namely that of helping adult survivors of child sexual abuse. It considers individual and group approaches to this, and in particular the important early stages of contact. It is probably unnecessary to justify the inclusion of a chapter on working with adult victims in the *Handbook*, since many child protection workers currently do involve themselves in this as a spin-off of their other work. However, if justification is needed, Liz Hall and Siobhan Lloyd point out that an understanding of the potential long-term effects derived from this work can be helpful in working with abused children and can improve our understanding of the nature of child sexual abuse and the ways in which children of different ages cope with the experience of abuse. The chapter also considers recent debates concerning false memory which is clearly relevant to working with adult survivors. The long-term effects of other forms of abuse are relatively neglected in research literature and in practice initiatives and, as Hall & Lloyd suggest, it seems likely that the needs of adult victims of such abuse are in many cases still unaddressed.

In the following chapter, that on out-of-home placements, June Thoburn (Chapter 27) provides a detailed review of research findings on the placement of children in residential care, foster care and with adoptive families, emphasising what they can tell us about how practice might be improved. She highlights the importance of assessment and decision-making about placements, and, linking with discussions in the earlier chapters in this section, discusses the provision of other services most likely to ensure that the short- and long-term needs of children are met.

In Chapter 28, which is new to this edition, Paul Dyson provides an important additional perspective to those offered in the first edition – that of the social services manager, who is responsible amongst other things for the provision of high quality child care services. As he argues, 'Translating a child-centred policy into practice in organisations in which child protection is a central issue is the particular task of managers'. This chapter is therefore an important addition to the *Handbook* because it provides a detailed first-hand account of the issues and difficulties faced by social service managers in fulfilling this complex task.

Finally, we conclude this section with a new chapter on training by Pat Walton (Chapter 29). In it she focuses particularly on post-qualifying social work education, but also discusses training within a multi-professional context, exploring the development of the notion of 'competence' and its application to vocational education and training for professionals. As she points out, the context, structure and delivery of social work education is under review, and a new post-qualifying award in child care is currently being piloted in England and Wales. This is an area therefore likely to see significant changes in the period ahead.

References

Hallett C 1995 Taking stock: past developments and future directions. In: Wilson K, James A (eds) The child protection handbook, 1st edn. Baillière Tindall, London

James A, Wilson K 1991 Marriage, social policy and social work. Issues in Social Work Practice 10 (1, 2): 92–111

Lynch M 1992 Child protection: have we lost our way? Adoption and Fostering 16 (4): 15–22

Partnership with parents

Stephanie Petrie, Brian Corby

**INTRODUC-
TION**

This chapter deals with the key issue of working in partnership with parents in child protection work, which became an increasingly important principle of practice in the 1990s. In the first section we examine some of the fundamental aspects of the notion of partnership. Second, we briefly review the way in which partnership with parents has been developed over time in child care social work from the formation of Children Departments in 1948 until the present day. Third, we examine the way in which the notion of partnership is used in current legislation and government guidance. Last, we examine research into the way in which partnership with parents is now being practised and, in the light of the preceding we make some practice and policy suggestions for working with parents.

The nature of partnership

Meanings

Although the word partnership is now commonly used, little attention has been given to its meaning and to whether it is a legitimate description of the relationship between professionals and service users. Arnstein (1969) suggested the following continuum for understanding the power relations between citizens and professionals. Arnstein considers partnership to involve a relatively high degree of power-sharing which goes well beyond helping, informing, consulting and cooperating activities.

8. Citizen control	
7. Delegated power	degrees of citizen power
6. Partnership	
5. Placation	
4. Consultation	degrees of tokenism
3. Informing	
2. Therapy	non-participation
1. Manipulation	

The idea that partnership involves a high degree of power-sharing is also argued by Jordan (1988):

Partnership ... implies a good deal more than cooperation. It implies a kind of pooling of resources, and fairly close integration of roles, as in the marital relationship, or in a commercial firm. It implies trust, and a good deal of potential or actual agreement on common goals, and the means of achieving them. (p. 30)

Jordan goes on to point out that there are many barriers to cooperation and, by implication, even more to partnership, including lack of trust, imbalance of power and differential access to knowledge and information.

These are important issues to bear in mind in relation to child care and child protection work with parents. The notion of partnership defined here suggests a relatively stable and trusting relationship with shared goals. Such a definition could well be used to describe some relationships between social workers and service users where issues of authority and control are less in evidence and where there is a genuine element of choice in the decision-making process, for example in relation to services for disabled people eligible to be budget holders for their own care by the provisions of the Community Care (Direct Payments) Act 1996. Indeed, in these situations, social workers work alongside service users who are able not only to state their preferences but also take control of the decision-making process.

However, the situation in relation to child protection work is somewhat different. First, the primary client is the child, and there may well be quite conflicting perspectives between the family adults and the professional workers as to the issues of risk and care. This may mean an absence of trust, particularly during the investigative stages of intervention. Second, the legal and administrative powers available to social workers during the course of a child protection investigation are greater than for almost any other social work task except perhaps for those carried out by social workers approved under the Mental Health Act 1983. Last, child abuse itself is a contested concept (see Parton, Chapter 1, and Butler, Chapter 9, in this volume), and, as Wattam (1999) points out, 'Perhaps the greatest impediment to the prevention of significant harm is the contested arena of what child abuse should be' (p. 327). In the light of these factors, it is hard to see how the parent–professional relationship could be seen as a partnership according to the definitions of Arnstein and Jordan.

Partnership as process

As will be seen later on in the chapter, however, partnership with parents in child protection work is in many ways an issue of process. It is clear from recent Government guidance (Department of Health (DOH) 1995a) and also from Government-sponsored research (Thoburn *et al.* 1995) that there is a recognition that partnership is a relationship to be aimed for rather than a right of parents upheld by legislation. Indeed, DOH (1995b) guidance identifies the four approaches to partnership as providing information, involvement, participation and partnership. It is acknowledged that these approaches are not sequential and may fluctuate over time. Furthermore, it is stressed that partnership is not an end in itself, but a means by which children are to be protected and their welfare promoted. It could be argued, therefore, that partnership in this sense is more a matter of rhetoric than reality. Despite this, it is clear that the term 'partnership' is used by the Department of Health to define a process of involvement which has previously not existed. In some senses the term 'partnership' is also being used in an exhortatory sense, to encourage child protection professionals to operate in a more consultative and less conflictual way than before.

History of partnership

Prior to the Children Act 1989

The place of parents in child welfare decision-making has had a long and varied history. Attempts both to involve parents and exclude them have swung like a pendulum, but with no consistent rhythm. For example, Dr Barnardo's view was that 'parents are my chief difficulty everywhere; so are relatives generally because I take from a very low class' (cited in Holman 1988). He reflected the nature of welfare provision in the latter half of the nineteenth century, which worked against any form of partnership as the parents of needy children were believed to be a pernicious influence on their offspring. By the late nineteenth and early twentieth centuries, things had changed somewhat. Ferguson (1990) clearly demonstrates that National Society for the Prevention of Cruelty to Children (NSPCC) inspectors were very much aware of the need not to alienate parents and communities in their efforts to protect children.

Post-war to the 1970s

The period immediately after World War II saw a significant change of attitudes towards poor parents. This shift was attributable to several key developments: the insights into the under-nourished and under-developed state of poor children evacuated from inner cities to the countryside; the development of ideas about the emotional ill-effects on children of separation from their parents, particularly by John Bowlby (1951); concerns about the standards of care for children provided by the state highlighted by the Denis O'Neill inquiry (Home Office 1945); and a post-war social consensus that a more liberal and humane welfare system was desirable (see Frost and Stein 1989).

As a result of these concerns, a specialist child care service was set up following the passing of the Children Act 1948, which had a particular remit to provide more child-sensitive services to children and families where breakdown was imminent or evident. The focus until the end of the 1950s was largely on providing good standard substitute care (particularly smaller residential homes for children and fostering), but increasingly it came to be realised that more resources needed to be deployed to prevent family breakdown in the first place.

New legislation passed in 1963 empowered local authorities to give assistance in kind to families, for the first time in cash, and by provision of social work support to prevent children coming into care. At this time there was a general consensus that the best place, certainly for younger children, was with their parents and that reception into care should be a last resort. Kinship ties (Fox Harding 1991) were seen to be all important. 'Maternal' deprivation (Bowlby 1951) was seen to be at the root of a wide range of personal and emotional problems and a key factor in the causation of juvenile delinquency.

However, despite these developments in thinking about the importance of the link between children and their families, two points should be noted. First, the numbers of children in care were not dramatically reduced during this period. Second, the social work approach to families was usually based on social casework derived from Freudian psychoanalysis where the worker was in the role of expert rather than partner (Yelloly 1980).

The 1970s to the 1980s

This consensus in relation to child welfare ideology began to shift in the 1970s as professional and public attitudes changed and conflicting perspectives emerged. These different perspectives were particularly evident in social work. One strand of professional practice was in the direction of generic neighbourhood teams and community-based services which were primarily family-focused and aimed at keeping children out of care. In contrast, those who wanted to retain a more specialist child care approach within this shift to genericism were questioning the predominance of 'kinship ties', particularly where this led to children languishing in care (Goldstein *et al*. 1973, Rowe & Lambert 1973). This took place in a changing social and economic context where the welfarist approach to poorer families was coming under challenge from right-wing groups, and theories about cycles of disadvantage and the need for more targeting of resources were being developed (Parton 1979).

However, perhaps the most important factor in questioning the hegemony of 'kinship ties' was that of the growing concerns being raised about baby battering (Kempe *et al*. 1962) and non-accidental injury to children. The publication of the report of the Maria Colwell inquiry (Department of Health and Social Security (DHSS) 1974) was a key event in this process. (The details of this inquiry are to be found in Corby, Chapter 13, in this volume). For the purposes of this chapter, it is sufficient to point out that this inquiry highlighted the potential dangerousness of some families for children and the inability of welfare-oriented professionals to provide adequate protection for them. The subsequent establishment of a more structured system for dealing with child abuse in 1974 and the passing of the Children Act 1975 reflected a considerable shift away from the broader family support approach which had characterised child care work since 1948. The focus was now clearly on the needs of children living with their parents to be protected from abuse and for those in care for any length of time to experience secure and permanent placements that excluded birth parents where necessary.

The 1980s to the 1990s

Social workers had found it hard to separate the needs of the child from those of the family as a whole, as the following criticism made in the course of the Lucy Gates inquiry in 1982 demonstrates:

The rights of parents appear to take precedence over the rights of children. There is confusion over what the rights of children are. There is currently strong pressure on professional workers to keep children with their parents at almost any cost.

(DOH 1991*a*, p. 5)

This and a whole series of other similar inquiries into child deaths in the 1980s (27 according to Corby *et al*. 1998) were significant in reinforcing the need for a greater child protective stance which paid less attention to the broader family situation than before. To some degree this approach was contradictory to the requirements of other developments taking place in the child care field. Both the 1984 Short report (House of Commons 1984) and a review of research published by central government (DHSS 1985) pointed to practice that did not sufficiently take into account parents' views and rights. However, it was not until the end of the 1980s that these criticisms found full voice following allegations of heavy-handed and inappropriate intervention into cases of intrafamilial sexual abuse (which had become a cause for concern for child protectionists in the middle of the decade) in Cleveland. The resulting inquiry report (Butler-Sloss L.J. 1988) particularly condemned the treatment of parents during these investigations. Among its recommendations were the following:

■ Parents should be given the same courtesy as the family of any other referred child. Parents are entitled to know what is going on, and to be helped to understand the steps that are being taken.
■ Parents should always be advised of their rights of appeal or of complaint in relation to any decisions made about them or their children.

- Parents should not be left isolated and bewildered at this difficult time.
- Social services should always seek to provide support to the family during the investigation.

The current situation

The Children Act 1989

The main professional debates in relation to child protection prior to the Children Act 1989 came from those who favoured a stronger child protective focus and those in favour of supporting families to care for their own children. Although not incompatible or mutually exclusive, they often became polarised and both themes were evident in the pressure for legislative change (Dickenson *et al.* 1991). The Children Act 1989 was drafted to deal with the tension that exists between the rights of children to be protected and the rights of children and their parents to their own family life. Local authorities were given increased powers attached to orders, but at the same time their powers were curtailed through strict time limits and more rights of challenge.

The Act therefore offers a framework within which parents have a place:

Parents should be expected and enabled to retain their responsibilities and remain as closely involved as it is consistent with their child's welfare, even if that child cannot live at home either temporarily or permanently.

(DOH 1989, p. 18)

Although the Act promotes a new model of parenthood through the concept of 'parental responsibility' (Part 1 (2)(3)), this is not a simple concept (Eekelaar 1991). Parental responsibility itself is defined as a set of rights and duties which more than one person (not necessarily the biological parents) can share; the local authority does not automatically acquire it when looking after children; and it is a life-long responsibility that nothing short of adoption can terminate.

The word partnership, however, does not occur in statute and is not defined, although it is frequently referred to in Department of Health publications accompanying the Children Act. As has been shown, there is considerable potential for different assumptions to be made about what this might mean in practice. Part III of the Act spells out the sort of assistance parents might expect if they are experiencing difficulty bringing up their children. However, the effectiveness of this development is crucially dependent on proper resourcing, which so far does not seem to have taken place (Tunstill 1997).

Although the Children Act 1989 pointed to the need for greater involvement of parents than before in all court processes and orders including child protection, it did not greatly clarify the appropriate level of parental involvement in the provision of child protection services. The difficulty involved in achieving clearer guidance in this field should not be underestimated:

Child protection is the area where family participation leads to most anxiety and where the term partnership is most stretched. When an agency takes a decision to intervene through court proceedings, partnership may seem a meaningless concept. Power is very much concentrated on one side.

(Family Rights Group 1991, p. 18)

In these circumstances, therefore, it may be better to think of partnership in child protection decision-making more in process terms as described in the Introduction, i.e. as a process that begins with information, involvement and participation before leading, ideally, to the status of partnership, which involves a sharing of power (Social Services Inspectorate (SSI) & DOH 1992).

Partnership with parents: research findings

Pre-1989 studies

The issue of the use of authority and the need to work democratically has been a perennial issue for social work from its inception. The terminology used to describe this debate has shifted over time. Care and control were terms used in the 1960s and early 1970s. Rights terminology came into being in the late 1970s and empowerment and anti-oppressive practice are terms that dominated the 1990s. Prior to the 1970s, despite the commitment of social work to self-determination and respect for persons, there was little research into the consumer's view of being at the receiving end of social work intervention, and therefore little evidence from that perspective to help determine the extent to which there was some degree of power-sharing or, at the least, sharing of views.

Early research indicated by and large that there was a great deal of disagreement between social workers and parents about desired outcomes (Mayer & Timms 1970). Rees (1978) found considerable evidence of confusion, uncertainty and even fear being sometimes felt by clients in their contacts with social workers. Sainsbury et al. (1982) found that social workers and their clients were often working to different agendas. This was particularly apparent where issues of social control were the context in which the interaction was taking place, a finding supported by Rees & Wallace's (1982) research review. They drew attention to the fact that suspicion or fear were common amongst people with child care difficulties: 'This is particularly the case amongst clients who associate social work departments with law enforcement agencies and courts ... No matter how caring a children's department, it always potentially has the power to be coercive' (pp. 31–32).

In contrast, studies by Sainsbury (1975) and Fisher et al. (1986) described practice that was experienced by family members as helpful. In the former study, practical help, genuineness and straight-talking were valued by service users. In the latter, the following was most appreciated: a 'cards on the table' business-like approach, a consistent showing of concern and an exhibited desire for their involvement in the decisions and activities of care (DHSS 1985, p. 29).

Post-1989 studies

Until the studies sponsored by the Department of Health in the late 1980s following the Cleveland inquiry, there was very little research into parents' views about being at the receiving end of child protection investigations. This is hardly surprising given the pressure on social workers not to get distracted from protecting children by focusing on the needs of the family as a whole, a view which, as we have seen, was dominant throughout much of the 1970s and 1980s. Small-scale studies by Brown (1984) and Corby (1987) were among the few that sought the parents' perspective in child abuse investigations in this period. Most parents felt that the process was stigmatising and painful, and most felt very ill-informed about the process and their rights within it (Prosser 1992).

This lack of knowledge from the consumer perspective was transformed by the DOH research which, in the wake of Cleveland and the controversies there, not surprisingly placed great reliance on parents' (and children's) views. The studies by Farmer & Owen (1995), Cleaver & Freeman (1995), Sharland et al. (1995)

and Thoburn *et al.* (1995) provide particularly good evidence of the impact of child protection investigations on those at the receiving end. The main findings are discussed more fully in the following section. It is worth noting here, however, two of the key findings which specifically relate to working in partnership with parents:

1. Where parents were more involved in participating in the process, this did not seem to result in their children being placed at greater risk.
2. Openness was appreciated and the early impressions of social work intervention were crucial to the development of relationships and a good interactive atmosphere later on in the process.

Apart from the DOH research, there have been, as mentioned earlier, several studies of parental participation at child protection conferences. As has been seen, such participation, while not unknown previously, was largely established following the publication of the 1991 *Working Together* guidelines (DOH 1991*b*). Lewis *et al.* (1992) review many of the studies. Some are positive about parental participation, finding that both professionals and parents consider the arrangements to have benefits. Others have found that participation, from the parents' viewpoint, has in fact been minimal (Corby *et al.* 1996). Much depends on the level of partnership being considered. Most parents seem to feel that the system is at least a more open one than before and that they are informed to some degree of what is taking place. On the other hand, very few feel that their contributions have had much impact on the final outcomes.

There has been relatively little research into the later stages of child protection interventions. Corby & Millar (1997) sought the views of a small number of parents about their involvement in the child protection system over an 18-month period following investigation. They found that parents who felt alienated in the early stages of the process were still unhappy at this later stage, thus confirming the findings of Farmer & Owen (1995). Calder (1990, 1991) has looked at the working of core groups, which were established at the end of the 1980s to enable key professionals, parents and children to implement plans agreed upon at the child protection conference (see later). Certainly they offer greater potential in theory for working in partnership with parents than do child protection conferences because of the smallness of scale, greater informality and the fact that they take place later in the child protection process.

Developing partnership in child protection in the 1990s

Many of the ideas about working in partnership with parents in child protection, while influenced by its general tenor, have been developed outside the Children Act 1989. As a result of the Cleveland inquiry, the Department of Health issued new guidelines for agencies involved in child protection investigations (DOH 1991*b*). It is notable that these guidelines were far more positive about the notion of involving parents in the child protection process than was true of preceding guidelines. For instance, those issued in 1986, following the report of the Beckford inquiry, expressly prohibited the attendance of parents at child protection conferences (DHSS 1986). In the 1991 guidelines, it is stressed that parental (and child) attendance at conferences should be the norm and that only in exceptional circumstances following a ruling by the chair of the conference should parents be excluded. The 1991 guidelines also required that social workers should consult with parents in writing reports for conferences and that parents should be shown them prior to the conference being held.

The notion of involving parents more fully in the follow-up to conferences was introduced in draft guidelines published in 1988 (DHSS & Welsh Office 1988) where the term 'core group' was coined. Throughout the early 1990s, however, the main focus was on the involvement of parents and (to a lesser extent) children in child protection conferences. This was seen as the key arena for partnership to be demonstrated and was the area of activity most thoroughly researched (see next section).

The main drive for developing partnership with parents, however, came from the more broadly-focused research, sponsored by the Department of Health following Cleveland, referred to in the preceding section. In all, 20 studies were initiated and published individually. They were also summarised in a publication entitled *Child Protection: Messages from Research* (DOH 1995a) and implications for child protection policy and practice were distilled from their findings. The main findings of these research projects in relation to working in partnership with families were as follows:

1.   The child protection system acted like a giant sieve, taking in a wide range of referrals about a plethora of issues concerning the care of children, ranging from concerns about the demeanour of children at nursery through to allegations of incest. In only 15% of these families were children registered as being at risk of significant harm, and the remainder received minimal intervention and service provision. Services were centred on children and their families who had been placed on the child protection register (Gibbons *et al.* 1995).

2.   Parents at the receiving end of child protection investigations experienced them as difficult and stigmatic forms of intervention. Many parents felt that they were being unfairly labelled as child abusers. To their mind, child abuse was equated with serious physical assaults and sexual abuse, not with problems with parenting (Farmer & Owen 1995).

3.   There were too few attempts to engage parents in the child protection process either by giving adequate information or by enabling participation at child protection conferences. There was little evidence of working in partnership with parents (Thoburn *et al.* 1995).

In *Messages from Research* it was shown that most children subject to child abuse inquiries come from poor families and there was a need for a shift of focus towards meeting their needs rather than the previous emphasis on more directly observable forms of child mistreatment such as physical and sexual abuse. Earlier, Bebbington & Miles (1989) had shown how indicators of poverty and deprivation were highly correlated with the entry of children into local authority care. They showed that children of mixed racial parentage were two and a half times more likely to enter care than white children (see also Phillips, Chapter 7, in this volume). In terms of styles of intervention, *Messages from Research* argued that there was a need for a more engaging and supportive approach, i.e. a need for greater partnership with parents. The emphasis should be on working with parents to enhance the development of their children rather than to concentrate so much on protecting their children from them.

The late 1990s saw further developments in this respect. There was much reframing of what had previously been considered to deserve the label of child abuse and a move towards treating it in a qualitatively different way from before (see Parton, Chapter 1, in this volume). By redefining many of what previously had been termed child protection referrals as concerns about children in need, and by redefining the process of engagement as assessing children in need (as opposed to carrying out child protection investigations), the aim was both to reduce stigma and direct more resources to meet the needs identified. Current draft revisions of the 1991 *Working Together* guidelines (DOH 1991*b*) and of the 1988 assessment tools (DOH 1988) were distributed in the autumn of 1999 (DOH 1999*a*, 1999*b*) reflecting these shifts in thinking. In these documents there is far greater emphasis on working in partnership than previously and considerable concern to ensure broad-based assessments and interventions. Child abuse is seen as one of a series of concerns about families that might be referred, not necessarily the focal one in all cases. Indeed, both documents seem to be very wary of using the term child abuse at all, so far has the shift in thinking changed.

Implications of research for practice

Carrying out assessments/investigations

The framework for investigating child abuse/child care concerns put forward in the recently published draft guidelines on investigations (DOH 1999*a*) and assessment (DOH 1999*b*) provides a different approach to developing relationships with parents.

As has been noted earlier, research shows that understanding the family's point of view and honesty about the nature of the power relationship are appreciated by those at the receiving end of investigations. This is crucially important in cases where there are serious concerns about a child's welfare as a result of severe physical abuse or neglect. The notion of working in partnership with parents in these circumstances at this early stage may be unachievable. There may be considerable conflict and resistance to intervention in some cases. The focus must remain on the child and the child's welfare, and workers may need to exercise their authority in a way that precludes any power sharing with parents. This message has been a constant theme of many inquiries into cases where children have died as a result of abuse (see for instance Doreen Aston, London Boroughs of Lambeth, Lewisham & Southwark 1989; and Sukina, Bridge Child Care Consultancy Service 1991). The most that can be achieved in these circumstances is reasonable communication and an atmosphere of being non-judgemental. It is also important to be aware that the interaction between service users and child protection professionals at this stage can have an important effect on work at later stages (Farmer & Owen 1995).

In cases where it is clear who has abused the child, the child's protection needs are best served by working closely with the non-abusing parent. In situations involving serious intra-familial sexual abuse, however, as Hooper (1992) has noted, it should not be assumed that the non-abusing parent (usually the mother) will immediately believe her child, and allowance needs to be made for this. In some cases the non-abusing parent will continue to disbelieve and in these circumstances, as with cases of serious physical abuse and neglect, there may be considerable conflict between parents and professionals.

It is clear from *Messages from Research*, that the bulk of child care referrals do not involve serious allegations of abuse. They result from concerns about low standards of care often in families experiencing a range of pressures. It is clear in these situations that there is potential for developing a more supportive, partnership-based approach. Research shows that it is important to get parents to identify their own needs in such situations and to make a careful assessment of how their needs and those of their children can best be met. This entails involving parents in the decision-making process. Research (Sainsbury 1975) also shows that practical help, as well as psychological support, is particularly appreciated in these circumstances.

It should be stressed that working openly and supportively in these early stages of intervention (particularly where serious abuse is involved) depends considerably on the strength of inter-professional cooperation (see Corby, Chapter 13, in this volume).

Decision-making at conferences

There can be little doubt about parents' wishes to be involved in key decision-making forums about their children: 'Above all most parents wish to participate in decisions about their children and to be included as important partners in negotiations' (DOH 1991b, p. 47).

The 1990s saw considerable developments in this respect and it is now the norm for parents to be invited to child protection conferences. The Family Rights Group/NSPCC (1992) produced a manual to assist in ensuring that such participation is conducted in a positive and as far as possible, power-sharing way. According to research findings (Lewis *et al.* 1992), professionals largely perceive this involvement to be beneficial in meeting the children's needs. As noted before, parents' perceptions have been interpreted in different ways by research and there is some disagreement about the extent to which they have actually participated in the process. There can be little doubt, however, that most parents are glad that they have attended conferences even if they have found them to be difficult experiences. There is clearly no going back in this respect.

However, it is important that parents do not gain false expectations about the extent to which they will have the opportunity actively to participate at such meetings. Child protection conferences are required to be held within 15 days of the initial investigation and this is often still too early to do little more than continue to lay the foundations for future work in partnership with parents (see McCallum & Prilleltensky 1996). It should also be noted that the structure and format of child protection conferences (as well as the timing) make working with parents problematic, however sensitive the handling of situations by those involved. Essentially, child protection conferences have been mechanisms for child protection professionals to share their concerns, to make judgements about degrees of concern and to plan to reduce risks. Parental participation has been grafted on to this forum and because of this does not particularly enhance the development of partnership (Corby *et al.* 1996).

The late 1990s have seen the growing use of Family Group Conferences (Marsh & Crow 1998) based on the New Zealand model (Connolly 1994), and do involve more active power-sharing with parents and the extended family. Whether these will augment or replace child protection conferences is an open question.

Ongoing work

As has been continually stressed, the real potential for working more in partnership with parents lies in the period after the initial investigation and assessment stages, though again as has been repeatedly emphasised, what happens in these stages is crucially important in preparing the ground for later work. It should also be noted that many families where child abuse allegations are made are often already receiving family support services. A child protection investigation may alter that relationship considerably, and for some time. Nevertheless, it is in everyone's interest to be clear and honest about the abuse issues. Children must be protected from harm, parents have rights to information so that they can, if they wish, challenge decisions, and social workers need to be clear about their accountability, roles and tasks.

Core groups, referred to above, can be important forums for working in partnership with parents. Rather belatedly the potential of these groups in this respect have been more fully recognised by the Department of Heath in its recently published draft guidelines on inter-agency work in child protection (DOH 1999a). They stipulate that core groups should be held within 10 days of the child protection conference – thus it is important to recognise that the first meeting of this group still takes place relatively early on in the process. Nevertheless, as has been noted earlier, the core groups do have potential for working with parents more constructively and supportively than in conferences because of their relative intimacy. It is also worth noting that in cases where serious abuse is involved, the function of monitoring the progress of parents may need to take precedence over other activities.

Children in care

Approximately 3000 children per year come through the child protection system and are accommodated by local authorities (DOH 1995a). Some of these may need to remain in care for long periods. Some are accommodated for short periods to help families through periods of stress and difficulty in a preventive capacity. In both these cases, there is a real need to work in partnership with parents.

Research shows that even children who spend long periods in care eventually live with one family member or at least re-establish contact and receive some practical help from their parents (Stein & Carey 1986, Farmer & Parker 1991). Research has also consistently shown the benefits for children of maintaining contact with parents while in care (Rowe *et al.* 1984). The value of such contact with regard to the identity of the child is enshrined in the requirement to take into account racial origin, cultural and linguistic background and religious persuasion when looking after children (see s.22 Children Act 1989). Parents can provide continuity of love and identity. They can be the guardians of history, culture and religion and they can be a watchdog on behalf of their child's welfare. There are many parents and family members who can and want to play a greater part in their child's life, even if they cannot provide full-time care and, with careful thought, it is nearly always possible to ensure that they have a significant voice in many decisions affecting their children, e.g. routines, clothing, hairstyles, education, leisure pursuits and health matters.

Encouraging parents to retain as much responsibility as they can may create other problems, however. Carers may feel they are being asked to perpetuate child care practices that are less successful than their own, or to respond to parents for whom they have little respect. Other agencies may be left feeling confused as to who has the main responsibility for the child. Previewing such consequences with those likely to be involved and continuing to review the partnership in practice in an open and clear manner is the only way to ensure quality care for children.

Despite these problems, it is clear that in situations where children are 'looked after' by local authorities (whether short- or long-term) when parents and family continue to play a part, children do better, and therefore that parents and families are a resource that no agency can afford to discard.

Relatives and partners

In an increasing number of cases, it should be noted that children are placed with relatives. In most cases such placements are beneficial, though the Tyra Henry case (London Borough of Lambeth 1987) points to the dangers of over-reliance on relatives without paying careful attention to the dynamics of the extended family network. Nevertheless, it is essential that children's real (as opposed to notional) families are acknowledged and involved and that we do not restrict ourselves to partnership with biological parents only. We cannot therefore always make assumptions about how many partners there will be, or even if there will be more than one partnership simultaneously or sequentially.

When identifying partners to work with, it is also important to be alert to power imbalances within the immediate family, particularly in situations involving domestic violence. Social workers and other child protection professionals may need, on occasion, to be actively partisan and form an open and stronger partnership with one parent in order to safeguard the welfare of the child, rather than adopting an even-handed approach.

Working with other professionals

Issues in relation to inter-agency coordination and inter-professional cooperation are dealt with in detail elsewhere in this volume (see Corby, Chapter 13, in this volume). It is noted there that the new emphasis on family support may provide some challenges for professionals who have taken many years to develop effective working relationships across professional boundaries under the more child-protectionist ethos. Hence there is added importance in stressing here that effective partnerships with parents depend on shared understandings and practices between different agencies. Agencies need to agree on some issues: their operational definition of partnership; who constitutes the family; acceptable ways of sharing information with families; how to deal with aggression and threats to workers.

Rights of challenge

The extent to which parents should be more actively encouraged to assert their rights to be more fully involved in the child protection process is an interesting one. To a large degree, parents do not have any obvious rights within the child protection system itself because it does not carry the full force of law, though breaches of the Government *Working Together* guidelines are legally challengeable. It is clear that they normally have rights of attendance at child protection conferences, but the nature of that involvement is less obvious. They may, according to the new draft guidelines, take advocates to the conference with them, but it is stressed that 'the conference is primarily about the child and while the presence of the family is normally welcome, those professionals attending must be able to share information in a safe and non-threatening environment' (DOH 1999a, para. 5.56).

As has already been seen, parents have acquired some rights in the Children Act 1989 in terms of emergency proceedings, court procedures, and in relation to the care system. It is clear that they should be actively encouraged to exercise the rights they have in these areas through advocates. Parental advocates (whether friends, relatives, or workers from another agency such as the Citizens' Advice

Bureau) should be able to arrange good legal advice, support any use of the complaints procedure, organise transport, assist with changes to benefit, explain any documents, attend meetings alongside parents and access any necessary translation. They must feel able to do this whether or not they believe the parents have abused their children, and they must be able to avoid being drawn into any other role by families or other professionals. Using advocacy in this way clearly has implications for child protection professionals working in partnership with parents. Nevertheless, the need to exercise rights is a crucial one at this stage and is often outside the capacity of the social worker whose prime responsibility is the protection of the child.

Conclusions

At the end of the 1990s, the notion of working in partnership with parents was seen to be of central importance in child protection work and is increasingly being required by central government guidelines. We have stressed throughout that, in our opinion, the aim of achieving partnership with parents in child protection investigations may be too ambitious. Partnership suggests lack of conflict and power-sharing of a kind that has not often been found to be possible, particularly in the early stages of such work. Nevertheless, recent research has shown that there are large areas of child protection work where the main problem is not related to serious abuse but the need for family support. In these circumstances, it is clearly appropriate that child protection professionals work much more in conjunction with parents to help find the best solutions to family problems and their children's needs. At the same time, however, social workers have to remain vigilant about the needs of children for protection, despite the statistics. The issue of getting the balance right still remains.

Acknowledgement

The authors wish to acknowledge Adrian James' contribution to the original chapter on which this revised version is based.

Annotated further reading

Department of Health (DOH) 1989 The care of children: principles and practice in regulations and guidance. HMSO, London
A useful summary of the main principles of the Act drawn together in a series of operational statements.
Department of Health (DOH) 1991*a* Child abuse: a study of inquiry reports 1980–1989. HMSO, London
An overview of the lessons learned from the main child abuse inquiries from 1980 to Cleveland. Although specific inquiries are difficult to locate, due to layout, it does draw together key messages for all agencies, including the failure to work constructively with parents and other family members.
Department of Health (DOH) 1991*b* Patterns and outcomes in child placement. HMSO, London
A compilation of research into care outcomes for children, including results of studies on the pattern of entry into care, impact of care on the health and educational achievement of children, decision-making in case conferences, and partnership with parents and carers. An excellent and illuminating publication with worksheets attached.
Department of Health (DOH) 1991*c* Working together under the Children Act 1989. HMSO, London
Practice guidance for child protective inter-agency working, including parental involvement, issued shortly after the implementation of the Children Act 1989. The tone is optimistic particularly in relation to partnership with parents.

Department of Health (DOH) 1995 Child protection: messages from research. HMSO, London
This is a compilation of 20 research studies looking at aspects of child protective practice. The thrust of the evidence suggests that the balance between child protection and family support services sought by the Children Act 1989 was not evident in practice. These studies have been very influential in more recent developments attempting to refocus practice on children's needs rather than simply characterising enquiries as child abuse investigations.

Department of Health (DOH) 1999 Working together to safeguard children. Consultation draft. The Stationery Office, London
These are the most recently published guidelines for child protection professionals. They strongly emphasise the need to view child protection within a family support context.

Frost N, Stein M 1989 The politics of child welfare: inequality, power and change. Harvester Wheatsheaf, New York
An interesting analysis of the concept of childhood from early times to date and society's changing response to children and their needs. Of particular importance when considering our current concept of partnership with parents are the shifts in child welfare policy since the end of World War II.

Parton N (ed) 1997 Child protection and family support: tensions, contradictions and possibilities. Routledge, London
This book provides a series of thoughtful chapters on the shift in thinking in the 1990s on the balance between child protection and family support.

Thoburn J, Lewis A, Shemmings D 1995 Paternalism or partnership? Family involvement in the child protection process. HMSO, London
This book presents research carried out in the early 1990s into the way in which parents were involved in the child protection process by professionals. It highlights a range of operational issues, including lack or inappropriateness of agency policy as well as practice issues.

References

Arnstein S 1969 A ladder of citizen participation. American Institute of Planners Journal 35: 216–224

Bebbington A, Miles J 1989 The background of children who enter local authority care. British Journal of Social Work 19 (5): 349–368

Bowlby J 1951 Maternal care and mental health. World Health Organization, Geneva

Bridge Child Care Consultancy Service 1991 Sukina: an evaluation report of the circumstances leading to her death. The Bridge Child Care Consultancy Service, London

Brown C 1984 Child abuse parents speaking: parents' impressions of social workers and the social work process. School of Advanced Urban Studies, University of Bristol, Bristol

Butler Sloss Lady Justice E 1988 Report of the inquiry into child abuse in Cleveland 1987. Cmnd. 412. HMSO, London

Calder M 1990 Child protection core groups: participation not partnership. Child Abuse Review 4: 12–13

Calder M 1991 Child protection core groups: beneficial or bureaucaratic? Child Abuse Review 5: 26–29

Cleaver H, Freeman P 1995 Parental perspectives in cases of suspected child abuse. HMSO, London

Connolly M 1994 An act of empowerment: the Children, Young Persons and their Families Act 1989. British Journal of Social Work 24: 87–100

Corby B 1987 Working with child abuse. Open University Press, Milton Keynes

Corby B, Millar M 1997 Parents' view of partnership. In: Bates J, Pugh R, Thompson N (eds) Protecting children: challenges and change. Avebury, Aldershot

Corby B, Doig A, Roberts V 1998 Inquiries into child abuse. Journal of Social Welfare & Family Law 20: 357–376

Corby B, Millar M, Young L 1996 Parental participation in child protection work: rethinking the rhetoric. British Journal of Social Work 26: 475–492

Department of Health (DOH) 1988 Protecting children: a guide for social workers undertaking a comprehensive assessment. HMSO, London

Department of Health (DOH) 1989 The care of children: principles and practice in regulation and guidance. HMSO, London

Department of Health (DOH) 1991a Child abuse: a study of inquiry reports 1980–1989. HMSO, London

Department of Health (DOH) 1991b Working together under the Children Act 1989: a guide to arrangements for inter-agency cooperation for the protection of children against abuse. HMSO, London

Department of Health (DOH) 1995a Child protection: messages from research. HMSO, London

Department of Health (DOH) 1995*b* The challenge of partnership in child protection: practice guide. HMSO, London

Department of Health (DOH) 1999*a* Working together to safeguard children. A guide to inter-agency working to safeguard and promote the welfare of children. Consultation Draft. The Stationery Office, London

Department of Health (DOH) 1999*b* Framework for the assessment of children in need and their families. Consultation Draft. The Stationery Office, London

Department of Health and Social Security (DHSS) 1974 Report of the committee of inquiry into the care and supervision provided in relation to Maria Colwell. HMSO, London

Department of Health and Social Security (DHSS) 1985 Social work decisions in child care: recent research findings and their implications. HMSO, London

Department of Health and Social Security (DHSS) 1986 Child abuse-working together. A draft guide to arrangements for inter-agency cooperation for the protection of children. HMSO, London

Department of Health and Social Security (DHSS), Welsh Office 1988 Working together. A guide to arrangements for inter-agency cooperation for the protection of children from abuse. HMSO, London

Dickenson D, Stainton-Rogers W, Roche J, Jeffrey C 1991 The Children Act 1989: putting it into practice. Open University Press, Milton Keynes

Eekelaar J 1991 Parental responsibility: state of nature or nature of the state. Journal of Social Welfare and Family Law 1: 37–50

Family Rights Group 1991 The Children Act 1989: working in partnership with families. Family Rights Group, London

Family Rights Group, NSPCC 1992 Child protection procedures: what they mean for your family. Waterside Press, London

Farmer E, Owen M 1995 Child protection practice: private risks and public remedies: decision-making, intervention and outcome in child protection work. HMSO, London

Farmer E, Parker R 1991 Trials and tribulations: returning children from care to their families. HMSO, London

Ferguson H 1990 Rethinking child protection practices: a case for history? In: The Violence Against Children Study Group (eds) Taking child abuse seriously. Unwin Hyman, London

Fisher M, Marsh P, Phillips D, Sainsbury E 1986 In and out of care: the experiences of children, parents and social workers. Batsford, London

Fox Harding L 1991 Perspectives in child care policy. Longman, Harlow

Frost N, Stein M 1989 The politics of child welfare: inequality, power and change? Harvester Wheatsheaf, New York

Gibbons J, Conroy S, Bell C 1995 Operating the child protection system: a study of child protection practices in English local authorities. HMSO, London

Goldstein J, Freud A, Solnit A 1973 Beyond the best interests of the child. Free Press, New York

Holman R 1988 Putting families first: prevention and childcare? Macmillan Education, London

Home Office 1945 Report by Sir Walter Monckton on the circumstances that led to the boarding-out of Dennis and Terence O'Neill at Bank Farm, Minsterley and the steps taken to supervise their welfare. Cmnd 6636. HMSO, London

Hooper C 1992 Mothers surviving sexual abuse. Tavistock, London

House of London Commons 1984 Children in care, Vol. 1. Second report from the Social Services Committee. Session 1983–1984. HMSO, London

Jordan B 1988 What price partnership? Costs and benefits. In: James A, Scott D (eds) Partnership in probation, education and training. Central Council for Educational and Training in Social Work (CCETSW), London

Kempe C, Silverman F, Steele B, *et al.* 1962 The battered child syndrome. Journal of the American Medical Association 181: 17–24

Lewis A, Shemmings D, Thoburn J 1992 Participation in practice: a reader. University of East Anglia, Norwich

London Borough of Lambeth 1987 Whose child? A report of the public inquiry into the death of Tyra Henry. London Borough of Lambeth, London

London Boroughs of Lambeth, Lewisham and Southwark 1989 Doreen Aston report. Lambeth, Lewisham & Southwark ACPCs, London

McCallum S, Prilleltensky I 1996 Empowerment in child protection work: values, practices and caveats. Children and Society 10: 40–50

Marsh P, Crow G 1998 Family group conferences in child welfare. Blackwell, Oxford

Mayer J E, Timms N 1970 The client speaks. Routledge, London

Parton N 1979 The natural history of child abuse: a study in social problem definition. British Journal of Social Work 9: 431

Prosser J 1992 Child abuse investigations: the families perspective. Evaluation Unit, Westminster College, Oxford

Rees S 1978 Social work face to face. Edward Arnold, London

Rees S, Wallace A 1982 Verdicts on social work. Edward Arnold, London

Rowe J, Lambert L 1973 Children who wait. British Association for Adoption and Fostering, London

Rowe J, Cain H, Hundleby M, Keane A 1984 Long-term foster care. Batsford/BAAF, London

Sainsbury E 1975 Social work with families. Routledge & Kegan Paul, London

Sainsbury E, Nixon S, Phillips D 1982 Social work in focus: clients and social workers' perceptions in long-term social work. Routledge & Kegan Paul, London

Sharland H, Jones E, Aldgate J, *et al.* 1995 Professional intervention in child sexual abuse. HMSO, London

Social Services Inspectorate (SSI), Department of Health 1992 Partnership with families in child protection: a practice guide. HMSO, London

Stein M, Carey K 1986 Leaving care. Blackwell, Oxford

Thoburn J, Lewis A, Shemmings D 1995 Paternalism or partnership? Family involvement in the child protection process. HMSO, London

Tunstill J 1997 Implementing the family support clauses of the Children Act 1989: legislative, professional and organisational barriers. In: Parton N (ed) Balancing child protection and family support: tensions, contradictions and possibilities. Macmillan, London

Wattam C 1999 The prevention of child abuse. Children and Society 13: 317–329

Yelloly M 1980 Social work theory and psychoanalysis. Van Nostrand Reinhold, New York

Individual work with children

Margaret Crompton

**INTRODUC-
TION**

You are mistaken if you think we have to lower ourselves to communicate with children. On the contrary, we have to reach up to their feelings, stretch, stand on our tiptoes.

(Korczak 1925; in Lifton 1989, p. 172)

The Central Council for Education and Training in Social Work (CCETSW) *Guidance Notes* for teaching about child care in the Diploma in Social Work (DipSW) courses emphasise that, 'The Children Act 1989 requires that the wishes and feelings of children should be considered in all decision-making. The Cleveland inquiry report (1988) gave the profession a salutory reminder about the importance of treating children as people, not objects.' Maintenance of 'that perspective of the child as client' requires development of 'skills in communicating directly and honestly with children, young people and adults, recognising the need to take time and not to compel … clients to talk' (CCETSW 1991, p. 18).

The implications of regarding the child as a client and of direct, honest and unpressured interaction must form the base of any work with children, together with avoidance of labelling by symptom. Only attention to the whole, individual child by the whole, individual worker can lead to communication. Whatever the agency and context of the interaction, it is essential to respect children and to be clear about the purpose of contact for *each* child.

The Utting Report found that 'Looking after [children living away from home] would be easier and much more effective if we really heard and understood what they have to tell us' (Utting 1997, p. 7). Ensuring that children are *heard* and *understood* requires practitioners really to *listen*, and not to substitute mechanistic procedures (Smedley 1999, p. 114).

A nursery nurse, in a voluntary agency specialising in help for abused and neglected children, summarises thus:

If you centre on the whole child she goes away from the sessions as a stronger person with increased confidence because she knows what's going on. If you centre totally on the abuse, on what actually happened, where is the rest of the child? You can give the child the impression that only the abuse is important.

(Crompton 1980, p. 12)

There are many kinds of abuse and many reasons for referral. The observable scars of children who have been subject to physical abuse (including neglect and sexual assault) are accompanied by wounds to the emotions, mind and spirit. Children also suffer invisible assault, unaccompanied by visible clues but nonetheless desperately needing careful attention from adults. Physical and sexual abuse attract far more attention than cognitive, emotional and spiritual abuse.

The main focus of this chapter is an introduction to some ways of communicating with children, including an account of work with a 10-year-old boy. Material is largely drawn from texts focusing on work with children who have been referred to agencies because of observed abuse. However, the aim of the chapter is to discuss individual work with children who have, as part of their experience of life, suffered abuse, as distinct from 'abused children'.

Emphasis is on straightforward, uncluttered, simple methods and approaches. Children and workers have neither time nor energy for elaboration and the most effective interactions are those in which child and adult *meet*, with minimal accessories, material or verbal. This is exemplified by the work of Madge Bray (co-founder of Sexual Abuse: Child Consultancy Service (SACCS)) who describes the essence of her approach as 'simplicity':

It is based on a willingness to receive, at the child's own pace, whatever it is that the child wishes to impart. As the adult she listens, responds and sets the boundaries ... She sits on the floor with a toybox and creates an environment where play is the natural medium, of communication.

(Boyle 1997, p. x)

The chapter is organised in three main sections:

1. The professional background to individual work
2. Some methods of communication
3. Work with a 10-year-old boy.

The professional background to individual work

The idea of working with, and not only on behalf of, children is far from new. Kastell (1962), Winnicott (1964) and Holgate (1972) were among influential writers and teachers in the UK, while in the USA the texts of Axline and Oaklander were first published in 1947 and 1964, and 1969 (new edition in 1978) respectively. Social workers in field and residential agencies understood the importance of play and the skills of listening, seeing, waiting and communicating. It is irritating to workers who are still far from decrepit to read of 'new emphasis on the concept of "communicating with children"' (Wells 1989, p. 45). Stevenson (1991) regrets that the CCETSW guidelines 'could not have been available earlier before innumerable wheels all over the country were reinvented!' (p. 5).

However, Stevenson (1991) emphasises the need for continuing efforts towards good practice, not least because of deficiencies in social work training which has lacked rigour and placed too little emphasis on 'knowledge and well-researched evidence ... Because a social work qualification is a licence to practise measurable standards should be set and adhered to' (p. 5). Decisions about individual work, regarding philosophy, models of human development and intervention, and efficacy of such intervention, should be well-founded (CCETSW 1991, p. 10). Boyle notes that 'skills in communicating with children are not taught as a matter of course' (Boyle 1997, p. xii).

Training should be a respected specialisation, with academic and practical work on many aspects of childhood, including the history of politics and philosophy in the legislation of education, employment, religion, health and social welfare, together with the day-to-day culture of school, leisure, fashion, family and peer group. Students should spend time in playgrounds and discos and read teen magazines and children's literature (Crompton 1992, pp. 5–6). Familiarity with a range of models of development and behaviour, and of approaches to helping is also essential. Thompson & Rudolph (1988) provides an excellent introduction.

Communicating with children requires professional rigour, including clear definition of the purpose and aims of every interaction. Stevenson's (1991) comment, 'Prompted in particular by concern about sexual abuse, social workers have rushed to observe children's play with little open discussion of the justification for the inferences drawn' (p. 6), illustrates the confusion of undertaking action without a sound philosophical grounding.

The decision to offer helping interaction to an individual child requires careful thought, understanding of what such interaction might entail, and commitment by both worker and agency, before the offer is made. O'Hagan (1989) is anxious that focusing on the individual may 'exacerbate the crisis generated by the disclosure' (p. 116), and Furniss (1991) points out that seeing children individually is not automatically synonymous with individual counselling or therapy. Disciplined definition is required, with an understanding of possible difficulties for workers (Stone 1990).

Moore (1992), whose chapter 'Face-to-face work with the abused child' is down-to-earth and useful, is clear that, 'An abused child has the right to be the primary client, to be facilitated in a face-to-face way, to make sense of what has happened and, in spite of the trauma, helped to become a survivor' (p. 127). She advises that:

What we can offer is warm, friendly, personal help, aimed at enabling [the children] to come to terms with themselves and their actual situation ... The only way for an abused child is forwards. We must help them understand and mature through the awful experience ... The role of a worker is to help children get in touch with the suffering part of themselves: to reassure them that they are understood and respected, so that they can move on, leave the baggage behind and start living for themselves.

(Moore 1992, pp. 130–131)

Such help cannot and should not erase memories of 'awful experiences'. Moving on involves the whole person in the real world, where the 'actual situation' and the problems of life have to be met again and again. The most important aim is to develop strength with which to face and manage challenges and suffering.

However, as Bagley & King (1990) note in their review of therapeutic philosophies, 'many children do not receive treatment for the traumas that child sexual abuse involves, during their childhood years. These principles of healing are equally relevant for "the hurting child" who may still be part of the adult personality' (p. 133).

Glaser & Frosh (1988) note that individual work may accompany, replace or succeed time-limited group experience and comprise contact with 'a professional, usually their social worker, teacher or counsellor' (p. 146). Decisions about what kind of help can be offered depend not only on an assessment of what should be available, but also of agency resources, and may be quite arbitrary. Workers should be clear about constraints.

The purpose of providing opportunities for communication directly between children and professionally caring adults may be simply defined as 'assessment' and 'help'. 'Assessment' includes, for example, all activities leading to writing reports, making recommendations to courts and planning for future accommodation. Tasks include gathering information, communicating to children information about possibilities and constraints, learning about feelings, perceptions, preferences and plans. 'Help' comprises provision of an environment conducive to developing self-awareness, confidence, self-esteem and the ability to trust wisely, to make realistic plans and decisions, and to form relationships that contribute to the well-being of all involved. Tasks include helping children to recognise and manage external realities (past events, present accommodation, future relationships) and inward experiences (memories, perceptions, feelings), and to cooperate in forming realistic plans. It is important to be clear about the primary purpose of interaction, particularly when considering such communicative activities as those reviewed in the second part of this chapter.

The implications of such concepts as self-esteem need analysis (see Roberts 1993). Trust, too, should be carefully considered (Cooper & Ball 1987, Crompton 1990, Doyle 1990, Furniss 1991). (References to Doyle are to 1990 edition; please note comment to 2nd edn. 1997 in Annotated Reading, below.)

Another word used frequently and loosely is 'therapy'. It is not always clear whether practitioners and authors associate 'therapy/therapist' with their original connotations of disease and healing. More important is the need to be clear about the distinction between 'therapeutically informed intervention' by social workers and long-term therapeutic work which requires more specialist skills. Therapy within social work interactions should not be confused with psychotherapy (Glaser & Frosh 1988, Doyle 1990). A distinction should also be made between this and such specialisations as art, drama, music and play therapies. Wilson *et al.* (1992) differentiate between 'the use of play in play therapy and in activities ... which are used by an adult to explain, clarify, prepare or for other purposes work on an area which the adult has identified as one of concern', defined as 'play-related communication' (p. 13).

Professional rigour requires semantic and conceptual precision. If individual, group or family-based help is available, the reason for choosing one approach rather than another should be clear. The exclusive attention of one adult offers the best chance of a peaceful, private and relaxed period, away from the immediate pressures of family relationships or identification in a group with a label, and the child can use this kind of interaction freely.

Workers' principal skills must be *really* to *see* and to *listen*. This necessitates leaving all fears and assumptions behind, and endeavouring to engage with the world of the child, both internal and external. Smedley (1999) considers that 'We will not reach children unless we can convey to them our openness to understanding their deep hurt, and we cannot do this if we deny our own pain' (p. 114). Moore advises: 'Communication is a reciprocal giving and receiving of thoughts and feelings. The worker's body posture and tone of voice must convey empathy and understanding' (Moore 1992, p. 132). Mearns & Thorne (1988), following the Rogers, Person-centered model, define *empathy* as 'a continuing process whereby the counsellor lays aside her own way of experiencing and perceiving reality, preferring to sense and respond to the experiences and perceptions of her client' (Mearns & Thorne 1988, p. 39). *Empathy* is a popular and overused word. The concept is useful but should be approached with care. It is easy, for example, to confuse it with sympathy or with recognition of a similar experience in the worker's own life, or to become dangerously immersed in the child's feelings (see also Crompton 1992).

One boy, named Adam, for example, felt so much pain, hopelessness and fear during a session that he 'stood up, wanting to throw himself through the window to the conservatory glass roof beneath'. The practitioner 'felt his fear and reflected this. I stayed seated, and quietly talked to him about how I wanted him to be safe'. Adam could later give clear advice about interviewing someone who was suicidal, including, 'you listen to him, try to do what he says, do your best. If you can't do it, explain why ... make sure he's safe ... remember the kid is scared, nervous' (Smedley 1999, p. 122).

The endeavour to engage so intimately with children's inner lives carries with it the danger of intruding on their privacy. Care should be taken to avoid 'pressing the bruise' or expecting too much response (if any). Even when respecting the right not to speak, it is easy to stimulate thoughts and feelings that are difficult and painful and that continue to have an impact long after the end of immediate contact between child and worker (Crompton 1991).

Children often give clues that they do not wish to pursue a particular line or activity; moving to another toy, running around, changing the conversation. This is in itself a form of communication. Workers should notice the triggers to withdrawal and judge whether the reaction is to the particular topic or activity, perhaps associated with some memory, or to a communication by the worker.

Pressing too hard for overt responses may lead to distortion, even lying. Conversely, apparent failure to respond may mask unexpressed internal activity or alterations of behaviour elsewhere. Dorfman (1951) writes of an aggressive and abusing 13-year-old boy who spent most of his regular and protected hour ignoring her. After ten sessions, he was told that although the hour was saved for him, he need not continue to attend. His response was, 'Whaddya mean, not come any more? I'll come till the cows come home!' His behaviour outside the worker's room had greatly improved. Only to the worker did he give no overt hint of the positive use to which he put the unpressured hour with her (Dorfman 1951, pp. 244–245).

Respect for *privacy* and non-intrusion is essential but Doyle (1990) notes that avoidance of discussing abusive activities may result from the inability of adults to tolerate children's pain. Interviews may remain superficial and 'the child left feeling that he or she has been involved in something so dreadful that it cannot be discussed. Children should be allowed to talk about the abuse and examine what it has meant for them' (Doyle 1990, p. 34). Only real attention to individual children, including *waiting* for their own timing, enables them to respond as they wish.

An aspect of privacy demanding special care is *confidentiality*, which cannot be guaranteed, perhaps because a worker fears that the child client, or other children, may be in danger. Children should be 'assured that only people who are in a position to help either them or other children will be allowed to know what the child does or says in a session' (Doyle 1990, p. 42). Some authorities suggest that confidentiality may represent a potential danger, mirroring the secrecy that characterises child sexual abuse cases (Glaser & Frosh 1988). It is most important to give children clear information about any limits to confidentiality, including, for example, whether any other staff member knows about interactions between child and worker and, if the worker should be unavailable at any time or leave the agency, whether colleagues know about the child's situation, feelings and attitudes. Such clarity can offer good experiences of honesty and plain dealing by the worker, and opportunities to exercise choice and control about speaking and keeping silent.

Danger, or at least confusion, may be represented by the physical privacy of one-to-one work for children whose experience of private engagements with adults has entailed abuse. Some writers suggest that workers risk seductive behaviour and allegations of abuse by children but Doyle (1990) regards the latter as unlikely, because 'few youngsters tell lies about sexual abuse'. However, workers should be alert to the possibility of misunderstanding by children whose experience of adults has not led to the development of wise trust, and children should not be exposed to feeling 'isolated and trapped' with workers (Doyle 1990, pp. 35, 39).

Nonetheless, common sense, good training, professional discipline and efficient agency organisation should ensure that such problems, confusions and dangers are prevented, and that every child for whom it is appropriate has the opportunity for individual, protected, private contact with a worker.

Smedley (1999), discussing transcripts of interviews with children, 'found the same message for social workers ... in all stages of child protection work,' articulated by Lisa: 'Social workers should try to understand what children are really trying to say, explain any questions the children have, and if they feel left out they should be made to feel important, wanted and loved'. Adam praised his satisfactorily listening social worker – 'I've got big shields around me now' (pp. 117, 118).

Some methods of communication

This discussion is necessarily selective and brief. No reference is made to such electronic aids as videos and computers, and the main focus is on work with the minimal material facilities usually available to workers, including drawing and writing equipment, books and a car. The most important constituents of communication are the individual people concerned, within time and space dedicated to the child.

Choice of activity and equipment is negotiated between child and worker, having regard to both preferences and explained, understandable constraints. For example, when working with a 10-year-old boy, without access to any room, my age and abilities precluded communication via football or swimming but we were able to share simple art work and walking. Equipment was kept in a carrying box which I took to every meeting and gave to him at the end of our contact. Shelter was provided by a café and my car. Cooperation in developing an activity may help to increase self-confidence and, thus, strength in managing everyday life.

Although some reference is made to 'therapy', examples illustrate activities which may be undertaken by non-specialist (but trained) workers. For example, a chapter on play therapy follows (p. 423), but there are innumerable ways in which play, interpreted very broadly, can be used as both a vehicle and an environment for communication by non-specialist practitioners.

Bannister (1989) is one of many writers to stress that workers should not seek to interpret the process and/or product of children's creative activity, for not only may such interpretation 'be incorrect or irrelevant' but, most important, 'the child has expressed feeling and, may be, found a solution' (p. 84; see also Oaklander 1978, Crompton 1992, West 1996).

Although the phrase 'face-to-face with children' is often used of direct work, play activities essentially provide opportunities for interaction without being face-to-face, so that eye contact need not be sought or forced, and verbal conversation may play only a small role.

Agencies sometimes produce packs of ideas for play activities. However, such material can be useful only as a reference base to stimulate creative development by individual practitioners and children.

The environment

A satisfactory physical and psychic environment, including safety and privacy, is essential. Whether meetings take place in playrooms or cafés, hospital wards or cars, workers are themselves part of the environment. For example, clothes should be appropriate for sitting on the floor, painting, cuddling or walking. It is important not to insult children by dressing in a slovenly fashion. Dress should reflect care and respect. It may even be possible to avoid wearing colours which are known to be particularly disliked by an individual child.

Anxiety about laddering tights or creasing trousers may be regarded by children as anxiety about being with them, for workers' feelings also contribute to the environment of the interaction. If adults are exhausted, anxious, unhappy, angry, depressed or ill, energy available for the children is limited and they may sense the emotionally charged or depleted atmosphere. Similarly, if adults are fit and fully able to concentrate on the children, the emotional environment will be clearer and more spacious.

Workers with abused children may communicate their feelings about the abuse too; for example, anger towards the abusers, horror about the events and sympathy with the children. It may at times be preferable to postpone a contact than to expose a child to the feelings of the worker.

Yet postponement itself can be perceived as rejection or evidence of the child's lack of worth. Meticulous courtesy and attention to punctuality and reliability are essential aspects of the total environment and the messages given and received. Children should not be kept waiting or let down because 'something has come up'. Khadija Rouf (1989) writes that she:

... got a social worker, Sue. She was okay but because our family had gone past crisis point she never came round. That is to do with big caseloads, I know, but we did *all* need someone to talk to ... [Workers should] remember that a lot of children are on their own. Don't let them down. If you arrange to go out, then go out. If you say you'll be in court, then for God's sake be there. Abused children have been let down enough. (pp. 9–10)

Attention should be given to the duration of interactions. Respect for the whole child includes recognition that life continues outside the playroom. The child may have other appointments, friends waiting or a favourite television show which will be missed if workers do not honour agreed stopping as well as starting times.

Enthusiastic work with a boy led to extended hours spent in the sitting room of the foster home. In one case, belated recognition that this delayed teatime and kept the family from the television led to better discipline and timekeeping by the worker. Beginnings and endings of not only individual sessions but also the entire period of contact are especially important (Crompton 1990).

Contacts should never be interrupted by telephone calls or enquiries from colleagues. Discussions with the agency director or court appearances would not be interrupted for the worker to take a message. Working with children requires concentration and continuity.

The physical environment is in itself a form of communication, indicating to children attention to their welfare. Some agencies provide well-stocked playrooms where workers may ensure a period of uninterrupted ownership of protected space. Many workers create defended space, for example, in 'empty broom-closets and in the back of gymnasiums' (Shapiro 1984, p. v).

It may help children's sense of being individual and cared-about if workers keep their materials in separate, particular bags, indicating that they are not just other 'cases'. Attention to materials is important; for example, folders used for life story books could be chosen in the child's favourite colours. Shopping together is not always possible, so care shown by a worker in demonstrating choice on behalf of the child is beneficial.

A personal set of coloured pencils, which only the child has a right to use or not to use, may offer some sense of control. If the favourite colours are constantly used, while others are neglected, children can see how their own choices affect the world, even in the form of only one coloured pencil. No other child is interfering and workers can protect this aspect of the child's environment by keeping the containers and equipment themselves and bringing them, regularly and intact, to appointments, thus indicating that the individual child is remembered and respected during the intervals between contacts. Similarly, children may keep their own equipment. This offers opportunities for them to demonstrate control and the ability to protect important possessions. The equipment can become a symbol of the continuity and reliability of contacts with workers.

Protecting and respecting material property that children share with workers indicates respect for, instead of abuse of, children. It helps to establish wise trust and encourages children to feel that, through those material extensions of themselves, they have worth.

Much important communication occurs indirectly through such aspects of everyday life as clothing and food (Crompton 1990). Respect for a child's personal preferences and cultural traditions, for example, dietary and clothing requirements, is essential and lack of such respect can be a form of abuse (Ahmed *et al.* 1986, Gardner 1987, Crompton 1998).

A nurse, for example, expressed exasperation that she was expected to obtain a special meal for a Muslim baby whose religion forbade her to eat pork. The nurse considered it to be acceptable to feed the child pork because, 'since the food was mashed up, the parents would not know what she had eaten, and the baby would certainly be unaware of the contents of her dinner' (Crompton 1998, p. 163).

Kenward (1989) illustrates the powerful symbolism of food for Anna (8 years old): the availability of food had 'been dependent upon her being sexually co-operative'. When her foster mother offered her food, Anna said, 'I'm hungry and I want it. I can't make my hand take it'. The foster family helped, partly by giving Anna control of serving food. Offering, receiving and sharing food can provide opportunities for children to exercise choice and control, and to experience ordinary routines of social interaction (see also Crompton 1990, chapter 10).

Anxiety can be raised in a child who feels unable to conform to adult expectations of everyday behaviour. Kenward (1989) quotes John (11 years old), following a visit to new foster parents: 'I liked them very much but they didn't know how I am inside ... I don't know what they want me to do or how to do it and I'm afraid in case I make them angry and they hurt me' (p. 32). Such clear expression of inner confusion is rare and illuminating.

Whatever the physical environment and activity, workers themselves define the immediate environment. On a walk, for example, the adult provides a boundary within which the child may choose the path, the speed, whether to stop and look down a rabbit hole or run across a field, leaving the worker behind. The child's freedom is safely within the context of the contact with the worker. Such freedom is not abandonment or lack of caring and boundaries are not arbitrary obstacles. Workers are the providers of space, time and interest. They set limits and ensure that doors are safely closed, so that there will be no interruptions. The environment must be non-threatening and safe, offering opportunities for choice, control, stimulus and peace.

Art

Workers do not have to be skilled artists to share artistic activity with children. Inadequacy may even be helpful if a child can discover and demonstrate greater competence than an adult, maybe taking the superior role of teacher. Simple, cheap materials are easily transported for spontaneous use. Drawing, painting and modelling provide opportunities for absorbing and relaxing activity. Children who have been subject to the stresses of abuse and investigation may find respite in a holiday from words, within space and time provided by a non-pressurising adult. Clues about feelings may be implied through choice of subject, colour, materials, use of space, concentration and response to making a mess, and it is interesting to note what is done with the product. For example, a picture may be given to the worker, taken home to a parent, treasured or destroyed.

Materials need not be used for obviously creative purposes. A nursery nurse noted that a 5-year-old used clay to dunk in a bowl of water, saying, 'I'm drowning the clay', soon after her sister had been accidentally drowned in her presence (Crompton 1990, p. 42).

Sharing artistic activity may help to relieve tension, for example, when awaiting a court appearance or on a journey.

Drawing may be included in making life story books with children (see below). An artistically unskilled worker may manage at least matchstick people or may be able to draw simple outlines to be coloured in, at will, by the child, or the child may draw all the pictures. Shapes of houses, people, animals, cars and so on can easily be cut from sheets of coloured paper and stuck onto paper or card. Very young children can be fully involved in choosing colours, gumming, choosing the position for shapes, and older children can also draw and cut. Pictures can be cut from magazines but young children may not appreciate the difference between photographs of models and of themselves: an attempt to teach a young boy about his life as a baby, using a photograph from an advertisement, led to confusion as he thought the picture was of himself.

Allan (1988), Bannister (1989) and Jones (1992) discuss drawing by children who have been sexually abused, including useful illustrations (pictorial and narrative) and analysis of method.

The rosebush-guided fantasy, based on Stevens (1971), is a method of encouraging self-expression through drawing and verbal exposition. Children are invited to imagine themselves to be rosebushes, then to draw and explain the picture. Allan (1988) comments that it 'may be a useful screening device for detecting children who have been or are being sexually abused', but advises great caution and specialised training and supervision (pp. 82–83). (Since this is a specialised discussion by a Jungian psychoanalyst, readers are recommended to study the original text.)

Oaklander (1978), using a Gestalt approach, writes of Gina (8 years old) who, suffering from much anxiety, said, 'I can grow easier if I don't have roots; if they want to replant me it will be easier. I always have buds'. Her adoptive parents had separated, causing much anxiety for the child. Oaklander found the rosebush work very helpful to Gina.

The same technique was used by Seymour (1990), a social worker, with Trevor (10 years old) who had been removed from home because of neglect and, following the end of an adoptive placement, awaited a 'permanent family'. Trevor's rosebush, like that of Gina, had no roots: they 'would not grow because nobody took care of it'. However, there were 'lots of thorns on it so that it would hurt anyone who tried to touch it' (pp. 1, 10; see also Crompton 1992).

Workers interested in this technique are advised to refer to Oaklander (1978) and Stevens (1971). Further discussion of art as a communicative activity can be found in books by Crompton (1980, Chapter 7, 1992, Chapter 9).

Music

Music may be overlooked as a communicative activity, especially when workers are shy about their own abilities. Musical instruments may be too large to transport but equipment in playrooms and residential units could include percussion, piano or keyboard, recorders and guitars, and a cassette/record player. Many cars are equipped with radios and cassette players.

Music may contribute to the total communicative environment; for example, children or workers may choose some recorded music to accompany an activity. Workers should be aware of the impact of such choices. A child might use a very noisy disc to overwhelm or distract the worker, or might respond with distress to the worker's choice of some melody intended to be calming. A piece of music or a sound may have important resonances which stir memories (possibly disturbing). A child who has suffered abuse may respond with anxiety to a record which was popular during the period of abuse or a favourite of the abuser, or even played during sexual or violent episodes and/or assaults on the emotions and spirit. Choice of background music offers children some control and a ground for negotiation about duration and volume.

Children may like to play instruments alone, perhaps finding relief and release in pounding a drum or piano, or finding relaxation in devising apparently formless, meditative melodies. The presence of the worker is important, protecting space, time and activity, and demonstrating acceptance and attention.

Playing an instrument or singing may be shared by child and worker and can bring relaxation and enjoyment, also providing opportunities for children to demonstrate abilities which can attract praise and encouragement for further development, invaluable when self-respect has been demolished.

Listening to music together can demonstrate the worker's ability to attend to the child, without pressure on the child to buy that attention with words (answering questions, offering revelations) or actions (collusion in abusive acts).

Words may be included in the form of songs, composed by the child or in the form of recorded or sung music, offering a clue to the child's feelings. Laurel, after confinement in a secure unit for unruly behaviour, chose to play again and again a record with words of loss and bewilderment. She did not seek to converse with the quietly attentive adult but recognition of the presence of that adult suggested that the choice of record was made partly in order to express something about herself (Crompton 1992).

Dance offers opportunities for relaxation, expression of feeling, concentration on the music or shared enjoyment and a break from the need for speech. Further discussion of music may be found in books by Crompton (1980, Chapter 6, 1992, Chapter 10).

Stories

Telling a story can provide an environment of comfort, particularly if the child can be cuddled. The child, too, may be the storyteller. Luke (6 years old) would lie on the settee in his foster home. While not very articulate, at these times he would tell a story about a recent experience, the words tumbling out with great feeling as he relaxed. When these stories were carefully written out, his rapidly spoken words and lively tales helped Luke gain a sense of himself existing in some relationship to the past, present and future. Also, he learned that the stories were of enough value for an adult to listen, write out between sessions and return to him. Joint illustrations used matchstick figures and outlines which Luke could colour in, as well as his own drawings (Crompton 1992).

Marion Burch (1992) has drawn on her experience as mother to five adopted children and 30 years fostering to produce a guide, *I Want to Make a Life Story Book*, which includes a model for such a book, photographs, stories and other ideas.

Bray includes the whole of 'Jessica's Story', beginning, as all good stories do, 'Once upon a time ...'. She sets the scene for writing the story, sitting with Jessica on her knee. The little girl says:

'Do you want to write? Do you like to write me a story?'
'Yes, I do.'
'But how will you know it's me?'
'I'll try to get it as close as I can.'
Jessica nodded pensively.
'I don't cry, do I, Madge? Will I cry in my story? I haven't cried, ever.'
'No, then probably you won't cry in your story.'

(Bray 1997, p. 168; the story is on pp. 169–184)

Bray concludes: 'I have often written stories for children which paralleled their own life experience in order to help them make sense of distortion in their lives' (p. 184).

Redgrave (1987) includes a substantial, practical and illustrated discussion of life story books, warning against routine and the unimaginative imposition of such an activity. Donley (1975) advises that the product of life story, or any other, activity belongs to the child and that social workers should beware of themselves becoming attached to such products. Crompton (1980, 1992) discusses communication through both life stories and other forms of narrative. Oaklander (1978) includes sections on writing, poetry and books. Allan (1988) describes serial story writing with a physically abused adolescent (pages 199–211).

Printed books may be useful as aids to communication but, as with any pre-packaged material, there are difficulties. Non-fiction books about feelings or experiences may be dull and/or confusing. Reading a story about experiences similar to the child's own may be reassuring demonstrating that the child is not unique and that feelings about such experiences are known to other people. However, published stories usually have neat plots and endings, whereas real experience is continuing and complex. Adults should not expect 'identification' with fictional characters.

The most influential books are usually those chosen by the individual child and it is useful to be aware of children's favourite or least favourite texts. Responses may be very different from those expected by adults. As a child, I avoided looking at illustrations of a menacing genie, an exploding witch, and a little naked boy floating down a stream alone. These represented terrifying power and powerlessness to the child, but to adults they were only illustrations of charming stories.

Published material may most usefully form an aid to relaxation and to learning about ways of managing the challenges of life through the eyes of other people. However, a programme of planned and guided reading may be devised, aiming to give support and modify behaviour, and known as *bibliotherapy* (Marshall 1981).

Bibliographies of focused texts are sometimes produced by libraries. Mills (1988) reviews fictional treatment of sexual abuse. Thompson & Rudolph (1988) include a bibliography of fictional texts about sexual and other abuse.

Particularly interesting and potent aspects of story telling are found in myths, legends and fairy tales. Apparently simple stories may hold different meanings for different individuals. A black American boy (8 years old) told the tale of 'Missy Red Riding Hood', wagging an admonitory finger with great glee. Polish students found the message of that story and of *Snow White* to be that they should not trust people. Yet for Julia (8 years old), who had suffered from severe neglect by her mother, 'Snow White provided an opportunity to enact the part of the wicked (step)mother, "Only in this story, she doesn't win", Snow White is queen' (Hunter 1987, p. 28). *Rapunzel* represented comfort and security to an American 5-year-old when he learnt that his grandmother, who often cared for him, was to enter hospital. Bettelheim (1976) suggests that he learnt, 'That one's own body can provide a lifeline', just as Rapunzel's hair was used as a ladder: 'if necessary, he would find in his own body the source of his security' (Bettelheim 1976, p. 17). A girl who had problems with body images was helped through *The Ugly Duckling* (Bannister 1989).

Janusz Korczak regularly told the children in his orphanage (many of whom had been abused by physical and/or emotional assault or neglect and, in pre-war Warsaw, were certainly socially abused and religiously oppressed) such old tales as *Puss in Boots*. He considered that, 'children who feel worthless in a society that doesn't value them, who feel angry and powerless because their parents ... can no longer protect them, need to believe that there are magic forces that can help them overcome their difficulties'. (Nazi occupation is far from being the only condition necessary for children to feel unvalued, angry and powerless.) Such traditional tales, full of difficulties and obstacles requiring perseverence and strength of will, were 'close to life' (Lifton 1989, p. 74). (Further discussion of myths and stories may be found in Crompton 1992, Chapter 7; Crompton 1998, Chapter 15.)

Drama

Drama (including role-play) is perhaps one of the most difficult and potentially dangerous methods and, I suggest, should not be used by non-specialist workers without opportunities for consultation. The feelings and memories stimulated may have repercussions for both child and worker. For example, the experience of wielding power when playing a role may be frightening for a powerless child, and new ideas about family relationships may be stimulated but not expressed, leaving a child in a state of bewilderment.

Bannister (drama therapist, psychodramatist and social worker), writing of work with sexually abused children (1989), describes how Michelle (7 years old), whose father had died, revealed that he had sexually abused her. Through acting based on *The Lion, the Witch and the Wardrobe* (Lewis 1950), she began to gain strength and autonomy. She took the parts of, first, a child who rescues the Lion, and then the Witch, 'a very powerful person who had control over everyone'. After this, she could take the role with which she really identified – the Lion, whom she played as 'strong and brave and able to help others'. When his friends had rescued him, 'they thanked him for allowing himself to be caught because this protected them' and they 'admired Michelle's strength and power and also her kindness. The Witch was dead so the Lion dug a hole and buried her. Michelle's healing had begun' (Bannister 1989, p. 94; see also Bannister 1998).

This recalls the *Snow White* theme explored by Julia with psychotherapist Margaret Hunter. Julia could explore aspects of her feelings and history by enacting roles from the story, including that of the stepmother (see Stories above) (Hunter 1987).

A toy may provide a third ear and voice through which child and worker may communicate. May (6 years old) wanted to name a large glove puppet 'May' but was dissuaded by her social worker, who felt that three-way conversations in which two participants had the same name would be confusing. May then chose her own second name and the puppet became 'Jessie'. Jessie became a regular participant in conversations, was always physically, even if silently, present, and at times behaved in such ways that May accused her of being naughty and put her outside the door (Crompton 1990). The worker sometimes felt in danger of losing control and noted, 'don't let materials run away with you – I felt the glove puppet begin to take me over, began to lose focus on the child and to enjoy the game too much' (p. 97).

A nursery nurse, Elaine, also recorded role-playing interaction was difficult and disturbing. Selma (6 years old) attended a voluntary agency weekly, with the aim of learning strategies for coping with her bizarre and neglecting mother. Although doing well at school and in good physical health, Selma appeared to be emotionally abused. During the fourth session, she began to act as mother to a doll and Elaine took the role of Selma, who then 'became' her own mother. They walked to a pile of teddies at one end of the playroom:

Selma/mother had been very aggressive but now she changed her whole voice and manner and asked Elaine/Selma 'would you like a present?' in a very soft stroking way. She gave Elaine/Selma all the teddies, then took her to the other end of the room to give another, enormous bear. Elaine/Selma said, 'I can't carry it'. Selma/mother immediately became annoyed, 'you will have it. I've bought it for you'.

Elaine/Selma found the difficulty was in coping with the 'gentle mum'. She felt frightened and puzzled: 'what have I done that's made her nice?' She waited for aggression to return, to be punished for the Selma/mother's being 'nice'.

Selma did not want to leave the role of mother and had enjoyed the power and control. Both she and Elaine 'needed a great deal of debriefing and cuddling'. Elaine wondered whether it had been a good idea to give her that taste of control, and she was also aware that 'Selma had let Elaine in on her world and feelings but then had to go home again to all the real stresses' (Crompton 1990, pp. 12–13). Elaine was well supported by a colleague with whom she could share such anxieties. Such work should not be undertaken unless consultation is available. (See also Ryan & Wilson (2000), who describe the way in which a young girl, Diane, devises during therapy a series of role plays to explore her difficult experiences with her birth family. They include a section on practice issues in responding to these spontaneous role plays.)

Spirituality and religion

When working with any individual, of whatever age, practitioners should be clear about their own, and their clients', concepts of being a whole person. For many people, the self comprises not only body, mind and emotions but also spirit. Many also hold some religious belief and fulfil religious obligations. It is therefore essential to recognise the importance of spiritual and/or religious elements of children's life and experience.

Smedley (1999, p. 114) considers that a frequent consequence of abuse is impairment of children's cognitive, emotional and spiritual development.

The CCETSW Training Pack *Children, Spirituality and Religion* includes a Social Work Practice Unit on 'Abuse and Neglect', with stimulus material and such questions as 'Can experience of abuse have a bad effect on children's spiritual welfare?' and 'if you have a strong religious belief, can you help children express anger against, and disbelief in, a deity?' (Crompton 1996, pp. 4:25–29).

Crompton devotes a substantial section of *Children, Spirituality, Religion and Social Work* to discussion of 'Spirituality, religion, abuse and neglect', including material on 'Abuse associated with religious and ritual practices' (Crompton

1998, Part 4, pp. 139–178). She considers that all abuse entails abuse of the spirit, however this is defined. A social worker, for example, suggested that 'the spirit can be abused if … children are constantly "put down", their fantasies rejected or adults are intent on making them pliable and obedient'. She 'visualised the body language of children who have been abused as "dragged down, slumping, exuberance crushed"' (Crompton 1998, p. 144).

Anxiety about, or hostility towards, religious beliefs and affiliations can hinder communication between practitioners and children. Kate, a social worker, was with a colleague when a girl told them that she had become a Christian. The colleague later confided, 'I'm glad you were there – I wouldn't have known how to respond'. Yet, surely, practitioners constantly receive information about terrible and distressing experiences (Crompton 1998, p. 152).

Attachment to a religious organisation can contribute to development of well-being. A girl who had been sexually abused by a family member later chose to be baptised into a Church and said that she had never expected to feel so loved again. She was coming to realise that the abuse had not been her fault, and that God and other Christians could love her (Crompton 1998, p. 152).

The wisdom of religious traditions can strengthen and inform practice. For example, Aliya Haeri bases her counselling process for recovery from abuse 'on a model of the self according to the Qur'an, Islam and Sufism'. The five-stage recovery process includes 'Affirming the child's innocence', 'Release by re-living the experience', 'Healing the whole person', 'Empowering the client to see justice done' and 'Liberation through unity'. Counselling may include diet and excercise, expression of anger and prayer. Crucially, 'It is not enough to counsel the client through the trauma alone, but also to treat her at the same time on the levels of the body, emotions, mind, soul and spirit as a unified human being'. The client is helped to 'visualise herself as whole and in well-being. By taking this decision, she takes responsibility for her healing and creates her own reality' (Haeri 1998, pp. 98, 99).

Work with a 10-year-old boy

This account of work with Mark (10 years old) illustrates some of the ideas mentioned above.

Mark was a member of a family in which sexual abuse had taken place and had been placed in a series of short-term foster homes. I was employed as an 'extra' social worker to help him emerge from the 'fog' in which he seemed to live, learn about the events that had brought about the break-up of his home and prepare for a so-called 'forever' home. Although not the direct victim of physical abuse, as a sibling, his life was irrevocably changed, for example, because of his removal from home. I was engaged to offer intensive, weekly, time-limited contact, in co-operation with the regular social worker. Contacts were substantial, usually about 90–120 minutes.

My aims were to offer Mark a structure of protected and reliable space and peacefulness, time that was all his own and interactions in which he had my whole attention. I hoped that we could really *meet* each other and that he could show me how, if at all, I could help him. There was no reason why he should like or trust me, or even give me his time. There was no reason why I should be able to make contact with him. My one guideline was *wait*, combating the urge to be seen to be successful within a short period of time (in the same way that workers are beset by pressures to produce results within set times by senior officers, case conferences and court schedules).

Since most of our meetings were after school, when Mark was tired, it was particularly important to find ways in which we could be relaxed and have a place of our own. We had no access to an office or playroom but found a hospitable café. When Mark moved to yet another short-stay foster home, we found a river bank where we could park in privacy and he could choose one of several walks and activities. He could either walk with me or run ahead, he could share his discoveries, we could watch a ship together or walk peacefully apart.

Mark was never greedy. In the café he never asked for extra food or drink but relished his two weekly milkshakes. He had choice and (with money I gave him) ordered the refreshments – an opportunity to gain social confidence too.

We worked hard. Every week, Mark dictated a story about recent events and I wrote, fast and illegibly. Then he drew an illustration, demonstrating ability and enjoyment. He taught me to draw such impossible objects as a bicycle, enjoying both his own achievements and the satisfaction of his superior skill (particularly important for a child with poor self-image). This pattern emerged from our first meeting when, on a walk, we had an adventure with a goose which became an excellent story and illustration when we next met. We thus immediately had shared experience and continuity.

Between meetings, I wrote out the week's story very carefully, using coloured pens or the word processor. My care and the continued existence of the story demonstrated that Mark himself had continued to exist for and with me and that his words had substance and were worthy of my time. With his own pictures, the stories built into a book recording the important events of his life. Finding a beautiful feather, getting lost, visiting a park – everyday events which had been important in themselves – became the focus for communication between us and were records of his past.

Darker aspects were regarded in the same way. When Mark wanted to discuss the abuse events and the reasons for his own removal from home, he asked his regular social worker for an explanation. At our next meeting, we wrote down this part of his story. Remembering that children should not feel defined by abuse or any other event or symptom, writing the story demonstrated that Mark's life included, but was not confined to, this aspect of his history.

His scattered parents and siblings could be gathered with stories, descriptions and drawings, helping Mark to decide how he foresaw his future, whether to be placed with a sibling or alone, and in what kind of family and place.

A whole day was spent visiting the scenes of his early life, including the maternity hospital and court. When a site on which he had loved to play and of which he had vivid memories was found to have been tarmacked and fenced by high wire, he asked, 'Why do things have to change?' We called at the museum to which Mark had gone on a recent school outing, and the castle, where he bought presents for his foster family and himself – his own choice was a cuddly toy (which, with a similar gift from his mother, became both a useful focus for and the medium of discussion of painful subjects, and a comforter). Writing, drawing, meals, silence and fun contributed to this important day.

Mark and I looked forward to seeing each other. I think he gained confidence, control, a sense of continuity and of himself. However, I felt that I failed him. The social services department failed to provide a 'forever' home. I had been asked to visit weekly but, after 5 months, at a distance of 40 miles, mileage was abruptly axed. When telling Mark that I could no longer visit him, I selfishly allowed my own anger and frustration to show and Mark, not understanding that my feelings were not directed at him, withdrew and asked, 'Can I go now?' If I had realised and controlled my self-absorption, it might have been better to have ended the day's contact early than to give Mark his full time, but spoil it. I would have valued support for myself, but I worked from home and did not wish to bother Mark's busy social worker.

We said goodbye in McDonald's, Mark's choice. I gave him all the materials we had used during our meetings and a strong carrying case, demonstrating that I had kept his possessions safe and that those aspects of his life which they represented were now in his own keeping. I had taught him to trust me and to enjoy being himself. It was important that in parting he should not feel abandoned, lest all my care become only another form of abuse.

We used physical activity, storytelling, writing, drawing, sending and collecting postcards, food, drink, car rides, toys, visiting places, conversation, explanation and silence. I tried to respect Mark's privacy and to be sensitive to his non-verbal messages, to be clear, straightforward and honest, and to give Mark opportunities for choice, control and the development of self-confidence. Everything was important for its own sake and I was (usually) careful to avoid interpretation traps.

It was frustrating that I could not complete the work for which I had been contracted. Mark had been abused at second hand by his family, and in effect by the failure of the department to provide appropriate care. The financial cost was a small price for the attempt to help a hurt and bewildered child and more resources should have been available routinely (including, perhaps, the use of part-time, experienced specialist workers to undertake this kind of intensive time-limited contract). Working with Mark was not a luxury but there are many 'Marks' for whom no such help is available.

Conclusion

This survey of individual work with children has, of necessity, been swift and superficial. Nonetheless, it is hoped that readers will consider the questions raised, slowly and in depth.

One of the main strands has been the importance of achieving and maintaining good standards of practice based on well-focused, substantial training, and supported within equally well-focused agencies. Clarity of thought, demonstrated through, for example, precision of language, definition of role and task, and self-knowledge, is combined with loving care for every individual child.

Children must not be labelled by symptom or experience. Effective help can be offered only by a whole, individual worker to a whole, individual child, taking into account the whole life of the child, together with the resources and constraints of the agency.

Really *meeting* a child may be helped through many kinds of communicative activity, but no materials or techniques can produce communication if the worker has no wish, or skill, to engage in such interactions.

Shared activities can offer opportunities for children to develop strength and confidence, to experience achievement, choice and control, and to share unstressed time with an adult who does not threaten or pressure and who gives reliable and courteous attention.

Annotated further reading

Aldridge M, Wood J 1998 Interviewing children: a guide for child care and forensic practitioners. Wiley, Chichester
While this text focuses on interviewing children during investigation of alleged abuse, the material has relevance to wider contexts of working with children. The authors (specialists in language acquisition and disorders) discuss children's language development with chapters on, e.g:

- 'Asking questions' (pp. 107–145)
- 'Children's language and development' (pp. 146–187)
- 'Interviewing children with special needs' (pp. 188–217).

Armstrong H (ed) 1991 Taking care: a church response to adults, children and abuse. National Children's Bureau, London
A practical guide to helping non-professionals to develop awareness of, and ways of responding to, abuse in various manifestations.

Bannister A (ed) 1998 From hearing to healing: working with the aftermath of child sexual abuse, 2nd edn. Wiley (with NSPCC), Chichester
A collection of papers focusing on some unusual aspects of working with children e.g:

- '"To all the flickering candles": dramatherapy with sexually abused children', Di Grimshaw (pp. 35–54)
- 'Young children who exhibit sexually abusive behaviour', Carol Day & Bobbie Print (pp. 118–141)
- 'Therapeutic issues in working with young sexually aggressive children', Anne Bannister (pp. 142–151).

Brandon M, Schofield G, Trinder L (with Stone N) 1998 Social work with children. Macmillan, Basingstoke
A useful general text introducing numerous aspects of working with children, e.g. child care policy, children's rights and the Children Act 1989, and the developmental framework. Three chapters are of particular relevance to practice with children who have been abused:

- Chapter 3: 'The Voice of the Child in Practice', which introduces 'Key factors: Legal context; Agency context; A place to work; Knowledge; Skills; Relationship; Honesty; Genuineness, warmth and empathy' (pp. 69–73).
- Chapter 4: 'Working with Children in Need and in need of Protection' (pp. 95–117), which includes a summary of 'Principles underpinning work' (pp. 103–105) based on guidance in Department of Health publications *Working Together* (1991) and *The Challenge of Partnership* (1994). Emphasis is on 'Children as active participants' (pp. 100–102), advising that 'Children and young people … need to be fully informed and involved without bearing additional responsibility' (p. 111).
- Chapter 6 'Children looked after by the Local Authority' (pp. 141–165) including, e.g. 'Making sense of the past and the present' (pp. 153–162); 'Participation in decision-making' (pp. 162–165).

Bray M 1997 Sexual abuse: the child's voice: poppies on the rubbish heap, 2nd edn. Kingsley, London.
The author, a social worker, trainer and therapist, co-founded SACCS (Sexual Abuse: Child Consultancy Service) and 'Leaps and Bounds', which comprises five houses and two smaller units providing for 30 children. Her book, first published in 1991, comprises powerful accounts of work with children in the form of stories that 'honour and celebrate the remarkableness of each child's capacity for survival and healing' and explore 'the meaning of these discoveries' (page xx). The author's own experience and beliefs enrich both the immediacy and depth and of this essential reading.

Butler I, Williamson H 1994 Children speak: children, trauma and social work. Longman/NSPCC, Harlow.
The authors argue that both childhood and child abuse are social constructs, created and maintained by adults.

- Chapter 3 'Children talking' (pp. 47–65) discusses interviews with children and young people, partly to learn about their perceptions of 'their worst experiences to date in their lives' (p. 50). 'Only by listening to the *meaning* imputed to such experiences by the young people concerned can those seeking to support them secure a measure of understanding of how they are affecting them' (p. 64).
- Chapter 4 focuses on 'Adults listening' (pp. 66–85).

Butler I, Robert G 1997 Social work with children and their families: getting into practice. Kingsley, London
A 'self-tutor' with, e.g. information segments and exercises. Unit 6 on 'Child abuse' (pp. 138–158) notes as Objective 3: 'Consider appropriate responses to abuse' (pp. 152–153) and lists 'Listen; Be supportive; Don't judge; Don't make promises you can't keep; Don't dither'.

Crompton M (writer/ed) 1997 Children, spirituality and religion: a training pack. Central Council for Education and Training in Social Work, London
This substantial pack is designed for use in formal training programmes or by individuals/small groups, and is suitable for practitioners in all areas of working with and on behalf of children. Material includes commissioned papers on seven religions and on spiritual development, focusing

on children/young people. 'Social work practice units' (Part 4:2) includes 'Abuse and neglect' (pp. 4:25–4:29) with material on:

- 'Spritual abuse and neglect'; 'Effects of physical and sexual abuse'; 'Caring for children who have been abused'; 'Abuse associated with religious practices'.
- 'Communicating about spirituality and religion' (Part 5, pp. 5:1–5:28) includes material and practice suggestions on 'Storytelling'; 'Talking about religion'.

Crompton M 1998 Children, spirituality, religion and social work. Ashgate, Aldershot
This text introduces numerous aspects of spirituality and religion in relation to children/young people, including rights; day-to-day implications of religious observances; spiritual well-being and distress. Of particular relevance to working with children who have been abused are:

- 'Spirituality, religion, abuse and neglect' (Part 4, pp. 141–180).
  - Chapter 11: 'Abuse and neglect' (pp. 141–155) 'explores associations between abuse/neglect and spiritual well-being' in the context of the UN *Convention on the Rights of the Child* (1989); reference is made to, e.g. 'Responses to religious teaching'.
  - Chapter 12: 'Abuse associated with religious and ritual practices' (pp. 157–180) introduces ideas about: 'Intentional abuse'; 'Abuse informally associated with religious organisations'; 'Oppression, persecution and sectarianism'; 'Abuse intentionally associated with ritual practices'; 'The needs of practitioners'.
  - Chapter 15 offers ideas about communication through 'Stories, myths and legends' (pp. 217–234).

Doyle C 1997 Working with abused children, 2nd edn. Macmillan/British Association of Social Workers, Basingstoke
Clear, straightforward ideas and advice to practitioners includes: Section 3 'Individual work with children' (pp. 41–62) with numerous sub-sections, e.g. 'The helping process' (pp. 53–62) which includes, 'The expression of emotion'; 'Positive messages'; 'Protective work'; 'Ending individual work'.

Kennedy M 1995 Submission to the National Commission of Inquiry into the Prevention of Child Abuse. Christian Survivors of Sexual Abuse (CSSA), London
This report provides invaluable material about children who have been abused within a religious context, e.g. by ministers of religion, or when children abused by their fathers have been taught that God is a loving Father. Many responses by survivors are supplemented by comments on e.g. fear, forgiveness and guilt and there are ideas for expressing their pain, anger and hurt to the deity in the form of special liturgies and worship (p. 26).

Milner P, Carolin B (eds) 1999 Time to listen to children: personal and professional communication. Routledge, London
This thoughtful collection of papers illustrates how the authors, drawn from a wide range of settings, 'use time to listen to children on matters that concern them and decisions that affect them … to enable children to learn an understanding, respect and responsibility for themselves, plus a respect and understanding for others' (p. 2).

- Part III: 'At work with children', includes 'Child protection: facing up to fear' (Chapter 7) by Barbara Smedley (pp. 112–125) in which perceptions of, and work with, several children who have been abused are described.
- Part IV: 'Listening creatively', introduces different modes of communication, including practice examples:
  - Chapter 10: '"I'm going to do magic …" said Tracey: working with children using person-centred art therapy', Heather Giles & Micky Mendelson (pp. 161–174).
  - Chapter 11: 'Listening to children through play', Carol Dasgupta (pp. 175–187).
  - Chapter 12: 'Listening: the first step toward communicating through music', Amelia Oldfield (pp. 188–199).

Patel N, Naik D, Humphries B (eds) 1998 Visions of reality: religion and ethnicity in social work. Central Council for Education and Training in Social Work, London
This compilation offers information and examples of aspects of religion and ethnicity essential for social work practice. Most relevant for work with children who have been abused is: 'Overcoming abuse: an Islamic approach' by Aliya Haeri (pp. 97–101).

Sinason V (ed) 1994 Treating survivors of Satanist abuse. Routledge, London
This book of papers by practitioners in a range of fields explores many aspects of a controversial subject. One paper with particular relevance to practice with children is: 'Fostering a ritually abused child', Chapter 10, by Mary Kelsall. Russell had been severely physically abused and later

described horrific experiences of ritual abuse. With the help of a psychotherapist, his foster parents hold on to the deeply disturbed boy (pp. 94–99).

Thompson C L, Rudolph L B 1999 Counseling children, 5th edn. Brooks/Cole, Belmont, California
An excellent fundamental text with well-organised, well-written accounts of models of counselling and approaches to working with children. Substantial summaries include lively vignettes of the originators (e.g. William Glasser, Fritz Perls, Carl Rogers) and notes on 'The nature of people', 'Theory of counseling', 'Counseling methods', a case study, 'Research and reactions', and references for every approach. 'Counselling children with special concerns' includes sections on 'Child abuse' and 'Child sexual abuse'. A bibliography of fiction and other books written for children includes references to 'Child abuse'.

References

Ahmed S, Cheetham J, Small J (eds) 1986 Social work with black children and their families. Batsford/BAAF, London

Allan J 1988 Inscapes of the Child's world: Jungian counselling in schools and clinics. Spring Publications, Dallas, Texas

Axline V 1947 Play therapy: the inner dynamics of childhood. Houghton Mifflin, Boston

Axline V 1971 Dibbs: in search of self. Penguin, Harmondsworth

Bagley C, King K 1990 Child sexual abuse: the search for healing. Tavistock/Routledge, London

Bannister A 1989 Healing action – action methods with children who have been sexually abused. In: Wattam C, Blagg H, Hughes J A (eds) Child sexual abuse: listening, hearing and validating the experiences of childhood. Longman/NSPCC, Harlow, pp. 78–94

Bannister A (ed) 1998 From hearing to healing: working with the aftermath of child sexual abuse, 2nd edn. Wiley (with NSPCC), Chichester

Bettelheim B 1976 The uses of enchantment: the meaning and importance of fairy tales. Thames and Hudson, London

Boyle S 1997 Introduction. In Bray M (ed) Sexual abuse: the child's voice: poppies on the rubbish heap, 2nd edn. Kingsley, London, pp. vii–xiii

Bray M (ed) 1997 Sexual abuse: the child's voice: poppies on the rubbish heap, 2nd edn. Kingsley, London

British Association for Adoption and Fostering (BAFF) 1989 After abuse: papers on caring and planning for a child who has been sexually abused. British Association for Adoption and Fostering, London

Burch M 1992 I want to make a life story book. University of Hull, Department of Social Policy and Professional Studies, Hull

CCETSW 1991 The teaching of child care in the Diploma in Social Work: guidance notes for programme planners: improving social work education and training, No. 6. CCETSW, London

Cooper D, Ball D 1987 Social work and child abuse. Macmillan/BASW, Houndmills

Crompton M 1980 Respecting children: social work with young people. Edward Arnold, London

Crompton M 1990 Attending to children: direct work in social and health care. Edward Arnold, Dunton Green

Crompton M 1991 Invasion by Russian dolls: on privacy and intrusion. Adoption and Fostering 15: 31–33

Crompton M 1992 Children and counselling. Edward Arnold, Dunton Green

Crompton M 1996 Children, spirituality, and religion: a training pack. Central Council for Education and Training in Social Work, London

Crompton M 1998 Children, spirituality, religion and social work. Ashgate, Aldershot

Donley K (1975) Opening new doors. British Association for Adoption and Fostering, London

Dorfman E 1951 Play therapy. In: Rogers C R (ed) Client-centred therapy: its current practice, implications and theory. Constable, London, pp. 235–277

Doyle C 1990 Working with abused children. Macmillan/British Association of Social Workers, Houndmills

Feminist Review 1988 Family secrets: child sexual abuse. No. 28, Spring

Furniss T 1991 The multi-professional handbook of child sexual abuse: integrated management, therapy and legal intervention. Routledge, London

Gardner R 1987 Who says? Choice and control in care. National Children's Bureau, London

Glaser D, Frosh S 1988 Child sexual abuse. Macmillan/British Association of Social Workers, Houndmills

Glasgow D 1987 Responding to child sexual abuse: issues, techniques and play assessment. Mersey Regional Health Authority, Liverpool

Haeri A 1998 Overcoming abuse: an Islamic approach. In: Patel N, Naik D, Humphries B (eds) Visions of reality: religion and ethnicity in social work. Central Council for Education and Training in Social Work, London, pp. 97–101 (first published in *Open Mind* 1994, 69, June/July)

Holgate E 1972 Communicating with children. Longman, London

Hunter M 1987 Julia: a 'frozen' child. Adoption and Fostering 11 (3): 26–30

Jones D P H 1992 Interviewing the sexually abused child: investigation of suspected abuse. Gaskell/Royal College of Psychiatrists, London

Kastell J 1962 Casework in child care. Routledge and Kegan Paul, London

Kenward H 1989 Helping children who have been abused. In: British Association for Adoption and Fostering (ed) After abuse: papers on caring and planning for a child who has been sexually abused. British Association for Adoption and Fostering, London

Lewis C S 1950 The lion, the witch and the wardrobe. Penguin, Harmondsworth

Lifton B 1989 The king of children. Pan, London

Lindsay G, Peake A (eds) 1989 Child sexual abuse: educational and child psychology, Vol. 6(1). The British Psychological Society, Disley

Marshall M R 1981 Libraries and the handicapped child. André Deutsch, London

Mcarns D, Thorne B 1988 Person-centred counselling in action. Sage, London

Mills J C 1988 Putting ideas into their heads: advising the young. Feminist Review 28: 162–174

Milner P, Carolin B 1999 Time to listen to children: personal and professional communication. Routledge, London

Moore J 1992 The ABC of child protection. Ashgate, Aldershot

Oaklander V 1978 Windows to our children: a gestalt approach to children and adolescents. The Center for Gestalt Development, New York (first published in 1969 by Real People Press, Moab, Utah)

O'Hagan K 1989 Working with child sexual abuse. Open University Press, Milton Keynes

Patel N, Naik D, Humphries B 1998 Visions of reality: religion and ethnicity in social work. Central Council for Education and Training in Social Work, London

Redgrave K 1987 Child's play: 'direct work' with the deprived child. Boys and Girls Welfare Society, Cheadle

Roberts J 1993 The importance of self-esteem to children and young people separated from their families. Adoption and Fostering 17 (2): 48–50

Rogers C R (ed) 1951 Client-centred therapy: its current practice, implications and theory. Constable, London

Rouf K 1989 Journey through darkness: the path from victim to survivor. In: Lindsay G, Peake A (eds) Child sexual abuse: educational and child psychology, Vol. 6(1). The British Psychological Society, Disley, pp. 6–10

Ryan V, Wilson K 2000 Case studies in non-directive play therapy. Jessica Kingsley, London

Seymour C 1990 Counselling children. Unpublished paper. Durham University, Centre of Counselling Skills, Durham

Shapiro L 1984 The new short-term therapies for children: a guide for helping professionals and parents. Prentice-Hall, New Jersey

Smedley B 1999 Child protection: facing up to fear. In: Milner P, Carolin B (ed) Time to listen to children: personal and professional communication. Routledge, London, pp. 112–125

Stevens J 1971 Awareness: exploring, experimenting and experiencing. Real People Press, Moab, Utah

Stevenson O 1991 Preface. In: CCETSW (ed) The teaching of child care in the Diploma in Social Work: guidance notes for programme planners: improving social work education and training, No. 6. CCETSW, London, pp. 5–7

Stone M 1990 Child protection work: a professional guide. Venture Press, Birmingham

Thompson C L, Rudolph L B 1988 Counseling children. Brookes/Cole, Belmont, California

Utting W 1997 People like us: the report of the review of the safeguards for children living away from home. The Stationery Office, London

Wattam C, Blagg H, Hughes J A (eds) 1989 Child sexual abuse: listening, hearing and validating the experiences of childhood. Longman/NSPCC, Harlow

Wells J 1989 Powerplay – considerations in communicating with children. In: Wattam C, Blagg H, Hughes J A (eds) Child sexual abuse: listening, hearing and validating the experiences of childhood. Longman/NSPCC, Harlow

West J 1996 Child centred play therapy, 2nd edn. Arnold, London

Wilson K, Kendrick P, Ryan V 1992 Play therapy: a non-directive approach for children and adolescents. Ballière Tindall, London

Winnicott C 1964 Child care and social work: a collection of papers written between 1954 and 1962. Codicote, Welwyn

Winnicott D W 1971 Therapeutic consultations in child psychiatry. Hogarth, London

22 Non-directive play therapy with abused children and adolescents

Virginia Ryan

INTRODUCTION

Current professional interest in play therapy has been heightened by the need for more effective help for the increasing numbers of abused children and adolescents requiring therapeutic interventions. Professionals are also increasingly aware of the seriousness of many abused children's emotional difficulties, which are likely to need more intensive treatment. One particular approach, non-directive play therapy, seems to be a viable and non-intrusive method of working with abused children and adolescents (Wilson *et al.* 1992, Ryan & Wilson 1996, West 1996).

This chapter will give an overview of this method of play therapy. The relevance of non-directive therapy within statutory settings will then be discussed. Child protection concerns, care decisions and court proceedings including children as witnesses, are all important considerations at referral for therapy and during therapeutic interventions. The last part of this chapter will present a case example of non-directive play therapy with a 13-year-old girl who was sexually abused. It will illustrate the ways in which the therapist, carers and social worker all helped to work within their specified roles to meet the emotional needs of this adolescent.

An Overview

The most significant way in which non-directive play therapy differs from other play interventions and therapies is in its non-directive nature. The choice of issues, and the choice of play contents and actions in the playroom, is determined by the child rather than by the adult. Non-directive therapists are trained to establish certain basic limits to behaviour in the playroom, yet the atmosphere in the playroom is intended to be relaxed and non-threatening to children and adolescents. Therapists have adult responsibility for physical and emotional safety, for care of the materials and the room, and for time limits. With abused children and adolescents it is even more important that limits are set clearly and consistently, and that therapists themselves recognise and respond appropriately to the changing emotional needs of the child during therapy.

Non-directive play therapists assume that children and adolescents will instigate therapeutic changes and achieve therapeutic insights for themselves. Therapists facilitate these changes without overt directions, suggestions or interpretations. Instead, therapists develop close helping relationships in which children's feelings and thoughts are reflected and responded to, and in which therapists use their own feelings and thoughts within relationships with children in therapeutic ways. Children and adolescents can therefore use both the playroom environment and the therapist to resolve their chosen emotional difficulties at their own pace and in their own manner. Some children may choose to use dramatic play as their primary means of communication and change in the playroom, other children may use the clay or cars and soldiers. Still other children and adolescents may choose to primarily talk and sit quietly with the therapist. In particular cases, for example with children who have serious attachment difficulties, the therapist may decide with the child, carer and social worker to include the carer in play therapy sessions directly. In other cases, sibling pairs or group therapy may be the preferred option.

Historically, non-directive play therapy was developed in North America by Axline (1947, 1987), who adapted Rogerian client-centred therapy with adults to child therapy (Rogers 1951). Children's play had already been established in psychodynamic practice by Klein and A Freud as the primary medium for therapeutic help with children (Wolff 1986). Axline, and to a lesser extent other practitioners (e.g. Moustakas 1953, 1959, Ginott 1961) relied heavily on clinical examples to explain the practice of non-directive play therapy. They did not specify its procedures or develop its theoretical underpinnings rigorously. This aprocedural and atheoretical stance was a deliberate one on their part. Early practitioners believed this stance was needed to counteract what they saw as the rigid and convoluted theorising of psychoanalytically trained child analysts and the simplistic and prescriptive stance of behavioural therapists. Non-directive play therapy did not evolve into a major, recognised school of therapy with closely specified techniques during this period. Currently, non-directive play therapy as an intervention method is being developed further in North America, most notably by Landreth (1991) and Guerney (1984), and in Britain by Wilson *et al.* (1992) and Ryan & Wilson (1996).

Approved training programmes for play therapists, including non-directive play therapists, are offered in different countries and two international professional organisations for play therapists, emanating from North America, are well established. These organisations offer international membership and international and national conferences. Within Britain in the last decade play therapists have developed into an accredited progression. They now have recognised national professional qualifications and are required to practise within the ethics and code of practice set out by the British Association of Play Therapists (BAPT). In order to ensure competent practice, employers and referrers now check the current professional status of play therapists with the BAPT registration of full members. Yearly play therapy conferences, a newsletter, play therapy information packs and other training opportunities are also being offered (see contact address at the end of this chapter).

Until recently, non-directive play therapy in Britain seemed to have been practised in relative isolation at child guidance and child treatment centres by a variety of professionals. There also seemed to be a tendency to drift into other therapeutic techniques and into direct work with children, while attempting to remain 'child-focused'. The practice of non-directive play therapy has been enhanced in recent years with the introduction of an accredited post-qualifying training course in non-directive play therapy at the University of York, which can be followed by a further period of academic study for an MA and PhD for qualified students. This course offers the advantage of close supervision during training and the development of trainees' practise in a single therapeutic method. While incorporating other therapeutic techniques, qualified play therapists are consistent and skilled in remaining non-directive. Three other play therapy courses also are currently approved by the BAPT (see end of chapter for address of the University of York course).

Wilson and I, in our writing on non-directive play therapy, have tried to develop the theory of non-directive play therapy by setting it within the context of current child development theory and research, including the way in which symbolic play serves an adaptive function in normal development (Wilson *et al.* 1992, Ryan & Wilson 1996). Using a broadly adaptive model, play is conceptualised as serving the function of assimilating personally important experiences for normally developing children into their existing mental structures, called schemas. For troubled and abused children these schemas, which are likely to be poorly developed and/or distorted, are enabled to become more developed and more flexible with the therapist's help during play therapy interventions.

We have also updated non-directive play therapy practise in several ways. First, we have looked at the place of individual child treatment within a wider systemic framework (e.g. Wilson & Ryan 1992). Second, we have discussed the role of non-directive therapy within statutory requirements, including the usefulness of therapeutic assessments in identifying children's needs, wishes and feelings in civil court proceedings (Ryan & Wilson 2000*a*, 2000*b*). We have also argued that non-directive play therapy, by remaining within the child's metaphors and issues, is suitable for pre-trial interventions with child witnesses in criminal courts (Ryan & Wilson 1995*a*). Third, we have demonstrated that other therapeutic techniques, such as structured exercises, and certain psychodynamic and cognitive behavioural techniques, can be modified and incorporated into a non-directive play therapy approach (Wilson *et al.* 1992, Ryan & Wilson, 1995*b*, Cigno & Ryan 1998).

Research in play therapy is not yet well developed. There appear to be several reasons for this. Play therapists seem to prioritise practice before research in their professional lives; case studies and applications of these studies to practice issues are most common. Earlier research in play therapy exists, but generally does not have tightly specified process and outcome measures (Guerney 1984). This difficulty is held in common with more general child therapy research. Child therapy, including non-directive play therapy, was found to be generally effective with troubled children, based on meta-analysis of studies in this field, but methodological problems often existed in these studies. Now, research in child therapy is turning to more carefully defined subgroups within clinical populations, such as children with conduct disorders, then evaluating specific interventions and outcomes for such groups (e.g. Kazdin *et al.* 1990).

Research studies in non-directive play therapy are beginning to increase and are reported most frequently in the *International Journal of Play Therapy*, which is linked to membership in one of the existing international professional organisations. This reported research in play therapy is an encouraging start and ranges from practice issues, such as therapists' opinions on limit setting, to training issues and to process issues within therapy sessions themselves with children and adolescents. However, much further research is needed, including investigating key issues such as the efficacy of play therapy for different clinical populations (e.g. the impact of class, gender and ethnicity on play therapy interventions) and many other process issues. Of particular concern for this chapter, definitive process and outcome research on non-directive play therapy for children and adolescents within statutory settings remains scant. But because the field of play therapy, including non-directive play therapy, is now maturing and requiring a higher level of post-qualifying professional training, this advancement will very likely contribute to generating support for and interest in more adequate and extensive evaluative research. At the University of York, for example, we have begun a research programme evaluating shorter-term interventions in non-directive play therapy with trainee therapists (Wilson & Ryan 1998).

Broader policy considerations

As discussed above, non-directive play therapy allows children and young people to address issues of their choice and to restructure their internal mental schemas at their own pace, within the relaxed environment of the playroom. When practised by a qualified therapist, it is a more global approach to therapy than other more limited interventions, such as programmes on the enhancement of self-esteem, or behavioural programmes. Non-directive therapists do not target specific maladaptive behaviours, but assume that children choose to focus on the issues troubling them for themselves. For this reason it seems more suitable for children within statutory settings, who often have multiple emotional difficulties.

Another strength of the non-directive approach is that it enhances choice within the playroom, and thus serves as an antidote to abused children's experiences in which abusers removed age-appropriate choices from the children they abused. And by staying within the child's play metaphors and communications, children who often have had multiple professional relationships that focused on verbal exchanges (e.g. investigative interviews, discussions about moving with their social workers) are allowed the freedom to choose to play rather than to be required to talk through their emotional difficulties with an adult.

All therapeutic interventions with abused children, including non-directive play therapy, must be practiced alongside consideration of child protection issues. Individual therapeutic intervention with children cannot protect them adequately if their environments are currently abusive. Indeed, in such cases, individual therapeutic interventions are contraindicated and child protection issues must take priority. There are several reasons for this. First, children who are already scapegoated or identified as the sole problem in abusing families may be further scapegoated by being singled out for an intervention. Second, children may be unable to make substantial therapeutic changes because their emotional energy needs to be channelled primarily into emotional and physical survival. Third, if children do make therapeutic changes, despite these obstacles – say by becoming overtly angry when abusing parents make unreasonable demands on them – children may put themselves at greater risk of harm in an already abusing environment. And fourth, children will often compare the therapist and therapeutic relationship with other significant relationships. If children's intimate relationships with their carers are already seriously inadequate and cannot meet their needs, or if the relationships are unsafe, the children may become overly and unrealistically attached to the therapist. The therapeutic relationship will then tend to be misused by children to fulfil needs which can only be adequately met for them on a daily, long-term basis by carers (Glaser 1991, Wilson *et al.* 1992). Therefore, for individual therapeutic work to be safe and productive, children's environments must, at the very least, be minimally adequate and stable for the fulfilment of their physical and emotional needs.

The practice of non-directive play therapy also has relevance for care decisions and court proceedings concerning children. Often it is through individual sessions that are utilised freely, rather than in sessions directed by an adult's agenda, that children's current concerns and the intensity of these concerns are discovered. This information is of great importance in making care decisions and in presenting evidence in court based on the Children Act 1989. Evidence from non-directive play therapy sessions can be quite different from, but as equally valid as, evidence derived from other means, such as direct questioning and family assessments (Ryan & Wilson 1995*a*, Ryan & Wilson 2000*a*, 2000*b*). While the contents of play therapy sessions must be kept as confidential as possible, important themes emerging in the sessions will usefully inform care decisions concerning the child. Evidence of further abuse of already abused children may also emerge in non-directive play therapy sessions (see 'Non-directive play therapy with abused adolescents' below). This in turn will further inform care decisions and the necessary protection of the child.

Finally, there is currently professional concern about the conflict between meeting the therapeutic needs of children when court proceedings require that children give evidence in court, and simultaneously meeting legal requirements for non-contamination of the child's evidential statements. Therapeutic interventions are not automatically ruled out for child witnesses in the UK, but they are at the court's discretion. There has been grave legal concern over contamination of evidence especially in sexual abuse cases where children are often the only other witnesses to events besides the accused. Therapy has sometimes been disallowed because of legal concern that children's evidence will be contaminated by a therapist's suggestions and interpretations. As discussed above, non-directive play therapy differs from psychodynamic and directive approaches because it does not use interpretation in its practice. The therapist instead keeps to the metaphors and symbols used by children to reflect their ongoing feelings. Non-directive therapists employ therapeutic suggestion in a much more curtailed and circumspect way than other therapeutic methods (Ryan & Wilson 1995a). Most importantly for the child's therapeutic needs, this method – more than any other therapeutic method – enables the child to set the pace for examining painful current material and memories. As well as addressing the child's best interests by providing therapeutic help as soon as possible, research also seems to demonstrate that children who have been traumatised by damaging personal experiences make better witnesses if they have been able to examine and work through on an emotional level their 'worst moments' prior to giving evidence concerning these events (Pynoos & Eth 1984). Non-directive play therapy therefore has the advantage with child witnesses of preserving the child's own perceptions of these traumatic events. The child's evidence in court is not invalidated by undue therapeutic suggestion, directions or interpretations. And most crucially, the child will be able to receive therapeutic help immediately, rather than having therapy delayed for some time until after a criminal trial.

Child abuse and non-directive play therapy

Turning from the advantages of employing non-directive play therapy in statutory settings, non-directive play therapy, as stated above, is effective with abused children and adolescents because it is directed at the underlying emotional damage they have sustained. The short- and long-term emotional effects of abuse on children and adolescents within a family context have already been discussed in an earlier chapter (see Hanks & Stratton, Chapter 5, in this volume). Although these effects will vary, and even though a number of abused children do seem to recover from their abusive experiences (Finkelhor 1992, Hall & Lloyd 1993), the experiences themselves are inevitably emotionally damaging to children's development (Wilson *et al.* 1992). Also, it is generally recognised that children who have been abused need increased levels of care either from their own families or from their new caregivers (Downes 1992, see also Thoburn, Chapter 27, in this volume). These increased levels of care often extend to children's relationships with professionals in positions of authority, such as teachers and social workers. Abused children often make greater demands on professionals' as well as carers' capacities for limit setting, appropriate physical and emotional closeness, and individual attention, even after the abuse has stopped.

Abused children, as mentioned earlier, have developed damaged, overly accommodating emotional responses to abusive experiences – responses such as passivity, peer aggression and regression to less mature levels of functioning, to name a few. This is because children's responses to ongoing abusive experiences result in relatively permanent mental schemas on all three cognitive, motor and emotional levels of functioning. These schemas mentally represent, not only children's carers but simultaneously represent internally the most fundamental aspects of children's own schemas about the self as well. Personally significant interactions, then, always involve the development of schemas concerning the self *and* significant others. Abused children's overly accommodating responses will necessarily involve disturbed personal schemas concerning both the self and carers. Repeated abusive experiences, or even one traumatic experience, may lead children to develop strongly negative or conflicting personal schemas about themselves and significant others. A highly compensatory environment after removal from as abusive one may not be sufficient to enable a child to abandon these previously adaptive, persistent mental schemas, or to transform them into more positive ones. Children often need an intensive, corrective experience such as non-directive play therapy in order to re-enact their emotionally damaging experiences on a symbolic (mental) level. The symbolic materials and activities in the play room and the therapists skills in developing a helping relationship which suits each individual child may be needed.

Sexually abused children or adolescents, for example, may have developed a mental schema which contains strong feelings of fear and anger towards their carer along with other positive feelings of trust and affection. The cognitive component of this schema may also contain discrepancies concerning parents who treat the child as an adult sexual partner and yet restrict that child's freedom is taking on a parental role in other ways. Relatively permanent cognitive explanations – usually deliberately fostered by the abusing adult (see Wyre 1991) – such as 'I am unusually sexy, that's why my father/mother can't help being sexually attracted to me' may develop. Motor level conflicts are also common: sexual abuse involves parts of children's bodies, usually both children's intimate body parts as well as body parts such as the hands and mouth which are normally involved in non-sexual activities. Children will have difficulty assimilating their abnormal sexually abusive bodily sensations and motor responses into existing motor schemas involving normal motor experiences. Take a motor schema related to physical care: a child having their hair brushed by the carer, for instance, would usually have developed a motor schema for hair-brushing associated with feelings and personal experiences of nurturance. But in sexual abuse, hair-brushing for this child may have emotionally powerful sexually abusive connotations as well.

Non-directive play therapy is of particular value for abused children and adolescents who have sustained this kind of emotional damage. Non-directive play therapy gives them time and privacy to address these deeper mental levels of personal experiences using symbolic play, accompanied by the therapist's focus on reflecting children's ongoing feelings. Symbolic play, as stated above, is a natural vehicle children use to assimilate and express their personal experiences. Abused children actively direct their own process of symbolic re-enactment of personally meaningful experiences, thus automatically individualising and personalising the play therapy sessions for themselves.

Another feature of abuse, that is its co-existence with other forms of abuse, is also addressed in this way. Very often the separate effects of neglect, emotional, sexual and physical abuse may be difficult to unravel (see Chapter 5 in this volume). Because of its highly individualised approach, non-directive play therapy can readily adapt to whatever additional issues emerge during therapy for the child. Besides the possibility of other forms of abuse, it is likely that children will also be able to symbolically recreate and explore the 'worst moments' in their traumatically abusive experiences (Pynoos & Eth 1986). These personally traumatic experiences may include the sudden, inexplicable abandonment of the child during a special, happy outing arranged by the usually abusive parent, or in another case, a child finding out that the abusing parent had lied to the child about the child's much valued toy being stolen when, in fact, the parent had deliberately sold the toy and kept the money herself. Abused children often understate the extent of their abuse initially. The extent of their abusive experiences may be discovered in non-directive play therapy. (The implications for child protection issues when further abuse is disclosed in therapy are discussed in the section, 'Non-directive play therapy with abused adolescents' below, and in Wilson *et al.* 1992.)

Returning to symbolic play, this type of play necessarily involves all the motor, emotional and cognitive levels of functioning together for children, thus enabling them to integrate and rework all these levels of abusive experiences. Furthermore, besides an immediate symbol children may be consciously aware of, there may be many more remote or more threatening meanings to a symbol of which they are unaware. Because children determine the contents and issues of play therapy sessions, they are able to give symbolic expression to thoughts and experiences which are less threatening to them, but which also connect with and activate more threatening schemas. In this way, non-directive play therapy does not raise children's anxiety by dealing directly with highly self-threatening experiences or by dealing directly with the coping mechanisms children have developed to protect themselves from anxiety, such as denial, dissociation or displacement. Children break down their own barriers to self-threatening experiences with the help of the therapist's reflections, using the natural and fundamentally non-threatening activity of play.

Non-directive play therapy, therefore, is based on real choices of content and issues which are made by children rather than by the adult therapist. This feature of the non-directive method is especially important in work with abused children. Control over the child's important personal experiences has been exercised abusively by the adult carer to meet the adult's emotional needs for power, aggression or sexual gratification, and not to fulfil the child's own needs. By the reintroduction of choice over personally meaningful experiences in non-directive play therapy, the lack of choice and previous adult coercion is directly counteracted. When abused children or adolescents have control over the content of their sessions and the pace of therapeutic change, their compliant or reactive mental schemas and overt behaviours that were developed in response to adult demands are minimised. As a result, children's awareness of their own personal thoughts, feelings and responses is enhanced. Additionally, because the therapist follows children's activities, thoughts and feelings and reflects these back, children begin to realise that their own external and internal actions during the sessions are of importance to the therapist and, therefore, must be of value internally as well.

In practising non-directive play therapy, therapists are trained to subordinate their own needs and emotions to the child's. But therapists are also trained to be consciously aware of internal emotions, especially those generated in the therapist by specific interactions with the child. These emotional reactions, which must be separated from personal and private emotions by the therapist, are then used by the therapist to help clarify and give primacy to the child's expressed feelings.

This general subordination of personal emotions, thoughts and needs by the therapist is a necessary part of the practice of non-directive play therapy and particularly necessary when working with abused children. It is an artificial enhancement of a feature of a normal adult–child nurturing relationship. The subordination of adult needs to those of the child in normal development, for example, the adult waiting to eat until the hungry child has been fed, is made workable because the adult parent's primary need, is for caring for their child (Erikson 1963). But a recurring feature of abusive experiences for children is that this normal adult–child relationship pattern has been damaged, and adults have put the fulfilment of their own emotional and physical needs before those of their children. This helps account for the extreme adaptations and vacillations observed in abused children's emotional reactions. In normal development, children's needs are adequately met and they gradually learn to wait and to subordinate some of their own needs to others' needs. But abused children often over-subordinate their own needs to others, or else become desperate and frantically out of control in an attempt to have their own needs fulfilled. Even when their needs do begin to be met in a more appropriate manner, abused children often retain a learned fear that these needs will remain unmet.

In non-directive play therapy the therapist participates in sessions at the child's pace and direction with great predictability, thus subordinating their own adult needs. But at the same time the therapist maintains an adult guiding role. The therapist needs to respond congruently with appropriate, healthy adult responses to abused children's expressed behaviours, thoughts and feelings. For example, if a sexually abused child attempts to thrust some playdough down the front of a therapist's trousers, the therapist must respond congruently by saying that the therapist would not feel comfortable because that place is private and stop the child's action. But at the same time, the therapist needs to help the child express these feelings and perhaps perform these actions in a more socially acceptable way, say to a doll.

The above example illustrates that although the overall emphasis in non-directive play therapy is permissive and child-centred, it is essential that therapeutic limits are established by the therapist in their adult role. Indeed, both therapeutic limits and emotionally healthy adult responses are an essential component of this approach. In these adult interactions with the child, the therapist enables the child to develop emotionally healthy responses to necessary adult limits on the child's behaviour. More generally, the therapist also makes more understandable and predictable to the child normal adult–child interactions (Ryan & Wilson 1995*b*). In this way, an abused child is able to correct previously self-destructive and antisocial adaptations developed in response to abusive experiences.

The practice of non-directive play therapy therefore entails creating an enhanced play environment in which the toys and materials provided are conducive to symbolic play (see Wilson *et al.* 1992, for a further discussion of the appropriate setting and equipment). This equipment remains the same at each session. The sessions themselves take place at the same time each week, for a predetermined time period, usually for an hour's duration. We have suggested that a short-term, time-limited intervention, say ten sessions to begin with, with a review and the possibility of ten more sessions is a workable arrangement. (Again, see Wilson *et al.* 1992, for an extended discussion of preparation and planning issues.) For more seriously damaged children and adolescents, more sessions may be required. Often, too, these very damaged children may need therapeutic input at key future points in their lives, say at adolescence or when changing schools, or moving from a shorter-term foster placement to a permanent home.

This regularity of time and place is adhered to in order to promote an emotionally troubled child's relaxation and confidence in a strange environment. More important still, the therapist, in addition to the environment, must convey familiarity easily to the child in their initial sessions. The therapist needs to communicate appropriate responsiveness to the child through their friendly, yet non-directive and non-intrusive stance during each session (Ryan & Wilson 1995*b*).

In summary, the practice of non-directive play therapy can be characterised as follows:

- Careful preparation and planning, to promote children's confidence in trusting themselves to therapy.
- The development of a trusting, accepting relationship with the child.
- The reflection of the child's feelings by the therapist in a non-threatening manner.
- The use of feelings congruently by the therapist to reflect back to children appropriate responses to their expressed behaviour and feelings.
- The establishment of appropriate therapeutic boundaries.

Working therapeutically within statutory settings

An important consideration in setting up and engaging in play therapy with abused children and adolescents is ensuring that all those involved in their care work together to provide a milieu which enables therapeutic progress. Often birth parents, foster carers and residential workers, if children and adolescents are in local authority care, and the key social worker are important figures in supporting therapeutic interventions. This chapter has already argued that children in abusive home environments may be put at further risk if therapy is offered under those conditions. Highly unstable and/or unsuitable care arrangements also were discussed as inappropriate for a referral for therapy. Play therapy cannot insulate children from abusive care. Nor, sadly, can it compensate for inadequate and emotionally neglectful care environments (Ryan *et al.* 1995).

As well as needing a relatively stable and emotionally available attachment figure for emotional well-being, children and adolescents referred for therapy have additional emotional needs. They often become worried about the unfamiliar relationship they are expected to develop with the therapist, a normal reaction to beginning therapy. In addition, abused and neglected children's anxiety is heightened considerably due to maladaptive parent–child relationships stemming from their previous care history. Acutely troubling thoughts and feelings may emerge during the course of play therapy sessions, and children's and adolescents' behaviour may deteriorate in the shorter-term when emotionally difficult issues are being addressed. Patience and hope are required by experienced and sensitive carers at these points in therapy (Ryan & Wilson 1995*b*, 1996).

Children and adolescents may also begin to change emotionally by making small changes in their behaviour and self-concept at home and at school. Understanding the significance of such changes, and being responsive to small but meaningful changes, are essential from carers in order to promote therapeutic progress. Carers therefore need flexibility and understanding of underlying emotional issues of children and adolescents in their care. The social worker and therapist are needed to help carers understand the essential role that caring for children plays during therapeutic interventions. Carers in turn will give valuable information and insight from their own relationships with children to the social worker and therapist. Regular meetings to review progress and to inform one another of key themes emerging in therapy, while respecting confidentiality, are crucial. Therapists and social workers also rely on carers to inform them of key events in children's everyday lives.

Carers, whether birth parents, foster carers or residential workers, may all need additional support, not only from the therapist and key social worker, but also from other professionals such as managers, workers from voluntary agencies and foster support workers, in order to take an active participatory role in therapeutic change, rather than remaining passive observers (Ryan & Wilson 1996). Carers may also be asked to play a more direct role in the play therapy sessions themselves by the therapist, as mentioned above, particularly when very young and traumatised children attend play therapy, or where children and adolescents exhibit severe attachment problems (Ryan 1999).

We have argued elsewhere that all adults need to be clear about their different roles and tasks:

> The therapist is there to help resolve conflicts, create understanding and lessen fears; an attachment figure to enable the child to establish and maintain a sense of identity and well being by providing stability, affirmation of self and a sense of belonging ... The social worker has the overall role of coordination and management [of the case].
>
> (Ryan *et al.* 1995, p. 134)

Social workers may themselves work therapeutically with various family members, such as the parental couple in the child's birth family. They also may offer appropriate direct work to the child in coordination with the therapist conducting the child's play therapy sessions. There may also be a need for increased practical support from the social worker, including transport to therapy for the child and carer, and increased guidance to carers on behaviour management and on promotion of therapeutic changes.

Therapists initially help carers and social workers at referral to understand their therapeutic role and the aims and practise of non-directive play therapy. For carers and social workers unfamiliar with play therapy, visual material in conjunction with explanations from the therapist may be beneficial (see details on a training video at the end of this chapter). Therapists also provide help with therapy-related issues in children's and adolescents' home and school environments, and help both the carers and the social workers integrate children's needs and new responses expressed during therapy into everyday life.

Non-directive play therapy with abused adolescents

Before illustrating the practise of non-directive play therapy within a statutory setting with a 13-year-old sexually abused girl, the appropriateness of this technique with adolescents will be discussed. Some practitioners state that children aged 12 and over of normal intelligence are unsuitable for non-directive play therapy. Case studies for early adolescence are seldom documented in the play therapy literature; an adult counselling relationship is advocated instead. The suitability of non-directive play therapy for older pre-adolescent children has also been questioned and a different, more realistic set of games and activities is often made available by play therapists for this age group (Guerney 1984, West 1996).

We have discussed this issue at some length elsewhere, (Wilson *et al.* 1992, Ryan & Wilson 1996), arguing that non-directive play therapy is both an effective and theoretically justifiable therapeutic method with troubled adolescents. Briefly, non-directive play therapy can help an adolescent to integrate earlier childhood experiences, present concerns and future, more adult concerns into the adolescent's developing sense of unique personal identity. Children and adolescents who have been abused have particular problems in integrating experiences that have been abusive into an emotionally healthy sense of self, as discussed above. When their personal mental schemas have been arrested or distorted, abused adolescents find it difficult to rework schemas of their childhood selves and apply them to emotionally healthy ways of functioning in more adult relationships. Not only will their earlier emotional development have been damaging, and parental role models unhealthy ones, but abused adolescents may also have developed difficulties in peer relationships and difficulties in their desire and ability to integrate into wider adult society in an emotionally healthy manner.

Non-directive play therapy can be used to help abused adolescents integrate emotionally damaging experiences into their current identities. In order to work effectively with this age group, however, certain practice issues must be considered throughout. While a few more highly structured materials may be desirable for this age group, most materials should still lend themselves to unstructured symbolic activities and play. As with younger age groups, materials (such as art materials, puppets and staging) should be selected that can be used at the highest potential level of adolescent functioning as well as materials that can be used for much younger, regressive play. Both types of materials should be made freely available for the adolescent's use. Adult-sized furniture also immediately demonstrates to the adolescent that the room is used by a range of ages to both sit and talk in and to play in. These preparations are needed for adolescents because the therapist must be aware of an adolescent's heightened sensitivity and negative reaction to being treated only as a child. At the same time, as with younger children, the therapist must enable the adolescent to feel a sense of permissiveness in the room which extends to whatever thoughts, activities (or non-activities) and materials adolescents themselves choose. Older children and adolescents can be given the choice of attending progress meetings and therapists can offer to outline the themes they intend to discuss beforehand during the play therapy sessions themselves.

Furthermore, concerns over privacy and confidentiality are often greater for adolescents than for younger children. A private room without any outside interruptions and which is not overlooked is particularly necessary for adolescents, who may be more self-conscious of other's reactions to their sessions and will only manage to engage freely with the materials and therapist in private. Another related area of concern to the adolescent may be anxiety about peers' and other outside adults' interest in therapy sessions, and others' possible misuse of this information by teasing or labelling the adolescent as different or deranged. Again, the therapist must be sensitive to arranging sessions at times which minimise this potential intrusion (for example, lunch-time or after school). With abused children and adolescents, however, privacy may be an even more sensitive issue. Too much privacy in one-to-one interactions may be reminiscent of abusive experiences, or may direct an adolescent's attention too painfully to the large discrepancies in their other significant adult relationships. In these cases, individual therapeutic intervention may not be possible, and other interventions may be more appropriate initially, such as group work or family work.

Another important related concern is the extent to which the therapist can assure the adolescent that the content of sessions will remain private. (It is essential, however, that abused children and adolescents are given permission explicitly by the therapist to reveal whatever contents of sessions the child or adolescent chooses to others. Otherwise, again, the therapeutic relationship may too closely mirror a previously abusive one.) It is impossible, and indeed misleading, for therapists to guarantee complete confidentiality. All therapists must consider issues of confidentiality because of their professional obligation to report disclosures of abuse made within therapy sessions. Added considerations for therapists working in statutory settings include the kind of communication to establish with the carer, the type of information from sessions which will be shared with a referring agency through case conferences and reports, and the level of detail to reveal in court proceedings (Wilson *et al.* 1992, Ryan & Wilson 1995*a*).

While younger children may have more difficulty understanding the circumstances under which the therapist must discuss their sessions with others, adolescents are usually able to understand these issues. However, adolescents may also feel a heightened need for confidentiality from the therapist. And abused children and adolescents in particular may want complete confidentiality, having often been previously subjected to different forms of threats and coercions by abusing adults to ensure the secrecy of the abuse, and thus the abuser's freedom from detection and punishment. This need for security and exclusivity can be generalised to any close relationship with an adult, including individual therapy.

It is imperative, then, that the therapist discusses confidentiality issues and recording procedures with adolescents (and with young children, in keeping within their understanding) at the beginning of their time together. If this discussion is omitted, adolescents may falsely believe, in keeping with their needs, that the therapist is offering complete confidentiality. Adolescents may then be less guarded and, justifiably, feel betrayed when the therapist must report general sessional themes or specific abusive incidents to others. With abused adolescents (and children) mistrust of adults or overly trusting responses are already likely to be a crucial feature of their emotional difficulties. The therapist will increase this emotional damage if issues of confidentiality are not addressed honestly and sensitively from the start.

Using non-directive play therapy with a sexually abused adolescent

Patricia was 13 years old at the time of referral for play therapy sessions. Her initial appearance was of a self-assured, verbally aggressive and articulate older adolescent. She was physically mature, attractive and careful about her appearance. Patricia had disclosed sexual abuse by her uncle and later by her step-father as well, but she was disbelieved and blamed for the resulting investigation by her family, which included her mother, step-father, 16-year-old sister and 6-year-old half-brother. Patricia's extended family had already been investigated for sexual abuse. From the case notes on file, the atmosphere in these related families seemed to be highly sexualised, with a blurring of adult–child role boundaries and a failure to maintain sexual boundaries between generations.

When Patricia began to attend play therapy sessions, which took place for an hour once a week over a 3-month period (15 sessions altogether), she had been separated from her family and placed in foster care because of the continuing risk to her of sexual abuse. Several key themes which were important to Patricia emotionally emerged during her play therapy sessions. These themes illustrate many of the points raised earlier about the value of non-directive play therapy in working with abused adolescents and children. Two important themes for Patricia in her sessions, to be discussed below, include: the therapist's trustworthiness; and the reworking of childhood memories and distortions of bodily image arising from sexual abuse. The way in which therapists work within statutory settings also will be illustrated. (For a more extended discussion of these themes, see Ryan & Wilson, 1996.)

Theme one: the therapist's trustworthiness

A key theme for Patricia throughout her sessions was whether the therapist was a trustworthy and reliable adult. This issue seemed to have strong emotional salience for Patricia because of her emotional development within an abusive family atmosphere. She shared her family's mistrust of and anger with any professional in a role of authority and was particularly vehement about social services' interventions which investigated sexual abuse. Patricia repeatedly blamed social services for removing her from home, yet she also began to express surprise during her sessions that her statements about sexual abuse had been believed by professionals in spite of her family's denials. Another conflict for her was that while she desperately wanted to return home, and later in therapy expressed a longing to return to her pre-school existence within her family, she was at the same time deeply hurt by her family's rejection of her. In the process of therapy, Patricia began to consciously acknowledge to herself that her family often distorted information given to her, to other family members and to professionals, as well as keeping secret from her much about the extended family's complicated and disturbed relationships. Patricia's growing ability to examine her family's attitudes was made possible by the permissive atmosphere of her sessions, but also by the therapist's predictable and caring responses to Patricia's verbal statements and the therapist's reflection of Patricia's quickly changing and conflicting feelings. Patricia seemed to use the therapist as an anchor for thinking about her family and herself.

Confidentiality was an important, recurring theme for Patricia and an important element in the development of a trusting relationship with the therapist. Patricia tested out with the therapist the confidentiality of her sessions with other professionals, often aggressively challenging the therapist on whether her social worker would be informed of what she was doing in the sessions. Towards the end of their sessions together, when Patricia's level of trust in the therapist had increased, she confided in the therapist that she had not earlier told the therapist about several of the dangerous games she had been playing with peers because she had enjoyed having secrets from the therapist. Besides, she was certain that the therapist would have told her social worker or the police. The therapist reflected Patricia's feelings that it was fun to feel more powerful early on by having secrets from adults who were trying to know just about everything about you. The therapist also acknowledged that Patricia was right. The therapist as an adult would have tried to prevent Patricia from seriously harming herself and others, and she may have had to tell others.

Patricia also spent an inordinate amount of time talking about other younger children who used the room. While this was related to Patricia retrieving her childhood memories, which are discussed below, she also seemed both intrigued and challenged by the therapist's rule of confidentiality regarding other children's use of the playroom. Patricia returned to this topic often, used a variety of persuasive arguments, and even resorted to a younger child's wheedling tone in her attempts to test out the therapist's resolve in keeping this rule. The therapist repeated that she must maintain silence, thus enforcing a necessary therapeutic limit, and she also reflected Patricia's varied feelings, including a genuine interest and concern for the younger children and a belief that if she was persistent, the therapist would weaken and do something the therapist felt was wrong. Patricia's use of more abstract thinking on this issue allowed the therapist to reflect Patricia's feelings back to her at each occurrence, to subordinate her own feelings of harassment to Patricia's need to adopt extreme means in an attempt to weaken the therapist's resolve, to state her own position to Patricia clearly and to give reasons for her position that Patricia at 13 years old could understand. Using this non-directive approach, Patricia actively engaged in a process common to normal adolescence, but usually engaged in with lesser intensity. That is, Patricia was in the process of examining and understanding her own values and how these differed from both the values of the therapist and the values of her own family. The therapist for Patricia, therefore, represented the adult world of values in a very direct sense, and Patricia gradually developed a somewhat grudging trust in the therapist.

Theme two: the reworking of childhood memories and distortions in bodily image resulting from sexual abuse

While the first theme seems to rely heavily on non-directive counselling skills rather than play therapy *per se*, it is important in understanding Patricia's progress in therapy to note that from her first session onwards Patricia was purposeful in choosing an activity to perform with her hands while she talked. Patricia seemed to have no difficulty accepting the play setting or materials as appropriate for her age. (Her initial worries instead centred on her own use of the materials, which she considered to be inept and 'babyish', and on being ridiculed by peers for needing therapy at all.) She decided to use the clay and spent her early sessions, and a few sessions towards the end of her 15 sessions, modelling in this medium. Her early work in clay consisted of forming simple clay figures and using her hands to work them into smooth curves and then squeezing them shapeless again as she concentrated on verbal exchanges with the therapist.

After her initial play with the clay as an adjunct to her conversation, Patricia began to concentrate more intently on her ongoing activity using her hands, and her verbalisations lost prominence. Motor activities and sensations became central, and Patricia began to cover her hands completely with smooth wet clay, allowing it to harden before washing it off and restoring her hands to their usual clean, well-manicured condition. The therapist reflected Patricia's feelings and hypothesised to herself (and not to Patricia, as a psychodynamic therapist may have done) that perhaps Patricia was beginning to rework on a motor and affective level using symbolic means, the abusive masturbatory experiences she had disclosed during her earlier investigative interview. Along with the clay, Patricia also began to use the playdough in the room and to remember several happy times in her earlier childhood when she had enjoyed similar play and felt well looked after by her mother.

Following these play sequences, Patricia began to experiment with finger paints, first covering her hands with bright, vivid colours and then coating them repeatedly with more colours until they turned stickily dark brown. This process of covering her hands in thick layers of sticky paint lasted for several sessions, with Patricia using her whole body in a diffuse, sensual way. The therapist reflected Patricia's feelings of how good the process felt at the beginning; but then Patricia never stopped there and had to make her hands messier, even though they weren't as nice as at the beginning. She also reflected Patricia's disgust with her transformed hands by the end of her play, followed by her anxiety over needing to quickly make her hands perfect again.

Patricia's actions became less frantic and of shorter duration as she continued to rework what appeared to be her abusive experiences on this symbolic level. The therapist made occasional reflections, but Patricia, while continuing her activities without constraint, did not herself verbalise her feelings and actions during this time. However, she did verbally express great concern that the therapist would keep the paints ready for her use as long as she needed them. After several sessions, however, Patricia had finished completely with the finger paints and chose to return to her earlier medium of clay. This intense play sequence with finger paints paralleled changes in Patricia's appearance. She became more casual in her dress, decided to change her hairstyle and generally looked younger and more similar to other young adolescents.

By reworking her abusive experiences on a motor and affective level in symbolic play, Patricia seemed to have transformed her previously distorted mental schemas involving her body and its actions into more appropriate ones.

Statutory considerations in Patricia's therapy

In this chapter, general considerations of the therapist's role in working with other professionals within statutory settings have been outlined. This section illustrates the ways Patricia's therapist worked in partnership with her carers and other professionals involved in her life.

Patricia's social worker, Matthew, had been given leave by the court to release court papers, including chronologies and witness statements, to the therapist before she began her therapeutic work. She also had received a letter of instructions from the court agreed by all parties involved in ongoing care proceedings that she would provide a report on Patricia's therapeutic progress and recommendations for her future therapeutic needs after ten weekly sessions with Patricia.

The therapist read the court documents released to her prior to her referral meeting with Matthew. At their meeting the therapist familiarised Matthew with her method of therapy and requested an additional document on an earlier psychiatric assessment of Patricia. They had a preliminary discussion of practical arrangements for therapy, including the time of day suitable to Patricia, the therapist and her foster carers, who would be asked to accompany Patricia to her sessions. Matthew discussed his ongoing involvement with Patricia's family, which currently was of serious concern to him. His numerous attempts to engage Patricia's mother in actively cooperating with him in protecting her children from the possible abusive relationship they had with her partner had, he considered, been largely unsuccessful. Her mother was hostile to him and viewed his requirements of supervised contact by herself and her partner with Patricia as coercive, as his witness statement described.

Matthew had already informed the therapist in their initial referral conversation that Patricia's foster placement was stable, potentially long-term, and seemed to be meeting her physical and emotional needs adequately. However, her future remained uncertain, since it was dependent on the outcome of her care proceedings. During their referral meeting, Matthew elaborated on the relationship Patricia had developed with her carers. She seemed, in his opinion, relatively accepting of their care in the shorter-term; however, she had stated to him at regular intervals that she wanted to return to her mother's care.

The therapist clarified her own position as a professional who was outside statutory responsibility for Patricia's care, but that any serious child protection concerns arising from her sessions with Patricia would be clearly mentioned to Patricia herself and reported to him immediately. She outlined for him her proposed meetings: with Patricia's mother, with the foster carers in which she requested Matthew's attendance, and with Patricia herself in the presence of her foster carers prior to beginning her work. The therapist proposed monthly progress meetings with herself, Patricia's mother and the social worker, if Patricia's mother seemed able to develop an alliance with the therapist and was accepting of Patricia's need for therapy. Monthly progress meetings were also arranged for the therapist with the foster carers and social worker. Other options, such as the possibility that it would be beneficial for Patricia to attend some of the progress meetings, that meetings with Patricia's school may be useful, and that her foster carers' link worker in the fostering team be included at times were also discussed. These options would be reviewed with Matthew after the therapist's initial meetings.

The therapist's initial meeting with Patricia's mother appeared to preclude the development of a cooperative relationship between the therapist and her mother at this stage in court proceedings. The mother stated that she and Patricia were coerced into being involved with the therapist by social services and that it would do no good. It was Patricia's lies and defiance which were the issue, not any emotional problems. The therapist attempted to redefine Patricia's problems, but her mother was not receptive to this alteration. The therapist also explained her role as external to social services and Patricia's mother forcefully replied that the therapist needed to support her request to social services for unsupervised access to Patricia. When the therapist empathised with the mother's feelings but felt unable to support the mother's request, the mother completely refused to consider further meetings with the therapist.

The foster carers were, on the other hand, very eager to be involved in Patricia's therapy, immediately understood the need for Patricia to have their emotional support before and after therapy sessions, and were interested in developing their understanding of important emotional issues for Patricia. They also stated that Patricia might want to be included as part of these meetings, but wondered if she would be able to tolerate the social worker's presence. The therapist planned to discuss this with Patricia during their session prior to the first scheduled progress meeting, after she had established an initial therapeutic relationship with her.

Patricia's foster carers became an important link for her between her therapy sessions and her day-to-day life with them. Patricia initially refused to attend progress meetings, but wished to know the exact details of the first meeting. The therapist and foster carers willingly shared these with her, as they had agreed at the meeting, and Patricia chose to attend the later progress meetings. She became able to tolerate the tension engendered in her by Matthew's presence at these meetings, with the help of her foster carers and her therapy sessions. The options of including the foster link worker and school in these meetings was not taken up, since the social worker and foster carer maintained adequate working partnerships with them. The adults agreed that Patricia would have found widening the number of adult professionals attending their progress meetings an added complexity and difficult to cope with easily.

Summary

Non-directive play therapy is an effective method of intervention for children and adolescents who have been abused. Because the method is non-directive, during sessions children themselves direct the issues and contents to be explored in symbolic play. As discussed above, symbolic play is a normal means children use to express highly personal, complex emotional experiences. In non-directive play therapy sessions, children's abusive experiences are reworked into healthier patterns of responses on all mental levels (i.e. emotional, cognitive and motor levels) of functioning simultaneously. This reworking of experiences by children using symbolic play occurs within the context of a trusting, permissive atmosphere that the therapist and child have established. This relationship, while permissive, is also kept within the therapeutic limits needed by the child.

Adolescents in non-directive play therapy will commonly combine symbolic play with verbalising to the therapist, who needs to employ non-directive counselling skills more intensively for older age groups. A core skill in working with both children and adolescents is the therapist's ability to reflect the child's or adolescent's feelings during sessions in an accurate, yet non-threatening manner. The therapist must also have developed a coherent, personally meaningful and viable theoretical framework for therapeutic practice, as outlined in this chapter, to allow the use of personal feelings congruently in making appropriate, emotionally normal responses to the child's or adolescent's expressed behaviour and feelings.

Conclusions

This chapter has argued that non-directive play therapy provides practitioners with a theoretically rich and coherent system of therapy based on developmental principles. This feature, along with its non-coercive and non-intrusive nature, provides the rationale for using non-directive play therapy as a preferred method of therapy with abused children and adolescents. However, more definitive research on process and outcome issues in non-directive play therapy, particularly in statutory settings, is urgently needed.

It is important that qualified play therapists who have active membership in their professional organisations nationally (and internationally) are employed in working with this vulnerable group of clients. In addition to employing skilled and qualified professional play therapists, the effectiveness of such interventions is dependent upon non-abusive, relatively stable and responsive care environments. Professionals and carers all have vital roles to coordinate in play therapy interventions. It was also argued that non-directive therapy, by being sensitive to age-related issues, can be an effective intervention for adolescents as well as children. To illustrate this method of therapy for young people within statutory settings, a case example of a sexually abused young adolescent was presented and an illustration of this was given through a case example of work with a young adolescent who had been sexually abused.

Professional organisation (including training information)

British Association of Play Therapists (BAPT)
PO Box 98
Amershan
HP6 5BL.
Telephone/fax. 01179 860390
Email: BAPT11@hotmail.com
MA/Diploma in non-directive play therapy (BAPT approved)

Department of Social Policy and Social Work
University of York
Heslington
York YO10 5DD
Telephone: 01904 432 629
Fax: 01904 433 475
(This programme may also lead on to further study and registration for a PhD.)

Annotated further reading

Axline V 1971 Dibs: in search of self. Ballantine Books, New York
A moving account of a young boy's experience in non-directive play therapy.
Axline V 1987 Play therapy, revised edn. Ballantine Books, New York
A general introduction to play therapy including Axline's eight principles.
Carroll J 1998 Introduction to therapeutic play. Blackwell Science, Oxford
A well-written and accessible introduction to this topic for professionals interested in the use of play. There is a chapter on non-directive play therapy which gives a general overview of this approach.
Guerney L F 1984 Client-centred (non-directive) play therapy. In: Schaefer C, O'Connor K (eds) Handbook of play therapy. Wiley and Sons, New York
An overview of research theory and practice.
Rogers C 1951 Client-centred therapy. Constable, London
Roger's explanation of client-centred therapy, as well as Dorfman's application of his approach to play therapy.
Ryan V, Wilson K 1996 Case studies in non-directive play therapy. Baillière Tindall, London (Reissued 2000 by Jessica Kingsley, London)
Ryan V, Wilson K 2000 'Playing Matters'. Department of Social Policy and Social Work, University of York, York
This video is intended for play therapy training and as an aid to carers and professionals in understanding non-directive play therapy, with an accompanying booklet. Illustrations of non-directive techniques with untroubled children and carers are provided.
West J 1992 Child-centred play therapy. Edward Arnold, London
A recent practical guide to working with children in non-directive play therapy.
Wilson K, Kendrick P, Ryan V 1992 Play therapy: a non-directive approach for children and adolescents. Baillière Tindall, London
An updated extension of theory and practice in non-directive play therapy.

References

Axline V 1971 Dibs: in search of self. Ballantine Books, New York
Axline V 1987 Play therapy, revised edn. Ballantine Books, New York
Cigno K, Ryan V 1998 Making therapy work for children using non-directive play therapy and cognitive–behavioural therapy. Paper presented at the 28th Congress of the European Association for Behavioural and Cognitive Psychotherapists, University of Cork, Ireland
Crittenden P M 1992 Children's strategies for coping with adverse home environments: an interpretation using attachment theory. Child Abuse and Neglect 16: 329–343
Downes C 1992 Separation revisited: adolescents in foster family care. Ashgate, Aldershot
Dunn J 1988 The beginnings of social understanding. Basil Blackwell, Oxford
Erikson E H 1963 Childhood and society. Norton, New York
Finkelhor D 1992 Child sexual abuse: recent developments in research. Paper presented at 'Surviving Childhood Adversity Conference', Trinity College, Dublin

Ginott H 1961 Group psychotherapy with children: the theory and practice of play therapy. McGraw-Hill, New York

Glaser D 1991 Therapeutic work with children. In: Wilson K (ed) Child protection: helping or harming. Papers in Social Policy and Professional Studies, No. 15. University of Hull, Hull

Guerney L F 1984 Client-centred (non-directive) play therapy. In: Schaefer C, O'Conner K (eds) Handbook of play therapy. Wiley and Sons, New York

Hall L, Lloyd S 1993 Surviving child sexual abuse: a handbook for helping women challenge their past. Falmer Press, London

Harris P L 1989 Children and emotion. Basil Blackwell, Oxford

Kazdin A E, Bass D, Ayas W A, Rodgers A 1990 Empirical and clinical focus of child and adolescent psychotherapy research. Journal of Consulting and Clinical Psychology 58 (6): 729–740

Mahrer A R, Nadler W P 1986 Good moments in psychotherapy: a preliminary review, a list and some promising research avenues. Journal of Consulting and Clinical Psychology 54 (1): 10–15

Moustakas C 1953 Children in play therapy. McGraw-Hill, New York

Moustakas C 1959 Psychotherapy with children: the living relationship. Harper and Row, New York

Pynoos R, Eth S 1984 The child as witness to homicide. Journal of Social Issues 40: 87–108

Pynoos R, Eth S 1986 Witness to violence: the child interview. Journal of the American Academy of Child Psychiatry 25 (3): 306–319

Rogers C 1951 Client-centred therapy: its current practice, implications and theory. Constable, London

Ryan V 1999 Building attachments: how play therapists help children develop loving relationships. Keynote address, British Association for Play Therapists 7th Annual conference, Leicester

Ryan V, Wilson K 1993 Non-directive play therapy: therapeutic intervention with children and adolescents. In: Bradley G, Wilson K (eds) The family, the state and the child. Papers from the Four Nations Conference. Department of Social Policy and Professional Studies, University of Hull, Hull

Ryan V, Wilson K 1995a Child therapy and evidence in court proceedings: tensions and some solutions. British Journal of Social Work 25: 157–172

Ryan V, Wilson K 1995b Non-directive play therapy as a means of recreating optimal infant socialisation patterns. Early Development and Parenting 4 (1): 29–38

Ryan V, Wilson K 1996 Case studies in non-directive play therapy. Baillière Tindall, London (Reissued 2000 by Jessica Kingsley Publishers, London)

Ryan V, Wilson K 2000a Conducting child assessments for court proceedings: the use of non-directive play therapy. Clinical Child Psychology and Psychiatry 5 (2): 267–279

Ryan V, Wilson K 2000b Using non-directive play therapy for court proceedings: our response to Turner's legal commentary. Clinical Child Psychology and Psychiatry 5 (2).

Ryan V, Wilson K, Fisher, T 1995 Partnerships in therapeutic work with children. Journal of Social Work Practise, 9 (2): 131–140

Schmidtchen S 1986 Practice and research in play therapy. In van der Kooij R, Hellendoorn J (eds) Play, play therapy and play research. Swete and Zeitlinger, Lisse

van der Kooij R, Hellendoorn J. (eds) 1986 Play, play therapy and play research. Swete and Zeitlinger, Lisse

West J 1996 Child-centred play therapy, 2nd edn. Edward Arnold, London

Wilson K 1993 The healer and the carer. Community Care 978: 27

Wilson K and Ryan V 1998 Individual child therapy and its impact on parenting skills. Paper presented at the 28th Congress of the European Association for Behavioural and Cognitive Psychotherapists, University of Cork, Ireland.

Wilson K, Kendrick P, Ryan V 1992 Play therapy: a non-directive approach for children and adolescents. Baillière Tindall, London

Wolff S 1986 Childhood psychotherapy. In: Block S (ed) An introduction to the psychotherapies, 2nd edn. Oxford University Press, Oxford

Wyre R 1991 Working with sex offenders. In: Wilson K (ed) Child protection: helping or harming. Papers in Social Policy and Professional Studies, No. 15, University of Hull, Hull

Helping to prevent abuse: a cognitive–behavioural approach with families

Katy Cigno

In 1982, Sheldon wrote that it was impossible for practitioners to open their mouths or put pen to paper without making others despise them for having got it wrong. This was because social workers and other professionals were looking for the approach to end, or encompass, all other approaches. This attitude to practice simplifies – dangerously so – the therapeutic task, particularly with regard to working with vulnerable people, as in child protection. A comparable view was more recently expressed in a paper on direct work with children (Ronen 1993).

Fortunately, we have moved some way since then. For example, the mention of the word 'behavioural' no longer arouses such frequent hostility in social work circles this side of the Atlantic. The careful incorporation of research on the place of cognition in determining which behaviours are likely to be repeated has helped widen the appeal of a cognitive–behavioural approach (Sheldon 1995, Cigno 1998). The question to ask is not 'which approach?' but 'what evidence is there that this or that approach works, in specified circumstances, with this client with this problem?' (Cigno & Wilson 1994).

The aim of this chapter is therefore to consider the circumstances in which a cognitive–behavioural approach, using social learning theory, can be useful in helping to protect children by preventing abuse through improving child–parent interaction, parenting skills and behaviours of children and parents. This emphasis on prevention is advocated by Cohn & Daro (1987) in their review of the research on treatment effectiveness, and the issue has been re-addressed by Hollows & Wonnacott (1994). The emphasis on supporting families in order to prevent deterioration in their circumstances and protect children is a current key issue and the focus of much government policy (e.g. Department of Health (DOH) 1998a). Re-focusing on children in need as an effective way of preventing abuse and neglect is also the focus of the Dartington Research Unit's review of what works in child protection (DOH 1995).

Some concepts associated with social learning theory and a cognitive behavioural approach have been incorporated into the Children Act 1989 (see below). Some have informed recent social work practice and education, as in the current emphasis on observable competencies in the Central Council for Education and Training in Social Work's Paper 30 (CCETSW 1991, 1996). Teachers and health visitors have also long been aware of the importance of positive reinforcement and modelling in child development and skill acquisition. Ronen (1994), while commenting that social work was founded upon a psychodynamic approach, writes:

Social workers have always been concerned with effective treatments, the definition of clear goals and the clarification of client needs. These features link social work to cognitive–behavioural therapy. (p. 273)

In short, there is now too much evidence of the effectiveness of behaviourally based approaches (Sheldon 1986, Macdonald *et al.* 1992) for these not to be part of a practitioner's repertoire (Hudson & Macdonald 1986, Sutton 1994, 1999, Webster-Stratton & Herbert 1994, Cigno & Bourn 1998).

The current policy context of intervention

Some key concepts, which have emerged to inform the policy context of social services, social work, health and education of the late 1980s and 1990s are:

- Clarity and openness, verbally and in record-keeping
- Service user empowerment
- Partnership with service users, other professionals and agencies
- Setting goals, monitoring and evaluating services
- Protecting vulnerable people as priority
- The need for practice to be evidence-based.

Examples of legislation that set out guiding principles for practitioners and incorporate such concepts are the Access to Personal Files Act (1987), the Children Act 1989, the National Health Service and Community Care Act 1990 and the Carers (Recognition and Services) Act 1995.

The idea of client or patient access to files initially aroused opposition from both the medical professional (Timmins 1987) and other practitioners and officials (Cohen 1982, Hennessy 1988) who were unused to promoting an open agenda with service users and who were often unclear as to who, in fact, was the client and in whose interests the records were kept (Cigno & Gottardi 1988, 1989). The same writers found that the more task-centred practitioners were clear on these issues and had, prior to the legislation and preceding Government circulars, worked openly on problem-solving and behavioural goals with their clients, many of whom were parents. More recent research has shown that parents involved in child protection investigations prefer social workers and others to be honest and direct with them (Hepworth & Larsen 1990, Sutton 1994, 1999, DOH 1995). The Data Protection Act 1998 strengthens users' rights.

The Children Act 1989 and the National Health Service and Community Care Act 1990 both stress the need for contracts, or working agreements, with clients. In the case of the former, however, this is implicit rather than explicit, but the Department of Health's document *Working Together* (DOH 1991) and the new guidance (DOH *et al.* 1999: note the replacement of 'protect' with 'safeguard') spell this out more clearly. The use of contracts is long established in behavioural work (Sheldon 1995). It is clear from both these Acts that practitioners are to carry out careful, detailed assessments (essential in cognitive–behavioural work) and empower clients by, for example, getting them to participate in writing records ('needs-led' user profiles, in the case of the National Health Service and Community Care Act).

The notion of partnership with parents for the benefit of the child is, again, implicitly incorporated in the Children Act 1989 (Herbert 1993). It is, however, elucidated in such documents as *Protecting Children* (DOH 1988), *The Care of Children* (DOH 1989) and *Working Together* (DOH 1991, DOH *et al.* 1999). These guidelines also stress that the child's interests are paramount.

The last few years have seen the issue of powerful statements and guidance concerning social services and working in partnership with other agencies, particularly the health services, and professionals. The White Paper *Modernising*

Social Services (DOH 1998*b*) included a mandatory implementation timetable for service directors and councillors. The White Paper was preceded by *Quality Protects* (DOH 1998*c*), aimed at ensuring quality services for vulnerable children in the social care system, and by the *Looking After Children* (LAC) materials issued with the same aim (see Parker *et al.* 1991). All these documents stress the need for clear goals and performance measures; and for working in partnership with children and their carers.

Cognitive–behavioural workers have always been aware that intervention in the home, however well planned and child-centred, will fail unless the parents or carers are informed and involved (Herbert 1987*a*, Corby 1993, 2000, Webster-Stratton & Herbert 1994). This is because they are important mediators for many types of intervention, and in any case spend far more time with their children than the practitioner.

In sum, a cognitive–behavioural approach would appear to incorporate the principles of good practice embodied in current legislation and policy affecting service users and, more particularly, families. In addition, because of its lack of mystique and its objectives of working with clients on specific, agreed goals, it is arguably also both ethical and anti-oppressive (Cigno & Bourn 1998).

Effective intervention: research and practice

The intention here is not to address every area where a cognitive–behavioural approach might be adopted. Space precludes this. Instead, the discussion will focus on specific, important and well-documented areas where the use of this approach has been particularly successful in work with families where risk to the child's well-being or safety has been identified. These include:

- Working with families on child–parent interaction where child behaviour problems have been identified
- Training for parents, particularly to help them cope better where children have severe behavioural problems or where parents have difficulty in controlling their anger
- Intervention where the child is failing to thrive.

Writers and therapists in these areas are from different helping professions, publishing monographs and articles in a variety of professional journals. As might be expected, however, psychologists have been at the forefront in research on behavioural intervention in families (e.g. Herbert 1987*a*, 1987*b*, 1989, Gibb & Randall 1989, Webster-Stratton & Herbert 1994). Nurses have also made important contributions to the case study literature on child abuse (e.g. Gilbert 1980). Important texts on behavioural family therapy and enhancing coping skills have been written by a psychiatrist and colleagues (Falloon 1988, Falloon *et al.*, 1993). Social workers have also, particularly recently, produced case study research in child care (e.g. Bunyan 1987, Bourn 1993, Cigno & Bourn 1998), while Sutton (1979, 1987, 1994, 1999) is one of a group with a background and qualifications in both social work and psychology writing on theory and practice in a variety of settings, including child abuse, neglect and parenting. The importance of early intervention to help children in need and improve their life chances is the subject of a study by social work academics Macdonald & Roberts (1995).

Mention has already been made of the importance of working openly in partnership with families. However, a research study (Thoburn *et al.* 1991) indicated that, sadly, few practitioners fully involve and inform family members in child protection work. The authors conclude that policies aimed at client participation and empowerment are unlikely to be effective unless workers make constant, concerted efforts to involve the family in the process of protecting children. Corby (2000) also concludes that programmes that empower and include parents are likely to be more effective.

Theoretical principles

The advantage of a social learning approach as a framework for effecting change is that working closely with family members to whose actions and words close attention is paid and who are considered partners in therapy is intrinsic to anti-oppressive intervention. As Sutton says, in a useful statement which includes both a definition and evaluation:

> Social learning theory comprises a large body of concepts which, happily, are recognised by researchers in the disciplines of both psychology and sociology. It concerns how children and adults learn patterns of behaviour, as a result of social interactions, or simply through coping with the environment ... it suggests how to focus upon the practical rather than the pathological, upon people's strengths and potentials rather than upon their weaknesses or shortcomings, and upon how to empower those with whom we work.
>
> (Sutton 1994, pp. 5–6)

Cognitive–behavioural therapy (CBT), as the name implies, is aimed at altering patterns of behaviour and thinking about behaviour which is dysfunctional and therefore requires the practitioner to focus on the detail of interactions between parents and children. Consequently, a useful and simple starting point for assessments is usually an ABC (antecedents, behaviour, consequences) analysis of these interactions. Briefly, the questions to ask when using such an analysis in assessment are:

Antecedents
- What are the circumstances in which the behaviour takes place?
- What happens just before the behaviour in question?

Behaviour
- What is the actual behaviour?
- What does the child/person do?

Consequences
- What happens immediately after the behaviour?

Parents, and children where possible, are encouraged to look at the relationship between the three as well as to look at established patterns of behaviour. Webster-Stratton & Herbert (1994) give many short examples of using the ABC format in family assessment. An example of the use of this format in child protection practice is given in the following section.

Working with families in the home

There is now a substantial body of studies evaluating behavioural and cognitive–behavioural intervention with families in non-clinical settings. What is striking about them is their careful, detailed, descriptive approach, attention to method, recording and use of observable criteria for success. Earlier studies contrast behavioural intervention with the prevailing psychodynamic approach. For example, Petts & Geddes (1978) point out essential differences and evaluate, by means of a chart and a descriptive account, the results of teaching child management to single-parent mothers as part of a strategy to improve family life. Seheult (1985) discusses the use of parents as their children's therapists and emphasises the importance of relieving stress which the whole family suffers when a child exhibits severe behavioural problems.

Therapeutic benefits to the pre-school child and the alleviation of family stress are also discussed by Bidder *et al.* (1981) who, from a medical school child health department, carried out a series of home interventions with nine children where there were similar problems to those reported by Bunyan (1987) and Bourn (1993), whose case studies are discussed below. Theirs was a carefully designed study which used a control group and aimed at achieving results over a short period. They found that the 'treated children' improved considerably, their behaviour becoming similar to those of the control group children after four to five visits. At 6 months, the improvements were maintained. They conclude that 'brief behavioural intervention has considerable potential and is reasonably economical in terms of staff time' (Bidder *et al.* 1981, p. 21).

Increasingly, programmes are multidisciplinary and multi-faceted. Research has shown that practitioners need to pay attention to many factors in the family's environment and networks, using an ecological approach (Gambrill 1983, Gambrill & Stein 1994). Specific interventions should be undertaken within a framework of the use of other resources (e.g. a family centre or a nursery – see Cigno 1988, Gill 1989, Cigno & Wilson 1994) and a warm rapport (Hudson and Macdonald 1986). Gill, a social worker working with health visitors, reports a high level of parental satisfaction with support groups where participants were actively involved in devising and implementing strategies for change appropriate to them (Gill 1989), a phenomenon well-known to those of us who work in and with family centres.

An example of such a multidisciplinary, multi-agency, multi-faceted approach is given by Carter *et al.* (1981). A teacher, social worker and educational psychologist successfully intervened in the case of Alan, a 10-year-old boy who was glue-sniffing, aggressive and truanting. His parents had attempted to control his behaviour by physical punishment. They used a contract with the boy and his parents (see also Webster-Stratton & Herbert 1994, for examples of contracts), targeted positive reinforcement and paid particular attention to working with the family to devise a strategy for maintaining improvements after programme termination. All targeted behaviours improved – for example, Alan began attending school again – but the authors claim only modest success and observe that 'time will tell' if the maintenance strategies devised will be effective.

In three articles, Ronen (1993, 1994, 1998) discusses direct therapeutic cognitive–behavioural intervention with children, mainly from a social work point of view. She is concerned with, among other matters, crucial issues of child involvement and careful choice of target and approach for intervention. She discusses important misconceptions about the selection of treatment methods; for instance, that the child who is lacking in verbal skills and has many problems is usually referred for long-term, dynamically oriented play therapy, while the child 'who suffers from a specific deficiency or problem and wishes to eliminate it is referred to short-term behaviour therapy' (Ronen 1993, p. 593). Echoing aspects of what is stressed elsewhere in this chapter, she urges practitioners to carry out careful assessments in order to find out where best to intervene and with which method, referring the child to another therapist if necessary.

Finally, two case studies describe the use by practitioners working in social services departments of the ABC format outlined earlier. Bourn (1993) gives an account of an intervention in the home where two children were put on the Child Protection Register after over-chastisement by the mother. The central problem was identified as child non-compliance and defiance towards a mother who was lacking in child-management skills. Bourn's analysis of $4\frac{1}{2}$-year-old Scott's problem behaviours includes the following.

Antecedents
- Background of poor housing and socio-economic disadvantage
- Active, restless child
- Non-compliance worse at home and with mother, during the week
- Mother tired and busy
- Scott refuses to eat breakfast or get dressed
- Mother gives unclear instructions, then demands immediate compliance with the implicit or actual threat of aversive consequences, e.g. 'Pack it in! Now!'

Behaviour
- Scott fails to comply
- Twirls around with his trousers on his head instead of getting dressed
- Swears at mother.

Consequences
- Mother makes threats which she is unable to carry out
- If punishment given – e.g. if Scott sent to his room – he amuses himself there
- Mother 'gives up', or over-chastises child in attempt to control him (adapted from Bourn 1993, pp. 488–489).

Intervention included specifying the rules for positive reinforcement; using role-play in the settings where the behaviour was likely to occur to enable mother to practise how to reinforce Scott positively, both materially and socially; and getting mother's partner to encourage and socially reinforce her for using the programme (see Bourn 1998 for an updated version of this case study).

Another useful example of an ABC analysis followed by behavioural intervention is given by Bunyan (1987), where a child at serious risk of abuse presented problems of defiance, aggression, destructiveness and sleep irregularity. Both Bourn and Bunyan stress the importance of thorough assessment. In both accounts, the intervention was aimed at increasing child compliance, improving parental management skills, reducing aversive interaction between parent and child using positive reinforcement (e.g. by praise, hugs, a sticker, small material rewards) and parent training.

The reported results are encouraging. In both families, there was a positive improvement in the child's behaviour and an increase in parental self-esteem and management skills as charted and observed by the practitioners. Bunyan followed up at 6 months and Bourn at 11 months. The results in both cases showed that the improvements in the target behaviours had been maintained, there was no symptom substitution, and the parents were relieved and more relaxed.

Parent training

Many practitioners and carers will have seen the BBC Panorama film showing examples of the adverse consequences for children of parents' inability to control a young child's behaviour (Panorama, BBC, 23 September 1996). The programme strongly reinforced the message that the prognosis for those children whose parents were unable to cope with a child's perceived 'misbehaviour', including non-compliance, was poor, even resulting in the removal of the child from home and later offending behaviour. On the other hand, the film provided evidence of the success of parent training in those families where the parents were able to use in the home the techniques demonstrated and rehearsed in the group.

It is often difficult to separate parent training from a 'working with families' approach described above, since it is often used as a strategy in family-centred interventions such as those considered in the previous section. However, Herbert (1987*b*, 1989) and Webster-Stratton & Herbert (1994) give many examples of parent training, which they refer to as a parent–therapist collaborative process. They include a review of the literature in this area as well as a detailed account of group work with parents.

Scott & Stradling (1987) and Scott (1989) have also carried out group parent training programmes in two connected areas: with parents of children with severe behavioural problems, and with parents who cannot benefit from such training, largely because they have difficulty in controlling their anger. The authors observe that the training can also work with individual parents. Scott's programme is based on six to eight sessions which include discussion, direct teaching of behaviours, role rehearsal and homework assignments. He stresses the importance of feedback and making sure that principles and instructions are understood. Where anger is a problem, parents can usefully be taught to relax before starting training (Barth *et al.* 1983).

Scott uses 'before and after' measures to evaluate how well new behaviours are learned, as well as a control group. Evaluation takes place at 3 and 6 months via home observation and role-play tests. He reports a significant decrease in frequency and intensity of child behaviour problems, and in parental depression and irritability (Scott 1989). Whiteman *et al.* (1987) also report good results from cognitive–behavioural intervention aimed at reducing anger in parents at risk of abusing their child. Scott *et al.* (1995) are also continuing their cognitive–behavioural work with adult survivors of childhood sexual abuse.

Webster-Stratton & Herbert (1994) and Sutton (1999) stress the significance of empowering parents and giving them self-confidence in training sessions. It is also important to make sure that parents will have support and reinforcement for good parenting once the sessions are over, such as monthly 'booster shots' with the therapist. Many practitioners and researchers in this field refer to Patterson's (1976) earlier work, on which they base their intervention. Patterson also reported that parent training is an effective way of changing a child's disturbed behaviours. Frosh & Summerfield (1986) review the effectiveness of parent training, stressing that such intervention has an educative as well as a treatment role, a point which could be made of much cognitive–behavioural therapy. Sutton's (1998) handbook on parent training makes these points as well as providing a detailed, user-friendly guide to working with carers to improve their child care skills and hence their child's welfare.

As community care policies are implemented, involving the emptying of hostels for adults with learning difficulties (many of whom came originally from long-stay hospitals), increasing attention has been given to the ability of such adults to cope in the community, even with the help of social services support workers. More particularly, there has been a focus on the ability of those who choose to have children to provide 'good enough' parenting. Dowdney & Skuse (1993) ask whether parents with a learning disability (they use the still current American term 'mental retardation') display competent parenting, and, if not, whether they can be taught parenting skills. This is an important area attracting increasing attention in terms of both research and practice. They report that the small amount of research so far available on the subject is conflicting, and that there are many factors to take into account. However, they conclude that intervention, within a relationship of rapport and trust, is usefully directed at teaching basic caregiving and play skills.

Where there is neglect or abuse, behavioural programmes can improve parenting. The authors suggest that imitating role models is a good way to acquire skills, which should be broken down into small steps (in a way similar to Portage methods used in families where there is a child with a learning difficulty; see, for example, Lloyd 1986). Non-specific counselling in this area of work is not useful. The authors go on to say that training needs to be long, rewards are effective for establishing and maintaining behaviours, and that more success is obtained where the goals are clear and individualised.

Booth & Booth (1993) also review the research evidence in their study of 20 families where one or both parents have learning difficulties. Their conclusion is that parenting skills can be improved by training, despite some reservations about the focus of North American research and the (largely unmet) need for long-term skill reinforcement. They rightly consider the place of parent training and behaviour modification techniques generally in a broad environmental context, which often discriminates against people with a learning disability. Practitioners are urged to take note when planning intervention that 'good parenting' models are necessary in order to be able to learn good parenting; and again, the work in this field needs a long-term commitment. These messages for practitioners are crucial.

Intervening where a young child 'fails to thrive'

Major research into cases of failure to thrive has been undertaken by Iwaniec and colleagues and reported in two parts (Iwaniec *et al.* 1985a, 1985b). Part I considers psychosocial factors and Part II describes the intervention. A detailed description of the characteristics of such a child is given (see also Budd 1990). Briefly, in cases of failure to thrive, the child is below average height, thin with a large stomach, cold to the touch, intellectually and speech delayed. The child can also appear sad and lethargic, refuse to eat and often vomits.

The intervention of Iwaniec and colleagues, based on social learning theory, has essentially three parts to it. It is often preceded by teaching the mother how to relax, since mothers of failure-to-thrive children tend to be tense and anxious. The workers:

- Use modelling, role rehearsal and advice to restructure the way in which the mother feeds the child (how to touch, smile and talk to the child at mealtimes)
- Gradually work to improve mother–child interaction on a wider front (e.g. in play), involving other members of the family, including the father
- Concentrate on positive parent–child interactions; give frequent and regular support to the family (e.g. by telephone calls as well as visits) in order to give positive reinforcement to the mother for her efforts.

The writers stress that the child also needs to go to nursery school as an added safeguard. Physical aspects of the child's well-being need constant control. Intervention is terminated only when the practitioner has observable evidence that the child's health and development have improved. An average intervention lasts 10 months. Immediate and long-term evaluation have shown positive results.

Herbert's case study of a 2-year-old twin suffering from failure to thrive follows similar lines (Herbert 1987a). He refers to theories of operant and classical conditioning to explain the child's behaviour, as well as theories of depression and learned helplessness (Seligman 1975) to explain the mother's behaviour. The child in the study had been hospitalised five times because of feeding problems and weight loss. With such serious threats to health, very careful monitoring and evaluation was essential. As well as self-monitoring by the mother and evaluation by the therapists, follow-up assessments by a paediatrician, nutritionists and health visitors were used to confirm progress, underlining the importance of multi-agency work, combined with the utilisation of community resources.

The work on failure to thrive was further developed by Iwaniec (1987). She continues to carry out research in this area (Iwaniec 1998) as well as focusing on the hitherto somewhat overlooked areas of emotional abuse and neglect (Iwaniec 1995). The emphasis is on helping children, their parents and the whole family through multi-modal intervention which includes cognitive–behavioural therapy.

Summary of key issues

Working under the Children Act 1989 often poses a dilemma for practitioners: how to work in partnership with parents *and* keep the child's interests central to the intervention; how to work with families in a non-stigmatising way where children are in need *and* protect children. Here, the notions of thorough assessment, careful monitoring and evaluation of intervention should help. Inspection after inspection continues to highlight the low standards of assessments and other key components of family work which are integral to a cognitive–behavioural approach. One such report (Social Services Inspectorate (SSI) 1997) identified that, even where assessments took place, 'they were poorly coordinated and lacked structure or analysis' and '[t]here was a major lack of skills and knowledge among social workers about conducting assessments' (p. 42). Further, as this chapter has underlined, in cases where the welfare of a child is of primary concern, a combination of techniques and services may be used to advantage, but the outcome criteria must be *observable*. That is, the practitioner is looking for positive behaviour change in the child and parent or carer; visible and audible improvement in child–parent interaction; and, in cases of failure-to-thrive, improvement in the appearance, weight, height and general health of the child. Practitioners need to become keenly observant of detail as well as conscious of the importance of the wider environment in assessment. The effects of the new assessment framework (DOH 2000), which attempts to take into account new evidence on effective practice with children in need, will take some time to become apparent.

There is a need for open approaches in which clients can understand and participate, where family members feel empowered by being treated as individuals. The use of a written contract to state precise goals parents need to achieve, desired reciprocal behaviour patterns between a child and his or her carers (as in 'contingency' contracts) and/or responsibilities of clients and practitioner (as in 'service' contracts) can seem coercive if badly drafted (as many are) by those with insufficient training, yet they are widely used in child protection and parenting skills groups. In experienced hands, however, such a document is the clear, honest result of negotiation. It will make clear to parents and others, in simple language, what they need to do to make the child safe; how to improve child–parent interaction; what resources are available to support them in this (e.g. practitioner home visits, toy library, play group); when the contract will be reviewed; and what the consequences are for non-compliance of the responsible adults. (For further comments on the use of contracts in cases of child abuse and neglect, see Sutton 1994, pp. 215–216, and pp. 174–175 for an example of a contract adaptable to many situations in one-to-one and family work; for helping a distressed child who soils, see Sutton 1999, pp. 286–287 and pp. 297–230 for principles of making agreements with parents; for rules for writing contracts, see Herbert 1993, pp. 172–173.)

It is particularly important in cases where parents feel they are failing in some way with their child that their views and feelings are carefully attended to, and that they are clear about the goals they need to achieve in order to demonstrate 'good enough' parenting. In some cases, service users need to know what they have to do in order *not* to be involved in intervention!

Gambrill's (1981) checklist for behavioural intervention in child abuse and neglect, although apparently basic, is still pertinent today and thus worth repeating. It provides a summary of key points to bear in mind, but also provides useful guidance for practitioners working with children and families about how to prevent abuse occurring. The checklist appears below in an abbreviated form.

1. *Looking as well as talking.* Direct observation of parent–child interaction is essential. Identify specific behaviours, their antecedents and consequences. Assess in natural settings, such as the home and school.
2. *Looking rather than inferring.* Do not presuppose particular associations between behaviour and environmental events. Directly observe interaction.
3. *Being specific rather than global.* Identify specific objectives – what should be done, by whom, in what situation, with what frequency, duration or intensity? Describe clearly what assessment and intervention procedures are to be used.
4. *Practising in addition to talking.* Arrange for clients to practise new behaviours at home.
5. *Focusing on overt behaviour.* Identify observable outcomes against which progress can be measured.
6. *Measuring rather than inferring progress.* Identify objective and subjective measures of progress. Identify clearly what the desired outcome is.
7. *Taking advantage of available resources.* Find out what the intervention costs in terms of time, effort and materials. Use resources already available and find out about suitable training material through publishers' lists, etc.
8. *Training material for clients.* Use self-help manuals, written rules, instructions, reminders, pamphlets, tapes (adapted from Gambrill 1981, pp. 18–20).

Conclusion

Practitioners have a duty to do their best for their clients, especially for those, like young children, who cannot demand a service for themselves. Unless workers keep themselves well-informed – for example, through reading and seminars – and make efforts to increase their skills through practice under supervision, then values expressed in such terms as 'anti-oppressive practice', 'working together' and 'empowerment' will be meaningless. Children and parents have a right to competent assessment and intervention.

There are many approaches described in the literature for working with children and families. It should not be a question of choosing a favourite and sticking to it unquestioningly throughout one's professional life. First, the empirical evidence must be considered: how successful is this approach, with which people, with which problems? Has the approach or the service been evaluated at all? As a Royal College of Nursing report on nursing and child protection revealed, there is a 'worrying lack of coordination' in the wake of the National Health Service purchaser–provider split; a danger of service fragmentation, putting children at risk; and 'haphazard, inadequately planned, inconsistent services [which were] neither evaluated nor monitored' (Friend & Ivory 1994, p. 3). Concerted efforts by largely government-funded initiatives and evidence-based projects over the last few years are seeking to address these deficits with carefully designed research and dissemination strategies of 'what works' (see, for example, the examination of child care initiatives by Bullock *et al.* 1998).

Second, in each particular case, we 'start where the client is' looking at their priority needs. In the field of preventing child abuse, this must mean that our concern is to make improvements in the family situation so that the child is safe from harm, is able to play, go to school, enjoy contact with carers, etc. As Sutton (1994) points out in her review of intervention evaluation in child abuse, 'the research in this area should make us cautious' (p. 113). Nevertheless, we know that early intervention to help troubled children with behaviour problems, low self-esteem and feelings of anxiety, and to help parents cope with their child's behaviour without the use of emotional and physical punishment is both therapeutic and effective, given the inescapability of differing personal perceptions, to paraphrase Sutton (1994, p. 5).

The evidence suggests that a multi-faceted, multi-agency approach where, for example, parent training is one of several services families receive, is more likely to lead to success. Moreover, concentrating on protecting children by preventing abuse happening or escalating is a better way of tackling the problem and is certainly more beneficial to children and families. The evidence also makes it clear that social learning theory and cognitive–behavioural intervention can make a significant contribution to the effectiveness of strategies for working with children and families.[1]

Annotated further reading

Cigno K, Bourn D (eds) 1998 Cognitive–behavioural social work in practice. Ashgate, Aldershot

The editors take a case study approach in order to bring practice alive. Chapter 1 gives an overview of research, theory and practice. Six of the subsequent chapters cover work with children and young people in a variety of settings, including the residential sector.

Iwaniec D 1995 The emotionally abused and neglected child. Identification, assessment and intervention. John Wiley, Chichester

It is now clear that emotional abuse and neglect have long-lasting effects and very often accompany physical abuse. Dorota Iwaniec's book is a detailed exposition of the subject, including failure to thrive. The work is relevant to all child care professionals.

Sutton C 1999 Helping families with troubled children: a preventive approach. John Wiley, Chichester

As usual, this writer takes a multi-agency, multidisciplinary approach to helping children, emphasising that a commitment to preventive measures and support is effective in relieving unhappiness in children and stopping or alleviating further harm. Social learning theory and its practice applications are clearly explained.

Webster-Stratton C, Herbert M 1994 Troubled families – problem children. Wiley & Sons, Chichester

The subject is child conduct disorders. The authors discuss family-based approaches and assessment, with an emphasis on working with parents. Part 1 is concerned with understanding child conduct

---

[1] Many behavioural and cognitive–behavioural practitioners compile their own material. One useful, published booklet is *Seven Supertactics for Superparents* by Wheldall *et al.* (1983). The Centre for Fun and Families also provides material to help families (for further information, see Neville *et al.* 1995).

disorders and their impact on the home and community, while Part 2 offers a detailed guide for therapists. There are many case examples and discussions of specific behavioural procedures, such as the use of 'time out' and contracts.

References

Barth R P, Blythe B J, Schinke S P, Schilling R F 1983 Self-control training with maltreating parents. Child Welfare 62 (4): 313–324

Bidder R T, Gray O P, Pates R M 1981 Brief intervention therapy for behaviourally disturbed pre-school children. Child: Care, Health and Development 7: 21–30

Booth T, Booth W 1993 Parenting with learning difficulties: lessons for practitioners. British Journal of Social Work 23: 459–480

Bourn D F 1993 Over-chastisement, child non-compliance and parenting skills: a behavioural intervention by a family centre social worker. British Journal of Social Work 23: 481–499

Budd J 1990 Falling short of the target. Community Care 15 November: 12–13

Bullock R, Gooch D, Little M, Mount K 1998 Research in practice: experiments in development and information design. Dartington Social Research Series. Ashgate, Aldershot

Bunyan A 1987 Help, I can't cope with my child: a behavioural approach to the treatment of a conduct disordered child within the natural home setting. British Journal of Social Work 17: 237–256

Carter B, Low A, Winter S 1981 A technology to replace an art. Community Care: 20–21

Central Council for Education and Training in Social Work (CCETSW) 1991 Rules and requirements for the Diploma in Social Work. Paper 30, 2nd edn. CCETSW, London

Central Council for Education and Training in Social Work (CCETSW) 1996 Assuring quality in the Diploma in Social Work. Part 1: Rules and requirements for the DipSW, 2nd revision. CCETSW, London

Cigno K 1988 Consumer views of a family centre drop-in. British Journal of Social Work 18: 361–375

Cigno K 1998 Cognitive–behavioural practice. In: Adams R, Dominelli L, Payne M (eds) Social work: themes, issues and critical debates. Macmillan, Basingstoke, Chapter 15, p. 184

Cigno K, Bourn D (eds) 1998 Cognitive–behavioural social work in practice. Ashgate, Aldershot

Cigno K, Gottardi G 1988 Il diritto dell'utente all'informazione e alla riservatezza: l'accesso dell'utente alla documentazione del servizio. La Rivista di Servizio Social 4: 33–56

Cigno K, Gottardi G 1989 Open files and data protection: serving the client's best interests? International Social Work 32: 319–330

Cigno K, Wilson K 1994 Effective strategies for working with children and families: issues in the provision of therapeutic help. Practice 6: 285–298

Cohen R N 1982 Whose file is it anyway? National Council for Civil Liberties, London

Cohn A H, Daro D 1987 Is treatment too late: what ten years of evaluative research can tell us. Child Abuse and Neglect 11: 433–442

Corby B 1993 Child abuse: towards a knowledge base. Open University Press, Milton Keynes

Corby B 2000 Child abuse: towards a knowledge base, 2nd edn. Open University Press, Milton Keynes

Department of Health (DOH) 1988 Protecting children: a guide for social workers undertaking a comprehensive assessment. HMSO, London

Department of Health (DOH) 1989 The care of children: principles and practice in regulations and guidance. HMSO, London

Department of Health (DOH) 1991 Working together: a guide to arrangements for inter-agency cooperation for the protection of children from abuse. HMSO, London

Department of Health (DOH) 1995 Child protection: messages from research. HMSO, London

Department of Health (DOH) 1998a Supporting families: a consultation document. The Stationery Office, London

Department of Health (DOH) 1998b Modernising social services. The Stationery Office, London

Department of Health (DOH) 1998c Quality protects. Transforming children's services. Social Care Group. The Stationery Office, London

Department of Health (DOH) 2000 Framework for the assessment of children in need and their families. The Stationery Office, London

DOH, Home Office, Department of Education and Employment, National Assembly for Wales 1999 Working together to safeguard children. A guide to inter-agency working to safeguard and promote the welfare of children. Consultation draft. The Stationery Office, London

Dowdney L, Skuse D 1993 Parenting provided by adults with mental retardation. Journal of Child Psychology and Psychiatry 34: 25–48

Falloon I R N 1988 Handbook of behavioural family therapy. Guilford Press, London

Falloon I R N, Laporta M, Fadden G, Graham-Hole 1993 Managing stress in families: cognitive and behavioural strategies for enhancing coping skills. Routledge, London

Francis J 1994 Cruellest cut of all. Community Care 7 April: 14–15

Friend B, Ivory M 1994 Fragmentation leads to chaos. Community Care 17 March: 3

Frosh S, Summerfield A B 1986 Social skills training with adults. In: Hollin C R, Trower P (eds) Handbook of social skills training, vol 1. Pergamon Press, Oxford

Gambrill E 1981 The use of behavioural procedures in cases of child abuse and neglect. International Journal of Behavioural Social Work and Abstracts 1: 3–26

Gambrill E 1983 Casework: a competency-based approach. Prentice-Hall, New Jersey

Gambrill E, Stein J D (eds) 1994 Controversial issues in child welfare. Allyn & Bacon, Boston

Gibb C, Randall P 1989 Professionals and parents: managing children's behaviour. Macmillan Educational, Basingstoke

Gilbert M T 1980 Child abuse: a behavioural approach. Nursing Times November: 828–831

Gill A 1989 Putting fun back into families. Social Work Today 20: 14–15

Hardiker P, Barker M, Exton K 1989 Perspectives on prevention. Community Care 'Inside' 7 December: i–ii

Hennessy P 1988 Secrecy: the virus in the bureaucrats' blood. The Independent 4 July: 4

Hepworth D, Larsen J 1990 Direct social work practice: theory and skills, 3rd edn. Wadsworth, Belmont, California

Herbert M 1987a Conduct disorders of childhood and adolescence: a social learning perspective, 2nd edn. Wiley & Sons, Chichester

Herbert M 1987b Behavioural treatment of children with problems: a practice manual, 2nd edn. Academic Press, London

Herbert M 1989 Discipline: a positive guide for parents. Basil Blackwell, Oxford

Herbert M 1993 Working with children and the Children Act. British Psychological Society, Leicester

Hollows A, Wonnacott J 1994 Protected by prevention. Community Care 30 April: 22–23

Hudson B L, Macdonald G M 1986 Behavioural social work: an introduction. Macmillan Educational, Basingstoke

Iwaniec D 1987 Assessment and treatment of failure-to-thrive children and their families. Behavioural Social Work Review 8 (2a): 9–19

Iwaniec D 1995 The emotionally abused and neglected child. Identification, assessment and intervention. John Wiley, Chichester

Iwaniec D 1998 Treating children who fail to thrive. In: Cigno K, Bourn D (eds) Cognitive–behavioural social work in practice. Ashgate, Aldershot

Iwaniec D, Herbert M, McNeish A S 1985a Social work with failure-to-thrive children and their families. Part I. Psychosocial factors. British Journal of Social Work 15: 243–259

Iwaniec D, Herbert M, McNeish A S 1985b Social work with failure-to-thrive children and their families. Part II. Behavioural social work intervention. British Journal of Social Work 15: 375–389

Lloyd J M 1986 Jacob's ladder: a parent's view of Portage. Costello, Tunbridge Wells

Macdonald G M, Roberts H 1995 What works in The early years? Barnardo's, Basildon

Macdonald G M, Sheldon B, Gillespie J 1992 Contemporary studies of the effectiveness of social work. British Journal of Social Work 22: 615–644

Neville D, King L, Beak D 1995 Promoting positive parenting. Arena, Aldershot

Parker R (ed) 1991 Assessing outcome in child care: the report of an independent working party established by the Department of Health. HMSO, London

Patterson G R 1976 The aggressive child: architect of a coercive system. In: Hamerlynk L, Hardy L, Mash E (eds) Behaviour modification and families, vol. 1. Brunner Mazel, New York

Petts A, Geddes R 1978 Using behavioural techniques in child management. Social Work Today 10 (5): 13–16

Ronen T 1993 Adapting treatment techniques to children's needs. British Journal of Social Work 23: 581–596

Ronen T 1994 Cognitive–behavioural social work with children. British Journal of Social Work 24: 273–285

Ronen T 1998 Direct clinical work with children. In: Cigno K, Bourn D (eds) Cognitive–behavioural social work in practice. Ashgate, Aldershot

Scott M J 1989 A cognitive–behavioural approach to clients' problems. Tavistock/Routledge, London

Scott M J, Stradling S G 1987 The evaluation of a group parent training programme. Behavioural Psychotherapy 15: 224–239

Scott M J, Stradling S J, Dryden W 1995 Developing cognitive–behavioural counselling. Sage, London

Seheult C 1985 Using parents as their children's therapists. Update 15 February: 309–318

Seligman M E P 1975 Helplessness. Freeman, San Francisco

Sheldon B 1982 Behaviour modification: theory, practice and philosophy. Tavistock, London

Sheldon B 1986 Effectiveness experiments: review and implications. British Journal of Social Work 16: 223–242

Sheldon B 1995 Cognitive–behavioural therapy: research, practice and philosophy. Routledge, London

Social Services Inspectorate (SSI) 1997 Inspection of assessment, planning and decision-making in family support services. Social Care Group. Department of Health, London

Sutton C 1979 Psychology for social workers and counsellors. Routledge, London

Sutton C 1987 A handbook of research for the helping professions. RKP, London

Sutton C 1994 Social work community work and psychology. British Psychological Society, Leicester

Sutton C 1998 Parenting positively: enhancing parenting skills, helping parents improve children's behaviour. Unit for the Study of Parent Education and Training, De Montfort University, Leicester

Sutton C 1999 Helping families with troubled children: a preventive approach. John Wiley, Chichester

Thoburn J, Lewis A, Shemmings D 1991 Family involvement in child protection conferences. Social Work Development Unit, University of East Anglia, East Anglia

Timmins N 1987 Doctors divided over patients' right to know' and 'Open files would spell the end of surgical witticisms'. Independent 5 May: 12

Webster-Stratton C, Herbert M 1994 Troubled families – problem children. Wiley & Sons, Chichester

Wheldall K, Wheldall D, Winter S 1983 Seven supertactics for superparents. NFER-Nelson, Windsor

Whiteman M, Fanshel D, Grundy J F 1987 Cognitive behavioural intervention aimed at anger of parents at risk of child abuse. Social Work 32: 469–474

24 Working with abusing families

Arnon Bentovim

In recent years, family work in child abuse has changed from a mainly psycho-dynamic approach to a much clearer concept of family work in a wider systemic context. The relationship between therapeutic work and statutory contexts has been clarified and developed in the work at the Hospital for Sick Children, Great Ormond Street, London, in Rochdale and elsewhere (Dale *et al.* 1986*a*, 1986*b*, Bentovim *et al.* 1988, 1996, Furniss 1990), and through the work of multi-systemic approaches (Henggeler 1999). The function of family centres, which traditionally provided little more than a holding environment, can now work in a far more structured and goal-oriented manner stressing aspects of responsibility, self-help, autonomy, strength and resourcefulness of families and family members (Asen *et al.* 1989).

Family work with abusive families has started to differentiate between families with physical abuse and neglect, and families where sexual abuse has occurred (Crittenden 1988, Stratton 1991, Hanks 1993, Kolko 1996). Work with families where children have been emotionally abused is less developed, and the focus is largely still on defining the core concepts involved (Crittenden & Ainsworth 1989, Erickson *et al.* 1989, Glaser 1993, Hobbs *et al.* 1993).

This chapter explores the role of family work and family therapy with families where child abuse has taken place. The first part of the chapter is concerned with all forms of child abuse and addresses a number of conceptual, planning and practice issues relevant to working with families where physical, sexual or emotional abuse or neglect has taken place. The second part focuses on child sexual abuse in order to highlight the specific considerations which need to be addressed and to allow the exploration of one area of child abuse in more depth. The chapter draws on an earlier chapter in the first edition of the *Handbook* by Furniss & Miller.

Within the first part of the chapter, the scene is set by a brief review of some of the relevant literature on family therapy and the links with child abuse. Next, some conceptual and planning issues are considered which relate to working with abusing families. These include: the differences between family therapy and consultation; the distinction between a family approach and a family therapy approach to family work with abuse; issues of motivation; indicators for involving the whole family; and the differing emphasis given to change and growth in work relative to the different forms of abuse and neglect. A range of practice issues relating to family work and family therapy for all forms of child abuse is then covered, and several family therapy techniques are described which can be useful in work with abusing families.

The second part of the chapter focuses on families where child sexual abuse has taken place. A distinction is made between child sexual abuse and other forms of abuse, highlighting the therapeutic importance of some key aspects of the family work which is required, including the evaluation of suspicion of child sexual abuse and the handling of disclosures, trauma work and work with siblings.

Family therapy as an intervention is then considered more specifically. The steps which need to be taken for effective family therapy are laid out, as well as a range of family therapy techniques which can be useful at different stages of work with families.

Child abuse and neglect

A brief look at the literature

This chapter is based on a systemic approach to working with abusing families. A systemic approach is based on systemic thinking which arose in the 1960s. Von Bertalanffy (1962) set out the principals of general systems theory in response to the then current dissatisfactions with a reductionist cause and effect tradition. The reductionist tradition attempted to explain complex multidimensional events in terms of simple cause and effect chains. General systems theory focused attention on pattern and form of the organisation of biological systems. This type of analysis was later extended to psychosocial systems including the family. A system is defined as 'an organised arrangement of elements consisting of a network on interdependent coordinated parts which function as a unit'. From a systems perspective the family was therefore seen as developing characteristic patterns and core ways of being and relating. Such patterns were thought to be carried forward in life and subsequent social contexts by family members.

Thus systems thinking encompasses a number of different issues, which include:

1.   A philosophy of observation which includes the context, as well as the object concerned. In child abuse, we conceptualise the way particular systems of relationships can give rise to problematic behaviour. But we also see that the way in which such problematic behaviour is defined in turn comes to organise what we see, and how family members and professionals relate to each other. The very recognition of child abuse as an entity followed the publication of Henry Kempe's seminal paper on the battered child in 1962 (Kempe *et al.* 1962). This formulation had the effect of defining the situation, and helping people conceptualise, understand and bring together many disparate observations to the entity we now recognise as child abuse in all its forms. This is described as a process of social construction which gradually helped professionals find a way of conceptualising the process to understand the true extent of abusive actions perpetrated against children in its many different forms, and in many different contexts.

2.   Systems thinking also encompasses an approach to treating problems in context, which includes the individual, the family and those concerned with them. Child protection is everyone's concern, all agencies and all professionals with a concern for children and the family, not just a single agency.

3.   Systems thinking has resulted in a number of methods of treatment, the best known being family therapy. There are, however, far broader implications for treatment using a systemic perspective.

Family therapy is a form of intervention that focuses on the whole family, including the relationships between family members, as the unit requiring attention. Family systems theory is used as a framework, both to make sense of the problems and difficulties encountered by individuals, subgroups or the family as a whole, and to shape the therapist's work with families. Family properties include the structure of the family, its boundaries, patterns and processes of communication, the relationship between different subsystems within the family and between the whole family and the outside world, family rules and belief systems, and the way the individual family members give meaning to their experiences (Bingley *et al.* 1984, Burnham 1986, Barker 1990).

The family can be seen as a group of persons related by biological ties and/or long-term expectations of loyalty, trust and commitment, and comprising at least two generations (P Loader, personal communication). There is a social expectation that the family performs certain functions and tasks. For example, the family can be seen as being expected to take responsibility for the physical and emotional well-being and socialisation of the children, and to provide for the maintenance of the emotional well-being and the personal growth of the adults. The tasks linked to the fulfilment of these responsibilities differ according to the various stages in the life cycle of the family, so that when children are young, for example, the focus is likely to be on physical safety and nurturing, whereas by adolescence the emphasis is shifting towards helping the children to establish themselves as relatively independent and secure adults (Carter & McGoldrick 1989).

The way in which families carry out these tasks varies greatly, because families are affected by the culture, ethnic group and religion to which the family belongs, their social and economic grouping, the balance of power within the family, and the values, attitudes, traditions and past experiences of adults in the family (Ahmed *et al.* 1986, Walters *et al.* 1988, Ahmad 1990, Perelberg & Miller 1990). All these dimensions influence how family members relate to each other and to the outside world.

These responsibilities, functions and tasks are carried out in a social context, and they are shared with other people and institutions such as the extended family and friends, and the wider framework of educational, medical, social services and social security and law enforcement services. These institutions provide a context for the family which is usually likely to be experienced by families as supportive and complementary, but which can be experienced as hostile and threatening, as is often the case with families where child abuse has taken place.

Family functions are underpinned by the particular character of the family. It is possible to assess the level of family health (Bentovim & Kinston 1991) by looking at family competence, the capacity to provide adequate care for children, the nature of discipline, the management of conflict and decision-making. These basic functions are underpinned by characteristics such as identity, sense of family togetherness, the quality of communication, listening, hearing, the alliances between family members both within the same generation and across generational boundaries. Assessments can be made both qualitatively and quantitatively, and a profile of family strengths and difficulties can be constructed (Bentovim & Bingley Miller 2000). A variety of approaches are used to stimulate family interaction, e.g. tasks and interviews, to help professionals make judgements which then help to act as a focus for therapeutic work.

Family therapists vary in the emphasis they give in their work to the different properties of the family as a system, and in this chapter we refer to a range of techniques from several different schools of family therapy. It may therefore be helpful to distinguish between some of these various family therapy approaches, although it is important to note that there is considerable overlap among them.

Structural family therapists work on creating change in the structure of the family system by paying particular attention to the boundaries around the different subsystems (parent–child, parent–parent, partner–partner, and so on) and the communication between them (Minuchin 1974, Fishman & Rosoman 1991).

The therapist initially seeks to 'join' the family and will then use a range of techniques to 'challenge' the family's usual pattern of behaving and communicating or, as Minuchin & Fishman put it, 'how things are done' (Minuchin & Fishman 1981). The therapist then actively works to provide the family with an experience of alternative ways of perceiving and experiencing family relationships and of behaving towards each other. The therapist reinforces any changes, thus 'restructuring' the family system into one more likely to enhance the development of family members.

Strategic family therapy focuses on devising strategies to solve the problems of the client or family (Haley 1976, 1980, Madanes 1982, Hayes 1991). A wide range of direct and indirect strategies are employed, one of which is to give the family tasks to carry out together between sessions. The tasks are designed to redefine the problem situation in the family and to shift the way the family organises itself. Problems are often framed in terms of the family (as a system) needing to find a way of negotiating a move (or transition) to the next stage of the family life cycle (Carter & McGoldrick 1989).

Systemic family therapy, as developed by the Milan group (Palazzoli *et al*. 1978, 1980, Boscolo *et al*. 1987), understands the problem presented by the family as an integral part of the system in which it occurs, and it is therefore regulated by the rules that govern that system. Thus, 'the way to eliminate that symptom is to change the rules' (Palazzoli *et al*. 1978). The Milan group initially emphasised the need for the therapist to remain 'neutral', although this has shifted more recently. The therapist, while avoiding taking sides with any part of the family, carefully gathers information about the way in which the family operates through techniques such as 'circular questioning'. This involves asking one family member about the relationship between two other family members, and then checking that perception. In this way, the therapist and the therapeutic team develop a picture of the myths and 'rules' that govern the family as a system, usually implicitly rather than explicitly, and the experience and meaning of family relationships for family members.

Interventions come in the form of statements offered to the family by the therapist which tie together the positive benefits or functions the symptom has for the family (reframing and positive connotation), with the negative price or 'sacrifice' the family has to pay to maintain it. Once the ambiguity around the 'symptom' has been identified, clarified and challenged, it is often unacceptable to the family to continue in their old pattern, and change takes place. Systemic family therapists, in common with some of the strategic family therapists, make use of tasks, rituals, paradox, metaphor and storytelling in their interventions with families (Campbell & Draper 1985, Boscolo *et al*. 1987).

While many family therapists focus their attention on working with the current pattern of communication and relationships in families (the 'here and now'), other approaches seek to unravel the influence of significant past events, experiences and relationships on current family relationships. The work of Byng–Hall (1973, 1990, 1995) links past patterns of attachment and authority structures to the family myths and scripts, attachment relationships and management of authority issues in the current family. A range of different ways of using genograms has been developed to highlight the pattern of inter-generational relationships (Satir 1967, 1972, Liebermann 1979, Carter & McGoldrick 1989). McCluskey (1987) has developed an existential approach to family therapy which focuses on the emotional life of the family, using a theme to anchor the work.

The focal family therapy workshop at the Hospital for Sick Children, Great Ormond Street, London, developed a format for integrating and assessing information about significant past events and relationships, the meaning given by individuals to these experiences, and the impact those meanings have on current family interactions and relationships (Bentovim 1979, Glaser *et al.* 1984, Bentovim & Kinston 1991). The focal formulation also enables the therapist to track and evaluate changes achieved during therapy (Furniss *et al.* 1983, Kinston & Bentovim 1983). McCluskey & Bingley Miller (1995) have combined focal family therapy and theme-focused family therapy to address the past in the present. Their approach gives adults the opportunity to re-edit the past and gives the children a voice to articulate their present concerns and feelings in relation to their experience of being in a family.

Recent developments in family systems theory have seen constructivist ideas coming to the fore (de Shazer 1984, 1989). The focus is on how individuals explain their experience to themselves by constructing a 'reality', or view of events, which is made up of elements of objective facts seen through the filter of that person's perception and experience of the world. Family therapists using a constructivist framework see the way in which family members construct their sense of reality as being integral to the distress or difficulties that bring them into therapy. The focus in therapy is to facilitate shifts in the constructed reality created in families, which in turn produce changes in their expectations and enactment of family relationships.

De Shazer's solution-focused therapy (de Shazer 1982) emphasises the solution to perceived problems and working with the self-organisation of the family towards realising that solution. It is future-focused, and looking at traumatic and salient past events in the life experience of family members is positively discouraged.

White & Epston (1990) also use a constructivist approach to separate the competent self from the problem saturated reality, a process described as externalisation. Children who are aggressive have to fight against 'Mr Temper', soiling children fight against 'sneaky poo'. He constructs a therapeutic narrative which seeks exceptions, looks for times when Mr Temper was beaten, enlists support from family to fight the battle. The victim or perpetrator of abuse is helped to fight the effects of abuse, and the abuser to battle and have the courage to overcome the impulses of the abuser within. The family coming together to fight the symptom has many echoes within earlier approaches, e.g. structural and inter-generational approaches.

In considering family work with abusive families, there has been a major critique of the traditional approaches described earlier in this review. Feminist thinkers such as Bograd (1988) pointed to the potential dangers in attempting to work conjointly with families where an abusive family member was organising family life and grooming children to become victims of their perverse interest and abusive action. Addressing such issues within a family context, it was feared, could result in secondary victimisation, retaliation, an increase in silencing and fear, and to be against the interests of children.

Restructuring the relationship between an abusive father and a terrified child seemed inappropriate when an approach which relies on the fact that the family context was one that was basically attempting to provide adequate care for family members, but where negative aspects of family character were hindering development for a particular child or the family as a whole. Thus it became essential to focus on the traumatic reality caused by abuse, and its impact on individual functioning and relationships. In introducing the theme of trauma organised systems (Bentovim 1995) it was pointed out that abusive events have traumatic effects on the lives of children, and repeated cumulative traumatic events cause increasingly severe effects on the emotional lives of those who are involved.

Those who were traumatising the child were part of the system that allowed them to maintain abusive action in secrecy. Other adults in the children's world were also caught in the process and involved in a system of secrecy, denial and blame. In the growing area of trauma therapy, Eth & Pynoos (1985), Figley (1990) and Herman (1992) stressed the need to work with the facts of abuse, the objective reality of traumatising events. Therapeutic work required the tracking of such details for each individual before there could be the possible integration for the family as a whole.

These different strands in the field of family therapy, with an emphasis on constructed reality and solution-focused therapy, on the one hand, and on trauma and trauma work, on the other, produce tensions and dilemmas in terms of practice for the clinician or practitioner working with abusing families. Experiences of authors over some years shows that an integrated approach that brings together both aspects of therapeutic work is crucial to effective work with abusing families. Therapists need to help families and individuals deal with the trauma they have experienced. Families also need to look at the relationship between the traumatic experiences they have had as individual family members and the solutions they have evolved as families, and at the impact of both on the way family members now relate.

Nevertheless, while the objective reality of the trauma of abuse is an essential focus for therapeutic work with abused children and other family members, it is also the case that the individuals concerned have had to make sense of their own experience, and they have constructed their own psychic sense of causality – the meaning they give to that traumatic experience. This 'constructed reality' of individual family members or the family as a whole, e.g. that abuse is harmless, the child's action evoked an abusive response, silence is best, may hinder the growth and development or recovery of the family members, and therefore require therapeutic intervention.

These new developments in family therapy have given rise to other significant tensions and dilemmas for practitioners working with abusing families. The psychologically and developmentally damaging effects of child abuse fuel the responsibility of social service and legal systems to evaluate the risk to the child and the actual harm resulting from child abuse and neglect, and to act on that assessment in their work with abusing families. It informs the need for them either to bring about change in the relevant patterns of family relationships, or to provide alternative care outside the family for the abused or at risk child.

This linear relationship between the family and the statutory agencies responsible for child protection work is, however, sometimes seen as incompatible with the therapeutic relationship between therapist and family in family therapy, where there is a greater emphasis on the need for the therapist to remain neutral and adhere to the concept of circular rather than linear causality, which some see as inevitably blurring the issue of individual responsibility. Thus, professionals have been concerned about using a family therapeutic intervention with abusing families because of these apparent tensions. Furniss (1990) introduced an integrated therapeutic and legal framework for working with abusing families (see also Bentovim *et al.* 1988, Sheinberg 1992, Sheinberg *et al.* 1994, Bentovim 1995), and this is further developed in this chapter.

In this chapter, we describe an approach to working with abusing families in a way that allows therapeutic work to progress within the legal framework of child protection without denying the reality of the abuse, splitting the professional network, or cutting across the work of the various professionals who form the child protection network or team around an abused child.

Conceptual and planning issues

Family therapy and consultation

The increased understanding of the context and greater clarity of aims of family work with abusive families has led to a clear distinction between family therapy that occurs as a result of a free contract between the family and the therapist, and conditional family work in the context of statutory decision-making. Family work with abusing families does not constitute therapy in the traditional sense. Family members do not come to therapy of their own free will, and the basic contract is not between therapist and family, but between therapist and the statutory agency, on the one hand, and between the statutory agency and the family, on the other.

This means that the basic rules of confidentiality do not apply, and therapists therefore need to distinguish carefully between therapy where these rules can apply and therapeutic work with abusive families as part of consultation to statutory agencies. Family work in child-abusing families can therefore only take place with close and open cooperation between therapist and statutory worker. Family therapists should not accept abusing families for 'therapy' independently of the professional child protection system, because this creates the danger of inducing damaging splits in the professional network between the therapist as the 'good person' and the statutory worker as the 'source of all bad things'.

All therapeutic work that therapists undertake with abusing families needs to relate to the requirements of decision-making processes by statutory agencies regarding the future of the family concerned. In that sense, family work with abusive families is part of a consultation process to social services departments or courts, in which the social services department or the court are the clients rather than the families. All therapeutic work needs to take place in the context of consultation with these institutions.

The nature of the therapeutic family work as part of consultation to social services and courts needs to be made explicit to the family, either by having the social worker present during family sessions or by referring explicitly to the link between therapist and statutory agencies. In a family session, we might therefore say, 'What would the social worker/the court say about the change you have achieved so far in these sessions? Do you think they would feel it is safe for your child to live with you again or not?' This sentence not only reminds the family of the context of consultation, it also helps therapists to remind themselves that any family work with abusive families is part of consultation and not traditional family therapy.

This distinction is indicated in Table 24.1.

Table 24.1
Therapy and consultation

Therapy	Consultation
Intervention directed towards:	
1. Family	Professionals
2. Relationships	Decision-making
3. Boundaries	Functions
4. Family conflicts	Conflict by proxy
5. Therapist is a free agent with respect to family (independent professional responsibility towards family)	Therapist is consultant in the service of other professionals and agencies (responsibility towards hierarchy of consulting institution)

A family approach and a family therapy approach to working with abusing families

A family approach uses a family systems theory framework to conceptualise the dysfunctional aspects of abuse at a family level and in the context of family relationships. Using a family systems perspective helps to keep the central family process and the child's need for carers in mind, while opening up the options for different, concurrent forms of therapy in addition to family sessions. It also provides a unifying rationale for the range of protection, care planning and therapeutic tasks that need to take place when attending to the welfare of the abused child and family.

Thus, a family approach to working with abusing families, in contrast to a family therapy approach, encompasses work on different levels using concurrent forms of therapy, including individual, group and family sessions as well as family–professional network sessions.

For example, with physical abuse and neglect, and even perhaps emotional abuse, in some less serious abusive situations conjoint family sessions may be the appropriate sole form of therapy; with sexual abuse, concurrent forms of therapy are always required. Abusers always need individual and/or group work focused on their abusive behaviour and cycles of abuse. Mothers who are non-abusing parents need individual help with the crisis of emotional turmoil, loss and practical problems that come with disclosure (Hooper 1992). The support of a group counteracts the isolation, disempowerment and low self-esteem associated with living in a family system shaped by the abuser's enactment of child sexual abuse as a syndrome of secrecy and addiction (Hildebrand 1988). Research on outcomes of treatment (Hyde *et al.* 1996, Monck *et al.* 1996) demonstrates the effectiveness of group intervention with women.

In cases of child sexual abuse, the aim of therapy for the child needs to be the therapeutic transformation from traumatic powerlessness to effectiveness, secrecy into privacy (Furniss 1990, Bentovim 1995). Although family sessions deal with the secrecy of child sexual abuse by the shared experience of disclosing the secret, thus creating a reality anchor, family therapy sessions alone do not give the child the necessary space to experience adequate privacy and to develop self-worth, self-respect, autonomy and individuation, i.e. to reverse traumatic effects, dysregulation of emotional functioning, and insecure attachments. This is achieved by individual sessions or group sessions which provide the individual space for self-experience (Wilson & Ryan 1994). However, individual and group sessions alone can transform the confidentiality of the individual or group session into renewed secrecy if concurrent family work does not guarantee a complementary domain of openness that keeps the abuse in the shared family domain.

The successful outcome of the concurrent use of different forms of therapy does not depend on the different forms of therapy alone, although individual and group work with sexually abused children using a cognitive–behavioural framework has been shown to be markedly helpful. Successful outcome depends on the willingness and the quality of cooperation between therapists, and on the ability of therapists to conceptualise their own form of therapy as part of a differentiated systemic framework of different concurrent forms of therapy.

Issues of motivation

Our skill needs to lie in knowing why abusing families are not motivated to be helped, and how we can motivate them to feel that they want help. The distinction between therapy and consultation in family work with child abuse underlines the fact that families are not primarily self-motivated to seek help as a result of emerging family problems. They are motivated to cooperate because of the danger of family break-up, and because of the openly stated preconditions for rehabilitation or for keeping their children at home.

The basically negative contextual framework of coercion in family work in cases of child abuse needs to be positively reframed by an explicit therapeutic contract stating openly the required aims and goals of family work. Some systemic approaches already make the development of the required aims and goals of treatment part of the treatment process itself. Questions like, 'What do you think needs to change in your attitude and behaviour towards your child in order for social services/the court to be satisfied that it is safe for you to continue living with your child?', or, 'What do you think social services/the court needs to know from you for them to trust your word when you say you are able to understand and satisfy the needs of your child without abusing them?' A systemic approach to family work can help to link issues of statutory responsibility and control with therapeutic aspects of required family functioning. The process of defining the aims for family work can help to motivate family members towards a wish for therapeutic change if we create a context where families take part and are co-responsible for the development of explicit, understandable, operationalised and detailed goals for therapy.

Indicators for or against involving the whole family

Family work needs to be considered in all forms of treatment of child abuse where rehabilitation is being contemplated. Rehabilitation can only be considered when there is a reasonable prospect for change which emerges following an initial phase of assessment. A *hopeful prognosis* requires that parents take dequate responsibility for abusive action where appropriate, there is a protective capacity within the family, e.g. a non-abusive parent who recognises that their partner has abused the child, and is prepared to protect the child over and above their relationship with their partner. There needs to be the possibility of a capacity for change in parents who have been abusive, with a willingness to work reasonably cooperatively with childcare professionals, and to accept the need for change even if it is with the motivation of maintaining children within the family context rather than the child being removed temporarily or permanently. There needs to be the potential for the development of a reasonable attachment and relationship between the parents and children, and appropriate therapeutic settings need to be available, whether on an out-patient basis, a day-care setting, or residential resource depending on the severity of abuse, and the nature of family difficulties and strengths.

The *prognosis is hopeless* for family work when none of these criteria are fulfilled. Situations arise where there is rejection of the child, a failure to take responsibility, the needs of parents take primacy over the needs of the children, a combative oppositional stance to professionals emerges, or psychopathology in parents (e.g. drug abuse, serious marital violence, or longstanding personality problems that may not be amenable to therapeutic work) or where there is complete inability or unwillingness to accept that there are problems. In such situations, family work has no place since the child will be persuaded to withdraw their statements or to become part of a process of maintenance of secrecy and denial.

Situations are of *doubtful progress* where professionals are not yet clear from the original work with the family whether the situation is hopeful or hopeless.

There is uncertainty whether there is adequate taking of responsibility, whether parental pathology is changeable, whether there is going to be willingness to work with care authorities and therapeutic agencies, or whether resources will be available to meet the extent of the problem.

As a result of such an assessment in the initial stage of work when disclosure of abuse has occurred, it becomes possible to be clear about which family member will be able to participate in family work, and at which stage. A good deal also depends on the assessment of the child. Children who are severely traumatised by physical, emotional or sexual abuse may be retraumatised through contact with an abusive parent, even when that parent is taking responsibility for their abusive action. In such situations it is often essential for the majority of work to be carried out either with the child individually, in groups, or with a protective parent, before any question of contact with the abusive parent is considered. Family work needs to be at its most intensive when rehabilitation is considered following parental involvement in individual and group work, either as protective parent or as an abuser dealing with abusive and violent action. Work involving the whole family then becomes far more of a possibility.

Practice issues

It is helpful to think of therapeutic work occurring in stages with different forms of family work being required at each phase:

1. Disclosure
2. Therapeutic work in a context of safety
3. Rehabilitation.
4. A new family phase.

Disclosure

Work in this phase needs to focus on the following main issues:

1. The extensiveness of re-abuse that has been perpetrated against the child(ren) must be clarified, and details established concerning the nature of abuse, its length, severity, context and who is responsible. Very often the initial presentation of abuse is the tip of an iceberg, and it is essential to ensure that sufficient time is given in a context of safety to ascertain how extensive the abuse has been, otherwise the nature of therapeutic work of the individual, and the family, will be underestimated.

2. There needs to be an assessment of the effect of abuse on the child(ren), the impact on children's capacity to attach themselves, and on their relationships. The extent of the traumatic impact and post-traumatic disorder on the child's sense of self and self-esteem as a result of traumagenic and dynamic effects must also be considered. Again, without such an assessment it is not possible to embark on the family aspect of the work as it would be very easy to underestimate the impact of abuse and the extent of therapeutic work required.

3. The degree of responsibility taken by the perpetrator of abuse needs to be assessed, as well as the fit between the perpetrator's explanation and the victim's account. Does this make sense? Is it possible to draw together the strands of what has happened to be able to plan a rational approach to work?

4. What is the attitude of the non-abusing caregiver? What is the degree of sympathy and belief in the victim's statement? What is the attitude towards the

perpetrator, whether that perpetrator is a young person within the family context who has abused a younger child, or a partner? Is it possible for the non-abusing parent to separate the needs they have from their partner to meet the needs of the child?

5.   What is the relevant family history of parents as individuals? Do they have a history of abuse themselves? What is their relationship history, the nature of present and past marital and parenting relationships with siblings and general functioning?

6.   What information can be gathered about the particular characteristics of the family in terms of communication, form of alliances, boundary formation and dealing with feelings? It may well be that such information can only be gathered through meetings with subsystems of the family as, in the absence of full knowledge and understanding of the extensiveness of abuse, responsibilities and protective capacities, it may not be appropriate to involve the abused child in family meetings at this stage. Motivation for help both by the child who has been victimised, and family members, needs to be assessed at this stage, and a balance achieved between protection and therapeutic work.

Treatment in a context of safety

During this phase there needs to be work where the victim is separated from the abusive context, whether this means the child living with a protective parent/family member, the perpetrator living separately, or the child living in alternative care. A good deal of the work during this phase is inevitably focused on the individual. Abuse-focused therapeutic work for victims, whether individually or within group contexts, is required to repair attachments, to manage emotional disregulation and develop a healing sense of self.

Disruptions of a child's attachment can be repaired through individual and group work. Individual therapists need to create a working alliance with the child or young person, to be consistent and reliably available, and to create a sense of safety. Group work fosters cohesion, belonging and identity, providing a sense of safety in the group to reverse the fears inherent in family life and to share support by substituting pleasure for pain. Family work can foster the development of secure attachments both in the phase of separateness and as the situation moves to the next phase of rehabilitation. Connections may be made through a caring parent, sharing and comparing their own experiences in their family with the child's experience. It is important that family therapy techniques such as reframing negative behaviour and positive connotation (giving apparently negative behaviour a positive meaning) connect children with family scripts and the experiences that parents have had growing up themselves. The process of 'externalising' distances abusive experiences from self and relationships, and strengthens and promotes bonds within the family with a protective parent. Later the sharing of experiences with the abusing parent which have been learnt from their own therapeutic work can help the child or young person feel part of the family context, rather than being blamed, excluded and scapegoated.

Therapeutic work with emotional dysregulation is aimed at reducing anxiety, developing a capacity to cope with emotional problems, and being able to effectively process experiences of abuse by sharing and exposing them with an individual therapist, the group contexts and eventually with family members. A variety of approaches are helpful to monitor arousal and foster containment. To be involved in such work, a protective parent needs to be able to be open to the experiences of the child, to be able to listen and share, and contain what may have been an extreme sense of terror, fear and powerlessness at the hands of the abusive parent. There needs to be the development of safe family care rituals to cope with sleeping difficulties, ways of coping with excitement, anger, sexualised behaviour and a modulation of the process to avoid retraumatisation.

For the child to develop a more *satisfactory sense of themselves*, they have to be helped to realise that behaviours defined as problematic – e.g. switching off, angry oppositional behaviour, fear and avoidance – are part of a survival strategy and are therefore strengths not weaknesses. Family work needs to be absolutely clear about the origins of blame, to help the child understand the way in which the abuser attributes abusive action to the victim rather than taking responsibility themselves. Where rehabilitation is a possibility, family work requires a carefully planned apology and taking of responsibility for abusive action. This must be more than the often brief acknowledgement that is possible in the earlier phases of work.

Rehabilitation phase

Rehabilitation requires that parents themselves confront their abusive behaviour. When both parents have taken part in abusive action they need to take on board the extensiveness of their abusive actions, to understand their origins and the process of abuse, and the damaging effect that this has had on the child. The apology session is a valuable component of part of a rehabilitation process. Questions that the child has about what has happened to them can be put to the abusive parent. Responses can be worked out with the therapists, and a joint meeting established where responsibility can be taken and victims freed from their own sense of confusion, guilt and attribution of abuse to their own actions.

Often, intensive couple therapy is going to be required because of the secrecy, and often associated violence between parents, before meetings involving the victim and siblings can be initiated. Permanent family structures are required where protection is uppermost.

Asen *et al.* (1989) indicate that in 30% of cases involving severe physical abuse, rehabilitation is not possible because of a failure to progress through such a process. In child sexual abuse in the Great Ormond Street series (Monck *et al.* 1998), 9% of children could be rehabilitated to the family, which included the abuser; 52% could live with a protective parent; and 37% could not live with any family members because of rejection or disbelief and needed a new family context.

New family phase

When a child cannot return home, intensive family work with a new family context is required, planning long-term care and preparation of a family for a child who has experienced extensive abuse. Sexually abused children may have a high level of sexual knowledge, may be prone to a sexual behavioural disorder, and may have an aggressive or victimising stance. There needs to be planning of a protective context within the foster family, and careful consideration of the appropriate mode of contact with the original family. Work with the foster family or alternative adoptive family is essential to maintain an appropriate supportive stance and to incorporate the victim into a new family context.

Child physical abuse

A recent review of the treatment of long-term sequeli of child abuse (Stevenson 1999) revealed how limited were the number of studies using a controlled design to evaluate treatment approaches with abusing families characterised by physically abusive actions. Two approaches seemed to describe satisfactory results: Kolko (1996) and Henggeler (1999)

Kolko

Kolko (1996) contrasted cognitive–behavioural treatment with family therapy and community care as a control. This study demonstrated that both cognitive–behavioural treatment and family therapy were effective.

Cognitive–behavioural treatment focuses on child and parent separately. The work with the parent has much in common with parent training approaches, shown to be successful approaches to physical abuse in other studies. The aim of the work is to implement parallel protocols addressing cognitive, affective and behavioural repertoires, clarifying family stressors, developing coping and self-control skills, and training in safety, support, planning and relaxation. Parents were trained in interpersonal affective skills, the use of social supports and assertion rather than the use of inappropriate punitive models. Parents' views of violence and physical punishment were clarified, self-control, anger management, and use of time-out reinforcement were all a part of the approaches used following well-known cognitive–behavioural approaches (see also Cigno, Chapter 23, in this volume).

The family therapy approach used an interactional/ecological model, with the aim of enhancing family functioning and relationships. The basic approach was to enhance the cooperation and motivation of all family members by promoting and helping them understand the nature of coercive behaviour, teaching positive communication skills and helping develop problem solving skills together as a family. There were three phases of work:

1. The *engagement phase*, which assessed structural roles and interactions, used a genogram to help clarify such roles. A variety of family tasks were used, and externalising approaches were used to help separate violent action from the 'real' life of the family. There was reframing of what seemed to be punitive action, or anger, as misplaced attempts to achieve control, togetherness and problem-solving. There was positive connotation of apparent disruptive behaviour as misplaced ways of helping family members pay attention to each other, and help achieve goals and enhance cooperation.

2. The *middle phase* of work reviewed the effects of physical force, and what it would mean for there to be a no violence contract for each family member. There was then training to use specific problem-solving skills and communication skills at home, building the capacities and skills of each family member.

3. The *termination phase* required the establishment of problem-solving skills and the development of family routines as an alternative to coercion or physical punishment.

A wide variety of tools were used to assess change, and there was significant improvement found both with cognitive–behavioural therapy and family therapy relative to community care. Of interest was that the use of family therapy was associated with the greatest reduction in children reporting their parents being violent towards them. Both the therapeutic approaches had a greater impact on children's externalising (aggressive) behaviour, the transmission of an aggressive style from parent to child, and on general parental distress. There was improved family cohesion and a marked reduction of conflict. There were far fewer further abusive incidents, children were far less anxious or aggressive, and the incidence of parental depression was very much lower. Parents felt less angry and thought about using force far less. Family therapy, in particular, helped in the identification of other significant family problems. It is likely that the approach advocated here of concurrent treatments would be most effective by bringing in the most helpful aspects of cognitive–behavioural work with individual children or parents, and bringing them together in a family-focused approach to reinforce such skills.

Henggeler

An approach that links with Kolko's interactional/ecological model is the multi-systemic therapy approach, e.g. Henggeler (1999). Although multi-systemic therapy has had its major focus with serious juvenile offenders, it has also been applied successfully to maltreating families. The principles of multi-systemic therapy include:

1. Understanding the fit between identified problems and the broader systemic context.
2. Therapy contexts emphasise the positive, and use systemic strengths as levers for change. Services are provided at times convenient to the family.
3. Interventions should promote responsible behaviour and decrease irresponsible behaviour among family members, and an atmosphere of mutual trust needs to be developed.
4. Interventions should be focused and action-orientated, targeting specific and well-defined problems, with families defining treatment goals and success.
5. Interventions should target sequences of behaviour within or between multiple systems that maintain identified problems.
6. Intervention should be developmentally appropriate.
7. Intervention should be designed to require daily or weekly effort by family members, and therapists need to earn family trust by their commitment to the family, and positive reinforcement of small gains.
8. Intervention effectiveness is evaluated continuously from multiple perspectives.
9. Intervention should be designed to promote treatment generalisation and long-term maintenance of therapeutic change by empowering caregivers across multi-systemic contexts. Self-defeating perception needs to be shifted to empowering beliefs.

This approach is very much in line with the one advocated in this chapter. The one study which compared parent training with multi-systemic therapy in maltreating families demonstrated improved parent–child interactions for a multi-systemic approach that was greater than parent training alone (Brunk *et al.* 1987). Thus the notion of concurrent work with family members from a multi-system perspective can be an effective approach in dealing with severe physical abuse. There are many parallels with emotional abuse and neglect.

Child sexual abuse

If physical abuse occurs as a result of perversion of punishment, then sexual abuse is a perversion of closeness and sexuality. Because of the nature of sexual abuse there is much more that is addictive and compulsive in the inappropriate sexual activities of the sex offender. Physical abuse may be seen as an impulsive act of attempted control and punitiveness triggered by the defiance or perceived defiance of the child. There are parallels in sexual abuse in that the sexual abuser describes themself as being helpless in the face of what they perceive as the sex-ualised signals and behaviour of the child. The notion of Trauma Organised Systems (Bentovim 1995) demonstrates that impulses are felt to be evoked by the victim. There is, in addition, a process of emotional congruence, sexuality with children being acceptable, and rationalisations that overcome boundaries to abuse a child and overcome the abusers' resistance are described (Finklehor 1984). Although this is a more elaborate process than physical abuse, there are many parallels, and indeed a strong association between the two. The child who is perceived as deserving punishment may also be perceived as deserving a sexual action perpetrated against them.

Extensive grooming of the child, and indeed of the family context, occurs as part of the process of abuse, so that the protective parent's capacity to care is undermined, the child feels blamed and responsible for abuse perpetrated against them, and is therefore silenced and adapts to the role attributed to them – a 'cor-rupting process'. Professionals who learn of inappropriate activities in a family are perceived by the abuser as misinformed, and prejudiced against the family rather than seeing abusive reality for what it is.

The first stage of work, *disclosure*, is often a prolonged and extensive piece of work requiring collaboration between social work, police and specialist inter-viewers with children and with adults. The complexity of legal contexts means that difficult decisions have to be taken about child protection action, criminal action, the likelihood of success of such processes, and the role of potential ther-apeutic work. The cost of taking responsibility often seems extremely high to the abuser. Indeed, in the Great Ormond Street research (Monck *et al.* 1996), fewer than 9% of abusers (both adults and older siblings) took full responsibility for abuse. Children perceived only a third of their maternal carers as truly believing them, a third disbelieving them, and a third feeling doubtful about whether sup-port was being afforded them or not. The state of the child (mental health indices, anxiety, depression, post-traumatic stress) is affected by the severity of abuse, as is whether the child perceives themself to be supported. To be an older female is often associated with being disbelieved by a mother who puts her need for her partner above the protection of the child, and parents come together in opposi-tion to authorities who are perceived as putting ideas in their child's head. The young person is thus doubly rejected.

In the Great Ormond Street treatment outcome study where the effectiveness of adding group work to a basic family professional treatment network approach was being tested, over half (60%) of the children were living apart from their original family at the time of referral, and had suffered separation not only from their parents, but also in many cases from their siblings.

Three-quarters of the perpetrators could not be included in the treatment either because they were in prison, had disappeared, or were taking no responsi-bility for abusive action. Mothers who had chosen to support their abused child frequently had to adjust to considerable changes: not only that abuse had occurred, but also to face the loss of a partner or another child, e.g. where a boy had been abusive to a younger sibling. There were emotional and/or financial implications of such changes, and there was continuing stress and uncertainty of impending court procedures. Children were involved in continuing high levels of disruption and change, a high level of involvement from child protection professionals as well as attempts to work therapeutically. It was a mark of success of intervention that children were able to return to a family member's care at the end of treatment.

Assessment and aims for treatment

The aims for treatment work where it was possible to involve the whole family or part of the family included the following:

Assigning responsibility for the abuse

It was felt that, given the considerable variability in responsibility expressed by family members at the outset (children blaming themselves, mothers blaming the child, parent abuser often denying the abuse) the following treatment aims needed to be achieved:

1. Father/mother/children need to acknowledge that abuse was the responsibility of the perpetrator, not the child.
2. Mother/father acknowledge their own responsibility for abuse, or for lack of availability to the child to be protective when applicable.
3. There needs to be evidence of the child's resolution of conflicted feelings towards the perpetrator and parents, i.e. instead of justifying the abuse through various distortions and rationalisations, the appropriate attribution of responsibility was taken.

Treatment focused on family relationships

1. Family members were able to express reasonable anger to each other in an appropriate non-destructive and non-scapegoating manner.
2. Family members could develop sufficiently open relationships for painful issues to be confided and shared between child and parents, and between the parents themselves.
3. Family allowed all members space to speak and listen to each other without scapegoating.
4. There was recognition of individual needs, appropriate to age.
5. Recognition of appropriate qualities in all family members, including each member recognising positive aspects of themselves.
6. Establishment and maintenance of appropriate generational boundaries.
7. Provision of adequate protection from further abuse to children.

Treatment focused on origins and effects of abuse

1. Recognition of potential and actual damage which might be the result of sexual abuse.
2. Parents show a capacity to help children with actual behavioural effects of abuse.
3. Recognition of damage caused to adults by abusive experiences in their own youth (where relevant).
4. Recognition by adults of need for help on an individual and couple basis, including specific help with sexual difficulties.
5. Ability of family and professionals to work together cooperatively.

Many of these treatment goals needed to be achieved in the first two stages through individual and group work whether with victims, protective parents or abusers, either young people or parental figures. (See Bentovim *et al.* 1988, Monck *et al.* 1996, etc. for details of individual/group work.)

Family treatment approaches to sexual abuse

Examination of a series of cases in the treatment outcome study (Monck *et al.* 1996) demonstrated that, although treatment of the family was a central part of the therapeutic programme, family treatment sessions were far more often held with parts of the family, e.g. the mother and victim. Increasingly it was likely that some time would be given to them individually, and in the few families where the offender had admitted responsibility for abuse, and where the mother wished to have some continuing relationship, there would be couple sessions or family sessions. Such contact occurred where the mother did not wish the offender to live with her or the children, but where she felt that it was in the interest of some or all of the children to have continued contact with their father or the offender.

It was usual for all family members to be seen during the evaluation period, but very young siblings were often not included in ongoing therapeutic sessions. In some families, older siblings showed marked resistance to attending and their mothers were not always able to persuade them to attend or convinced that it was appropriate to do so. In several families, children aged around 11 were most reluctant to include younger siblings aged around 8 on the grounds that they were afraid that the sibling concerned would gossip about the abuse and so bring more distress to the abused child. This anxiety was shared by the mothers on what seemed to be realistic grounds. Nevertheless it was important to work towards some inclusion of younger siblings in order to identify any help they might need in dealing with the sudden loss of a father or step-father. Responsibility was seen as lying clearly with the individual abuser, but it was felt essential to identify any elements in the family system which might have contributed to the vulnerability of a particular child(ren), or which might maintain an abusive context.

It was also recognised that even if there had not been a dysfunction in the relationship between mother and a female victim prior to the abuse and its disclosure, the disclosure itself might make the relationship more vulnerable because of the feelings of guilt, rivalry and responsibility, however misplaced. Relations following disclosure by male victims was often far less conflictual. During the initial crisis of disclosure the primary aims were to ensure appropriate protection for the victim(s) and any other children. This meant supporting them with court proceedings, both civil and criminal, and having the therapists involved actively in such proceedings as a therapeutic team service. Second, the therapist must try and prevent the family 'closing up' and so refusing or becoming unavailable for treatment. This is most likely to occur either if the family denied that abuse had occurred, or if they minimised the seriousness to such a degree that they refused professional help, insisting there was no risk of further abuse and no harmful sequeli to the child or family from the previous abuse.

During the crisis phase, offenders almost invariably denied the possibility of their abusing again, which was hardly surprising since none of them had received any treatment. There was only a partial admission of offences, and it was not possible to be clear whether denials of abuse that carried more severe penalties were made out of protective self-interest, or from a need to minimise and deny the offences even to themselves.

We noted three different family contexts where treatment was offered:

1. Those families where there was no change of membership because the abuser had left it forever prior to disclosure, and where the fact that the abuser had left the family had enabled the child to disclose abuse perpetrated against them.
2. Families who hoped to reintegrate the offender or the victim if they had been moved out.
3. Families who were new and where there was no intention to reunite with the offender.

Specific areas of work carried out at Great Ormond Street, London, are outlined below.

The process of clarification, taking appropriate responsibility and apology

The process of clarifying exactly what type of abuse has occurred, to whom, how extensively and who is responsible, needs to be a theme kept in mind throughout therapeutic work. Work with the abused child begins at the point of disclosure, and needs to be extended both during the initial diagnostic phase and during the phase of exposure in the individual/group therapeutic phase.

Perpetrators in treatment also need to acknowledge and share the extent of their abusive action, using victim statements as a key to their work. Both victims and perpetrators need to share with protective parents and with victims, acknowledging and attributing responsibility for abuse and failure to protect, and giving appropriate apologies.

Furniss (1990) has advocated the value of an early session where responsibility can be taken and the victim absolved from guilt and blame, and the potentially protective parent empowered to provide adequate care for the victim. Through this process, adequate boundaries can be established, and the abusive parent helped to take on a parental role that will require separation – preferably themself leaving the home, rather than the child. Furniss gives extensive guidelines to carry out such sessions. It was possible to explore this approach in the early phase of the Great Ormond Street Team when we carried out the initial diagnostic work.

The problem of this approach is twofold. It presupposes that during the initial phase of disclosure sufficient information is obtained from the child and that the perpetrator acknowledges sufficient responsibility to make such a session possible. Second, it presupposes that a multidisciplinary/multi-agency team is available to carry out the complex therapeutic task.

The structure of current child protective action usually means that police/social work professionals carry out initial investigation and assessments. The necessity for interviews following the guidelines in the *Memorandum of Good Practice*, and police statements means that early clarification/responsibility work is not feasible, and needs to take place once such processes have occurred. Referral to therapeutic services is made at a later stage, and as we saw in the Great Ormond Street research project, this brings about three problems: a high level denial by alleged perpetrators that abuse had occurred, disbelief by mothers, and the placement of children in alternative care. The scope for family clarification, taking adequate responsibility and apologising was more limited, and needed to take place at a later stage of treatment, when possible.

In work with perpetrators who do take adequate responsibility, acknowledging appropriate responsibility and apologising for harm caused to a victim can be a key moment in therapeutic work for the whole family, whenever it occurs.

Working on denial, minimisation and projection of blame

One of the continuing processes of family work at all stages is the constant revisiting of the issue of who is responsible for abusive action, resisting the desire to blame the victim, and minimising the extent of abusive action and its impact. One of the most helpful therapeutic approaches to dealing with denial, minimisation and projection of blame is to constantly ask the question, 'what would happen if there was no denial, if there was no minimisation, if the victim was not blamed?' What would the consequence be for a mother who is a non-abusing parent, if the abuser fully took responsibility for their action? Would there be any possibility of maintaining a relationship, or is there is necessary degree of denial for parents to maintain a relationship and function as parents? If the victim was not blamed, if the child were seen as being victimised, groomed, their ordinary childish sexual responses amplified and perceived as giving sexual permission when there was none, what would be the consequences? What would be the responses if a mother who is a non-abusing parent, instead of contending that they had no knowledge or information that abuse was going on, were to acknowledge that they had seen and were aware peripherally of abusive action? What would be the consequences? Would there be depressive, suicidal behaviour? An approach that positively connotes denial as a means of self-protection, and sees dissociation as a necessary defence before full acceptance, makes it possible to work with denial, minimisation and blame, even if this results in stress on the potential to relate, say between a mother and her children, or between parents in the early stages of work.

A sequence of hypothetical questions may need to be used to clarify the function of denial when abusive action is denied by a perpetrator. For instance, a parent or an older sibling who is alleged to have abused within their family context and who is denying this, may be asked what would be the consequences if they did recall that abuse had occurred. For instance, if they woke up one morning and became aware that the allegations made were true, that their own 'protective' dissociation had lifted and they discovered that they had indeed been responsible for abuse. They may be asked what their partners would say/think, what extended family members would say, what they themselves might do with such a realisation. Do they think they might be able to live with themselves, might there be a risk of suicide? Did they feel that this sort of behaviour was one which could be treated adequately? If responses are such that there may indeed be serious suicidal attempts, then again denial can be positively connoted. If there is a feeling that neither they nor any other family member believe that treatment is possible, then denial can be positively connoted because it means that if the court believes the child has been abused then they will be protected. If no treatment was possible then this would be the best outcome for the child. Perhaps at some level this is what the parents want professionals to do in order to protect their children from themselves.

Addressing abuse of power, powerlessness and empowerment

Research on factors that trigger abusive behaviour, and intense traumatic responses, e.g. flashbacks and visualisations, demonstrates the pervasive effects of the sense of powerlessness experienced by both perpetrators, victims and other family members. Powerlessness may result in the use of oppressive and violent strategies to resolve differences between parents, and between children and parents. A belief in powerlessness leads to an abdication of responsibility on the part of family members, or to constant power struggles to gain control. It is essential that work with individuals and in family contexts offers opportunities to develop appropriate non-coercive self-management, anger management, different ways of assertiveness and a contract of no-violence, as noted earlier in the treatment of physical abuse. There is often a need to track intergenerational patterns of abuse, coercive strategies, power-orientated approaches through genograms and through helping parents see that they have survived themselves, that strategies of inappropriate power use are part of the same scenario they have been subject to and have adopted as a dysfunctional coping strategy.

Work with guilt and rivalry in mother–child relationships

We found that guilt was one of the most prevailing feelings amongst both mothers and victims, particularly if they were female. Much of the treatment centred on helping families modify this, as much was unreasonably attributed. Offenders contributed actively, as the more they could engender it the more they shifted responsibility from themselves and avoided having anger directed at them. Where a mother wished the offender to return, and the victim did not, there was always a painful tension because of the conflict of need and wish. Both the victim and the mother felt guilty and contributed to continued or increased problems in communication between them. The children often felt let down and angry, yet because of their dependency it was difficult to show such feelings openly. There was anger on the mother's side that the child's needs could prohibit her meeting her own emotional needs. There was also a need to cope with feelings of jealousy, that their daughter had been 'another woman' for their partners, even when they themselves rejected the partner and were supportive and protective of the child. Adolescent daughters were particular sources of such jealousy rather than younger children, and this led to denial and rejection.

This was a difficult process to work with, but exposure and the child giving a full account of their abusive experiences often helped mothers understand the extent of traumatic memories and anxieties triggered by thoughts of meeting or seeing the abuser.

A similar process of guilt and anxiety occurred when, for instance, the abuser was a child who had abused a younger sibling. The mother was faced with her sense of push/pull between her feelings for both her children, yet she had to be protective of one, and excluding of the other. When the young person who was a perpetrator against a sibling had also been abused, for instance by a former partner, then the degree of pressure and anxiety on the parent was considerable. It is necessary to work with both the mother's victimised child and victimised perpetrator. The mother needs to deal with her own sense of guilt and her inability to be able to meet the needs of both her children adequately and balance this with her own needs. Children were often more able to forgive a sibling who had abused them if that sibling had also been abused. It was easier for mothers to facilitate an apology session and reconciliation between siblings where there was no betrayal by a partner.

Work on sexual feelings, beliefs and activities

One of the major problems presented by victims of sexual abuse is sexualisation, or major anxieties and inhibitions about touching of any kind. In family settings we would usually work with the mother and children together in order to try and ensure that the mother was actively enabled to help her child overcome confusions and learn appropriate boundaries for sexual behaviour. Learning appropriate touch, modesty and assertion skills could often be well carried out in groups with peers, but generalisation and reinforcement within family context was often an important teaching experience to consolidate what the child had learnt within group contexts.

Many mothers found this extremely difficult. Social norms and their own personal upbringing did not facilitate open discussion of normality of masturbation and childhood erotic pleasure. Group work for parents where such issues as approaches to sex education, understanding of how to help children with sexualisation problems and giving explanations of sexual matters was an important training ground for family work. Books and drawings were helpful tools in facilitating such work, and could be given to mothers to take home and continue work with children. Even older children and young adolescents found such publications very helpful. Unless there were young children close in age to the children who had been abused where work could be pursued as an educational task, we did not see this work as appropriate to share in a family context with all members of the family.

Parent–child work was particularly important when boys had been abused, and had also been exposed to a context of violence, rejection and aggressive male roles. The combination of grievance, and the eroticisation of anger can lead to a re-enactment of sexual abuse and needs to be handled at a number of levels – including the family.

Where mothers had been abused themselves and where this led to an inability to perceive inappropriate sexual activities going on within the family, or where there was extreme sensitivity to ordinary sexuality, such issues needed to be addressed both in individual and group contexts, as well as within the family context itself.

Focusing on blurred and confused role boundaries

There is a need to clarify blurred and confused role boundaries in family work with sexual abuse. A common grooming technique that blurs boundaries is for the abusive parent to create a partnership role with a child, giving them inappropriate authority, putting the parent into a childlike rejected role. Such inappropriate partnerships undermine the relationships between the child and the mother, maintain silencing and maintain a sense of blame and guilt. Parental roles and sex roles become confused, the child is organised into an adult partnership role, becoming the object of emotional and physical closeness, and there is a gradual transformation from the parent–child relationship to a partnership that is eroticised.

The individual work to enable adults and children to take on appropriate roles and to counter such pressures is an essential preliminary task before family work that reinforces appropriate boundaries. Techniques such as sculpting can help look at the relationships of family members whilst abuse was continuing, and demonstrates the process leading to a safe family context. Such work can only be carried through when family members have completed individual work and is an essential component of a rehabilitation programme that will include apology sessions, abusers taking appropriate responsibility, and sharing the ways in which abuse has been perpetrated and the ways in which the family has been manipulated and organised into allowing abusive behaviour to be maintained in secrecy.

In one family, for instance, the father was perceived as being on a totally different level to other family members – the authority, the controlling agent. Mother and children saw themselves at quite a different, lower level. The abuser described the way in which he used his position of authority to belittle and diminish the mother's sense of herself through criticising her sexuality. He was aware that she had been abused in childhood and had never revealed this to anyone except to himself. He rationalised her silence on the basis that she must have enjoyed her sexual experiences in childhood with the uncle, which was why she had never spoken about it. He then set up a highly punitive organising approach to his daughter. He was punitive, seeing her as bad and rebellious. Using this process of inappropriate authority he then secretly groomed then abused his daughter, demanding silence and continuing secrecy. He had grown up in a family where he had been subject to extensive physical abuse himself, and his father had a position of considerable authority, a role he took himself within the family context. Following a period of therapeutic work in groups for each of the individuals it became possible for the mother to assert her authority, for the father to move down to a more appropriate level, and for the mother to take the central role in the family, both protecting and negotiating the relationship between her children and her partner.

Loss and bereavement

Given that there was no proposal to reunite with the offender in many families, and that many had become single parent families without wishing to do so, therapeutic attention was paid to issues of loss and bereavement. In that area it was important to try and involve all family members since all children experience the change. Non-abused siblings sometimes felt the loss very differently from the victims, and there needed to be an acceptance of difference. Mothers often needed support in these situations, and in some families there was some active involvement of extended family members who might be supportive in a session. Mothers were encouraged and helped to share openly, either with extended family or friends in order to gain some social support.

Meeting of individual needs

Helping parents understand the impact of abuse on their children, in order to understand regressed behaviour, the aggression associated with powerlessness, the dissociation associated with traumatic phenomena such as flashbacks, re-enactments, depressed affect, fears and phobias, are an essential aspect of family work. Promoting communication, seeking solutions to problem behaviour, offering support and constantly linking the care professionals with the therapeutic needs of the family is an essential therapeutic task. There is no one set of techniques that are useful in every context. Techniques from structural family therapy may be used, getting parents and children to work through a problem to a solution. Apparently difficult behaviour may need to be connoted positively as examples of healing, frustrations understood as necessary processes towards change. Children need help to repair disrupted attachments, develop more satisfactory emotional dysregulation and reverse their negative sense of self. Abusive parents need help to face the nature of their abusive action, to understand its origins and the factors that maintain it, and how to prevent relapse and recurrence. Protective parents need to understand how the addictive needs of a partner can distort and destroy family life. These are all important elements which need to be confronted to create a healthy family life for those who are willing to undertake the long journey to health.

Annotated further reading

Bentovim A 1996 Trauma organised systems: physical and sexual abuse in families. Karnac, London

This text provides a systemic theoretical framework for understanding the impact of both physical and sexual abuse as traumatic experiences, which can organise individual, family and professional systems. In particular, he links sociological, social-interactional and systems perspectives which describe how family systems become organised around the trauma of family violence, and he goes on to give a systematic account of trauma organised systems associated with different forms of family violence. The need to break the denial process inherent in trauma organised systems is addressed and a focal model described which provides a systematic way of describing families and planning therapeutic work. The book is illustrated with numerous case examples and provides child protection professionals with a valuable framework for understanding and assessing families in which child abuse has occurred.

Furniss T 1990 The multi-professional handbook of child sexual abuse: integrated management, therapy and legal interventions. Routledge, London

This book makes a more direct link between child abuse and family therapy. It is a good resource for readers who wish to look in more depth at working with families where sexual abuse has taken place. Using a systems approach, Furniss considers child sexual abuse as a syndrome of addiction and secrecy which requires a multidisciplinary response. He presents an integrated approach to the management, therapeutic work and legal frameworks involved in the care and treatment of sexually abused children and their families, and shows how practical steps in therapy and management directly influence each other. The first part of the book outlines the principle ways and basic concepts used in dealing with child sexual abuse. The second part focuses on practical problems ranging from the evaluation of suspicion, the management of disclosure and inter-professional problems through to a wide range of treatment issues relating directly to working with abusing families. The theoretical and practice sections are cross-referenced, so that the reader can use the conceptual framework to inform their therapeutic work in a direct and specific way.

Glaser D, Frosh S 1993 Child sexual abuse. Macmillan, London

Danya Glaser and Stephen Frosh's very useful and accessible book is divided into two parts. The first part centres on understanding child sexual abuse and discusses the dimensions of child sexual abuse; ideas and research on sexuality and abusers; as well as the constellation of relationships, social circumstances and values that make it more or less likely that children are victimised. The authors also review the family systems model and offer a critique of its strengths and limitations. The second part, on therapeutic practice, addresses the management of suspicion and disclosure of child sexual abuse and the validation and decision-making process. It then focuses on therapeutic intervention, with the emphasis very much on practice. Glaser & Frosh are particularly helpful in linking up the overall aims of professional involvement with the specific therapeutic interventions that can be used to meet the needs of sexually abused children and their families, and they stress the need for a coordinated therapeutic approach.

Jones D P H, Ramchandani P 1999 Child sexual abuse: informing practise from research. Radcliffe Medical Press, Oxford

A research/evidence-based review of many aspects of work with child sexual abuse. Brings together recently commissioned research by the Department of Health in an accessible, clear and well-argued way. Essential to assist in developing practice, and to clarify the family role in work with sexual abuse.

References

Ahmad B 1990 Black perspectives in social work. Venture Press, London

Ahmed S, Cheetham J, Small J 1986 Social work with black children and their families. Batsford, London

Asen G E, Piper R, Stevens A 1989 A systems approach to child abuse. Child Abuse and Neglect 13: 45–58

Barker P 1990 Basic family therapy. Blackwell Scientific, Oxford

Bentovim A 1979 Towards creating a focal hypothesis for brief focal family therapy. Journal of Family Therapy 1: 125–136

Bentovim A 1995 Trauma organised systems: physical and sexual abuse in families. Karnac, London

Bentovim A, Davenport M 1992 Resolving the trauma organised system of sexual abuse by confronting the abuser. Journal of Family Therapy 14: 29–30

Bentovim A, Bingley-Miller L (2000) The assessment of family competence, strength and diffculties. Pavillion, Brighton

Bentovim A, Kinston W 1991 Focal family therapy, joining systems theory and psychodynamic understanding. In: Gurman A, Kniskerm D (eds) Handbook of family therapy. Brunner-Mazel, New York

Bentovim A, Elton A, Hildebrand J, *et al.* (eds) 1988 Child sexual abuse within the family. Wright, London

Bingley L, Loader P, Kinston W 1984 Research report: further development of a format for family description. Australian Journal of Family Therapy 5 (3): 215–218

Bograd M 1988 Power, gender and the family: feminist perspectives on family systems therapy. In: Dutton-Douglas M A, Walker L A (eds) Feminist psycholtherapies: integration of therapeutic and feminist systems. Ablex, Norwood, New Jersey

Boscolo B, Cecchin G, Hoffman L, Penn P 1987 Milan systemic family therapy. Basic Books, New York

Brunk M, Henggeler S W, Whelan J P 1987 Comparison of multisystemic therapy and parent training in the brief treatment of child abuse and neglect. Journal of Consulting and Clinical Psychology 55: 171–178

Burnham J 1986 Family therapy. Tavistock, London

Byng-Hall J 1973 Family myths used as a defence in conjoint family therapy. British Journal of Medical Psychology 46: 239–250

Byng-Hall J 1990 Attachment theory and family therapy: a clinical view. Infant Mental Health Journal 2: 228–236

Byng-Hall J 1995 Rewriting family scripts: improvisation and systems change. Guilford, New York

Campbell D, Draper R (eds) 1985 Applications of systemic family therapy: the Milan approach. Academic Press, London

Carter E, McGoldrick M (eds) 1989 The changing family life cycle: a framework for family therapy. Allyn and Bacon, Boston

Crittenden P 1988 Family and dyadic patterns of functioning in maltreating families. In: Browne K, Davies C, Stratton P (eds) Early prediction and prevention of child abuse. John Wiley, Chichester

Crittenden P, Ainsworth M 1989 Child maltreatment and attachment theory. In: Cicchetti D, Carlson V (eds) Child maltreatment: theory and research on the causes and consequences of child abuse and neglect. Cambridge University Press, Cambridge

Dale P, Davies M, Morrison T, Waters J 1986a Dangerous families: assessment and treatment of child abuse. Tavistock, London

Dale P, Waters J, Davies M, *et al.* 1986b The towers of silence: creative and destructive issues for therapeutic teams dealing with sexual abuse. Journal of Family Therapy 8: 1–25

de Shazer S 1982 Patterns of brief family therapy: an ecosystemic approach. Guildford, New York

de Shazer S 1984 Keys to solution in brief therapy. Norton, New York

de Shazer S 1989 Wrong map. Wrong territory. Journal of Marital and Family Therapy 15: 117–121

Elton A 1988 Assessment of families for treatment. In: Bentovim A, Elton A, Hildebrand J, Tranter M, Vizard E (eds) Child sexual abuse within the family. Wright, London

Erikson M, Egelend B, Pianta R 1989 The effects of maltreatment on development of young children. In: Cicchetti D, Carlson V (eds) Child maltreatment: theory and research on the causes and consequences of child abuse and neglect. Cambridge University Press, Cambridge

Eth S, Pynoos R S (eds) 1985 Post-traumatic stress disorder in children. American Psychiatric Association, Los Angeles, California

Figley C (ed) 1990 Treating stress in families. Brunner Mazel, New York

Finkelhor D 1984 Child sexual abuse: new theory and research. The Free Press, New York

Fishman C, Rosoman B 1991 Evolving models for family change: a volume in honor of Salvador Minuchin. Guilford, New York

Furniss T 1990 The multi-professional handbook of child sexual abuse: integrated management, therapy and legal interventions. Routledge, London

Furniss T, Bentovim A, Kinston W 1983 Clinical process recording in focal family therapy. Journal of Marital and Family Therapy 9 (2): 147–170

Glaser D 1993 Emotional abuse. In: Hobbs C, Wynne J (eds) Baillière's clinical paediatrics, vol. 1(1). Baillière Tindall, London, pp. 251–265

Glaser D, Frosh S 1993 Child sexual abuse. Macmillan, London

Glaser D, Furniss T, Bingley L 1984 Focal family therapy – the assessment stage. Journal of Family Therapy 6: 265–274

Haley J 1976 Problem-solving therapy. Jossey-Bass, San Francisco, California

Haley J 1980 Leaving home. McGraw-Hill, New York

Hanks H 1993 Failure to thrive: a model for treatment. In: Hobbs C, Wynne J (eds) Baillière's clinical paediatrics. Baillière Tindall, London

Hayes H 1991 A re-introduction to family therapy: clarification of three schools. Australian and New Zealand Journal of Family Therapy 12: 27–43

Herman J 1992 Trauma and recovery: from domestic violence to political terror HarperCollins, New York

Hildebrand J 1988 The use of group work in treating child sexual abuse. In: Bentovim A, Elton A, Hildebrand J, *et al.* (eds) Child sexual abuse within the family. Wright, London

Hobbs C, Hanks H, Wynne J 1993 Child abuse and neglect: a clinician's handbook. Churchill Livingstone, London

Hooper C A 1992 Mothers surviving child sexual abuse. Routledge, London

Hyde C, Bentovim A, Monck E 1996 Treatment outcome study of sexually abused children. Child Abuse and Neglect 19: 1387–1397

Jones D P H 1987 The untreatable family. Child Abuse and Neglect 11: 409–420

Kempe C H, Silverman FN, Steele BF, Draegmuller W, Silver HK 1962 The battered child syndrome. Journal of the American Medical Association 181: 17–24

Kinston W, Bentovim A 1983 Constructing a focal formulation and hypothesis in family therapy. Australian Journal of Family Therapy 4: 37–50

Kolko D J 1996 Individual cognitive behavioural treatment and family therapy for physically abused children and their offending parents: the comparison of clinical outcomes, Journal of Child Maltreatment 1 (4): 322–342

Lieberman S 1979 Transgenerational family therapy. Croom Helm, New York

Madanes C 1982 Strategic family therapy. Jossey-Bass, San Francisco, California

McCluskey U 1987 Theme focused family therapy. In: Walrond-Skinner S, Watson D (eds) Ethical issues in family therapy. Routledge and Kegan Paul, London

McCluskey U, Bingley Miller L 1995 Theme-focused family therapy: the inner emotional world of the family. Journal of Family Therapy 17: 411–434

Minuchin S 1974 Families and family therapy. Harvard University Press, Cambridge, Mass achussets

Minuchin S, Fishman W 1981 Family therapy techniques. Harvard University Press, Cambridge, Massachussets

Monck E, Bentovim A, Goodall G, *et al.* 1996 Child sexual abuse: a descriptive and treatment study. Studies in Child Protection. HMSO, London

Palazzoli M, Prata G 1992 Snares in family therapy. Journal of Marital and Family Therapy 8: 443–450

Palazzoli M, Cecchin G, Prata G, Boscolo L 1978 Paradox and counter-paradox. Jason Aronson, New York

Palazzoli M, Checchin G, Prata G, Boscolo L 1980 Hypothesising – circularity – neutrality: three guidelines for the conductor of the session. Family Process 19: 3–12

Perelberg R, Miller A 1990 Gender and power in families. Tavistock/Routledge, London

Satir V 1967 Conjoint family therapy. Science and Behavior Books, Palo Alto, California

Satir V 1972 People making. Science and Behaviour Books, Palo Alto, California

Sheinberg M 1992 Navigating treatment impasses at the disclosure of incest: combining ideas from families and social construction and family process. Family Process 31: 201–216

Sheinberg M, True F, Frankel P 1994 Treating the sexually abused child: a recursive multi-model programme. Family Process 33: 263–276

Stevenson J 1999 The treatment of the long-term sequeli of child abuse. Journal of Child Psychology Psychiatry 40 (1): 89–11

Stratton P 1991 Incorporating circularity in defining and classifying child maltreatment. Human systems. Journal of Systemic Consultation and Management 2 (3/4): 145–296

von Bertalanffy L 1962 General systems theory. Penguin, New York

Walters M, Carter B, Papp P, Silverstein O 1988 The invisible web: gender patterns in family relationships. Guilfrod, New York

White M, Epston D 1990 Narrative means to therapeutic ends. Norton, New York

Wilson K, Ryan V 1994 Working with the sexually abused child: the use of non-directive play therapy and family therapy. Journal of Social Work Practice 8 (1): 71–78

25

Group work in child protection agencies

Anne Bannister

The efficacy of groups in medical and social settings has been well documented by Moreno (1934), Foulkes & Anthony (1957) and, more recently, by Williams (1991) and Sanderson (1995). The further reading list gives other proponents and pioneers of group work in settings from a psychiatric hospital to a children's home.

An important task of a group in a child protection setting is to provide a safe place where clients may feel supported and may, if they wish, explore their own forbidden agendas. They may reveal mistakes, or make fresh mistakes, without being punished, and they may practise future behaviour or relationships without causing pain to existing family members. The worker can assess more easily clients' existing behaviour in a group, in order to encourage change, and the client may rehearse new behaviours where help is at hand to assess these.

Benson (1987) feels that the purpose of groups generally is to develop a sense of identity, to establish trust, to use power, to develop roles and values, and to create boundaries. When applied to child protection, the most relevant task from this list is probably to create boundaries. Many people who have suffered abuse, or who have become abusers, are afraid of the power of their feelings, which they have not been helped to contain by their carers as part of their normal development. The group can act as a therapeutic container that will allow expression of feelings in a safe way. Of course, the establishment of trust needs to occur first. Workers can use their power to empower members which, in turn, will lead to the development of a sense of identity and increased use of different roles and values.

Writing specifically about group work with children and adolescents, Dwivedi (1993) points to the fact that children and adolescents may find that groups more closely simulate the real world than one-to-one therapy. He reminds us of the power differential between adult and child and feels this is diffused in the group setting. He also points out the ability of the group to help children with their personal identity and to enable roles to be practised. For children who have been abused, this issue of their lack of personal power is crucial to their future development and behaviour. An abused child may need to be supported and empowered to a certain extent before being able to join a group. Once this is accomplished, however, the healing provided by the group may prevent years of suffering for both child and family.

Agencies, resources, policies

Resources in child protection agencies have always been limited. After the implementation of the Seebohm report in 1974, when several different agencies amalgamated to become a generic social services department, there was a concern that the specialised needs of specific groups were not being addressed and therapeutic groups were set up in an effort to meet these needs. The probation service, social services, child guidance clinics and other health departments set up groups (sometimes working inter-agency) for their clients who appeared to have similar problems. Self-help groups were also springing up at this time. These were usually supportive rather than therapeutic in nature.

Inter-agency cooperation is essential, especially if referrals are taken from several sources. Referring a client to a group run by another agency does not mean that responsibility ends for the referrer. The group member will receive most benefit if their worker is supportive (possibly providing transport or bus fares), as well as cooperative, in liaising with other family members if necessary. Cooperation across agencies can also be helpful in providing an accessible meeting place or facilities for groups with special needs.

It is sometimes thought that group work is very economical of staff resources since a number of people can be seen at one time. However, groups require careful planning, selection and assessment, recording and supervision, if they are to have a successful outcome and these processes are time-consuming. With practice, though, group workers do become more efficient at planning and selection, and at this stage the resource benefits may be felt in the agency.

One of the key functions of a group is to provide a place where members can experience a different way of interacting with others. They also have a ready-made setting for practising new ways of behaving. It is therefore vital that the group facilitators fully understand the dynamics of abuse. If the workers are new to group work, it is particularly important that they meet for several weeks (or longer) before the group starts with an experienced supervisor or consultant who can prepare them for the situations they are likely to face. This consultant should also be prepared to meet with them on a regular basis throughout the life of the group.

It is vital that an experienced person outside the group should provide a viewpoint to help the workers to understand the transferential feelings expressed by group members and the counter-transference experienced by the workers. In addition, the consultant can see how the co-workers react to each other and how their relationship is likely to impact upon the group. Sometimes an experienced person will run a group alone, but in the child protection field this is unusual. The reason is because workers need the support that a co-worker can provide, otherwise the personal stress can be too much to bear.

An experienced consultant will also help to monitor the power positions within the group as a whole. A group should never reflect the abusive situation with which its members may be familiar. Great care should be taken to ensure that the potential abuses of power within gender, ethnicity, disability, age, etc. are recognised by the workers so that group members can be encouraged to support and assist each other, rather than relying upon the workers.

Another potential conflict of power arises from the agency or agencies which are providing workers and premises for the group. Parents may feel oppressed in a group run by the statutory social services or National Society for the Prevention of Cruelty to Children (NSPCC), and the social worker facilitators may have a harder task to build trust. Likewise, young offenders may feel wary in a group run by the probation service. Nevertheless, these constraints may be used positively by group workers, and this is most likely to be effective in jointly run groups across the agencies. A psychiatric nurse and a social worker may be the most suitable people to run a group for mothers of abused children, for instance, and the presence of the social worker with statutory powers could be particularly helpful as a demonstration of how those powers could be used positively. It is vital, too, that the workers in a group for adolescent or adult perpetrators of abuse are very clear about the boundaries of the members' behaviour. For example, issues of current or recent abuse not previously known must be immediately addressed and child protection procedures instigated. Workers from the medical agencies would be strengthened by someone from the probation service; each agency could provide good 'modelling' for a discussion of boundaries, which could include the issue of 'care and control'.

The time spent planning a weekly group, preparing and running it, debriefing, recording and meeting with a consultant is likely to take up to 8 hours per week. It is unrealistic for workers to transport clients to groups because of the time involved. This also changes the group dynamics, since the group begins to function once two or more members are together, even on the journey to the group meeting. Consideration should also be given to the group setting, since some institutions (hospitals, police stations) can have unwelcome connotations for some members. This is not to say, of course, that highly effective groups cannot be run in a secure hospital or prison if the workers can use their skills to create a safe space where the members can address their forbidden agendas.

Initial planning

Population

The initial planning decision concerns the population with which one wishes to work, and this may be determined by need. The range of groups in child protection runs from children and adolescents who have been abused, through adolescent offenders, parents who have abused their children, non-abusing parents whose child has been abused, and adult survivors of abuse. Recently, young children who are abusing others have also been treated in groups. Groups for children and young people cannot be run without the full cooperation of their carers. Sometimes carers may be in parallel treatment groups (MacFarlane *et al.* 1986, Frey-Angel 1989, Breen 1994).

Workers

The next important decision concerns the group workers. I have already suggested that two workers are preferable to one, and that a consultant is also necessary. Unless the co-workers have previously worked together, they will need the consultant to help them look at their relationship before they begin.

Setting

The setting for the group is also important, and I would add to my previous comments on this that, where confidentiality is important, it is not wise for members to be drawn from one small geographical area. The place for the group would then have to be accessible from a wide area. Groups for young people should pay attention to the safety of their members, including travelling to the group. Agency transport is, therefore, preferable.

Size

It is usually considered that six to ten people is a suitable number for a group with two workers, and for children I would suggest the lower figure. Indeed for 5–10-year-olds, six may be a maximum figure for a therapeutic group, unless there are three workers.

Type

Groups may be 'closed', where members join together and leave together, or 'open', where some members may join and leave at different times. A closed group is usually more suitable for children and adolescents and those for whom confidentiality is vital. A 'slow open' group is a compromise for adolescents and adults. This type of group starts with a fixed membership, but may agree to take more members at certain intervals and for some members to leave at specific times. A group for survivors of abuse would probably benefit from being closed because of issues of trust. Some adult groups, especially in residential settings, can cope with a 'slow open' situation.

Length and duration

Time-limited groups are important to establish boundaries, especially for children. Many workers consider 12 weekly sessions to be ideal for young children. It is not advisable to have sessions less frequently than weekly for children. It may be that 20 sessions is a more realistic number in terms of measurable improvement in outcome. Certainly, for adolescents and adults it would be difficult to measure change in fewer than 16–20 sessions. An hour is a minimum length for a session; $1\frac{1}{2}$–2 hours is more realistic, including time for consuming food and drink. This is usually provided at the beginning or halfway through a session.

Singer (1989) reports that men who have suffered childhood trauma appear to need a longer period in a group before progress can be made and maintained. From 6 months to a year is suggested, with members sometimes rejoining the group after a break. This is longer than the 6 months suggested by some authors for groups for female survivors, but it may reflect a tendency in the USA for such groups to be continued for a longer period. For instance, a group in Ohio for health professionals who had been sexually abused in childhood extended over 56 sessions (Kreidler & England 1990).

Practitioners agree, however, that groups for adult sexual abusers cannot be effective unless they are continued over a considerable period. Although workers in Nottinghamshire (Cowburn 1990) describe short intensive 'courses' for sexual offenders, most workers (Erooga *et al.* 1990) agree that a year is a minimum time for such a group in the community. Short-term groups are sometimes run in prisons (Barnet *et al.* 1990), and since such groups are totally dependent on the duration of sentences and the availability of suitable clients, it may be that a short-term approach is the only viable one. The authors mentioned above (Barnet *et al.* 1990) were describing a group for women sexual offenders, and since there are far fewer women than men convicted of such crimes the availability of suitable group members may have been very limited. Colton & Vanstone (1996) describe male offender treatment groups lasting 15–20 weeks, meeting twice a week, in the prison setting.

Selection and assessment

It is important for the health of the individual client and of the group that prospective group members are carefully selected. It is true that participation in a group may have an immediate attraction for someone anxious to overcome feelings of isolation. In my experience, though, some people may be unable to function within a group without prior individual work (see Lewis & Gordon 1997). Attention paid during the planning stage to issues of selection can increase the possibilities for the group to become an environment that is safe and healing.

Assessment of individuals for suitability for inclusion in a group varies widely, depending on whether the group is therapeutic and to be attended on a voluntary basis, or whether membership of the group is part of an order through the criminal justice system or child care system which mandates an individual to attend. With scarce resources, it makes sense to include only members who are able to benefit fully and who have demonstrated during an assessment period that they can make some progress. This can usually be done by the co-workers carrying out one or two interviews to test the motivation and potential for change of each proposed member. Inclusion in an adult sex offenders community-based treatment group may need to be mandated, and the client should be prepared for a highly structured setting with space built in to measure change and progress.

In groups where attendance is voluntary, the idea of commitment to the group from members and workers should be introduced during selection. Unless a member is capable of some commitment, their presence could be unhelpful for the health and stability of the group.

Gender and sexuality

Groups offer an opportunity for people to learn different ways of relating to each other. A mixed-gender group may facilitate this best. A male and a female worker can also provide useful role models. However, in child protection treatment groups there are other important considerations. For example, female adolescent survivors of child sexual abuse need the support and safety of other girls and of women workers. I have some experience of groups for boys aged 8–11 who have survived sexual abuse, and also of groups for girls of a similar age. It seems to be important that groups for boys have co-workers who are male and female in order to reduce anxiety for boys who have been abused by men, and also to help them to look at their own worries concerning homosexuality. Young abused girls sometimes find it difficult to work on sexual abuse issues with male workers (unless they have had a male individual worker with whom they already have a good relationship and who has helped to prepare them for the group experience). However, in a recent mixed-gender group of 8–9-year-old sexually abused children, I found that boys and girls worked well with male and female co-workers (see case study in this chapter).

Age range

For adults, life stages may be much more important to consider than age, but for children and young people fairly narrow age ranges are preferable, with developmental rather than chronological age being considered. Groups containing siblings can cross the age barrier more easily. Janice Frey-Angel (1989) describes such a group for children in violent families, usually where the father is violent to the mother. The children's ages range from 3 to 12 years, and although they often replay their parents' abuse, they can practise different behaviours in the group. They may form supportive, age-related subgroups across family boundaries.

Ethnicity

Race and culture need to be addressed. Workers should be aware of their own limitations in this regard. In groups for children and young people, care must be taken in selection to ensure that one child is not isolated because of racial or cultural differences. With adults, this possibility could be addressed directly with the potential group members during the assessment interviews. A group for black and white sexually abused children is described by Marie Lebacq & Zaffira Shah (1989). They keep to a narrow age band (from 5 to 8 years), but they mix boys and girls and members include black Asian, black Afro-Caribbean and white children. All the children are also described as British. The group is led by a black and a white worker. Their consultant is white, and they feel that if a suitable black consultant had also been available this would have been particularly helpful to both workers. The issues with which a black consultant could have assisted include exploring techniques to help black children move on from believing they were sexually abused because they are black to an understanding that sexual abuse happens irrespective of race. This reminds us that children who have been sexually abused are especially sensitive to abusive environments and discriminatory behaviour. Lebacq & Shah conclude that children of this age can work in mixed-gender groups on abuse issues.

Homogeneity

Groups are usually formed because of some thread of experience that is common to all members. This should not, however, become too narrow. For example, in groups for survivors of child sexual abuse the inclusion of survivors of intrafamilial and extrafamilial abuse can add a richness to the group. The sense of identity created by the group is not necessarily undermined by different backgrounds. Mothers of abused children, for instance, can form strong group cohesion because of their shared experience, although their personal histories are very varied.

Support

A high level of support outside the group is essential for members of a therapeutic group. This may not be so important in a group formed simply to provide support. Many young people require a great deal of practical help, which may include being transported to and from the group and the provision of a 'listening ear', in order to process material that is brought to consciousness in the group.

Motivation

Assessing motivation depends very much on the type of group. Often adults with a shared stated problem are highly motivated to meet in groups, and they often have difficulty in ending their involvement. Motivation can be very low for young offenders who are forced into groups as a result of court orders. However, even in mandated groups, members can become highly motivated to remain and continue when they feel their needs are being met and where change is made possible for them.

Learning ability

This is particularly important to assess where groups have a formal structure with an educative input. Many rely on confrontational challenging of distorted cognitions, and group members have to be able to cope with this. Groups for members with learning difficulties would need to have a format more appropriate to their needs. For instance, the use of creative techniques such as art, drama and music could be emphasised instead of pursuits requiring literacy or numeracy.

Running the group

Although it is the responsibility of the group workers to plan carefully and to set the boundaries of their group, the workers must respect and trust the group to deal with any difficult dynamics that may occur. Benson (1987) likens this to the art of aikido, where the warrior never goes against his opponent's strength, but blends with and redirects the energy of the attacker. Benson continues with a helpful introduction to understanding group dynamics.

Workers have to be prepared to relinquish some of their power and control by trusting the group. This does not mean colluding with group repression of certain issues indefinitely, but it does mean respecting that the group may not yet be ready to address painful revelations.

Contracting

This trust of the group can be demonstrated by setting up a mutual contract with workers and members about confidentiality, commitment and caring for each other. It should also include an agreement to respect others, to be non-judgemental and to listen. If members are encouraged to contribute to the contract, this will set the tone for subsequent sessions. Groups for young children should also be approached in this honest and open way, so that members know why they are meeting. Members, including children, should be clear about the duration and structure of the group from the start.

Methods

Children

Young children who are sexually abusing others may benefit from a carefully structured group which uses the '12-step method' (MacFarlane & Cunningham 1990). This is an adaptation of the method used by Alcoholics Anonymous. MacFarlane & Cunningham (1991) also incorporate the 'sexual abuse cycle', as devised by Connie Isaac & Sandy Lane (1990). They demonstrate how a child can work through the process during which he moves from thinking of himself as a 'bad boy' to his actual sexually abusive behaviour. It is vital that the child's parents or carers also attend a parallel group where they too can work through (perhaps also with a 12-step method) their process of facing up to the problem, accepting help, not blaming others and recognising that they may need to look at their own behaviour.

It is important that young children should not be confined in a very small room, but also that they feel cosy enough to foster group bonding. The room should contain art materials, toys, etc., according to availability and the group workers' expertise. Setting group boundaries, including issues of confidentiality, is just as important for children as it is for adults. In fact, it is often more important because parents often feel that their children should not have 'secrets' from them, and children similarly feel that adults will automatically tell their parents what they have said. Exemptions to confidentiality, such as issues of a child abusing another child or damaging themselves, should not be avoided.

Each session should contain some educational material, and also some physical activity (even if it is only passing a squeeze round a circle), and each session should begin and end in ways which constitute a simple ritual that can be repeated each week. Educational input and physical activity must, of course, be sensitive to children with learning difficulties or physical disabilities. Naturally, no group member should be forced to talk about anything that has happened to them. It is enough that they acknowledge that they are part of a group which has suffered similar events. Most children will enjoy drama and role-play. All ages can have fun acting out their favourite fairy story or TV series. Older children will often spontaneously discuss the similarities in these stories with their own situation. For younger children, we can be sure that although the symbolism might not be overt, their expression of feeling as they rage against the 'monster' will be therapeutic.

Kinetic family drawings, making a collage of their family, or making a collage together which depicts the group, can be useful ways of working which children enjoy. Watching suitable videos together can also be helpful if plenty of time is allowed for discussion. Making up a story is a good exercise for older children. The worker starts a story and each group member adds a little to it.

Many children, both boys and girls, like to put on a puppet show, and animal puppets are useful in portraying all kinds of characters. Workers should take care when selecting puppets not to buy those that perpetrate racial or gender stereotypes (see case study, below, for the use of puppets in 'projective' play). Even young children can participate in simple 'guided fantasy' sessions, and older children often find these most helpful. In particular, practising the fantasy of 'a lovely safe place' can be helpful to a child who is troubled by frightening dreams or nightmares.

From about the age of 7 years, writing games and exercises can be used. Sometimes this can take the form of writing letters which are not sent, or sometimes simply writing down lists of 'things that I am good at' to aid self-esteem. Drawing the outline of male and female bodies and naming the parts can be part of simple sex education for children of this age. These children can also be encouraged to write poems or design posters to 'help other children with the same problems'.

Other authors have described useful techniques for working with sexually abused pre-adolescent children (Berliner & Ernst 1982, Corder *et al.* 1990).

Case study

The following is a description of a group for four young children who had been severely sexually abused. This group was set up as a pilot for part of a research project by the author, and was held on NSPCC premises.

The staff team

A small team of two NSPCC child protection workers (including the author who is a psychotherapist/social worker) and two local authority social workers collaborated on the venture. Two of the team members were male and two were female. Only two people ran the group on any particular day, while a third person sat in on the group, taking notes as an observer, and the fourth ran a parallel group for the mothers of the children. All the workers had training together (in a programme run by the author) before the group started and all the workers attended pre-group planning and post-group debriefing. A rota was drawn up so that the staff team were able to take the different roles of group leader or observer each week. A group analyst/social worker employed by NSPCC supervised the staff team.

The group members

The team had sought primary age children (boys and girls) who had been abused over a period of time by family members or friends of the family. It was likely that such children were suffering from complex post-traumatic stress disorder (PTSD) as defined by Herman (1998). The children, and their mothers, were seen for assessment, by one of the staff team, over two sessions. Staff were aware that sexually abusive behaviour is often ignored or condoned by adults (Bannister & Gallagher 1996) so the child's coping mechanisms were assessed to see if there was likely to be any danger to other children. The children completed B/Gsteem tests (Maines & Robinson 1988) to check their locus of control at this stage (internal and external) and also their self-esteem. We also looked at relationships with others, particularly attachment to carers, since this attachment is usually damaged in severe sexual abuse. It is important that young children undergoing group therapy are able to make some attachment (even if this is to a therapist). We asked the mothers to complete the Devereux Behaviour Rating Scale (Naglieri *et al.* 1993) so that we could see what they thought was problematic about the children's behaviour. We tried to ensure that the mothers (fathers were not available) were able to support the children during the therapy. We looked at development levels and agreed that we would take children from a fairly narrow developmental age band to facilitate group bonding. We had hoped for six children but finally started with four children (two boys and two girls) all aged 8 or 9.

Therapeutic methods

The staff team agreed to use creative therapy methods in this group. This included psychodrama, drama therapy, play therapy and some art therapy. One of the aims of the research project was to explore the child developmental theories of Moreno, who invented psychodrama, and Jennings, who developed dramatherapy and playtherapy. Moreno (in Fox 1987) suggested that a child's development comprises:

1. finding a separate identity
2. recognising the self
3. recognising 'the other'.

Moreno felt that children learn these stages of development largely through the actions of a parent or carer (or sometimes a sibling) who 'doubles' for that child by expressing the child's needs when they are not yet able to do so. In the second stage of development the parent 'mirrors' the child's feelings so that the child beings to understand the nature of emotions. In the third stage, parents, siblings and friends all assist the child in playing different roles, e.g. baby, younger sister, older brother, clown, 'quiet one', 'angry one'. All these behaviours develop naturally through play and can be replicated in psychodrama and in play therapy. Jennings (1993) has also suggested a developmental theory that builds on that of Moreno. She states that children develop through embodiment play (using the whole body or media such as clay or water) then through projective play (using puppets or dolls or small figures on which to project feelings), then through role play. In drama therapy and play therapy these developmental stages are replicated, often using metaphor and symbolism. For instance, puppets can be used to express emotions or needs and to play different roles (Carlson-Sabelli 1998).

Another aim of the research was to look at theories that suggest that child development is blocked, distorted or delayed by early traumatic experiences, especially sexual abuse. A psychiatrist, van der Kolk (1996), has suggested that traumatised people may be able to 'express their internal states more articulately in physical movements or in pictures than in words'. He suggests that traumatic events may be registered somatically or visually, rather than through the use of language. Most workers with abuse survivors know that abusers (who may be carers) distort their relationship with the child and actively denigrate more sup-portive relationships (see 'Four pre-conditions' in Finkelhor 1984). This, of course, damages the child's attachment processes to primary carers. A research hypothesis is that creative therapies can recreate developmental processes in a positive way, which may undo the damage caused to development by severe abuse. This is suggested by van der Kolk (1996) when he states that 'drawings and psychodrama may help such people to develop a language that is essential for effective communication and for the symbolic transformation that can occur in psychotherapy'. He goes on to say that group psychotherapy may be most effective in providing interaction and support.

Group process

The whole team met the children at the first session and shared information. The children decided on the group name – 'The Friendly Group' – and on the group rules or contract. They accepted the 'observer' role without difficulty, probably because the observer was always a team member whom they knew and trusted. The group followed the psychodramatic process of 'warm-up', 'action' and 'shar-ing'. The warm-up consisted of a game of tag where the 'wolf' had to catch the 'sheep'. They took turns at playing wolf and were very inventive about finding 'safe places'. This 'whole body' play was also typical of the embodiment stage of play. This was followed by puppet play in which the children chose an animal puppet and were invited to identify the feelings of the puppet. This, of course, was projective play, and was still part of the warm-up. Often, during this play, it was possible to identify problems that were carried through into the middle or 'action' section. At this point we had a break for a drink and a snack together, and infor-mal trust building continued during this. In the action section the children were offered different art media and were asked to express any feelings that had come up during the warm-up. There was a group consensus about the media to be used and, in the first sessions, clay and paint were chosen. These were most familiar from school. Soon they chose to play further with puppets and small figures and eventually, during this middle section, the group used the dressing-up clothes and created elaborate scenes which they acted out, with the help of the therapeutic team. The final part of the session was a sharing in which the children threw a ball to another child or worker and thanked them for specific things which they had appreciated during the session. They also collaborated in chanting a group slogan.

Test reports and ratings

Children

All the children registered 'low' on self-esteem in the B/Gsteem test assessment. After the 20 weeks of the group they all registered 'normal' or 'high'. Also on this test most of the children had registered a completely external locus of control in which they felt powerless in their lives. One child had an inappropriate internal locus of control which meant that he thought he had extensive powers to control others. At the end of the group there were changes showing that the majority were more able to protect themselves from further victimisation, and the boy with controlling behaviour was less inclined to bully.

Mothers

All the mothers rated their children's self-esteem and creativity higher at the end of the group than at the beginning. One mother, whose relationship with her child had been very difficult, reported much improvement. All the mothers rated their children's depression to be much less. Two mothers found their children's new assertiveness difficult to deal with.

Staff

The staff group noted how the children brought many themes of loss into their sessions. Loss is often an overwhelming component of PTSD and is usually accompanied by a need to mourn (Herman 1998). In puppet play the children expressed their losses and were able to mourn. Their loss of integrity and wholeness was also expressed through unnamed grief during the sessions. The progress from grief and mourning to expressions of strength and support was marked from about halfway through the 20 sessions. The final joint scene, played out by all the children with small figurines, was of an eagle who taught all the other animals to fly.

Discussion

The use of creative therapies with abused children has been well documented (Cattanach 1992, Bannister 1997, 1998, Hoey 1997, see also Ryan, Chapter 22, in this volume). Most of these descriptions refer to individual work. However, group work with abused children using educational or cognitive methods has also been well publicised (Reeker *et al.* 1997, Reeker & Ensing 1998). This pilot group sought to demonstrate that creative therapies with young sexually abused children, in groups, can also be effectøive and may have long-term benefits if it can be shown that damage to child development can be healed in this way. A further group is to be run shortly. One finding was that group therapy was more effective with children who had received some individual therapy first. It was also less effective with children who were still in the immediate aftermath of the sexual abuse disclosure. As expected, those children who benefited the most were those with good parental support. Unfortunately the group for mothers was not always well attended because of practical difficulties.

This project, at first sight, appeared not to be economical with human resources. However, the benefits for the staff team were greater than anticipated. All staff learned much from each other, and from the children, as well as from the initial training. The use of an observer (although originally for the purposes of the research only) provided the opportunity for 'live supervision' and thus for further learning. It is an economical way of receiving training if workers with different levels of experience are used.

Adolescents

Probation and social services departments have provided groups for young offenders to capitalise on the very powerful influences adolescent peers have on each other. One group is described (Bannister 1983) which used drama therapy to enable young people to act out their frustration and to help them to face the more serious side of their offending behaviour.

Despite the links established between physical and emotional abuse of children, and acting-out/violence in adolescence, there is little in the literature on the use of therapeutic, preventative groups with these children or young people, and it is their antisocial or criminal behaviour which is then the focus of group intervention. For example, adolescent acting-out in one of its most serious forms can be sexual assault on children, and group work has become a central component of the treatment of this population (Print & Morrison 2000).

Groups for teenage mothers have provided a good forum for education on health and parenting skills, and for some of its members a much needed source of support (Rosenwald 1989).

Blick & Porter (1982) suggest that open therapeutic groups can be effective with adolescent girl survivors of child sexual abuse, with well-established members facilitating the integration of newer members. However, this same group of young people may also benefit from a closed, time-limited group with therapeutic aims.

An essential difference in treatment of survivors and sex offenders is that the latter are normally resistant to change and wish to 'protect behaviour that provides a significant sense of empowerment and adequacy' (Ryan & Lane 1991). Adolescent survivors, on the other hand, come to group treatment desperately wishing to reduce their levels of fear, anxiety and sense of powerlessness. There are, however, some shared issues for these two client groups, one being the inability to trust, and change in this area must be a long-term goal for both groups.

Victim advocacy, which is also central to offender treatment, should be fostered in survivors, who are often lacking in concern for themselves.

The use of confrontation and support by peers is the basis of much offence-specific treatment in groups of adolescent sex offenders as described by Gail Ryan (Ryan & Lane 1991). Identifying antecedents, patterns of abusive behaviour and high-risk situations for individuals is met with less resistance when done by peers.

A strong motivating factor to remain in such a group can be the realisation that the young person has patterns similar to other offenders in the group, and Ryan believes this provides a source of hope for many young abusers.

Adults

Groups for adults may be mandated by the courts (as in groups for sexual abuse perpetrators) or be purely voluntary, run by the adults themselves (as in groups for adult survivors of abuse). They may also not be strictly mandatory, but members can feel pressured if they agree to attend a group for physically abusing parents (the sanction being that otherwise their child might be removed from home). Although mandates are often seen as anti-therapeutic by some agencies, there is evidence to show that a mandate to attend a group can help an offender to work through their level of denial. Superficial denials will already have been addressed in the selection and recruitment process. Obviously, no one can work with a person who totally denies their culpability, but most offenders have some cognitive distortion which enables them to live with the consequences of their behaviour. The compulsory element of a group and peer pressure exert force on the member to address these distortions (see Erooga *et al.* 1990).

Cognitive distortions are also used as coping mechanisms by survivors of abuse. The abuser passes on their own distortions to a child and 'grooms' the child to believe that they are responsible for their own abuse. The guilt that ensues is a result of that distortion and may protect a child from facing their own fear. In a group setting, members can recognise the unjustified guilt of others more easily than their own, and so can facilitate an understanding of the process for themselves as well as others.

Yassen & Glass (1984), discussing their model of group work with adult survivors of rape, suggest similarly that witnessing the irrationality of others' guilt feelings can help group members to identify and face their own guilt. They also point out that members of such a group can go through an early stage where they suggest that their own rape was 'not so bad' or 'worse than' that of another group member. They see this as an attempt to validate members' own experience and to determine whether the group will meet their needs. This kind of comparison may therefore be useful in helping a survivor to place their own abuse in context, and to have witnesses who accept the nature of their experience.

Women who have physically abused their children often feel isolated and are frequently unsupported by partners or relatives. A group can reduce isolation, overcome stigma, provide an opportunity to work through childhood trauma and a practical forum for education on child care matters (Bannister & Prodgers 1983). Such groups can work well on a 'slow open' basis. This type of group would be unlikely to be mandatory, and there may be little pressure to attend but, as with all groups, a contract must be agreed between workers and members about attendance, confidentiality, group language and respect. A crèche may be provided, and it is important that boundaries are not broken by mothers crossing over into the crèche, or by children invading the mothers' group.

Groups for mothers who have physically abused their children can often contain a very high proportion of women who have been sexually abused in childhood. Often the group is the first place where they are able to share this. The main aims of such a group would be to improve the relationship between mother and child through insight and catharsis (Bannister 1985). There may not be sufficient time for members to work in detail on their own abuse, but they may then be sufficiently empowered to join a group for adult survivors.

Summing up a review of the literature on group therapy with adult survivors of abuse, Sheldon (1998) states that all the authors agree that group work is particularly suited to addressing the issues of secrecy, mistrust, isolation, low self-esteem, shame and self-blame. She goes on to show that the group work approach has been extremely effective with women who have been sexually abused in childhood. She states that in her experience such groups should run for about 20 sessions, each session should last for $1\frac{1}{2}$ hours and should be 'closed' to new members. A new group is then started after a short interval, and some members may rejoin for a further 20 sessions.

Following the inter-agency model described earlier in this chapter, Sheldon, who is a psychotherapist, works with several other professionals from different backgrounds. She stresses the need for structure in survivors' groups, especially when they are just starting, but points out that this diminishes as the group progresses. She reminds us, however, that careful boundaries of safety remain the responsibility of the group facilitators.

Most groups for adults who have experienced traumatic childhoods take some time to develop trust and cohesiveness. However, the facilitators of a group for women who had been mistreated by pathological mothers (Roback *et al.* 1981) felt that their group bonded immediately. They considered that this was because no one before had ever appreciated what the members' lives had been like, in particular how their childhood experience of abusing mothers had led them to build conflictual relationships with abusing men in adulthood.

This reminds us of the long-term damage that abusive parents can cause to children, both male and female. Groups for males who have suffered childhood trauma are less well-reported, but authors (Singer 1989) report similar feelings of low self-esteem and difficulties in relationships amongst male survivors in groups.

There is very little in the literature to date on the necessity of male perpetrators of abuse receiving therapeutic work for their own experiences of childhood abuse. Most groups for perpetrators concentrate largely on the necessary behavioural treatment. Members learn about their own triggers for thinking about abusing and how to control their reactions. This is vital, but the work could perhaps be extended by running parallel groups for such perpetrators to work on their own trauma, whether it be physical, sexual or emotional. Sometimes, of course, this is done in individual therapy sessions, but it might be more productive for men who are already experienced members of their behavioural group to have another group as described. One of the main difficulties might be in keeping the boundaries of the two groups separate.

Mothers whose children have been sexually abused are often totally neglected by the child protection agencies who care for the children and by the agencies who treat offenders. Women in this situation are often desperate to talk to other women who have gone through, or are undergoing, this experience. Some authors (Print & Dey 1998) feel that groups for such women rarely suffice as the only form of therapeutic intervention. They feel strongly that individual work should be offered to women who have difficulty in coping with this almost impossible situation. It is particularly difficult for women who have been abused themselves, and such women may well need some intensive individual work following practical intervention and support provided by social workers. A group, however, can provide another dimension in empowerment for women who have felt severely disempowered in their lives. Print & Dey also point out that mothers are generally the most important agents in ensuring that their children survive abuse and remain protected. A group can provide the essential support that women need for this demanding task.

Problems

Difficulties with a group can begin at conception unless careful negotiation is carried out within the agency and between agencies if necessary. Receiving suitable referrals may be dependent upon a trusting relationship which referrers have with group workers, so time spent in building this will be rewarded. Equally, a group can be ruined by jealousies or misunderstandings between co-workers, and it is here that a good consultant is invaluable. A group member who feels they have joined unwillingly may become a saboteur, so assessment of motivation is important.

In the case of children and adolescents, it cannot be emphasised too strongly that parents or carers should be carefully prepared for the group and also supported for its duration.

The birth of a group can be difficult if group members feel workers have not been entirely truthful as to the scope of the group or its purpose. Emergencies such as the illness of a co-worker should be discussed in advance, so that decisions can be made about groups being run with only one worker. Planned absences for holidays, for instance, can usually be managed successfully if the group knows what to expect.

Often people continue their most accustomed role in groups. This could be the scapegoat or victim, the 'wet blanket', the 'controller', and so on. It is unhelpful, not only for that person, but also for other group members if this is allowed to continue for long. The most effective way to combat this is not to protect the scapegoat or discipline the controller, but to point out what seems to be happening and to allow the group process to take effect. In addition, group 'games' or exercises which give people a chance to practise other roles can be facilitating.

Group members who drop out may make the rest of the group feel rejected. They should be encouraged to compose a letter or to contact the members directly to sort out the problem. If the member does not return, the group will need to discuss the loss and to air grief and anger. Sometimes a group member may remain in the group but refuse to join in. The group workers should not use pressure to persuade the member to join in, but should try and encourage them to do so. If a facilitating move is not successful a discussion with the carer, in the case of a young person, or with the referrer may be helpful. If the problem persists it should be openly addressed within the group.

Closure may also be a problem for many groups in child protection. Often members will have suffered abrupt and traumatic endings to relationships and may have been advised to 'forget' parents or others who have abandoned them. Allowing members to work through their grief and anger about closure of the group is an important part of healing. Closing rituals are also necessary for each session of a group. Children may decide for themselves that a particular game will always be played at the end of a session. Adolescents may prefer to make a single statement to the group about their feelings at the end. Some adults may accept a physical closure such as standing in a circle with hands touching.

Co-workers should ensure that they discuss their own issues about endings with their consultant.

Some people find closure so difficult that they leave the group prematurely or they invent reasons why the group must continue beyond its allotted span. Again, premature departure can be explained to the group so that they do not feel abandoned and their sense of loss at the ending of the group can be acknowledged.

Most 'group problems' have occurred before within groups, and an experienced consultant can help to allay fears that one's own group is particularly difficult. The worker's self-esteem can easily be undermined, so the worker should allow sufficient time for preparation and debriefing, and be clear that this time is just as essential as the time spent actually running the group.

Summary and conclusion

Therapeutic group work has a history which brings together the work of the pioneers in medicine, sociometry and social work. It can be used with good effect in many populations in child protection agencies. It requires careful planning, both from the agency and the workers, and there is a multiplicity of methods which can be applied according to the skills and experience of the workers and the group. Problems can be recognised and overcome.

Reports of groups run by practitioners seldom contain much information about evaluation. This may be because it is difficult to measure progress in an objective way. Hiebert-Murphy *et al.* (1992) made careful evaluations of groups for girls from 3 to 12 years which showed improvement in functioning and behaviour on measured scales. In my own groups, I have used evaluation forms as described by Giarretto (1989), and also questionnaires which I have devised with colleagues. Groups for which I have acted as consultant have held post-group interviews for the purpose of filling in the evaluation forms. If this is done, care must be taken to advise members that this will be happening, otherwise some members may feel distressed to be contacted some months later. Dwivedi & Mymin (1993) give a thorough discussion of the literature on the evaluation of groups for adolescents and children, including the grid technique, assessment scales and self-report questionnaires. Benson (1987) reminds us that evaluation should be considered at the planning stage, and suggests that members should be encouraged to keep a group diary which could be used for a group evaluation.

Group work can be a successful mode of therapy for many people, but it is important to remember that some may need individual work first. Working with therapeutic groups can be frustrating and time-consuming. It can also be rewarding, for both members and workers, and extremely satisfying. In self-evaluations, the majority of members find groups to have been a nurturing, satisfactory experience which has brought long-lasting benefits.

Annotated further reading

Bach G R 1954 Intensive group psychotherapy. Ronald Press, New York
Describes a system of group development – helpful for a basic understanding of groups.
Benson J F 1987 Working more creatively with groups. Tavistock, London
A comprehensive practical guide to planning, running and ending a group, using many techniques such as Gestalt, psychosynthesis, psychodrama, art therapy, drama therapy, etc.
Bion W R 1961 Experiences in groups. Tavistock, London
Well-known theories on psychotherapeutic groups, basic to understanding process.
Brands D, Philips H 1978 The gamester's handbook. Hutchinson, London
Dozens of useful ideas for group activities.
Brown A 1992 Group work, 3rd edn. Ashgate, Aldershot
Brings the original 1979 edition up to date with new chapters on groups in residential settings and on the significance of race and gender in group work.
Dwivedi K N (ed) 1993 Group work with children and adolescents. Jessica Kingsley, London
A wide selection of chapters focusing on young people. The chapter by Dwivedi & Mymin is particularly helpful.
Ernst S, Goodison L 1981 In our own hands. The Women's Press, London
Full of empowering exercises and ideas for use in women's groups.
Lewis T, Gordon R 1997 Groupwork. In: Turning points: a resource pack. NSPCC, Chailey Heritage; Department of Health, Leicester
Groups for children, especially disabled children, are described.
Sanderson C 1995 Group treatment. In: Counselling abult survivors of child sexual abuse. Jessica Kingsley, London, ch 10 (1991, reprinted 1995)
Gives advantages and disadvantages of groups. Good section on problems.
Tuckman B W 1965 Developmental sequence in small groups. Psychological Bulletin 63: 324–399
A good explanation of how groups behave, 'forming, norming, storming and performing'. Reassuring to know your group's behaviour is probably not unique. Simplifies Bach's original system of group development.
Whitaker D 1985 Using groups to help people. Routledge, London
Broad scope, many kinds of group discussed. Particularly good on selection for a group, commitment of facilitators and problems when the group is ongoing. Hardly mentions consultancy, though.
Yalom I 1975 The theory and practice of group psychotherapy. Basic Books, New York
A basic text for understanding group dynamics and psychotherapeutic issues.

References

Bannister A 1985 Psychodrama with abusing parents. Community Care, November
Bannister A 1997 The healing drama: psychodrama and dramatherapy with abused children. Free Association Books, London
Bannister A (ed) 1998 From hearing to healing: working with the aftermath of child sexual abuse. John Wiley, Chichester (original published 1992, Longman, Harlow)
Bannister A, Gallagher E 1996 Children who sexually abuse other children. The Journal of Sexual Aggression 2 (2): 87–98
Bannister A 1983 Dramatic recovery. Social Work Today 14 (18): 14–15
Bannister A, Prodgers A 1983 Actions speak louder than words. Community Care 472: 22–23
Barnet S, Corder F, Jehu D 1990 Group treatment for women sex offenders. Groupwork 3 (2): 191–203
Benson J F 1987 Working more creatively with groups. Tavistock, London
Berliner L, Ernst S 1982 Group treatment with pre-adolescent sexual assault survivors. In: Stuart I, Greer J (eds) Survivors of sexual aggression: men, women and children. Van Nostrand Reinhold, New York
Blick L C Porter F S 1982 Group therapy with female adolescent incest victims. In: Sgroi S M (ed) Handbook of clinical intervention in child sexual abuse. Lexington Books, Lexington, Massachussats
Breen H 1994 Child sexual abuse: parent group leads to community and social action. Canadian Journal of Public Health 85: 381–384
Carlson-Sabelli L 1998 Children's therapeutic puppet theatre. Action, interaction and cocreation. The International Journal of Action Methods 51 (3): 91–112
Cattanach A 1992 Play therapy with abused children. Jessica Kingsley, London
Colton M, Vanstone M 1996 Betrayal of trust: sexual abuse by men who work with children. Free Association Books, London
Corder B, Haizlip T, Deboer P 1990 A pilot study for a structured, time-limited therapy group for sexually abused pre-adolescent children. Child Abuse and Neglect 14: 243–251

Cowburn M 1990 Work with male sex offenders in groups. Groupwork 3 (2): 157–171

Craig E 1990 Starting the journey. Groupwork 3 (2): 113–117

Dwivedi K N (ed) 1993 Groupwork with children and adolescents. Jessica Kingsley, London

Dwivedi K N, Mymin D 1993 In: Dwivedi K N (ed) Groupwork with children and adolescents. Jessica Kingsley, London

Erooga M, Clark P L, Bentley M 1990 Protection, control and treatment. Groupwork 3 (2): 172–190

Finkelhor D 1984 Child sexual abuse: new theory and research. Free Press, New York

Fox J 1987 The essential Moreno. Springer, New York

Foulkes S H, Anthony E J 1957 Group psychotherapy: the psychoanalytic approach. Penguin, Harmondsworth

Frey-Angel J 1989 Treating children in violent families: a sibling group approach. Social Work with Multi-Family Groups 12 (1): 95–107

Giarretto H 1989 Treatment and training manual. ICEF programme, California

Herman J L 1998 Trauma and recovery: from domestic abuse to political terror. Pandora, London (original published 1992)

Hoey B 1997 Who calls the tune?: a psychodramatic approach to child therapy. Routledge, London

Hiebert-Murphy D, De Luca R V, Runtz M N 1992 Group treatment for sexually abused girls: evaluating outcome. Families in Society (April): 205–213

Isaac C, Lane S 1990 The sexual abuse cycle in the treatment of adolescent sexual abusers. The Safer Society Press, Orwell, Vermont

Jennings S 1993 Playtherapy with children: a practitioner's guide. Blackwell Scientific, Oxford

Kreidler C, England D B 1990 Empowerment through group support: adult women who are survivors of incest. Journal of Family Violence 5 (1): 35–42

Lewis T, Gordon R 1997 Groupwork. In: Turning points: a resource pack. NSPCC, Chailey Heritage, Department of Health, Leicester

Lebacq M, Shah Z 1989 A group for black and white sexually abused children. Groupwork 2: 123–133

Maines B, Robinson G 1998 B/Gsteem: a self-esteem scale with locus of control items. Lucky Duck Publishers, Bristol

Macfarlane K, Cunningham C 1990 Steps to healthy touching. Kidsrights, Charlotte, North Carolina

Macfarlane K, Cunningham C 1991 Children who molest children. Safer Society Series. The Safer Society Press, Orwell, Vermont

Macfarlane K, Waterman J, Conerly S, *et al.* 1986 Sexual abuse of young children. Holt, Rinehart and Winston, London

Miller A 1983 For your own good. Faber & Faber, London

Moreno J L 1934 Who shall survive? A new approach to the problem of human interrelations. Nervous and Mental Diseases Publishing, Washington, DC

Naglieri J A, Le Buffe P A, Pfeiffer S I 1993 Devereux behavior rating scale – school form manual. Harcourt Brace, San Antonio

Print B, Dey C 1998 Empowering mothers of sexually abused children – a positive framework. In: Bannister A (ed) From hearing to healing. John Wiley, Chichester (orig. 1992 Longman, Harlow)

Print B, Morrison T 2000 Treating adolescents who sexually abuse others. In: Itzin C (ed) Home truths about child sexual abuse: influencing policy and practice. Routledge, London

Reeker J, Ensing D 1998 An evaluation of a group treatment for sexually abused young children. Journal of Child Sexual Abuse 7(2):

Reeker J, Ensing D, Elliott R 1997 A meta-analytic investigation of group treatment outcomes for sexually abused children. Child Abuse and Neglect 21(7): 669–680

Roback H B, Romfh H, Bottari M, Lutz D 1981 Group psychotherapy for adult women mistreated as children by pathological mothers. Child Abuse and Neglect 5: 343–349

Rosenwald P R 1989 Wee care: reaching teenage mothers and changing their lives. Children Today 28 (3): 28–30

Ryan G, Lane L 1991 Juvenile sexual offending, causes, consequences and correction. Lexington Books, Lexington, Massachusetts

Sanderson C 1995 Counselling adult survivors of child sexual abuse, 2nd edn. Jessica Kingsley, London

Sheldon H 1998 Working with adult female survivors. In: Bannister A (ed) From hearing to healing: working with the aftermath of child sexual abuse. John Wiley, Chichester, (original published 1992, Longman, Harlow)

Singer I 1989 Group work with men who experienced incest in childhood. American Journal of Orthopsychiatry 59 (3): 468–472

van der Kolk B A, McFarlane A C, Weisaeth L (eds) 1996 Traumatic stress: the effects of overwhelming experience on mind, body and society. Guilford, New York

Williams A 1991 Forbidden agendas. Routledge, London

Yassen J, Glass L 1984 Sexual assault survivors groups: a feminist practice perspective. Social Work (May–June): 252–257

26

Helping adult survivors of child sexual abuse

Liz Hall, Siobhan Lloyd

This chapter will examine a number of issues relating to work with adult survivors of child sexual abuse. It does not consider issues for adults who were abused in either a specific physical or emotional way, although it recognises that both of these forms of abuse often accompany sexual abuse. The long-term effects of these forms of child abuse have received rather less attention from researchers and writers on the subject, and it may be the case that survivors of these forms of abuse have not had their needs met to the same (limited) extent as survivors of sexual abuse. It is important at the outset to explore the reasons for including a chapter on working with adult survivors in a book that deals primarily with issues relating to children. There are two main reasons to consider. First, it is now recognised that childhood sexual abuse can have long-lasting psychological, emotional and physical consequences for a person well into adulthood (Browne & Finkelhor 1986, Russell 1986, Hall & Lloyd 1993, Kendall-Tackett et al. 1993). An understanding of these potential long-term effects can be helpful in working with children whose distress manifests in ways which, with hindsight, may provide clues to these consequences. Table 26.1 gives a summary of the long-term consequences. Many survivors of sexual abuse have also experienced other forms of abuse, which can compound their problems in later life. These long-term consequences are significant and they have facilitated the recognition that prevention and early identification of child sexual abuse should be a high priority for all health and social service agencies.

Second, through the process of disclosing their childhood experiences, adult survivors are improving our understanding of the nature of child abuse and the ways in which children of different ages cope with being repeatedly sexually abused. This pool of knowledge has broken the secrecy surrounding child sexual abuse and increased our awareness of major trauma in a child's life. This chapter concentrates on survivors who have been sexually abused by a trusted adult. Individuals who have experienced physical and emotional abuse and neglect suffer many of the same long-term consequences. These areas of child abuse are, however, less well researched. The majority of survivors currently seeking help are female, but an increasing number of male survivors are identifying themselves and literature is developing about them (Lew 1990). In the future, it is possible that an increasing number of male survivors will ask for help, as well as survivors, both male and female, who have been abused by women.

Recent research on adult survivors of child sexual abuse has continued to examine the long-term consequences of such abuse and to refine our understanding of the factors influencing the severity of these consequences. It has been shown that a history of child sexual abuse is associated with an increased use of medical services (Cunningham et al. 1988, Arnold et al. 1990, Felitti 1991) and psychiatric services (Shapiro 1987, Krarup et al. 1991, Waller 1991). A number of studies are also now beginning to clarify the relationship between aspects of the child's experience and the nature of the long-term consequences. For example, Wyatt & Newcomb (1990) showed that the nature and extent of the

Table 26.1

Summary of potential long-term consequences of child sexual abuse

Low self-esteem
Confusion

Emotional reactions:
 – guilt
 – anger and rage
 – sadness and grief
 – complete absence of emotional reaction

Depression

Anxiety problems:
 – generalised anxiety
 – panic attacks
 – specific fears and phobias
 – pronounced startle response

Isolation and alienation

Bad reactions to medical procedures:
 – hospital admissions
 – gynaecological procedures
 – dental procedures

Physical complaints

Sleep disturbance

Eating disorders
 – compulsive eating and obesity
 – bulimia
 – anorexia

Multiple personality disorder

Dissociative problems:
 – perceptual disturbances
 – flashbacks
 – nightmares/bad dreams
 – out of body experiences

Problems with trust

Victim behaviour
Further assault/revictimisation
General fear of men

Interpersonal difficulties:
 – in relationships with men
 – in relationships with women

Sexual problems:
 – impaired sexual arousal
 – difficulties with orgasm
 – lack of sexual motivation
 – lack of sexual satisfaction
 – guilt during sexual contact
 – vaginismus
 – pain during intercourse

Problems with touch
Parenting problems

Abuse of self:
 – self-mutilation and injury
 – suicide attempts

Substance abuse:
 – alcohol
 – drugs
 – transquillisers

Compulsive and obsessional problems

Under-achievement in education and occupation
Difficulty in sustaining positive experiences

long-term negative consequences for an adult were related to the closeness of the relationship between the child and the perpetrator, the severity of the abuse, the extent of self-blame and non-disclosure as a child about the abuse. Leitenberg *et al.* (1992) have further suggested that the abused child's coping strategies of suppressing and avoiding emotions are associated with poorer adjustment in adulthood.

There is now a growing awareness of the similarities in response to events which are 'outside usual experience' (Colodzin 1993), and there is a body of literature to support this (Herman 1992, Scott & Stradling 1992, Parkinson 1993). These events include bombings, air disasters, industrial accidents and, in relation to sexual violence, rape, sexual assault, child sexual abuse and domestic violence. They can lead to hypervigilence, an increased startle response, depression, general anxiety, dissociation and flashbacks, sleep problems and the development of 'survivor guilt'. These consequences are a normal response to these traumas and are summarised in the phrase 'post-traumatic stress disorder' but, as Colodzin points out, it is not always useful to think of the person's pattern of functioning as a disorder. He suggests that the phrase 'post-traumatic stress' is more appropriate because this makes it easier to concentrate on the person who has lived through something overwhelming rather than on the symptoms of a medically defined disorder. This encourages a focus on the healthy responses and survival mechanisms rather than on what is 'wrong' with the person.

Seeking help

Therapeutic work to overcome the effects of being abused as a child begins with a survivor's acknowledgement of the abuse. For some survivors, this acknowledgement is not possible for a number of reasons: the survivor may not remember the abuse; it is not the right time to disclose; the survivor does not feel safe enough with the helper or does not acknowledge that early experiences are having an effect on later life experiences. The survivor may, however, find that within the context of seeking help for another problem such as relationship difficulties, substance abuse or self-esteem problems, their history of sexual abuse emerges.

A survivor may come for help with a number of problems relating to the traumatic childhood experiences. Feelings of guilt, shame and helplessness, combined with fears of betrayal in close relationships may provoke a need to flee. The survivor can also fear disbelief, blame and rejection. From the outset, therefore, the helper should aim to establish an accepting relationship so that the survivor knows they are believed and taken seriously. For the helper, this may involve suspending any preconceived ideas about sexual abuse, actively listening to the survivor, responding with warmth, support and interest, going at the survivor's pace and respecting the survivor's right to remain silent about any issue.

The specific aims of the work will vary according to the needs of the survivor and the setting in which it takes place. General aims include enabling the survivor to talk about childhood experiences so that an understanding of the long-term effects is reached, facilitating the safe release of emotions, exploring any losses resulting from childhood, breaking the secret of the past and gaining an acceptance of it so that the future can be faced with more optimism and hope.

When survivors make the decision to seek help, they are making a first important step in coming to terms with their childhood experiences. It may have taken months or years to get to this point, and knowing what sources of help are available locally can be difficult. There are few specialist resources for survivors, but increasing numbers of helpers in statutory and non-statutory agencies are developing their work and training in this area.

In the statutory sector, family doctors are often the first person a survivor tells about childhood experiences. The doctor's reaction can determine whether further help is sought or made available. Referral can then be made to a clinical psychologist, psychiatrist, counsellor or psychotherapist working in the health service, or to a social worker or specialist worker in a voluntary agency. There are also therapists and counsellors in the private sector who work with survivors. Rape crisis centres and community mental health resources are also good local sources of help.

Professionals in nursing, social work, health visiting, community work, clinical psychology and psychiatry increasingly find clients disclosing a history of sexual abuse. It would not, therefore, be helpful to argue that only specialists in working with survivors are the most appropriate source of help. More realistic and helpful to survivors is training for these and other professionals; training which enables helpers to confront the difficult issues faced in working with survivors and building on skills which they already possess (Hall & Lloyd 1993). Training should, at the very least, include input on the reality of sexual abuse and challenging the myths about abuse. It should also address practice issues relating to disclosure.

Knowing what resources are available locally can be the most difficult part of the search for help, and, until the survivor has reliable information about local

Table 26.2
Questions to ask about sources of help

Can I refer myself?
If not, do I need to have a letter from my doctor?
Will notes be kept on my visits?
Who will see these notes?
Will information about me be sent to my doctor?
Can I see what is written about me?
Will I be able to get time off from work to attend for help?
Will I have to pay?
Are child care facilities available?
How regular will the sessions be?
How long will each session last?
Who will be present?
Where will we meet? (Hospital, own home, helper's office?)
Who else will my helper speak to about me?
Can I stop attending if it gets too difficult?
How will I know when it is time to end my contact?

resources, it is impossible to make an informed choice about an appropriate source of help. There are a number of questions which might be asked before deciding which route to pursue. These are listed in Table 26.2.

An additional, but no less significant, issue is that of the increased distress a survivor might feel once they start talking about their experiences. Relationships with partners, family members and their own children can all be affected. Child care issues may come to the fore, particularly if the level of distress reaches a point where the survivor becomes unable to provide adequate care. In these circumstances low self-esteem and a sense of failure can pervade, and in extreme circumstances children may need to be taken into care. It is hardly surprising that a survivor can feel as if he/she is doubly failing here, yet letting go of responsibility for others might be a significant part of their healing process.

A framework for working with survivors of child sexual abuse

In this section, key features of work with an adult survivor of child sexual abuse are considered, showing how they can facilitate the healing process and allow the individual to reverse some features of their childhood experiences. This framework fosters an understanding that links the survivor's experiences as a child with difficulties, strengths and resources as an adult. The key aim of the approach is to create a relationship between the helper and the survivor that acts as a partnership, using their collective resources to enable the survivor to come to terms with the past. It is important to start from the adult's childhood experiences and not to discount the very significant developmental effects that the experience of being abused may have had.

As a child who has been sexually abused grows into adulthood, feelings of powerlessness, lack of choice and control can continue, resulting in an expectation of betrayal by others. Issues of trust predominate and are obvious within a therapeutic relationship. The framework for therapeutic work should therefore address the key issues of power, choice, boundaries, understanding, attachment (Briere 1996) and trust. It is also necessary to consider issues relating to the silence and secrecy surrounding the abuse.

Power

Children have little or no power and are expected to obey the adult who is abusing them. The abuser, however, misuses the position of power and responsibility they have over the child. The helper is likely to be seen by the survivor as more knowledgeable, powerful, expert and important. This imbalance of power can reflect the survivor's view of authority figures and can also reinforce a lack of self-esteem. This is the reality of many therapeutic situations and, in order to redress this imbalance of power to some extent, the survivor's strengths, resources and courage should be acknowledged, valued and used within the helping situation. For example, if the survivor uses writing to describe feelings relating to the abuse and other childhood experiences, this can be used constructively to further an understanding of these emotional reactions. Ultimately, the survivor is the best judge of how he/she feels, even if the helper has to assist in finding the right words to describe these reactions.

The helper can empower the survivor primarily by listening, believing any disclosures about traumatic childhood experiences and showing acceptance without judgement. Acceptance by the helper should enable the survivor to begin to value his/her strengths and resources and to use them more constructively. In this way, the survivor can be empowered to take control and regain a sense of personal worth and power.

Choice and control

A child has little or no choice or control over what happens in an abusive situation, although the abuser may have led the child to believe that they did have a choice. The therapeutic framework can reverse this by providing choice over certain aspects of the helping situation. The most important relates to disclosure of details of the abusive experiences. Survivors should have choice about when, how much and to whom they choose to tell about the abuse. They often report feeling forced to tell a helper what happened to them as children, with no consideration given to the consequences this might have in terms of continuing contact after the disclosure and their possible need for support.

The gender of the helper can be very important because many survivors find it difficult to work with someone of the same gender as the abuser. For women who were abused by men, the initial choice is often for a female helper, but a male helper can have beneficial effects in learning to trust a man. This can have positive implications for relationships generally.

Other areas where the survivor can have choice relate to the location and timing of sessions with the helper and other people available for support. Some survivors, for example, prefer not to meet the helper in the helper's office. Others might not be able to ask for time off from work to attend regular sessions and prefer to organise the time during lunchtime or after work. Where possible, these preferences should be respected. The process of coming to terms with sexual abuse can be greatly facilitated if the survivor feels comfortable, unpressured and in control of the helping process.

Boundaries

Normal physical and emotional boundaries between adult and child are violated when an adult sexually abuses a child. This can leave a child with problems in developing a clear sense of boundaries. Within the helping situation, it is essential that clear boundaries are established, so that there is no danger of the survivor being victimised again by the helping situation. Boundaries relating to confidentiality, the length and frequency of sessions with the helper, and the level of support available between sessions should be established early and may need regular review, especially at times of crisis or when the survivor is involved in a period of disclosure.

It is also essential that boundaries relating to touch are agreed. Touch should be used with great caution and, if at all, in a limited way, only with the survivor's permission. Issues of gender are very important in this respect, and touch may be more acceptable, for example, from female helpers working with female survivors. Regrettably, some survivors have been sexually abused by their helpers (Armsworth 1989). Helpers need to be aware of any of their actions which might be felt by survivors to be in any way abusive. This clearly calls for a substantial degree of self-awareness. The issue of confidentiality should be discussed openly, with the survivor's wishes respected in this matter. Information about the agency's policy concerning confidentiality should be given so that the survivor knows what the guidelines are. It is also important to indicate how much of the content of sessions with the helper will be recorded and how much, when and with whom the survivor may be discussed by the helper in supervision and support meetings, in meetings with other helpers, or with members of the survivor's wider support network.

Problems relating to confidentiality may arise when a survivor is being seen by a number of different agencies, or by several members of a multidisciplinary team. In these situations, it is important to inform the survivor of any policies regarding confidentiality, particularly about any information that may have to be passed to another helper. The helper is responsible for drawing the boundaries clearly and for explaining them to the survivor.

Understanding

Children are unlikely to have any real understanding of what is happening during the abuse. They may have no words, concepts or knowledge to allow them to describe the sexual abuse – even to themselves. A child may have feelings that range from extremes of love and respect for the abuser to acute terror, pain and hatred.

An important aspect of the framework for helping adult survivors of child abuse is to facilitate an understanding of how the experience of being abused has affected them, both as a child and as an adult. This could include recognising the ways the child used to cope with and survive the trauma. Linking the abuse with adult difficulties should enable survivors to recognise the relevance of the abuse to their development and facilitate the process of coming to terms with it.

Part of this aspect of the framework could include helping the survivor to understand the helping process. Predicting and managing potential crises, difficult times and the effects of doing certain aspects of the work can be shared between the helper and the survivor. This is likely to help the survivor to use their resources and the resources of any support network, including the helper, to minimise potential problems. For example, if the survivor is about to do some disclosure work, the possible short-term effects and difficulties can be anticipated and relevant support sought during this time. Thus, the survivor is more able to be actively involved in the helping process and can make choices to maximise the success of the work.

Trust

When children have been sexually abused by adults, they have been betrayed by someone who should have been protecting them from harm and danger. One consequence of this is that survivors may expect to be betrayed or let down by people in authority. This is compounded if a survivor's confidence in another person has been betrayed as an adult. Many survivors come for help having had previous unsuccessful or unhelpful contacts with helping agencies. It is therefore important for the survivor to be given enough time to learn to trust the helper, and not to be pressurised to say more than they want to. Building trust takes time, and this process can easily be disrupted by situations that seem unimportant to the helper. For example, if the helper fails to return a telephone call, a survivor may find it difficult to trust the helper. Trust tends to be experienced as 'all or nothing' by survivors.

Breaking the silence and secrecy

A child is often unable to tell anyone about the abuse. The abuser may have used threats of violence or threatened the family. The child may also be unable to tell because of a sense of guilt and shame, or because there was no one to tell who might have believed. The child's coping mechanisms may complicate this further, as a child may deny, dissociate from, minimise or rationalise the abuse, so that telling someone becomes even more difficult. Finally, a young child does not have words and concepts to describe the abuse, thus making disclosure nearly impossible.

The burden of keeping the secret can cause many psychological and physical problems that can be resolved through talking about these experiences (Lister 1982). Disclosure requires sensitive handling and careful monitoring afterwards, as it can be both a liberating and painful process. Through disclosure, however, the survivor can discover that the abuser was responsible, that a child has a right to have protection and care from an adult, and that the emotional energy used to maintain the silence can become available for more positive use in adult life. Many long-term problems can be resolved through talking about the abuse within a sensitive and accepting environment. The helper will therefore have to be prepared to hear about the trauma of the abuse and its associated emotions, and be able to set aside preconceived ideas and myths about child abuse. For the survivor, being accepted by the helper when the helper knows 'the worst' can lead to a significant improvement in self-esteem.

By addressing these issues within the helping process, the survivor is helped to gain control and power over current problems, and they develop an understanding of the relevance of the abusive experiences to their development. It also facilitates acknowledgement of the survivor's strengths and resources and, perhaps for the first time, leads to feelings of being valued and respected. The legacy of sexual abuse and the burden of responsibility for the abuse can then be shifted to the abuser. Within this framework, a wide variety of therapeutic methods can be used to address particular issues. By starting with the child's experience, the helping process immediately gives the sexual abuse a central place in the work, thus allowing for the potential for resolution of traumatic experiences.

Adult survival strengths

One of the main resources available in coming to terms with the abuse are those personal resources and strengths developed by the survivor in order to survive the abuse. A useful starting point can be the confirmation of the strength and courage involved in surviving into adulthood and in seeking help. There is a continuum of coping behaviours used by survivors. At one end are strategies like alcohol and drug abuse, suicide attempts and other types of self-injury. At the other end, there are survivors who channel all their energies into being high achievers in education or employment. Some see their coping mechanisms as something to be ashamed of, and they may not wish to admit to them. It can also be difficult for the helper to confirm these strengths with the survivor when they are both working on difficult and painful memories and feelings.

Some coping mechanisms develop into clear strengths, such as becoming self-sufficient or being steady in a crisis. Others can develop into self-destructive patterns of behaviour. There are also behaviours which have both healthy and destructive aspects – high achievement in academic matters may secure a college place or a good job, but it may lead the survivor into becoming more socially isolated from other people as their energy is channelled into the pursuit of academic success.

The task for the helper here is to identify and examine the survivor's coping mechanisms, and to see which ones may still be useful in adulthood. For example, writing can be a useful way of expressing the pain of childhood or disclosing aspects of the abuse that are difficult to express verbally. Other examples include work, educational or family achievements.

In recent years, the resourcefulness of survivors has been shown in the growth of published material written by survivors themselves in the form of poems, autobiographical accounts, songs, letters and self-help books (Evert & Bijkerk 1987, Spring 1987, Finney 1990, Malone *et al.* 1996). These have been crucial in breaking the silence about child sexual abuse and in educating professionals about the experience and effects of abuse in a very direct, accessible way. This literature has also played an important part in enabling survivors to see that they are not alone in their experience, that other survivors have struggled with similar difficulties, and that recovery is possible.

The false memory debate

Any discussion on aspects of sexual abuse can trigger strong feelings and reactions. Walker (1998) wisely points out an enduring irony of the 1970s and 1980s where, on one hand, feminists accused professionals of denying the reality of abuse, with a resultant silencing of survivors, whilst at the same time social workers, in particular, were often charged with removing children from actually or potentially abusive homes without sufficient cause. In the 1990s the pendulum has moved to the other extreme with helpers villified for being over-zealous and 'planting' the idea of abuse where it has not occurred. The issue of 'recovered memories' is highly contentious and belies the fact that many survivors enter counselling with clear memories of abuse and others may recover memories whilst in therapy (British Psychological Society 1995). Walker (1996) also makes clear the importance of helpers taking great care not to be in any way suggestive to clients, not to use methods such as hypnosis and to handle all aspects of memory with great care. She says:

Whichever way the argument goes, the crux is that it is all in someone's mind: either the mistaken client's or the unscrupulous therapist's – someone must be fantasising somewhere. A convenient escape route for the perpetrator, with the counsellor and therapist too often becoming a handy fall guy, and another avoidance of the real issues of recognising the extent of abuse and the seriousness of its effects.

(Walker 1996, p. 60)

The complex nature of memory, in particular how it deals with the trauma associated with sexual abuse, is in need of further research in a way in which the results of laboratory experiments are not applied uncritically to the process of therapeutic work. Van der Kolk and his associates (Van der Kolk *et al.* 1996) have begun to examine the biological and physiological aspects of traumatic memory. A final word here – despite the continuing controversy surrounding false/recovered memory there is little indication that it has deterred adults who were sexually abused as children from seeking help to deal with issues from their past.

Case study

A case study provides a useful means to look at the application of this framework in practice, with a particular focus on the first session between the survivor and the helper.

Background

A 30-year-old woman – we shall call her Anne – attends a counselling agency for her first appointment. She was sexually abused as a child between the ages of 6 and 13 by her father, a successful businessman. He abused Anne at her home when her mother was out working night shifts as a nurse. He was physically violent to his wife and to Anne and her two younger sisters. Anne suspects that he sexually abused them too. She has never spoken about the sexual abuse to anyone. Her father died suddenly of a heart attack about a year ago, and the family have had problems in coming to terms with his death.

Anne works as a primary school teacher. She has a partner and two young children. Her oldest child – a daughter – has just started school. Anne's partner does not know that she was abused as a child, but Anne thinks he would not understand how she feels. Over the last 6 weeks, Anne has been having nightmares, increasing problems in going to work and difficulties in her sexual relationship with her partner. She told her general practitioner (GP) of these difficulties, but not about the abuse, and he suggested that she go to a counselling agency to talk over her problems. Anne feels that she will finally have to tell someone about the sexual abuse, as she is beginning to wonder if it is really the cause of her problems. She has misgivings about disclosing the abuse, particularly as she has no information about the helper she is to see. She is pleased to know that she will be seeing a woman.

First session

The helper encourages Anne to talk about what has brought her to the agency at this time. Anne tells her about current problems and a little of her family background. Anne does not feel pressurised and is surprised that the helper seems genuinely interested in her problems but does not come up with easy solutions that might have made Anne feel dismissed. Anne says that she was relieved to know that her helper would be a woman.

She decides that she has to tell the helper about the fact that she was sexually abused and that her nightmares have been about these experiences, many of which she has forgotten. The helper listens without appearing shocked, surprised or disgusted by this information. She asks if Anne wants to talk more about the abuse during the session and congratulates her for sharing this information, recognising the difficulty that Anne may have felt before telling her. Anne feels that she cannot say any more at this stage, but says that she would like to talk more on a later occasion. Thus, the helper gives Anne choice and respects her decision not to say more at this stage, giving her as much control as possible within the helping situation.

Before the end of the session, the helper summarises their meeting, placing Anne's initial disclosure about the sexual abuse as a very important factor in the difficulties that she is having. Anne feels considerably reassured that she is experiencing similar problems to others who have been sexually abused. From the outset, the helper facilitates an understanding of the relevance of the sexual abuse to Anne's difficulties, indicating that, if she wants, she can talk about the abuse when she is ready.

The helper offers Anne the opportunity to talk in further sessions about her problems, and about the abuse if she wants to. Anne agrees to this, and she is given choice in deciding the most appropriate time for her next session. They agree that they will meet for four further sessions before reviewing the situation. Each session will last for approximately an hour and will, where possible, be held in the same room as the initial session. Anne comments that she is glad to be meeting the helper in the agency's office, as this assures her of anonymity which is not available to her in her GP's surgery.

The helper discusses confidentiality with Anne and says that she discusses her work on a regular basis with a supervisor. She assures Anne that although she may discuss Anne's case with her supervisor, any personal details which could lead to her being identified will remain confidential. Anne is concerned that her employer will be able to find out that she is attending for help, but is reassured that this information will not be shared. She feels she would like her GP to know, however, and agrees that she would like to tell him about the abuse but may need the helper's support in doing this.

The helper stresses that Anne has a choice about how much and when she wishes to discuss the abuse, but that it will probably be helpful to talk more at some point. However, her right to remain silent will be respected. She also tells Anne that she may experience strong emotional reactions now that she has discussed the abuse and suggests that she might look at available sources of support for herself before she returns for the next appointment. Anne does not feel that her partner will be very supportive, but she has a good friend whom she has supported in the past. This person knows about Anne's appointment with the helper.

The helper has helped to establish the framework from the outset. She indicates that choice about the range of issues to be covered will rest with Anne. She indicates the boundaries to their sessions and is clear about confidentiality. She respects Anne's decision to disclose the secret of the abuse and indicates that further discussion of the abuse may be necessary. She also confirms the place that the abuse has in Anne's difficulties. Throughout, the helper acknowledges Anne's strengths in disclosing but does not pressurise her for further information. By listening and accepting Anne and not making light of her problems, she is validating Anne's experiences, and in so doing is empowering her to begin the process of recovery from the abuse.

Over the next year, Anne meets the helper on a regular basis, initially once a week and later at less frequent intervals. The focus of the work initially was to facilitate Anne's disclosure of her childhood experiences and to examine the effects of the sexual abuse on her as a child. She identified that she still blamed herself for the abuse and was encouraged to look at the lack of choice, power and control that she had over her situation as a child. She had previously underestimated the effects of the fear generated by her father's violence and her need to protect her mother from any further problems. Her self-esteem improved as she placed responsibility for the abuse on her father and when she felt able to disclose details of the abuse, the nightmares and flashbacks she had been experiencing diminished significantly.

Eventually, she was able to tell her partner of her childhood experiences and was surprised to discover that he had already suspected the fact, as he had witnessed her nightmares. Together, they were able to look at the effect it had on their sexual relationship with guidance and support from the helper and by reading a number of useful books.

By the end of the year Anne felt that she no longer needed to come to the agency and was proposing to discuss gradually her experience of abuse with her sisters. She had also made plans to educate her own children realistically about child abuse, and to discuss introducing a child abuse prevention programme with colleagues at the school where she worked.

Therapeutic contexts

A survivor needs to consider whether a one-to-one setting or a group context with other survivors would be preferred. At some stage, some work with other family members or with a partner may be requested. It is obviously preferable for a survivor to make use of resources located in the community, but sometimes an in-patient admission to a psychiatric hospital or unit may be necessary because the survivor is experiencing severe depression or suicidal feelings. Admission to hospital can give the survivor a period of rest away from the pressures of everyday life and a safe environment whilst difficult disclosure work is undertaken. There are a number of potential difficulties posed by a hospital admission, the main one relating to confidentiality and trust if the survivor is expected to talk to several members of staff about the abusive experiences.

One-to-one settings

Most survivors choose a one-to-one therapeutic situation, preferring the confidentiality and sense of security it offers. Waiting times for an appointment can be a problem, however, and this can sometimes leave the survivor feeling abandoned after having made the courageous first step in seeking help. There are a number of issues which can arise for both the survivor and helper in a one-to-one setting. It can establish a long-term trusting relationship with someone who believes the survivor, details of the abuse are confidential to one person, and the therapeutic work can be done at the survivor's own pace. Survivors can sometimes fear the intensity of the work. They can also be concerned with burdening the helper with details of the abuse, and this can result in protecting the helper from their pain. For the helper, on the other hand, there may be concerns about over-involvement or dependency on the part of the survivor.

Table 26.3
Group settings: advantages and limitations

Advantages	Limitations
Survivors share the burden of the abuse with others who have been through similar experiences.	Group setting may be too threatening for some survivors.
Emotional and social isolation is reduced when survivors realise they are not the only ones to have been abused.	Confidentiality may be more difficult to maintain.
It can help survivors to face the reality of what has happened.	Individuals may feel excluded or need more individual attention.
It can validate as normal a survivor's feelings of guilt, anger, grief, loneliness and other long-term effects.	Survivors may need more regular support than the group can offer.
More established members can acknowledge the progress they have made and can give hope to newer members.	Hearing about the experiences of others may be too painful.
Group can be a place of safety to express true feelings and emotions.	There may be a reluctance to participate in the group if the survivor feels he/she has not suffered as much as others in the group.

Survivors' groups

A survivor may decide to move on from an individual source of help to a self-help group whose members are survivors. Alternatively, a survivors' group can be the main source of help from the outset. Table 26.3 lists the main advantages and limitations of such groups.

Sgroi (1989) suggests that group members should plan to be seen individually by another helper outside the therapeutic group whilst the group is meeting. This, she suggests, will secure time for working through issues specific to the individual which have been triggered by the group experience.

Groups can be open-ended or closed, and there are advantages and disadvantages to each type. The former can provide immediate access when it is needed, and members at different stages can give each other encouragement and support. It is, however, difficult to build trust and to undertake planned work when group membership constantly changes. Variable attendance and issues relating to confidentiality are additional problems in open-ended groups.

Closed groups have the advantage of a more easily established climate of trust and greater ease in establishing and maintaining a group culture. Members can also get to know each other over a period of time, and can move on together from one issue to another. One disadvantage is the difficulty of leaving if the group is not meeting the needs of the individual. There are three types of survivors' groups:

Self-help groups

These are formed by survivors themselves, without the support of professionals or volunteers. They usually operate without a formal leader, and the main difficulties they face relate to maintaining continuity, boundaries and the powerful effects of hearing about the experiences of others before the survivor is ready for this. Their strengths are related to their immediate availability and the use of survivors' own strengths, resources and experiences to help each other.

Therapeutic groups

These are groups that are usually time-limited, more highly structured and facilitated by trained staff or volunteers. Potential members may be screened for membership, allowing the facilitator to assess the survivor's readiness for joining the group. The emphasis is on working together to understand, learn and move on from the experience of childhood sexual abuse.

Pressure/social action groups

Here, the emphasis of the group is on raising the public profile of the issue of sexual abuse. Organising such a group can be an empowering experience, and it is also a way of informing the local community about an issue of great social importance.

Working with partners

As more survivors seek help in dealing with issues from their past, a partner is often the first person a survivor tells about the abuse. This may be the result of feeling secure in a relationship, often for the first time; it can be the result of issues relating to pregnancy or children, or of difficulties which the couple experience in their relationship. It is not always possible, however, for survivors to work with their partners.

Partners themselves may need support during times of disclosure. They may find it difficult to understand the behaviour of a partner, and their relationship may experience significant change. There are three areas in which it can be helpful for partners to talk to someone: understanding the long-term effects of sexual abuse, gaining an understanding of the process of healing for the survivor, and consideration of the potential effects on the couple's relationship in the future. There are a number of helpful books which survivors can use with their partners, including *Allies in Healing* (Davis 1991) and *Outgrowing the Pain Together* (Gil 1992).

At some point, a survivor and their partner may wish to deal with the effects of the abuse on their sexual relationship. A useful book in this context is *The Sexual Healing Journey* (Maltz 1991). There are also agencies, for example Relate and some clinical psychology departments in healthcare trusts, that deal specifically with this area of work.

Conclusion

The partnership between survivors and their helpers has invoked a language to describe the child's experience in a way that has facilitated helpers to suspend any disbelief they might have, and to dispel any remaining myths about sexual abuse. If helpers can listen to and hear adults who tell them about their experiences as children, this can facilitate a true understanding of their experiences. Throughout the last decade, the voices of survivors heard in prose, poetry, song, letters and novels have provided a powerful testimony of painful childhood experiences. Despite advances in devising appropriate methods for communicating with children when there is a suspicion that they have been abused, it has been and continues to be adult survivors who convey a fuller knowledge of the child's experience. This can provide helpers with valuable information, and it provides a further justification, if one was needed, for working with adults.

Acknowledging the strengths of survivors in seeking help and working on issues from their past means taking a perspective that genuinely empowers the survivor and confirms that helpers acknowledge at the outset that the 'expert' view is that of the survivor, that survivors have power and control over the pace and depth of the work, and that helpers are facilitators and enablers rather than experts who 'help victims'. Survivors have many strengths, not least their courage in breaking the silence about sexual abuse. Although there may be times when survivors feel overwhelmed by the experience of recalling events they thought were long-buried, the trauma of sexual abuse can be resolved, and survivors can begin to lead happier lives without being haunted by its legacy.

Coming to terms with the experience of childhood sexual abuse can be a long process. Many survivors are now embarking on that process, and they show great determination and courage in their ability to recover. Working with survivors is likely to challenge helpers in a number of ways. Methods of working may need to be reassessed, and long-held assumptions about the nature of the family and the status of childhood may need to be questioned. As a result, helpers will hopefully be able to listen to survivors in ways that are more appropriate to their needs. Being creative in the work, ensuring that there is good support and supervision, evaluating the work in the light of progress, knowledge and experience, encouraging survivors to write about their experiences and always being aware of the difficulty for a survivor in disclosing details of the abuse are all-important. Working with survivors can be slow, exhausting, sad, angry, despairing and tense. It can also be exhilarating, exciting, energising and rewarding work.

<table>
<tr><td>

Annotated further reading

</td><td>

General books for working with survivors

Courtois C A 1988 Healing the incest wound: adult survivors in therapy. Norton, New York
A book for readers who are familiar with psychological concepts on the process of therapy with survivors.
Dinsmore C 1991 From surviving to thriving: incest, feminism and recovery. State University of New York Press, Albany
This book acknowledges the strengths of survivors in overcoming the trauma of sexual abuse. There are good sections on the issues for women who are lesbian, on therapeutic issues and the area of memory recall.
Gil E 1988 Treatment of adult survivors of child abuse. Launch Press, Walnut Creek
Looks at a wide range of issues, including prevalence, therapeutic work with survivors and specific issues including post-traumatic stress, multiple personality disorder and self-mutilation.
Hall L, Lloyd S 1993 Surviving child sexual abuse. A handbook for helping women challenge their past. Falmer Press, London
A practice manual written for survivors and helpers. Covers the long-term effects of sexual abuse, disclosure, therapeutic methods, themes in working with survivors, training and issues for helpers.
Nelson S 1987 Incest: fact and myth. Stramullion, Edinburgh
A classic – examines and refutes some of the commonly held myths about sexual abuse of children.
Walker M 1992 Surviving secrets: the experience of abuse for the child, the family and the helper. Open University Press, Buckingham
An excellent account of the process of therapeutic help using detailed case studies.

Personal accounts

Allen C V 1980 Daddy's girl. Berkeley Books, New York
A first-person account of the author's experience of being sexually abused by her father. Gives a good insight into a child's ways of coping and the effects of the abuse on her subsequent development.
Evert K, Bijkerk I 1987 When you're ready. Launch Press, Walnut Creek
A personal account of coming to terms with sexual abuse by a mother. Especially helpful for a survivor who uses regression as a means of reawakening memories.
Malone C, Farthing L, Marce L 1996 The memory bird. Survivors of sexual abuse. Virago, London

</td></tr>
</table>

Sisk S L, Hoffman C F 1987 Inside scars. Pandora Press, Gainesville
An account of a woman's recovery from sexual abuse by her father. Gives a good insight into the process of therapy from the perspective of the survivor and her helper.
Spring J 1987 Cry hard and swim. Virago, London
A personal account of a Scottish woman's journey in coming to terms with sexual abuse by her father. Describes the process of seeking and finding help with a social worker, along with the difficulties she encountered. A moving and readable account.
Wilson M 1993 Crossing the boundary. Black women survive incest. Virago, London
Looking at the situation of black women, the author focuses on the costs of survival and the strengths that sustain women. The book challenges the myth that sexual abuse is the norm in black communities.

Books written for survivors

Bain O, Sanders M 1990 Out in the open. Virago, London
A book for teenage survivors, written in a clear and readable style.
Maltz W 1991 The sexual healing journey: a guide for survivors of sexual abuse. HarperCollins, New York
A book for helping female and male survivors deal with the sexual problems that might result from the experience of sexual abuse.

Books for male survivors

Lew M 1990 Victims no longer. Men recovering from incest and other sexual abuse. Harper and Row, New York
This is a very helpful book.
Quinn P 1984 Cry out. Abindon Press, Nashville
Describes the abuse of a young boy and the consequences of the abuse in later life.

Books for partners and families

Byerly C M 1985 The mother's book. Kendall/Hunt Publishing, Dubuque A useful, clearly written account of issues for women who discover that their children have been sexually abused.
Davis L 1991 Allies in healing. Harper and Row, New York Full of information for partners and extended families of survivors.
Gil E 1992 Outgrowing the pain together. Launch Press, Walnut Creek
A little book for survivors and their partners.

References

Armsworth M 1989 Therapy of incest survivors: abuse or support? Child Abuse and Neglect 13: 549–562
Arnold R P, Rogers D, Cook D A G 1990 Medical problems of adults who were sexually abused in childhood. British Medical Journal 300: 705–708
Briere J 1996 A self-trauma model for treating adult survivors of severe abuse. In: Briere J, Berliner L, Bulkley J A, *et al.* (eds) The ASPAC handbook on child maltreatment. Sage, Walnut Creek
British Psychological Society 1995 Recovered memories: the report of the working party of the BPS. British Psychological Society, London
Browne A, Finkelhor D 1986 Initial and long-term effects. A review of the research. In: Finkelhor D (ed) A sourcebook of child sexual abuse. Sage, Beverley Hills, California
Colodzin B 1993 How to survive trauma. Pulse Station Hill Press, New York
Cunningham J, Pearce T, Pearce P 1988 Childhood sexual abuse and medical complaints in adult women. Journal of Interpersonal Violence 3: 131–134
Davis L 1991 Allies in healing. Harper and Row, New York
Evert K, Bijkerk I 1987 When you're ready. Walnut Press, Walnut Creek, California
Felitti V J 1991 Long-term medical consequences of incest, rape and molestation. Southern Medical Journal 84: 328–331
Finney L D 1990 Reach for the rainbow. Changes Publishing, Park City, Malibu
Gil E 1992 Outgrowing the pain together. Launch Press, Walnut Creek
Hall L, Lloyd S 1993 Surviving child sexual abuse: a handbook for helping women challenge their past. Falmer Press, London

Herman J L 1992 Trauma and recovery. Basic Books, New York

Kendall-Tackett K A, Williams L M, Finklehor D 1993 Impact of sexual abuse on children: a review and synthesis of recent empirical studies. Psychological Bulletin 113 (1): 169–180

Krarup G, Nielsen B, Bask P, Petersen P 1991 Childhood sexual experiences and repeated suicidal behaviour. Acta Psychiatrica Scandinavica 83: 16–19

Leitenberg H, Greenwald E, Cado S 1992 A retrospective study of long-term methods of coping with having been sexually abused during childhood. Child Abuse and Neglect 16 (1): 399–407

Lew M 1990 Victims no longer. Men recovering from incest and other sexual abuse. Harper and Row, New York

Lister E D 1982 Forced silence: a neglected dimension of trauma. American Journal of psychiatry 139: 872–876

Malone C, Farthing L, Marce L 1996 The memory bird. Survivors of sexual abuse. Virago, London

Maltz W 1991 The sexual healing journey: a guide for survivors of sexual abuse. HarperCollins, New York

Parkinson D 1993 Post trauma stress. Sheldon Press, London

Russell D E H 1986 The secret trauma: incest in the lives of girls and women. Basic Books, New York

Scott M J, Stradling S G 1992 Counselling for post traumatic stress disorder. Sage, London

Sgroi S 1989 Healing together: peer group therapy for adult survivors of child sexual abuse. In: Sgroi S (ed) Vulnerable populations. Evaluation and treatment of sexually abused children and adult survivors, vol. 2. Lexington Books, Cambridge, Massachusetts

Shapiro S 1987 Self-multilation and self blame in incest victims. American Journal of Psychotherapy 41: 46–54

Spring J 1987 Cry hard and swim. Virago, London

Van der Kolk B A, McFarlane A C, Weisaeth L (eds) 1996 Traumatic stress: the effects of overwhelming experience on mind, body and society. Guilford Press, New York

Walker M 1996 The recovered memory debate. In: New directions in counselling. Routledge, London

Walker M 1998 Feminist psychotherapy and sexual abuse. In: Sen I B, Heenan C (eds) Feminism and psychotherapy. Reflections on contemporary theories and practices. Sage, London

Waller G 1991 Sexual abuse as a factor in eating disorders. British Journal of Psychiatry 159: 664–671

Wyatt G E, Newcomb M 1990 Internal and external mediators of women's sexual abuse in childhood. Journal of Counsulting and Clinical Psychology 58: 758–767

27

Out-of-home care for the abused or neglected child: research, planning and practice

June Thoburn

**INTRODUC-
TION**

Developments in the provision of out-of-home care for children who have been abused or neglected mirror more general developments in child and family policy, law and practice. When the emphasis has been on the importance of the natural family, greater efforts have been made to provide residential placements and foster carers who will support the family at times of stress by providing good care for the children and facilitating positive contact with family members so that they can return home as soon as possible. When a child-centred approach has predominated, an emphasis on rescue and a fresh start has led to more resources being available for the placement of children with permanent new families, preferably for adoption. This chapter starts from the premise that this either/or approach to child placement is detrimental to children whose protection or other needs require them to be placed away from home.

Like other aspects of service for children at risk of abuse or neglect, out-of-home placement has benefited from lateral thinkers and creative and adventurous practitioners, but it has also suffered when the work of the pioneers has been translated in a rigid way into practice, and has been expressed in jargonised language which has inhibited evaluation and adjustment. The two most obvious terms to which this statement applies in placement practice are 'permanence' and 'drift'. In the 1970s and 1980s, first in America and then in Britain, even to ask for a clearer definition of these words when applied to individual children was seen as condemning them to a life of impermanence or further abuse. The reader of the statement, 'the plan is permanence' at the end of a court report was led to believe that to plan for permanence was to achieve it. Little was said about the risks inherent in placement for adoption, which had to be balanced against the risks involved in children returning home or remaining in long-term foster or residential care. As British research studies evaluated permanence policies, the balance shifted yet again with the implementation of the Children Act 1989, which instituted a phase of more careful planning for each individual child who cannot remain at home. The Department of Health's (DOH) introduction to the Children Act (DOH 1989a, p. 5) states:

The Act seeks to protect children both from the harm which can arise from failures or abuse within the family and from the harm which can be caused by unwarranted intervention in their family life.

This requirement to balance the consequences of different sorts of 'harm' arises from research findings which have shown that some children who were rescued' from their family homes were further harmed by the system that sought to protect them.

Other chapters in this *Handbook* have referred to research findings on the impact of abuse and severe neglect on the long-term health and well-being of children. The research findings discussed here on the outcome of a range of substitute placements indicate that 'love is not enough', that a substantial minority of children placed with loving and dedicated new parents will still need additional services if they are to overcome the harmful effects of their early experiences, and that a proportion will not totally recover and will remain emotionally vulnerable. The children who we most want to rescue are most vulnerable to the sort of adversities that can happen once they leave home, most obviously renewed abuse, multiple placements and leaving care at the age of 18 without a secure base to provide the support they will need as young adults. (See Triseliotis 1983, Bowlby 1988, Thoburn 1990, for detailed discussions of the concepts of 'a family for life' and a 'secure base'.)

In short, the early optimism of the 1970s and 1980s that, if restoration back home was not easily achievable, children could be placed successfully for adoption and thus be 'got off the books', has been shown in many cases to have been wishful thinking rather than a realistic appraisal of the child's long-term problems and needs. Even when strenuous efforts to prevent placement 'drift' are made, only a small minority of maltreated children are placed for adoption, and in a substantial minority of these cases the placements are not successful.

This chapter will summarise the research findings and place particular emphasis on what they tell us about how practice might be improved. It will highlight the crucially important tasks of assessment and making decisions about the type of placement and other services which are most likely to ensure that the short- and long-term needs of the child are met. A discussion of the role of task-centred carers in providing a safe, nurturing and stable environment for assessment is followed by a consideration of the alternative long-term options for those children who cannot safely return to live with their parents.

The literature on out-of-home placement

There is an extensive literature on the placement of children in residential care, foster care and with adoptive families. For the busy UK practitioner, the most useful sources are the Department of Health publications which accompanied the Children Act 1989. Guidance volumes 2 and 3 on family support and foster care placements, and volume 4 on residential care are based on the practice wisdom of the many writers and practitioners who have had an impact on what has become widely recognised as 'best practice'. *Principles and Practice in Regulations and Guidance* (DOH 1989*b*) summarises the principles which should underlie all family social work, including the placement of children away from their families of origin. The Utting (1997) report, the Government's response (DOH, 1998*b*) and the *Quality Protects* performance indicators (DOH 1998*c*) provide the most recent guidance for policy and practice to safeguard the welfare of children looked after away from their families. The British research that has been most influential is summarised in four DOH sponsored research reviews: *Social Work Decisions in Child Care* (Department of Health and Social Security (DHSS) 1985); *Patterns and Outcomes in Child Placement* (DOH 1991*a*); *Caring for Children Away from Home: Messages from Research* (DOH 1998*a*), and *Adoption Now: Messages from Research* (DOH, 1999). A review in preparation of post-Children Act research (DOH, in preparation) summarises 20 research studies, several of which report on cohorts of 'looked after' children.

The surveys by Rowe and her colleagues (Rowe *et al.* 1989) of the extent to which over 10 000 placements met the desired aims, Bullock and his colleagues (Bullock *et al.* 1993) of 875 children, most of whom returned home from care, and Thoburn & Rowe of 1165 placements with permanent new families (in Fratter *et al.* 1991) are complemented by a large number of smaller-scale studies which give a more detailed picture of child placement work in the UK. The results of a large-scale longitudinal study commissioned by the DOH of nearly 500 foster care placements are shortly to be published, (Sinclair, unpublished data). The review of adoption law and the working papers that led up to it provide a very helpful summary of the legal and administrative structures that underpin the placement of children with permanent new families, including placements for adoption (DOH 1992). Other overviews considering research evidence and the practice literature are those of Maluccio *et al.* (1986), which reviews the North American as well as the British literature, Thoburn (1994), Berridge (1996), Sellick & Thoburn (1996), Roberts (1993), Packman & Hall (1998) and Brandon *et al.* (1999) writing more specifically about foster care for children who have been abused or neglected. Triseliotis *et al.* (1997), Howe (1998) and Thoburn *et al.*(2000) review the research and child development literature on the outcomes of adoption. However, professionals who make recommendations about plans for specific children are advised to use these overviews merely as a starting point in the search for research literature that is relevant to any particular child, since the range of options to meet individual needs is wide, and some studies are more relevant to some types of need and placements than others. Over-simplification of research findings can lead to avoidable mistakes, the price of which will be paid by the children. I shall therefore consider the importance of assessing the needs of individual children, before considering the possible alternative placements that might be available to meet those needs.

Assessing the placement needs of children who cannot remain safely at home

When plans are being made for the placement of a child who cannot remain safely at home, the following questions have to be considered:

- What sort of placement?
- For how long?
- What will be the appropriate legal status for the placement?
- What sort of contact will be appropriate, where and with whom?
- What services, support or therapy will be needed by all those involved in the placement – the child, the carers and members of their own families, the original family members and relatives?
- What financial help and practical support will be needed to maintain the placement?

The answers to all these questions must come from a view about the long-term aims, which in turn have to be based on a painstaking and individually planned assessment process leading to a detailed statement of the child's needs and the ability of any of the adults who are currently a part of the child's life to meet those needs.

Professionals who are considering long-term plans for a child must have a clear idea of what they consider to be a successful outcome. It is worth noting that the review of adoption law suggests that any future legislation should stress the fact that the decisions taken at the time that adoption is being considered will have a lifetime impact on the child and other family members. Any placement must not only meet physical needs and offer protection, but must also meet the child's needs to give and receive love, feel secure and supported, and have the confidence to branch out and have new experiences. Professionals making decisions about children should have in mind the long-term aim of ensuring that as young adults they will have self-esteem and a positive self-concept which will allow them to make satisfying relationships and to provide in turn good enough parenting for any children for whom they may be responsible. Self-esteem grows out of mutual attachments to at least one parent figure – *a psychological parent* – who may be a birth parent or a substitute parent. Research has indicated that self-esteem is most likely to be enhanced if children have a *sense of permanence* in their relationships with their primary carers, and a *sense of identity*, and that these two must be kept in balance. Without a sense of permanence, the child will not feel secure enough to take the risks which go with new attachments, whether to new parents, siblings or friends. Without a sense of personal identity, which includes knowing and preferably being in contact with members of the birth family and important people from the past, racial and cultural identity, pride in appearance including skin colour, and being valued as the individuals they *are* and not measured against the persons their parents would like them to be, there is a risk that children will undervalue themselves in new relationships, or have the sense of being incomplete described by many adopted adults. Walby & Simons (1990) describe the groups they facilitated for adopted people who movingly talk about these feelings. Mary, whom I interviewed 6 years after she was placed at the age of 12 with a permanent foster family, considered that her new parents had given her a great deal, including stability. However, she left home on New Year's Eve just before her 18th birthday, leaving a note for her foster mother saying, 'Mum, I'm sorry, I can't be the person you want me to be' (Thoburn 1990).

The needs listed here are common to all children, but the way in which they are met will be peculiar to each individual child, including each member of a sibling group needing placement. One of the exercises in the Appendix of *Patterns and Outcomes in Child Placement* (DOH 1991*a*) offers a framework for listing each of the child's needs and considering the 'job description' for the carers who are most likely to be able to meet the needs identified. During this assessment process, it will be essential for those responsible for making plans for and with the child to be aware of research findings. There is no point in identifying the perfect placement if research suggests that it is unlikely to be successful given the particular circumstances of this particular child. A second best solution that is likely to be successful in at least some respects may be preferable to the ideal solution that is highly likely to break down.

Research findings suggest that information must be collected about the characteristics, personality, aptitudes and any particular disabilities, whether emotional, behavioural, learning or physical, of each child. The age of the child is another important dimension, since age at placement has been associated by several researchers with outcome, with children who are older when placed being more likely to experience placement breakdown. The third dimension is the relationship of the child with significant others. This will involve a consideration of the child's attachments.

The child may be well-attached, ambivalently attached or not attached to birth mother, birth father, step-parent, siblings, relatives or the present foster parents, and these relationships must also be carefully considered when planning a new placement. The assessment must also consider whether the people who are significant to the child wish the child to continue to remain where they currently are, to return to them or to be placed elsewhere, and, if they have parental responsibility, whether they will consent to a particular form of placement but not to another form of placement. This occurs most obviously when a parent who acknowledges that the child cannot return home will consent to a placement with a view to a residence order (guardianship order in some countries), but not to a placement for adoption. The Children Act 1989 requires that the child, and all those who have parental responsibility, be consulted and due consideration given to their views, wishes and feelings. Whilst the wishes of important people, including the child themself, may sometimes have to be overruled, it is desirable to avoid this if accommodating their wishes will not clearly be detrimental to the child's long-term well-being.

Having formed a picture of the child's needs and relationships, and having consulted all those whose wishes and feelings must be given due consideration (Children Act 1989, section 22 and the welfare checklist, section 1), those considering the child's placement will be in a better position to answer the key placement questions listed above. Before considering alternative long-term placements, the key role of short-term or bridge carers will be discussed.

Bridge placements

The pendulum swings in child care policy and practice have already been noted. The emphasis and the value placed on short-term, bridge or task-centred foster placements have increased or diminished with these swings. In the 1950s and 1960s, many writers emphasised the value of short-term foster placements as an essential part of a family support service. The official guide to foster care practice which resulted from a working group set up after the inquiry into the death of Maria Colwell (DHSS 1976) emphasised the particular skills and tasks of foster carers in facilitating good relationships between children and their natural parents. However, the concern about child abuse which followed that death and subsequent inquiries, together with a realisation that many children did not return to their natural families and remained in unplanned care (Rowe & Lambert 1973), led to a greater emphasis on the placement of children in care with permanent new families, and to a concentration on the skills of permanent family placement to the exclusion of skills in recruiting, training and supporting short-term foster carers. The exception to this was the creative thinking and positive practice which went into the recruitment, training and support of carers for teenagers, no doubt because the concern about child abuse at that period was rivalled only by concern about troublesome teenagers (Shaw & Hipgrave 1983, Hazel & Fenyo 1993, Hill *et al.* 1993).

The attempt to have a permanence policy without a well thought out and properly resourced foster care policy led to a new problem identified by the researchers whose work was reported in the Department of Health overviews. Drift, or lack of planning, ceased to be a significant problem, and was replaced by two equally serious problems: poor quality short-term foster care, which led to a succession of different placements while the child was awaiting a long-term placement; and poor and inflexible planning, which replaced a lack of planning. These two were inter-related, in that it is not possible adequately to assess the needs of children and undertake the work that is necessary with the parents, the child and the new family to prepare them for a permanent placement which is going to have a chance of succeeding, if the child is not in the interim period offered stable and skilled care by either residential workers or foster parents. More recently, researchers and social work theorists have paid more attention to children (especially adolescents) in temporary placements. Farmer & Pollock (1998) report on an important post-Children Act study of the early months in foster or residential care of a cohort of 'abused and abusing' children. Downes (1992) uses attachment theory to provide frameworks for understanding and helping troubled adolescents in foster care.

Rowe *et al.* (1989) identified the tasks of short-term or bridge carers as temporary care (including short periods of planned respite care to alleviate family stress); emergency placements – to offer a roof for a very limited period; preparation for long-term or permanent placement, whether back home or with a new family; assessment; treatment; and a bridge to independence. Utting (1992) identified similar tasks for residential care.

The Children Act 1989 encourages the provision of accommodation as an important part of family support, to be used alongside day care when families are under stress and children are suffering as a result. Packman & Hall (1998) demonstrate that there has indeed been a post-Children Act shift towards the greater use of accommodation (as opposed to court orders) in cases of child maltreatment. Brandon *et al.* (1999) in a study of 105 newly identified cases of significant harm or likely significant harm, find similarly. When parents or older children ask for such help, or social workers consider a child's needs are not being adequately met and the child is suffering significant harm or likely to do so without an out-of-home placement, an early discussion of the sort of care that may be appropriate will alleviate the need for emergency placements and allow for better planning in more cases. Introductions can then be made, agreements about placement carefully negotiated, and the trauma of the separation minimised. In some abuse cases, it is inevitable that emergency action is taken. However, even here it is possible to minimise the harm by providing care for the whole family, or perhaps 'crash pad' facilities in residential care or family centres, so that time can be taken for a more careful decision about the placement of the child, or indeed about whether an alleged abuser is willing to move out temporarily and can be offered help to find accommodation outside the home.

A series of smaller-scale studies of foster care, most notably those of Berridge & Cleaver (1987) and Westacott (1988), preceded the more comprehensive study of placements of Rowe *et al.* (1989). These authors studied a total of 5868 children from six English local authorities, who between them experienced over 10 000 placements between April 1985 and March 1987. They identified short-term placements which broke down without achieving their aims, and also those which were intended to be short-term but lasted longer than expected. Although 57% of the children had only the one placement in care, 8% had three or more during the 2-year period, and there were 38 children who had five or more moves. Six of these were aged under 5 years although most of those who had several moves were teenagers. Short-term placements had a lower breakdown rate than long-term placements, but the proportion breaking down (almost one in five in the Berridge & Cleaver study) is still alarming when one considers that they were only intended to last for up to 8 weeks. Few writers have measured outcomes other than placement breakdown for children who stay away from home for short periods. However, Packman *et al.* (1986) found higher satisfaction rates amongst parents whose children *were* temporarily accommodated than amongst those whose request for care was refused. Stalker (1990) has reviewed the mainly positive but some negative effects of respite care for children with disabilities, and Aldgate & Bradley (1999) describe and evaluate the (generally positive) impact of respite care for children whose families are under stress for reasons other than disability.

One explanation for those who were reported as staying too long in short-term foster care is that foster parents all too quickly come to see the children as 'theirs', and in subtle and unsubtle ways start to discourage contact between the parents and children, thus inhibiting the social worker's efforts to keep a space for child and parents in each other's practical and emotional lives.

What sort of placement?

Brandon *et al.* (1999) found that 65% of children at risk of maltreatment were placed in out-of-home care at some point during the 12 months after they were identified as suffering or likely to suffer significant harm.

Having already made the decision that a child may not safely remain at or return home, at least for the present, the alternatives will be placement with relatives or friends; foster family care; adoption or placement in some form of group care which may be a children's home, boarding education, or a larger foster home such as those provided by the Children's Family Trust (Cairns 1984).

A careful assessment should allow a decision to be made as to whether what is needed is a placement where the parent or parents will remain the 'psychological' parents, or whether new psychological parents are needed. Bullock *et al.* (1993) demonstrate that up to 90% of children will eventually leave care and return either to their parents or relatives. The majority do so within the first 6 weeks, and almost all do so within the first 6 months. This 'leaving care curve' has been misinterpreted to imply that if a child is still away from home after 6 months, they are unlikely to return and should therefore be placed for adoption. The majority of the long stayers are not infants who will easily be placed with a new family, but are older children, many of whom have behaviour problems, and who are likely to return to their first families or at least, after leaving the local authority's care, drift back to their home neighbourhoods.

If it appears that the child will not be able to return home in the near future, but that there is a good attachment between parent and child, a placement is needed where the carers will *supplement* the care of the parent. The parent will remain the main attachment figure, and the placement carers will need to be chosen for their skills in facilitating this. If such a placement is likely to last for a period of years, and especially if the child is quite young, it may be that the birth parents and the carers will *both* fulfil psychological parenting roles. (See Thoburn 1996, for a fuller discussion of the issues around 'dual' or 'multiple' psychological parenting.) This most often happens when a child remains with a relative such as a grandparent, but there are cases when dual psychological parenting is appropriate for lengthy periods of time with children in foster care. In some cases, assessment will make it clear that the child needs new psychological parents, either because there is no attachment or a very destructive or ambivalent attachment with the birth parents, or the child is young and it is not feasible for them to remain psychologically attached to two sets of parents. In that case, substitute parents will be sought. These will normally be adoptive or permanent foster parents, but on occasion a young person may have been so hurt by early experiences within a family that they will request a group care placement. Some small children's homes and group foster homes are able to offer psychological parenting within a group care environment. Some older children who have been sexually abused may feel safer in such an environment, and skilled and loving carers are sometimes able to help them develop trust and indeed form long-term relationships with them which may offer a secure base from which to launch out into adult life.

For how long?

Clarity is always needed about the approximate length of any placement, and this should be stated in the placement agreement. Where the situation is unclear, it is usually possible to estimate approximately how long might be needed for clarification. It is preferable in such cases to overestimate the time needed, and thus avoid a change of placement. If an older child has been harmed by earlier experiences, and assessment indicates that a permanent or long-term placement is needed, 18 months to 2 years is a realistic outer limit which allows for assessment followed by the search for the right placement and preparation for the move. Shorter time limits on task-centred placements merely result in unnecessary movements, as was demonstrated by Berridge & Cleaver (1987) and Cliffe & Berridge (1991) in their studies of the very much shorter-term foster placements favoured by some local authorities. If the intention is that the placement should be until the child is an adult, this should be clearly stated and recorded in the agreement. Brandon *et al.* (1999) found that just over half of the 68 children in their significant harm study who left home at any point during the 12-month follow-up period were back home after 12 months. Nearly a quarter had been adopted or were placed with adoptive families. All except one of the youngest children (a 5-year-old in unplanned foster care) were either at home or in a stable long-term placement. Stability was more difficult to achieve for those over 10 and still looked after.

What legal status?

The first option is for voluntary arrangements (accommodation is the terminology of the Children Act 1989) where parents retain full parental responsibility, but perhaps with the intention, if all are agreed, that the relatives or foster parents will make an application for a residence order once the child appears to be settled. In some cases where there is serious risk to the child, even though the plan might be to work towards rehabilitation, it may be appropriate for a residence order to be made at the onset of the placement to give legal security. This might also be appropriate if a parent is impulsive or suffers from a mental illness or an addiction associated with impulsive behaviour, or there is evidence from the past that an agreement may not be adhered to. Where there is evidence that a child is suffering or likely to suffer significant harm and an agreement cannot be reached to secure the child's placement in accommodation, or for the child to remain in a placement until a residence or care order is sought, it may be necessary to apply for an emergency protection or care order to secure the placement. If a permanent placement is being considered, the child may be placed directly under the Adoption Agencies Regulations, regardless of whether or not there has been a previous care order. Alternatively, the child may remain accommodated or in care as a foster child with the intention of an application for adoption or a residence order once the child is settled. Or the child may remain as a foster child, in which case it will be important to have a very clear agreement that this is intended to be a *permanent* foster placement, especially if the child is placed under voluntary arrangements (see Thoburn 1990, for a fuller discussion of the importance of ensuring that the child and the carers have a sense of permanence in such situations, and ways in which this sense of permanence can be facilitated). The Adoption Law White Paper (DOH 1993) proposes a more secure residence order which will convey the status of *inter vivos* guardian on the foster parents or relatives until the child is 18. No application for a revocation of the order will be permitted without the leave of the court, and the guardians will be allowed to make provision for guardians for the child in the event of their death.

What sort of contact and with whom?

The work of Millham *et al.* (1986, 1989) played a major part in emphasising the importance of continued contact for children who are looked after by the local authority, not only with their parents but also with siblings if they are not placed together, and with relatives and friends. These authors also summarise previous research on the subject. Research on 'open adoption' and the issues surrounding openness when children are placed with permanent new families is summarised by the writers in Mullender's edited book on the subject (1991), and by Fratter *et al.* (1991), Fratter (1996) and Grotevant & McRoy (1998). There are circumstances in which face-to-face (or even more rarely indirect) contact cannot be safely achieved or is not in the interest of the child, but these are exceptions to be decided in each individual case. Cleaver (2000) describes contact arrangements for 185 children in long- or intermediate-term placements after the implementation of the Children Act 1989. From a retrospective study of the records of 152 children and a prospective interview study of 33 children whose care cases were followed up for 12 months, she concluded that the proportions of longer stayers who had face-to-face contact with parents had not changed significantly since the implementation of the Act. Moreover, those who did have contact with at least one parent did so more frequently and regularly than was reported in earlier studies. From the prospective study they concluded that when children did not have contact there was usually a good reason for this. There is not sufficient space here to cite all the research evidence on contact with members of the birth family, whether or not the child is to return to them, but the cumulative findings can be summarised as follows. As far as I am aware, no large-scale study has concluded that face-to-face contact is associated with a higher risk of breakdown or other placement problems. One or two smaller-scale studies have pointed to problems resulting from specific factors such as inconsistency. Rowe *et al.* (1984) found that long-term foster children who appeared to be doing well were either regularly visited or had contact with parents at the start of the placement which had gradually diminished over time. Continued face-to-face contact with members of the birth family, especially birth parents, has been associated by one or more research studies with the following benefits:

- Increased likelihood of return home of the child (Fanshel & Shinn 1978, Aldgate 1980, Thorpe 1980, Bullock *et al.* 1993).
- A clearer sense of identity (Thoburn *et al.* 1986, Aldgate 1990, Kelly & McAuley 1995).
- Increased self-esteem in the child as they grow up (Weinstein 1960, Fanshel & Shinn 1978, Aldgate 1980).
- Increased well-being, including higher educational performance (Fanshel & Shinn 1978, Aldgate 1990, provided that the child also has a sense of permanence).

- A diminished risk of placement breakdown (Berridge & Cleaver 1987, Thoburn 1990, Kufeldt & Allison 1990, Fratter *et al.* 1991).

Other benefits of continued contact which have been pointed out by research studies of a more qualitative nature include the following:

- It offers continuity, in that the members of the birth family offer some continuity of relationships to those children who experience a series of different placements whilst in care. For this reason, it is especially important that contact is maintained when a child is changing placements.
- It may help in a crisis or with a contingency if a placement in care breaks down and no suitable placement is available. On occasion in such circumstances, a reassessment may lead to the conclusion that the child may safely return home. On other occasions, members of the family, perhaps grandparents or relatives, may provide a bridge placement until a new placement can be identified.
- Continued contact will provide 'a family for life' for the child. If the child does settle well and form attachments with a substitute family, they may have the benefit as an adult of two 'families for life' if contacts have been maintained with the first family. If the placement in care does not lead to a good long-term attachment and a secure base, family members who have not been able to meet their children's needs when young may be able to do so when they are young adults. The particular importance of siblings must not be forgotten, since the relationship between siblings is potentially even more long-lasting than is the parent–child relationship. This may apply to siblings born after the child left home, and there are many examples of siblings forming close friendships as adults, even if they never actually lived together as children.

The questions as to what sort of social work help and therapy will be provided and for whom will be discussed in more detail later in this chapter. Financial support can be available when appropriate through adoption allowances, residence order allowances, foster care payments, grants made under section 17 of the Children Act, settling-in grants and one-off grants, for example, if a child is particularly destructive.

In the next sections, the range of long-term placements which might be chosen following assessment are considered.

Respite, long-term shared care and placement with relatives

Sometimes parents will themselves request out-of-home care to tide them over particularly stressful periods in their lives, or residential therapy for a child whose behaviour is particularly difficult. In some cases, the family may be most appropriately supported by the provision of regular planned periods of respite care in the same foster home or residential placement. In other circumstances, the family may be linked with a foster carer or residential placement which will provide accommodation at times of stress, as when a parent suffers from a debilitating physical illness such as AIDS-related symptoms, or a recurring mental illness such as schizophrenia or clinical depression (see chapters by Fratter & O'Hara in Batty 1993, and Aldgate & Bradley 1999).

Mention has already been made of the importance of clarity about who is intended to play the psychological parenting role for a child living away from home. It has also been suggested that on occasions there will be dual psychological parenting. More often, however, the intention of using these options will be to maintain a strong attachment with the parents and other family members, including siblings. Longer-term shared care options are particularly appropriate when a parent and child are closely attached but there is danger to the child if they continue to live at home. It is often possible to arrange for visits home to be fully supervised, or for the adult believed to be a danger to the child to be out of the home when the child returns home for visits. If this is not possible, a comfortable environment is needed so that the non-abusing parent and child can spend extended periods of time together.

Long-term group care placements

In some cases, boarding education may be an appropriate way of maintaining the child's attachment to the natural parents. Some older children and their parents or step-parents are unable to live harmoniously together, but their fragile relationship can be maintained if they keep some distance between them, and may strengthen as the child becomes a young adult. In a study of 177 American adopted children with special needs, Nelson (1985) found that placement away from home or boarding education was a much valued service to adoptive families and made it possible for some placements under stress to survive. Grimshaw & Berridge (1994) studied boarding education for children with educational and behavioural difficulties. While they express concern at the potential risk of abuse of children placed in boarding education, they also note the positive role such provision can play in the lives of children and families under stress. Aldgate (1980) noted that some parents found it very difficult to visit their children in foster care and were more able to remain in touch if they were placed in children's homes. Rose (1990) describes the therapeutic community approach to young people with serious behavioural difficulties.

More recent research on children in residential care reports mixed results. Rowe *et al.* (1989) found that placements in children's homes were as likely to achieve their aims as foster care placements. However, Sinclair & Gibbs (1998) and Berridge & Brodie (1998) report more negative results. Berridge & Brodie found that specialist children's homes for children with disabilities appeared to plan more carefully and to be more successful in meeting the needs of the children than those caring from more mixed populations.

Long-term shared care in foster homes

When long-term shared foster care is the placement of choice, particular attention must be paid to ensuring that the birth parents and the foster parents get on with each other well enough to share the parenting of the child. In some cases, the child will remain in accommodation on a voluntary basis, in which case the parents retain full parental responsibility, and the placement agreement must spell out which responsibilities are delegated to the foster carers, and the actions that all parties will take as contingencies if the arrangements break down. It is often small things such as a change in hairstyle that can cause trouble between the two sets of parents, and creative social workers and skilled foster carers must think ahead to pre-empt such difficulties. Even when there is a care order, the Children Act 1989 requires that the parents are enabled to retain as much of their parental responsibility as possible, and that the authority only takes away that much of their parental responsibility necessary to secure the child's well-being.

The major British sources of information about the success of intermediate- or long-term foster care, residential placement and placement with relatives are found in the work of Rowe *et al.* (1984, 1989), Berridge (1985), Millham *et al.* (1986) and Bullock *et al.* (1993) on residential care, and Berridge & Cleaver (1987), Aldgate (1990) and Kelly & McAuley (1995). Some North American studies are by Fein *et al.* (1990) and Kufeldt & Allison (1990). Shaw & Hipgrave (1983) and Caesar *et al.* (1994) have described and summarised the research on special placement schemes for adolescents, which normally aim to prepare them for independence and often endeavour to build bridges for them with their natural parents and relatives. Schofield *et al.* (2000) provide detailed descriptions of patterns of attachment with their birth and foster families of 58 children newly placed with long-term foster parents. They review the important role played by long-term foster parents in meeting the needs of some of the most damaged children in care.

Most studies note that there is a higher breakdown rate of placements of teenagers, regardless of whether or not they are placed in specialist or profes- sional foster schemes, in 'ordinary' foster homes, in lodgings or in residential care. Berridge & Cleaver (1987), however, noted a high breakdown rate amongst youngsters aged 7–11 years. Placements in residential care are least likely to break down. However, Colton (1989) compared the nature of caring in special- ist foster homes and children's homes and concluded that, irrespective of the skills of the carers, those looking after young people in family environments are more able to be child-oriented than residential workers who can provide less indi- vidual attention. In their study of abused and abusing young people, Farmer & Pollock (1998) find similarly. However, they also point out that there are differ- ences between young people placed in foster care and those placed in residential care. The voice of the children and young people is included in most of these studies, but is reported more fully by Fletcher (1993). Although breakdown rates are quite high, many adolescents speak well of their residential and foster carers, and it should be noted that adolescents are in any case a group of people 'on the move'. Studies using outcome measures such as health and educational progress are reviewed by Roberts (1993). Ward (1995) describes the development of the 'looking after children' practice and management tools to encourage better prac- tice and monitor children's development and progress on seven dimensions of health and well-being.

Turning to the research in more detail, Rowe *et al.* (1989) compared the findings of their large-scale survey of foster placements with earlier studies. Twenty-seven per cent of the 194 children placed in long-term foster care during the first year of the study had experienced breakdown between 12 and 24 months later. The proportion for those aged under 4 was 4%, for those aged between 5 and 10 years 23%, but for teenagers over 30%, rising to 66% of those aged 16 or over. The authors concluded that two-thirds of the long-term placements were at least fairly successful. Most studies of educational progress of children in foster care have concluded that their education is negatively affected. However, Aldgate (1990) found that children in long-term foster placements were doing as well educationally, and in other aspects of their well-being, as were children who were on the social workers' preventive case loads but were not looked after by the local authority. They also note that increased well-being and satisfactory educational progress were associated with having a sense of stability and security within the foster home. The benefits of continued contact with members of the birth family have already been listed. Berridge & Cleaver (1987) found that more placements broke down if there was no contact, and Millham *et al.* (1986) showed how formal and informal barriers are often put in the way of contact, so that visiting is prevented or quickly tails off in the majority of placements.

To summarise, these studies, and the more recent Packman & Hall (1998) study of accommodation, show that the goalkeeping – 'care is bad for your health' or 'once they are in care, it is hard to get them back home' – attitudes and policies of the 1980s represented an over-simplification and must be adapted in the light of new knowledge. There is much in the studies to indicate how practice can improve to reduce the casualty rate even further, and to help identify the potential casualties, so that services (both when children are being looked after and when they leave) can be of a higher quality.

The fact that the majority of placements are reasonably successful should not, however, prevent us from recognising the extreme vulnerability of children who *do* become split off from their families of origin, and whose placements in care or for adoption are unsuccessful. Studies of homeless young people, and of young people in custody, indicate that a substantial proportion of these were originally abused, placed in care for their own protection and re-abused, or felt so unprotected or alone in care that they ran away and preferred to trust to their own devices (Biehal *et al.* 1995, Wade *et al.* 1998).

Placement of children from minority ethnic groups

Most studies also consider whether placements of black children are any more or less successful than those whose parents are both white. It is generally considered that black children are over-represented amongst children in care. Rowe *et al.* (1989) point out the dangers of over-simplification. Asian children are under-represented, and children, both of whose parents are African Caribbean, are over-represented amongst those in short-term placements but not amongst those in long-term placements. Children of mixed racial parentage, however, appear to be over-represented amongst all groups of children in care. These authors found no difference in the pattern of placement of children whose parents were black, white, or of mixed racial parentage. They were equally likely to be placed in foster homes or in residential care, although black 'looked after' teenagers were more likely to be placed in specialist foster homes. Nor, in that study, were black teenagers any more likely than white teenagers to be in penal establishments.

Placement with relatives

Rowe *et al.* (1984, 1989) and Berridge & Cleaver (1987) are the major sources of information about children placed with relatives. All three studies note that such placements are more successful, whether measured in terms of breakdown rates or in terms of successfully achieving placement aims, than placements with non-related foster carers or residential placements when like children are compared with like. The Children Act 1989 strongly recommends placement with relatives in appropriate cases, even though social workers tend to be cautious about making such placements when children have been abused or neglected. Brandon *et al.* (1999) found that relatives provided short- or long-term care for around one in five of the 105 children in their study of children at risk of 'significant harm', six of the 21 who were in permanent substitute family placements were living with relatives. Rowe *et al.* (1984) found that relatives were particularly good at keeping the child in touch with both sides of the family, as well as offering long-term stability and good parenting to the children in their care. The point made earlier about the importance of well-negotiated agreements must be stressed here also, so that the child *does* have a sense of stability and security and is not afraid of impulsive removal, and also in order to ensure that the child is kept safe from renewed abuse when in contact with any relatives who were implicated in the original abuse.

Permanent placement with substitute parents

It has already been noted that only a small proportion of the children cared for away from home will be placed with permanent substitute parents. In the study by Rowe *et al.* (1989), long-term placements accounted for nearly 10% of all foster placements. However, the six authorities studied only made 261 placements directly for adoption or as foster children with a view to subsequent application to adopt (fewer than 3% of the placements studied). Only 16 of the 450 children who came into care in the cohort study by Millham *et al.* (1986) were adopted or remained with their long-term foster parents until the age of 18 (3.5% of the total).

There have been many English language accounts of the permanent family placement of children in care over the last 20 years or so, both from practitioners and researchers. The American studies are summarised by Barth & Berry (1988) and Ainsworth *et al.* (2000) and the British research studies are summarised by Thoburn (1990), Sellick & Thoburn (1996) and Triseliotis *et al.* (1997).

The psychology of adoption

There have also been many studies over the years of the placement of infants for adoption which are also relevant to this volume, since some children are placed for adoption at birth if it is believed they are likely to be significantly harmed in the light of the experience of siblings. Space precludes a full consideration of the subject, but readers are referred to the work of Brodzinsky & Schechter (1990), who have brought together their own writings and those of other researchers and practitioners on the psychology and outcomes of adoption. Although care must be exercised when applying their conclusions to children adopted when older, these writers do throw light on the problems adopted children and their new families may encounter. Their thesis is that the adoptive family faces additional challenges which result from the loss experienced by the child, and the loss for some adopters of the child by birth which they had hoped to have – the 'double jeopardy' theory. Additional challenges will be there if the child carries the scars of earlier harm, and if the child is of a different skin colour or cultural background from the adoptive family (Thoburn *et al.* 2000). These writers join Kirk (1964, 1981) in postulating that successful adopters are those who accept the special challenges of adoptive parenting which make it different from parenting a child born to them. They consider that an adoptive family is a dual identity family, in that it has to incorporate the original family of the child conceptually, even if there is no actual contact. Accordingly, they strongly support some form of contact between the birth family and the adoptive family, even if this is only by way of letters and photographs, partly because this reminds the adopters that they have extra parenting challenges to overcome, and partly because it avoids the risks of the child fantasising and idealising the first family, or the sense for the adopters of 'sitting on a time bomb' and wondering if and when the child will wish to seek out the natural family and what they may find when they do so.

This adoption research gives clues about the sort of family who is likely to be most successful with a child who has been abused or neglected. Since they have to be comfortable with the child's first identity, it is especially important that they can empathise with the parent who was responsible for the abuse or neglect. A child whose parent is a known abuser is likely to need help in establishing a positive sense of self, and this will not be helped if the adopters or foster carers make it clear that they have a low opinion or condemnatory attitude towards the first parents.

Permanent placement of older children

Lowe *et al.* (1999) and British Agencies for Adoption and Fostering (1998, 2000), give detailed information on adoption policy and practice, and the numbers and ages of children being placed for adoption in the UK.

Within the last few years, several outcome studies of permanent family placement of older children have been published, and their findings are generally similar. Some, such as the study of 1165 permanent placements with families not previously known to the child, use placement breakdown within 3–6 years of placement as the outcome measure (Thoburn in Fratter *et al.* 1991). Other generally smaller-scale studies use a range of more subjective measures, such as the satisfaction or otherwise of the parents, the child, or other members of the family (Tizard 1977, Macaskill 1985, on the placement of children with a disability, and Thoburn *et al.* 1986, Rushton *et al.* 1988, Thoburn 1990). Thomas & Beckford (1999) provide important insights into the lives and opinions of 41 children who were placed for adoption when over the age of 5. Others use more objective measures, such as well-being scales, educational achievement or delinquency rates (see especially Rushton *et al.* 1988 and Quinton & Rushton 1998, for two particularly thorough studies of the well-being of children and changes in their behaviour during the early years of placement). A series of studies of the work of Lothian Social Work Department, which set up a specialist section to place children in care with permanent new families, combines survey methodology using breakdown rates as the outcome measure with detailed studies of a small number of the placements using a range of other measures (Hoggan & O'Hara 1988).

Some of these studies include children whose placement with a foster family with whom they were well established is confirmed as a permanent placement, whilst others only include new placements with parents who were previously unknown to the child. The first group are less likely to break down, since the new parents and child have already got to know each other before deciding that this should be a permanent placement (Lahti 1982, Fein *et al.* 1983). Other variables which may affect outcome are the age range of the children placed, the quality of the social work support and the agency policies. The percentage of placements that had broken down between 18 months and 6 years after placement in the large-scale survey of 1165 placements made by voluntary agencies was 22% (Fratter *et al.* 1991). However, it is not particularly helpful to have a global breakdown or success rate. All the studies identify the characteristics of the children which have an impact on the success or otherwise of the placement. Age at placement has been identified by all large-scale studies in Britain and America as associated with placement breakdown. Children who are younger and have disabilities might be hard to find families for, but once the family has been found these placements seem to be particularly successful. On the other hand, it is not too difficult to find families for sibling groups in the primary school age range, but these children do seem to be harder to parent than new families or social workers had anticipated. Around 22% of placements of 8-year-olds break down, and this rises to almost a half of the placements of 12-year-olds. One factor identified by most researchers as being associated independently with breakdown is that the child has been abused or neglected prior to the placement (Fratter *et al.* 1991). Gibbons *et al.* (1995), in a study of children who were physically abused or severely neglected when under the age of 5 years, found that 8 years later the well-being of those placed for adoption or in foster care was, on average, no higher than that of children who returned home, and lower than for a matched sample of children who had not been abused. Other factors associated with breakdown were the child being described as institutionalised, or behaviourally or emotionally disturbed. Several studies (Berridge & Cleaver 1987, Borland *et al.* 1990, Fratter *et al.* 1991) found that placements where there was face-to-face contact with the birth parents after the placement were either less likely to break down or it made no difference.

Children, both of whose parents were black, were no more likely to experience breakdown than children of two white parents, but those of mixed-race parentage were significantly more likely to experience placement breakdown. When variables such as age at placement were controlled for there was no difference in placement breakdown rates between those placed in ethnically 'matched' families and those placed trans-racially.

Thoburn *et al.* (2000) look in more detail at the long-term outcomes of 297 children of minority ethnic origin. Outcome measures of 51 of them included well-being, ethnic pride and self-esteem. On the basis of this detailed information provided by the adoptive parents and young people, the authors concluded that the requirements in the Children Act 1989 (re-stated in a 1998 clarification, SSI 1998) that children should be placed wherever possible with families of similar ethnic and cultural background is likely to be associated with more successful outcomes. However, if this is not possible, some white families can successfully parent black children if they are carefully selected, trained and supported.

In the full cohort of 1165 children, there was no difference in breakdown rate between those who were permanently fostered and those who were adopted. However, it should be noted that these children were all placed with the intention that the placement would be permanent, and the practice of the workers was aimed at giving them and the new parents a sense of permanence from the beginning of the placement. In that sense, they differed from long-term placements which at least early on were accompanied by uncertainty about the future. Gibbons *et al.* (1985) found that more of the children maltreated when under the age of 5 were in the higher well-being groups when placed with foster parents than with adopters. However, other smaller-scale, qualitative studies have found that higher levels of satisfaction among the children and higher educational achievement were associated with placement for adoption rather than foster care (Triseliotis & Russell 1984, Hill *et al.* 1989). Thoburn (1990), Bullard *et al.* (1990), Kelly & McAuley (1995) and Schofield *et al.* (2000) noted that there are a group of children who are closely attached to their original families and wish to have the security of knowing that they will remain with a substitute family but do not wish to give up their legal attachments to their first family. The conclusion to be drawn from the studies is that the decision about legal status should depend on the wishes, attitudes and temperament of all concerned, especially the child. The apparent cost advantage of adoption should not play a major part in this decision, since it is likely that a high proportion of maltreated children who are adopted will need support through adoption allowances, and the costs of long-term post-placement support are likely to be incurred whatever the legal status. In more complex cases in order to avoid unnecessary delay, there are advantages in seeking, concurrently, adoptive or permanent foster families, thus broadening the choice of families and making it more likely that the special needs of maltreated children be met.

Research studies differ in their findings about the sort of people who can successfully become substitute parents for children who have been abused or neglected. They agree in only one respect: that there is a high risk of failure if there is a younger-child in the family who is within 3 years of the age of the child being placed, particularly if this younger child is of pre-school age. Most studies find that more experienced and older parents are more successful, but some studies (Hart 1986, Wedge & Mantle 1991) have found that younger childless couples have been particularly successful with groups of siblings. Moving away from these more obvious characteristics, writers agree about the attitudes, personal characteristics and skills of substitute parents who are more successful, and these will be discussed in the next section. Successful substitute parents have a range of reasons for undertaking this task. Provided that they enjoy being with children, and enjoy a challenge, research does not point to clear desirable or undesirable motivation.

The task and skills of carers and those who support them

An overview of the social work task

There are several dimensions under which this work can be considered. Firstly, there are organisational decisions to be made about who will be primarily responsible for providing a social work service to the birth parents and their relatives, the child, and the carers and possibly members of their family. In some cases, it may be appropriate for the same worker to provide all these services. More often, a specialist worker will be responsible for the recruitment and approval process, and will support the carers or new parents whilst the worker for the child remains principally concerned with the child's welfare. If there is a conflict of interest between the child and the natural family, or strong disagreement about the plans that have been made, it will be appropriate for support to be offered to the parents by another worker or even another agency. The training, supervision and support needs of workers in group care settings are similar in some respects, but there are also differences. The emphasis here will be on those who care for children in their own homes.

It will be clear from the previous sections that the role of carers and, therefore, the skills and attributes needed are varied. Most obviously, carers fall into two groups: those who for a shorter or longer period or episodically will join with natural parents and social workers in caring for children in need; and those who will take on the prime parenting responsibility until the child becomes a young adult and beyond. The tasks of the social workers with these two groups are in many respects similar, but in other respects there are important differences. These tasks need to be considered in respect of the following stages:

- recruitment
- selection and preparation
- training
- matching the carers with the child
- preparing for the placement
- providing support and, when appropriate, therapy for the child, the carers and the natural parents when the child is in placement
- when appropriate, helping all those involved to ensure a smooth transfer back to the natural family or on to a new family.

Once approved, the Children Act 1989 requires that all foster families should be visited annually for the purposes of reviewing whether they are succeeding in undertaking the tasks they wish to undertake, with the sorts of children and families with whom they have skills and can empathise. The review is also an opportunity for them to discuss their training and support needs, and the adequacy of the support service they have received over the previous year. It is also an opportunity for the agency to monitor how effectively they have discharged their obligations to the children placed with them during the year and to their parents.

All children who are away from home in respite or bridge placements should be offered a dependable relationship with the social worker who is responsible for the child's care plan. This area of social work practice has now been well documented, and a wide range of practice guidance is available. The term 'life story work' is most frequently used to describe some of the work undertaken with children away from home, but a classic article first published by Claire Winnicott in 1966, and reprinted by British Agencies for Adoption and Fostering in 1986, is still the best statement of the principles and values which must underpin such work. Aldgate & Simmonds (1987), Redgrave (1987), Aldgate *et al.* (1989), Fahlberg (1990, 1991) and Ryan & Walker (1993) are all useful sources on working directly with children in placement about the circumstances of their lives.

Useful practice texts on social work practice in foster care are those on group work edited by Triseliotis (1988) and on the support of short-term foster parents by Sellick (1992) and Triseliotis *et al.* (1995). Hill & Shaw (1998) and Hill (1999) have selected articles from the journal *Adoption and Fostering* – many of which provide 'signposts' for practitioners. Sinclair and his colleagues report findings from their study concerning relationships between foster carers, family placement social workers and the children's social worker (Fisher *et al.* 2000).

Task-centred carers

While a few of those who take children into their homes to provide a service on behalf of the agency will care for only one child, perhaps a young relative or a child who will have periods of respite over many years, the majority of task-centred carers must be able to care for a range of children with a variety of needs. Matching is therefore only possible in the broader sense of a particular age group, or children with particular characteristics or disabilities. Enjoying the company of children and feeling comfortable with them is an essential prerequisite, as are flexibility, negotiation skills and non-judgemental attitudes. Since some children will be placed before it becomes clear that they have been abused, all task-centred carers must be able to understand and empathise not only with the child who has been abused, but also with the parent who was unable to protect the child or was the abuser. If these characteristics are present, it will be possible to provide training and support both before and during placements, so that the special needs of each child and family can be met (Thoburn 1991). Batty (1991), Macaskill (1991), Downes (1992) and Farmer & Pollock (1998) write specifically about the foster care task and the support needs of carers and children who have been sexually abused.

Substitute parents

When children are placed with the intention that the new parents will become the psychological parents, many of the qualities required of them and the skills of the social workers are similar. There are, however, important differences, most notably that permanent carers will usually care for only one child, and will be selected and matched specifically with that child. A broad range of skills is less important than the matching of their skills and needs with the needs and potential of the child to be placed. The art of making permanent placements appears to be in learning what the new parents have to give, and what they will expect in return, and matching these with what the child can give and needs and is willing to take from the new parent. It would thus be a mistake to place with a childless couple who want to love a child who will love them in return, a youngster who has been so hurt by earlier experiences that it is not at all obvious that the child will be able to become fully attached to them. Such a child will be more likely to settle with new parents who have already had the rewards of successfully parenting their own children, are motivated by a love of children and the desire to help a youngster in difficulties, and can accept that the youngster may never grow to love them in the same way that their own children have grown up loving them from their early months. Assessing and matching, then, are the major social work tasks in permanent family placement on which can be built the later work of supporting the new family. Permanent placement work differs from work with task-centred carers in the sense that a family approved to take a child on a permanent basis should not have a child placed with them unless the match seems an appropriate one. For that reason, an even wider range of families may be approved. Indeed, many successful substitute parents have been turned down by foster care or more traditional adoption agencies as being unsuitable.

Another difference lies in the nature of social work practice. Once a child has been placed, most researchers have concluded that it is most appropriate for the long-term support of the placement to be undertaken by the specialist who undertook the home study and approval work. At the time of placement, the person who is most likely to help the new family to develop a sense of commitment and permanence is the worker in whom the substitute parents already have confidence. Many adopters or long-term foster carers have talked to researchers about their nervousness when visited by the child's worker. Children also report being made anxious by a visit from the worker who has been responsible for moving them around in the past. Thus, the child's worker is best seen as a caring presence in the background who arrives at the time when the placement is reviewed, but otherwise leaves the support to the new family's worker (Thoburn *et al.*

1986, Thoburn 1990), or undertakes an agreed piece of work at the request of child, new family or the support worker.

The second of these studies which followed children through from their situation prior to placements to 6 years later found that therapeutic intervention in the early years when the child was settling in was not usually appropriate, although a continuation of the 'life story work', often undertaken jointly by the new family's social worker and the new parents, was particularly helpful at the appropriate moment. In the longer-term, however, perhaps in the 3rd, 4th or 5th year after placement, when the new family felt established as a family, therapeutic intervention often became necessary with those children who had suffered abuse or neglect. It was sometimes appropriate in these circumstances for the therapeutic intervention to come from an agency other than the one that had made the placement. However, Howe & Hinings (1989) and the workers at the Post-Adoption Centre note that therapists must address themselves to the special nature of adoptive families.

Allegations of abuse in foster family care

Many children who have been abused are vulnerable to renewed abuse, whether physically, emotionally or sexually, and some children who have been abused in the past may make reference to abuse which may be misinterpreted as having been inflicted by the foster carer (Nixon 1997). Great sensitivity is needed when investigating allegations or suspicions of abuse when children are in foster care. It has been noted by some practitioners and foster care support groups that the incidence of unsubstantiated suspicion, and false allegation, is higher when children are in foster care. Procedures for investigating allegations must be followed but, as when children are living with their original families, they should not be removed without careful planning unless this is absolutely necessary for their protection. This is especially so if the placement is planned as a permanent substitute placement, and the child is becoming attached or is already attached to the new parents.

Summary and conclusion

This chapter has emphasised that removal from home of a child who may be in need of protection may solve one set of problems but makes the child vulnerable to a new set of hazards. It has also referred to research findings which suggest that if temporary or permanent removal *does* become necessary, a course has to be steered between excess optimism and excess pessimism about the outcome for the child.

A succession of studies on permanent family placement and on the impact of abuse or severe neglect on children have indicated that it is the lucky or the temperamentally resilient minority who remain relatively unscathed. The majority will need more than replacement parent figures, no matter how much love they have to offer. Their fragile identities will require skill as well as love. If they cannot return safely home, their carers must work hard at understanding their past, and substitute parents must incorporate it into the life of the new family. Direct contact with members of the first family will usually be the best way of doing this, but a two-way exchange of letters and photographs may sometimes have to take the place of direct contact, sometimes for only temporary periods.

For those who help and support the children, their first families, their temporary carers or new families, the keys to success are good planning which adapts to the needs of each situation; imaginative and sensitively negotiated agreements and an adequate supply of 'bridge' carers with choices between family and group care settings. Above all, children need carers and professional workers who will go on fighting on their behalf but who can live with uncertain outcomes and the lack of tidy solutions.

Annotated further reading

The literature has been reviewed in the body of the chapter, and there are no shortcuts when considering placement for a particular child. For the child protection worker wishing to get to grips with the issues the most useful texts are as follows:

On the principles underlying child placement and reviewing the research

Bullock *et al.* 1993; Department of Health (1985, 1989*b*, 1991*a*, 1999); Berridge (1996), Sellick & Thoburn (1996); Thoburn (1994).

On short-term placements

Berridge & Cleaver (1987); Farmer & Pollock, 1998, Millham *et al.* (1986); Rowe *et al.* (1989); Sellick (1992); Triseliotis *et al.* (1995).

On residential care

Department of Health (1991*a*, 1998*a*); Grimshaw & Berridge (1994); Rose (1990); Utting (1992).

On placement with relatives

Berridge & Cleaver (1987); Bullard *et al.* (1990); Rowe *et al.* (1984, 1989).

On permanent placement with substitute parents

Brodzinski & Schechter (1990); Fratter *et al.* (1991); Howe (1998); Quinton & Rushton (1998); Thoburn (1990); Thoburn *et al.* (2000); Triseliotis *et al.* (1997).

On social work practice with children who are looked after

Aldgate *et al.* (1989); Cleaver (2000); Downes (1992); Fahlberg (1990, 1991); Schofield *et al.* (2000); Triseliotis (1988); Triseliotis *et al.* (1995).

References

Ainsworth F, Maluccio A N, Thoburn J 2000 Child welfare outcome research in the United States, Britain and Australia. Child Welfare League of America, Washington

Aldgate J 1980 Identification of factors which influence length of stay in care. In: Triseliotis J P (ed) New developments in foster care and adoption. Routledge and Kegan Paul, London

Aldgate J 1990 Foster children at school: success or failure. Adoption and Fostering 7 (2): 38–45

Aldgate J, Bradley M 1999 Supporting families through short-term fostering. The Stationery Office, London

Aldgate J, Simmonds J (eds) 1987 Direct work with children. Batsford, London

Aldgate J, Maluccio A, Reeves C 1989 Adolescents in foster family care. Batsford, London

Barth R, Berry M 1988 Adoption and disruption: rates, risk and responses. Aldine de Gruyter, New York

Batty D (ed) 1991 Sexually abused children – making their placements work. British Agencies for Adoption and Fostering, London

Batty D (ed) 1993 HIV infection and children in need. British Agencies for Adoption and Fostering, London

Berridge D 1985 Children's homes. Basil Blackwell, Oxford

Berridge D 1996 Foster care: a research review. HMSO, London

Berridge D, Brodie I 1998 Children's homes revisited. Jessica Kingsley, London

Berridge D, Cleaver H 1987 Foster home breakdown. Basil Blackwell, Oxford

Biehal N, Clayden J, Stein M, Wade J 1995 Moving on: young people and leaving care schemes. HMSO, London

Borland M, Triseliotis J, O'Hara G 1990 Permanency planning for children in Lothian region. University of Edinburgh, Edinburgh

Bowlby J 1988 A secure base. Tavistock, London

Brandon M, Thoburn J, Lewis A, Way A 1999 Safeguarding children with the Children Act 1989. The Stationery Office, London

British Agencies for Adoption and Fostering (BAAF) 1986 Working with children. BAAF, London

British Agencies for Adoption and Fostering (BAAF) 1998, 2000 Children adopted from care. BAAF, London

Brodzinsky D, Schechter M (eds) 1990 The psychology of adoption. Oxford University Press, Oxford

Bullard E, Malos E, Parker R 1990 Custodianship: a report to the Department of Health. University of Bristol, Bristol

Bullock R, Little M, Millham S 1993 Going home. Dartmouth, Aldershot

Caesar G, Parchment M, Berridge D, Gordon G 1994 Black perspectives on services for children and young people in need and their families. National Children's Bureau, London

Cairns B 1984 The children's family trust: a unique approach to substitute family care? British Journal of Social Work 14: 457–473

Cleaver H 2000 Fostering family contact. The Stationery Office, London

Cliffe D, Berridge D 1991 Closing children's homes. National Children's Bureau, London

Colton M 1989 Dimensions of substitute care. Avebury, Aldershot

Department of Health (DOH) 1989a Introduction to the Children Act 1989. HMSO, London

Department of Health (DOH) 1989b Principles and practice in regulations and guidance. HMSO, London

Department of Health (DOH) 1991a Patterns and outcomes in child placement. HMSO, London

Department of Health (DOH) 1991b The Children Act 1989: guidance and regulations, vols 2, 3 and 4. HMSO, London

Department of Health (DOH) 1992 Review of adoption law: a consultation document. HMSO, London

Department of Health (DOH) 1993 Adoption: the future. HMSO, London

Department of Health (DOH) 1998a Caring for children away from home: messages from research. Wiley, Chichester

Department of Health (DOH) 1998b The Government's response to the children's safeguards review. The Stationery Office London

Department of Health (DOH) 1998c Quality protects. Objectives for social services objectives for children. DOH, London

Department of Health (DOH) 1999 Adoption now: messages from research. Wiley, Chichester

Department of Health and Social Security (DHSS) 1976 Foster Care: a guide to practice. HMSO, London

Department of Health and Social Security (DHSS) 1985 Social work decisions in child care: recent research findings and their implications. HMSO, London

Downes C 1992 Separation revisited: adolescents in foster family care. Ashgate, Aldershot

Fahlberg V 1990 Residential treatment: a tapestry of many therapies. Perspectives Press, New York

Fahlberg V 1991 A child's journey through placement. Perspectives Press, Indianapolis

Fanshel D, Shinn E B 1978 Children in foster care: a longitudinal study. Columbia University Press, New York

Farmer E, Pollock S 1998 Sexually abused and abusing children in substitute care. Wiley, Chichester

Fein E et al. 1990 No more partings. An examination of long-term foster family care. Child Welfare League of America, New York

Fein E, Maluccio A N, Hamilton V J, Ward D E 1983 After foster care: permanency planning for children. Child Welfare 62 (6): 483–558

Fisher J, Wilson K, Gibbs I, Sinclair I 2000 Sharing the care: what foster carers want from Social Workers. Child and Family Social Work (in press)

Fletcher J 1993 Not just a name: the views of young people in foster and residential care. National Consumer Council, London

Fratter J 1993 Positive options planning scheme. In: Batty D (ed) HIV infection and children in need. British Agencies for Adoption and Fostering, London

Fratter J 1996 Adoption and contact: implications for policy and practice. British Agencies for Adoption and Fostering, London

Fratter J, Rowe J, Sapsford D, Thoburn J 1991 Permanent family placement: a decade of experience. British Agencies for Adoption and Fostering, London

Gibbons J, Gallagher B, Bell C, Gordon D 1995 Development after physical abuse in early childhood: a follow-up study of children on child protection registers. University of East Anglia, Norwich

Grimshaw R, Berridge D 1994 Educating disruptive children. National Children's Bureau, London

Grotevant H D, McRoy R G 1998 Openness in adoption: exploring family connections. Sage, New York

Hart G J 1986 Entitled to our care: a study of an adoption agency placing children with special needs. University of Salford Department of Sociology and Anthropology, Salford

Hazel M, Fenyo A 1993 Free to be myself: the development of teenage fostering. Human Service Associates, London

Hill M (ed) 1999 Signposts in fostering. British Agencies for Adoption and Fostering, London

Hill M, Shaw M (eds) 1998 Signposts in adoption. BAAF, London

Hill M, Lambert L, Triseliotis J 1989 Achieving adoption with love and money. National Children's Bureau, London

Hill M, Nutter R, Giltinan D, *et al.* 1993 A comparative survey of specialist fostering in the UK and North America. Adoption and Fostering 17 (2): 17–22

Hodges J, Tizard B 1989a Social and family relationships of ex-institutional adolescents. Journal of Child Psychology and Psychiatry 30 (1): 77–97

Hodges J, Tizard B 1989b IQ and behavioural adjustment of ex-institutional adolescents. Journal of Child Psychology and Psychiatry 30 (1): 53–75

Hoggan P, O'Hara G 1988 Permanent substitute family care in Lothian – placement outcomes. Adoption and Fostering 12 (3): 35–39

Howe D 1998 Patterns of adoption. Blackwell Science, Oxford

Howe D, Hinings D 1987 Adopted children referred to a child and family centre. Adoption and Fostering 11 (3):

Howe D, Hinings D 1989 The post-adoption centre: the first three years. University of East Anglia, Norwich

Kelly G, MacAuley C 1995 Foster care in Northern Ireland. British Agencies for Adoption and Fostering, London

Kirk H D 1964 Shared fate. Collier-Macmillan, London

Kirk H D 1981 Adoptive kinship: a modern institution in need of reform. Butterworths, Vancouver

Kufeldt K, Allison J 1990 Fostering children fostering families. Community Alternatives: International Journal of Family Care 1 (17): 1–17

Lahti J 1982 A follow-up study of foster children in permanent placements. Social Service Review. University of Chicago, Chicago

Lowe M, Murch M, Borkowski M, *et al.* 1999 Supporting adoption. British Agencies for Adoption and Fostering, London

Macaskill C 1985 Against the odds. Adopting mentally handicapped children. British Agencies for Adoption and Fostering, London

Macaskill C 1991 Adopting or fostering a sexually abused child. British Agencies for Adoption and Fostering, London

Maluccio A, Fein E, Olmstead K A 1986 Permanency planning for children: concepts and methods. Tavistock, London

Millham S, Bullock R, Hosie K, Haak M 1986 Lost in care. Gower, Aldershot

Millham S, Bullock R, Hosie K, Little M 1989 Access disputes in child care. Gower, Aldershot

Mullender A (ed) 1991 Open adoption. British Agencies for Adoption and Fostering, London

Nelson K A 1985 On the frontier of adoption: a study of special-needs adoptive families. Child Welfare Leagues of America, Washington

Nixon S 1997 The limits of support in foster care. British Journal of Social Work 27: 913–930

Packman J, Hall C 1998 From care to accommodation: support, protection and care in child care services. The Stationery Office, London

Packman J, Randall J, Jacques N 1986 Who needs care? Social work decisions about children. Blackwell, Oxford

Quinton D, Rushton A 1998 Joining new families: adoption and fostering in middle childhood. Wiley, Chichester

Redgrave K 1987 Child's play: direct work with the deprived child. Boys and Girls Welfare Society, Cheadle

Roberts J 1993 Abused children and foster care: the need for specialist resources. Child Abuse Review 2: 3–14

Rose M 1990 Healing hurt minds: the Pepper Harrow experience. Tavistock, London

Rowe J, Lambert L 1973 Children who wait. Association of British Adoption Agencies, London

Rowe J, Cain H, Hundleby M, Keane A 1984 Long-term foster care. Batsford, London

Rowe J, Hundleby M, Garnett L 1989 Child care now – a survey of placement patterns. British Agencies for Adoption and Fostering, London

Rushton A, Treseder J, Quinton D 1988 New parents for older children. British Agencies for Adoption and Fostering, London

Ryan T, Walker R 1993 Life story books. British Agencies for Adoption and Fostering, London

Schofield G, Beek M, Sargent K 2000 Growing up in foster care. British Agencies for Adoption and Fostering, London

Sellick C 1992 Supporting short-term foster carers. Avebury, Aldershot

Sellick C, Thoburn J 1996 What works in family placement. Barnardos, Barkingside

Shaw M, Hipgrave T 1983 Specialist fostering. Batsford, London

Sinclair I, Gibbs I 1998 Children's homes: a study in diversity. Wiley, Chichester

Social Services Inspectorate (SSI) 1998 Circular on adoption. The Stationery Office, London

Stalker K 1990 Share the care. Jessica Kingsley, London

Thoburn J 1990 Success and failure in permanent family placement. Gower/Avebury, Aldershot

Thoburn J 1991 Permanent family placement and the Children Act 1989: implications for foster carers and social workers. Adoption and Fostering 15 (3):

Thoburn J 1994 Child placement: principles and practice, 2nd edn. Arena, Aldershot

Thoburn J 1996 Psychological parenting and child placement. In: Howe D (ed) Attachment and loss in child and family social work. Avebury, Aldershot, pp. 129–145

Thoburn J, Murdoch A, O'Brien A 1986 Permanence in child care. Basil Blackwell, Oxford

Thoburn J, Norford L, Rashid S P 2000 Permanent family placement for children of minority. Jessica Kingsley, London

Thomas C, Beckford V 1999 Adopted children speaking. British Agencies for Adoption and Fostering, London

Thorpe R 1980 The experiences of children and parents living apart: implications and guidance in practice. In: Triseliotis J P (ed) New developments in foster care and adoption. Routledge and Kegan Paul, London

Tizard B 1977 Adoption, a second chance. Open Books, London

Triseliotis J P 1983 Identity and security in adoption and long-term fostering. Adoption and Fostering 7 (1): 22–23

Triseliotis J (ed) 1988 Group work in adoption and foster care. Batsford, London

Triseliotis J P, Russell J 1984 Hard to place: the outcomes of adoption and residential care. Heinemann and Gower, London

Triseliotis J P, Sellick C, Short R 1995 Foster care: theory and practice. Batsford, London

Triseliotis J P, Shireman J, Hundleby M 1997 Adoption: theory, policy and practice. Cassell, London

Utting W 1992 Children in the public care. HMSO, London

Utting W 1997 People like us. The Stationery Office, London

Wade J, Biehal N, Clayden J, Stein M 1998 Going missing: young people absent from care. Wiley, Chichester

Walby C, Symons B 1990 Who am I? Identity, adoption and human fertilisation. British Agencies for Adoption and Fostering, London

Ward H (ed) 1995 Looking after children: research into practice. HMSO, London

Wedge P, Mantle G 1991 Sibling groups and social work. Avebury, Aldershot

Weinstein E 1960 The self-image of the foster child. Sage, New York

Westacott J 1988 A bridge to calmer waters. Barnardos, London

28

Child protection: the manager's perspective

Paul Dyson

Paul Dyson

INTRODUC-TION

All work with children and families should retain a clear focus on the welfare of the child.
(Department of Health (DOH) 1999*a*)

The protection of children from harm is a difficult job; this simple fact can too often be forgotten in the daily management of social care and health agencies. Even more so can it be forgotten at times of crisis, when a child has been harmed or killed and there are the inevitable inquiries. Many organisations are involved in protecting children and, with the exception of the National Society for the Prevention of Cruelty to Children (NSPCC), child protection is often a small element of their overall work and responsibilities. All would doubtless agree with the contention that children have a right to be protected from harm. Yet the catalogue of child abuse enquiries since the 1974 death of Maria Colwell in the UK (see Corby, Chapter 13, in this volume), and for that matter in other countries (for example Belgium in the late 1990s) indicates some of the difficulties faced by those charged with protecting children.

It is the joint task of employers, managers and practitioners to ensure that the child's welfare is paramount. It is a focal theme of this chapter that the child is at the core of the manager's role, albeit the tasks vary from those of the practitioner. It is all too easy for children to be lost in the pressures that are faced in running large, complex health or social care agencies.

The death of Maria Colwell led to the most public enquiry since the death of Denis O'Neil in 1944, into the cause of a child's death. The report (Department of Health and Social Security (DHSS) 1974) placed managers centre stage. The practice of individual workers was critically examined but, as the report, stated:

What has clearly emerged, at least to us, is a failure of system compounded of several factors ... A system should so far as possible be able to absorb individual errors and yet function adequately.

(DHSS 1974, p. 86)

It is unequivocally the task of managers to develop strategically and manage operationally those systems. This chapter analyses that management task, and examines policy issues facing managers.

Review of relevant literature and research

The literature on child protection addresses the role of managers through advice and guidance from government, the analysis of 'what has gone wrong', and through research.

Most of the organisations involved in child protection are large, complex and multi-purpose, with a range of organisational cultures reflecting that diversity. Child protection agencies have to develop a common understanding, strategic direction and guidelines and procedures. These tasks were enshrined in the first edition of the Government's guidelines on inter-agency cooperation for the protection of children, *Working Together under the Children Act 1989* (Home Office *et al.* 1991). They are reinforced and expanded in the recent edition, *Working Together to Safeguard Children* (DOH 1999a). It is *Working Together*, more than any other publication in recent times, that has set the context of managing child protection by giving government guidance on inter-agency working focused on the Area Child Protection Committee (ACPC). It is clear that ACPCs should include senior managers from the main agencies, and the latest edition speaks of the need for ACPC programmes of work to be endorsed at senior level.

Working Together is issued under section 7 of the Local Authority Social Services Act 1970 which lays a duty on local authorities to comply with guidance unless local circumstances indicate exceptional reasons that justify a variation (DOH 1991). The intention is clear: senior managers should lead on child protection, a message highlighted by the Social Service Inspectorate (SSI 1997). The key body for inter-agency work is the ACPC, and each agency contributes to an integrated approach to meeting children's needs. Child protection in the 1970s and 1980s was dominated by a series of high profile cases and subsequent very public enquiries which generated a feeling amongst both practitioners and managers of being 'damned if you do, damned if you don't'. Agencies, their managers and their staff were, and remain, in the frontline. There are high expectations but also concerns about failure, and managers have to balance the support, and indeed the protection, of staff against the need for transparency and accountability.

This is not an issue that is well explored in the literature, but Reder *et al.* (1993), argue that there is a need to move away from a blame culture into one that examines the issues, offering an analysis that enables both practitioners and managers to develop an understanding of the processes that have led to the failure of the child protection system, as well as its successes and how it might be improved. The inquiry into the Cleveland affair (Butler-Sloss L. J. 1988), and before it the two inquiries into the deaths of Jasmine Beckford (London Borough of Brent 1985) and Kimberley Carlile (London Borough of Greenwich 1987), were defining reports, dealing as they did with the dual issue of perceived over-reaction in Cleveland and a failure to protect in the cases of Beckford and Carlile.

These reports, along with others (DHSS 1982, DOH 1991), indicated that agencies were not meeting the challenge of child protection. This state of affairs, combined with an emerging analysis from commentators (e.g. Thorpe 1994) that the broad range of the needs of children were not being met, has led to a renewed focus on protecting the most vulnerable children and providing support to their families. The Department of Health commissioned an array of research studies that were summarised in *Child Protection: Messages from Research* (1995). Using evidence from the research studies, *Messages from Research* queried whether the balance between 'child protection and the range of supports and interventions available to professionals is correct' (p. 54).

Since its publication, agencies have been faced with increasing pressure to develop their family support services. The literature, from both research and Government, has concentrated on achieving the balance between protection and family support. Parton *et al.* (1997) sought to analyse the issues for managers and practitioners in a book that contains much advice and insight for managers as they consider their child protection tasks. Not least, they highlighted the importance of the assessment of risk which, if it is to be of benefit, must centre on the child. In the process of refocusing services, managers must ensure that there is a robust risk-assessment strategy that leads to sound decision-making. This must be a consistent process that is evidence-based and provides a framework for referral to family support services, rather than triggering the child protection process inappropriately. If supportive interventions are offered to families, then risk must be identified and made explicit. The authors suggest that in Britain, in the decade following the Cleveland affair, child abuse has no longer been seen or understood in essentially medico-legal terms but that:

Signs of abuse have been replaced by what we call a regime of signification where notions of 'high risk' now both constitute the metaphor for child abuse and characterise the focus for the work itself.

(Parton *et al.* 1997, p. 218)

There are, however, inherent tensions and ambiguities in policy and practice terms arising from this regime of signification. For example:

- the concerns with both over- and under-intervention
- the way in which child protection has become contested in ways never previously evident (e.g. arguments within the medical profession as to the significance of signs and symptoms, and their relevance for indicating the presence of child abuse)
- the recognition of sexual abuse; an issue which touches a range of sensitivities not evident in earlier concerns about physical abuse and neglect.

The authors conclude that these factors have led the child abuse debate into new, problematic areas. For example, they query how cases of child abuse can be differentiated when the broad signs and symptoms '... associated with it seem to characterise normal families and to typify adult–child relations' (Parton *et al.* 1997).

This analysis poses challenges for managers. The late 1990s has seen the emergence of the performance culture (DOH 1999*b*), which has developed a framework for monitoring the public sector through national performance indicators. The problematic nature of the child abuse debate makes the identification of indicators more difficult, a factor that might well sit uncomfortably with the emerging culture. This is because it is a culture that sometimes appears to seek answers to unproblematic questions so as to produce performance indicators that managers, wanting to improve the standing and services of their organisations, understandably drive their organisations to attain.

Parton *et al.* (1997) also highlight the importance of managing risk through well-defined risk-assessment techniques, which must become the core of the professional task in child protection if the balance between protection and support is addressed. It is the task of the manager to develop risk-assessment processes and to ensure that they are evaluated. Managers are at the helm of organisations and the onus rests on them to create the space and time for practitioners to undertake these tasks. The importance of staff having space to reflect cannot be overemphasised because risk assessment is a daunting process and a child's and family's future may rest on it. Unfortunately, however, the problematic nature of child protection has led many social workers, health visitors, teachers and doctors to feel that their situation can, at crunch times, be one of 'low warmth high criticism', to parody *Messages from Research*, and not one of support. All too frequently the human resource issues arising for staff and middle managers working across agencies in child protection can be ignored.

In the UK, 1997 saw another watershed – the election of the New Labour Government and Tony Blair as Prime Minister. The Government adopted a policy of modernisation that has generated the need to concentrate on the big picture, as well as the detail, and brought extra tensions for managers, especially in health and social services.

Modernising Social Services (DOH 1998*a*) sets out Government expectations. In the introduction, Frank Dobson (then Secretary of State), wrote of his determination to have a system of 'health and social care which is convenient to use, can respond quickly to emergencies and provides top quality services'. The White Paper has a chapter devoted to child care and sets high expectations for both support and protection of children in society. The emphasis is clearly on providing high quality services across the whole range of child welfare. In this huge agenda, there is a real danger of losing sight of the need for the protection and support of children, or of prioritising the holistic agenda at the cost of child protection. In this book, in a chapter about the role of managers, it is therefore appropriate that the strategic tasks of child protection are highlighted, without losing sight of the larger issues.

Modernising Social Services identifies the large-scale social agenda. It is children of socially excluded families, of the poor and of ethnic minorities that are over-represented on child protection registers and in the looked after children population. Thus the Government's emphasis (DOH 1998*b*) on partnership, community safety, regeneration and other cross-agency initiatives has a clear contribution to make to child protection.

The manager in health and social care is faced with an increasing speed of change. *Modernising Health and Social Services* (DOH 1998*b*) reinforces the fact that the modernising agenda is a joint one for both Health and Social Services, standing alongside the demands of the emerging 'Performance Assessment Frameworks', exemplified in *A New Approach to Social Services Performance* (DOH 1999*b*). This consultation document sets out performance indicators for social services departments which are designed to improve the quality of services and will be used as a basis for publishing league tables of local authorities' performance (Flynn 1997). Inevitably, and rightly, all authorities want to do well and it lies at the heart of the managerial task to develop strategies to ensure the best performance. The social services performance framework includes 46 indicators, of which just three relate specifically to child protection. A local authority is performing well if there is a reduction in re-registrations, registration is for a shorter period and child protection reviews are completed within the established timescale. These are important aspects of the child protection system and are clearly linked to the development of an infrastructure of family support services. To achieve change for families requires extensive support services, however, and the pressure on managers to meet performance targets might lead to pressures on staff in the field to move families on without having achieved change or lessened risk. Such a managerial culture can therefore place great pressure on staff to meet organisational, rather than practice, goals.

Refocusing has costs in terms of extending resources, however. Waulby & Colton (1999) warn that statistics 'beg wider and more complex questions', arguing that crude interpretations of statistics are dangerous and must be avoided. They suggest, for example, that the balance of investment is moving away from the policies of family support, quoting the Chartered Institute of Public Finance Accountancy (CIPFA), which has revealed that the national costs of dealing with child abuse have risen in the UK at a rate of 1.2% above inflation. Cost is a factor on managers' minds at all times and, in a period of refocusing on family support services, such figures are challenging, especially when Government guidance and the research literature are highlighting the advantages of family support. Frost (in Parton 1997) redresses the balance by tentatively calculating the potential savings through the provision of family support services.

There is interesting research focusing on child protection services in Europe that suggests that British social work is perceived by its practitioners as being overly proceduralised and led by a managerial hardheadedness. The present performance culture may reinforce this view! Heatherington *et al.* (1997) researched child protection systems in eight European countries and sought to establish differences and common themes in the respective child protection systems. Interestingly, the emphasis on open non-stigmatised access to services in European systems, often with child abuse investigations not being the responsibility of the same agency offering family support, emerged favourably with British workers. The emphasis in Europe was on a more flexible continuum between support and protection. The authors suggest that there has been a longstanding difficulty in terms of families receiving support in the English system. This was identified in *Messages from Research*, and reinforced by the work of Gibbons *et al.* (1995), who illustrated that it is those children registered, and their families, who received significantly more services.

But Heatherington and colleagues analyse the reasons for this as being partly related to the development of eligibility criteria and thresholds, which they argue have become an English preoccupation and are essentially about keeping people out of services. *Modernising Social Services* comments:

Eligibility criteria are getting ever tighter and are excluding more and more people who would benefit from help.

(DOH 1998*a*)

Although this quote relates specifically to adult services it nonetheless has a bearing on all services. The comments of Heatherington, summarising the view of participants in the research from English social services departments, should therefore be heeded:

A farrago of legalism, proceduralism, managerialism, and more than a whiff of commercialism are the major elements which combine to deflect English social workers from sustaining a clear focus on the needs of the child and wider family in favour of procedural or legal rectitude and resource led managerial hardheadedness.

(Heatherington *et al.* 1997, p. 89)

The development of preventative services will help to avoid this 'farrago'. The literature reinforces the value of early intervention and wider access, along with partnership between agencies and families (see Petrie & Corby, Chapter 20, in this volume), The issue of inter-agency working is also well addressed elsewhere in this book (see Corby, Chapter 13), but a chapter devoted to the managerial perspective cannot avoid also considering this matter because managers hold the responsibility for the strategic planning of inter-agency work.

One of the best overviews of such issues is written by Hallett & Birchall (1992), an outstanding contribution to the field. Their work is concerned with the coordination of services and the nature of working together to protect children. It summarises the relevant literature and research and leaves no reader in any doubt as to both the necessity of working together and of its inherent difficulties. As the authors state in their introduction:

The phenomenon of child abuse which the professional network is commissioned to manage is profoundly problematic ... Equally important is the recognition that factors from the general field of organisational and interpersonal dynamics – agency function, compatibility and mutual understanding of techniques, professional acculturation and roles, personal and organisational power, status, gender – are all played out on this contentious material.

(Hallett & Birchall 1992, p. 3)

This quotation pinpoints many of the problematic aspects of working together. The Cleveland report identified the problems that can occur when key agencies cannot work together. In the concluding part of her report, Butler-Sloss L. J. (1988) highlights the lack of communication between agencies as a key reason for the crisis. Three years earlier, Parton (1985) had also highlighted the need for inter-agency working.

In 1999, New Labour again reinforced the need for partnership. Hallet & Birchall (1992) identify the nature of organisational and interpersonal dynamics and most managers reading the above quote will be only too well aware of the challenges behind that statement. Some of these difficulties are well illustrated by a recent publication by the Department of Health Social Care Group (1999), *Getting Family Support Right*, which examined the services of eight local authorities. The Inspectors found conflict in six authorities between health trusts and social services about how to provide a joint child and adolescent mental health service and there was little input from education professionals. In addition, the Inspectors found 'that in almost every authority inspected and in 40% of cases examined' (Department of Health Social Care Group 1999, para. 1.10) there were indicators of abuse and neglect that justified further assessment. Almost all families who were consulted expressed high levels of satisfaction. However, '... this success was often achieved without sufficient support from management' (p. 1).

Problems of inter-agency work and the effective management of the child protection system are highlighted in the work of Hallett & Birchall, the Maria Colwell report (DHSS 1974) and almost every other report into child abuse in the last 20 years of the twentieth century. The managerial task is to achieve genuine change that reduce some of the internecine conflict that seems to bedevil inter-agency work. Although interdisciplinary professional work at the practitioner level is often successful, the relationships between middle and senior managers can be complex (Butler-Sloss L.J. 1988), with a number of differences and disputes emerging, as well as substantive areas of agreement that may contribute to the welfare of children being lost.

Policy issues

Implications for managers

Inquiries describe the need for senior management to establish standards and monitor them, a process which effectively can fill the gap between a central policy and everyday practice.

(SSI 1997)

Translating a child-centred policy into practice in organisations in which child protection is a central issue is the particular task of managers. It is worthwhile restating that for most organisations in social, health care and the criminal justice system, child protection is a small proportion of their work. This section concentrates on the managerial task of integrating child protection into the wider strategic work of their organisations.

The day-to-day work of managers – for example, budget management, workforce planning (Utting 1997, Warner 1992), and setting strategic objectives – is of crucial importance to a sound child protection system. Workforce planning is particularly essential. Supporting and developing staff is one way to ensure that the balance of protection and support will be incorporated into practice. It also helps to avoid dangerous professional situations as reflected by the Department of Health (DHSS 1988) and more recently by Dent (1999).

All managers are responsible for developing coherent policies and practices that fit the diversity of the organisations involved in child protection, focusing on the needs of children and maintaining a range of services. As Denise Platt, Chief Inspector of Social Services, wrote in her 1999 Annual Report:

> What makes a significant difference to the performance of an organisation is the quality and competence of frontline managers ... [they] are the keystones of the organisation.
> (DOH 1999*d*)

Translating strategy into practice, maintaining quality of practice and developing knowledge and skills falls on these managers. Senior managers need to set strategy and create systems to monitor results. The evidence from research, the deluge of Government advice and the experience of managers working in the field underlines the fact that the development of child protection services is complex and requires managers to enable and motivate staff in their own agency, whilst also engendering inter-agency cooperation. This is a well-established difficulty that, as the Hallet & Birchall (1992) comment above illustrates, evokes many organisational and interpersonal issues. The need to have mechanisms to address cases of death and special interest, both within the organisation and jointly with others, adds to the complexity, as does the task of managing relationships with large organisations which have other complex responsibilities.

However, the understanding of the nature of child abuse remains problematic. The whole thrust of *Messages from Research* (DOH 1995) is that too much of the work undertaken comes under the banner of child protection, particularly highlighting the fact that many initial referrals alleging child abuse did not result in child protection conferences, let alone registration or, as importantly, the provision of services. There is therefore a need to provide a more balanced service for vulnerable children. Achieving this balance is the crux of the managerial task in the first decade of the millennium. The problematic nature of much of the subject matter makes the task daunting. *Messages from Research* clearly sets in train a refocusing on providing help and support to families alongside protection.

It is, perhaps, a cosy assumption for some in non-social service settings that focusing of services is solely a local authority role or that others have only a minor part to play. Nothing could be further from reality. The key strategic issue for mangers is that enhancing child protection requires enhancing family support services across *all* agencies. Child protection, whether it is work arising from registration, therapeutic interventions or the panoply of other activities involved, is a family support service. It is an inter-agency function that highlights inter- and intra-agency tensions, but engendering a culture that seeks protection through focused joined-up services is the objective.

Families in Focus (DOH 1998*d*) highlights policy and practice issues in the development of the child protection–family support continuum. Children in need will be better protected if families are given support through *early intervention* by *all* appropriate agencies. This does, however, raise issues of eligibility criteria and thresholds for services, as referred to above. Additionally, much more needs to be done to ensure that *the voice of the child is heard*. The sadness of this statement is that it needs saying at all since the duty to listen to children should be central to the professional ethos of all those involved in child care. Linked to listening to children is the *importance of using local knowledge* and *listening to families* who use services. Building meaningful structures for consulting with users and translating that into strategic thinking, so that policy and practice reflect the needs of the community, is important. *Monitoring and self-evaluation* also assures the quality of services provided. As agencies plan their children's services there is an emerging industry providing guidance, techniques and consultancy to monitor and evaluate services. Managers need to understand what works best for children and their families to ensure that at strategic and local level there is a consistent, effective evaluative framework.

Family support services and their relationship to child protection are at the core of the strategic development of child protection, as they broaden the opportunity to help families without losing sight of protection. There are, however, no simple nostrums to enable the development of family support. It involves resources. It takes time and space for children who are distressed and damaged to be heard, training for staff in interventive techniques, and for both managers and staff (Davies 1990) in their ability to examine their own work and actions. The task in meeting the challenge of providing both protection and family support is to build an organisation that is responsive to what is being said by children and their families, and that has robust risk-assessment procedures which enable statutory intervention when required.

Assessment and thresholds

Managers constantly have to address the issue of who gets a service and on what basis judgements are made about the allocation of resources to provide that service. Health and social care services in the public sector are involved in rationing, whether it is referred to as a National Health Service (NHS) waiting list or social services eligibility criteria. The evolving emphasis on family support services might challenge some well-established customs and practices, particularly in social services departments, about what are priority services. Traditionally a high priority is placed on the statutory duties of protection and care. As Heatherington *et al.* (1997) and Gibbons *et al.* (1995) highlight, however, families and children in the 'lower' priority categories do not always receive services.

If social services departments are to prioritise family support services, then families in many parts of the UK, who need but do not receive a service, will need to be provided with one. To implement an extensive family support service raises resource implications and, whether it is a case of reprovision or new money, prevention and support requires resources. Child protection has to be an integral part of the framework of family support services. If the findings of the Social Services Inspectors (Department of Health Social Care Group 1999) are replicated, then the development of family support services may also add to the burden of child protection services as further assessment of possible indicators of abuse are required. It is for managers to ensure that there are appropriate training and development opportunities for staff and that the agencies have a rigorous approach to assessment that is informed by research and best practice.

In the autumn of 1999, the Government published two documents for consultation: *A Framework for the Assessment of Children in Need and their Families* (DOH 1999c), and the new edition of *Working Together to Safeguard Children* (DOH 1999a). The *Framework* provides a structure for helping to collect and analyse information about children and their families, to assist agencies in ensuring that the most vulnerable receive a service. The intention is clear:

Effective collaboration between staff of different disciplines and agencies requires a common language to understand the needs of children, shared values about what is in the children's best interest and a joint commitment to improving the outcomes for children.

(DOH 1999c, p. ii)

Although primarily aimed at social service departments, the advice is for all agencies in the public and independent sector. It places a high priority on the joint planning of, and on the consistent and equitable implementation of, the assessment process. This, linked to good and effective planning, is a strategic task for managers. The new edition of *Working Together to Safeguard Children* clearly requires that assessment of all children in need – whether or not there are child protection concerns – should be undertaken using the new assessment framework.

However, there is confusion across agencies about the criteria used for triggering services. To agree these criteria is a complex business and balancing the allocation of resources in all agencies, in order to respond to allegations of abuse by providing support services which, if effective, should reduce the numbers of referrals of harm, is the real nut to crack. This will not be achieved without consistency in assessment frameworks.

Evidence suggests that such consistency is not there at present. Jones & Ramchandani (1999), commenting about research evidence in respect of the comprehensive assessment and planning in child sexual abuse cases, wrote:

Formal assessments were not the norm for many children who were considered sexually abused, although they were more likely in cases that were subject to conferences and formally registered. (p. 39)

Procedures and policies for assessment, care planning and intervention that are owned within and across organisations are necessary; they epitomise working together. Research evidence (Jones & Ramshandami 1999) challenges the assumption that all cases are appropriately assessed so the importance of the new framework and its implementation cannot be overemphasised, although its implementation might cause some tension in the competition for cash-limited resources. Assessments are of course the bedrock of child protection. Jones & Ramchandani (1999) comment:

Refocusing should not lead to a dismantling of the all-important protection services. Findings from this research on the numbers of children remaining unsafe and vulnerable despite intervention, emphasise this point. (p. 80)

Managers are faced with guidance, advice, regulation and research, and virtually instructed, at times, to follow all! When considering the development of child protection services, the senior manager will do well always to keep the diverse and complex needs of the child, the user of the service, in mind. An assessment framework that is implemented consistently (and there are good models published, e.g. Bridge Alert, from the Bridge Child Care Consultancy 1999) and whose results are monitored, will inform the planning and commissioning of services by mapping both outcomes and identifying unmet need. The importance of the corporate task of planning children's services and linking that planning to the activities of the ACPC will create a safer environment for children.

The strategic task of working together

There is a need for greater integration and closer links between social work and health, as well as other professions and agencies, because currently the needs of these children and their families are not being adequately addressed, dealt with or responded to.
(Jones & Ramchandani 1999, P. 81)

It is significant that these words were written in 1999, 25 years after the Maria Colwell report, which spoke of system failure, was published. There has been ample evidence of the difficulties of working across many agencies and, significantly, within agencies (DHSS 1982, DOH 1991, Hallet & Birchall 1992). A graphic example of the complexity of inter-agency working is illustrated by the report prepared by the Bridge Child Care Consultancy, into the death of a child, for Islington Area Child Protection Committee (Bridge Child Care Consultancy 1995). There were 30 operational units and the number of professionals was 'so high as to be unquantifiable' providing support to the family and child. Issues of communication, information flow, intra- and inter-agency tensions and professional demarcation all emerged. Inter-agency is used here to describe the more strategic activity of planning, commissioning and evaluating services across agencies. It is the arena in which much of child protection management occurs. Hughes (1998) suggests that inter-agency work is not the same as multi-agency work. She writes that inter-agency work requires all agencies to take responsibility for the problem, to subscribe to a common aim and evaluate in relation to that aim, to negotiate lead role(s) and move in and out of the lead as appropriate and finally, to consult with each other before developments are decided. These headings set an agenda for managers and identify the context in which tensions arise.

In 1998, the Government embarked on a series of major initiatives to encourage partnership across all health and social care organisations, including Quality Protects, an initiative to raise the standards of care, support and protection to children who are vulnerable and/or looked after (DOH 1998c). These initiatives are often tied to money, of course, in that agencies only receive finance if they evidence that they have met agreed targets (e.g. Quality Protects), and in many cases joint work is an identified performance indicator. The imperative for joint work is therefore crystal clear.

So why is it that issues of inter- and intra-agency working constantly arise, since we do not need more evidence to be sure that it is a real issue. The conclusion seems clear – that staff, and particularly managers, from the agencies involved sometimes find it very difficult, if not all but impossible, to work together. This is a frightening prospect for children suffering harm and in need of protection.

Balance is required, however, and not all multi-agency work is poor. There are countless examples of good practice, especially between practitioners, and there is an honourable record of multidisciplinary working (London Borough of Islington 1989, DOH 1999b). The key agencies involved in child protection are used to working together. Local authorities have well-established protocols with police forces for jointly investigating allegations of child abuse and the *Memorandum of Good Practice* (Home Office 1992) has led to many cooperative training ventures between police and social services. There is room for improvement, of course, and the example cited above from the Department of Health's review of family support services, about conflict between Health and Social Services over child and adolescent mental health services, is probably familiar to many practitioners and managers. Nonetheless, multidisciplinary practice is well-established. It is particularly the responsibility of ACPCs to develop joint training events which, perhaps, more than any other activity except practice, reinforces jointness. Inter-agency working is a skilled interpersonal task.

A manager's job consists of mostly interpersonal transactions, however, and Kakabadse et al. (1988) estimate that senior managers spend up to 80% of their time in oral communication with people inside and outside the organisation. Managers need to accept responsibility for, and develop their interpersonal skills to enable, inter-agency working. In the field of child protection, it is senior managers who comprise the ACPCs, and it is senior managers who undertake negotiations to set up planning groups, joint initiatives, Joint Investment Plans and so on.

But also it is senior managers who define and shape the uniqueness and identity of their own organisations and who create individual organisational cultures. Local authorities, health trusts, schools, police forces, to quote but a few, are all proud of their individual identities and want to maintain them within the multi-agency framework. It can be time-consuming and arduous to agree, implement and evaluate joint aims and objectives, and the tasks of developing organisations whilst also working together can lead to some degree of protecting organisational confidentiality and competition. It is therefore at least worthwhile considering that such dynamics may not be the best ingredients for encouraging the development of inter-agency working.

Nonetheless, senior managers spend a great deal of time meeting each other. Certainly if good relationships and effective inter-agency work was directly proportional to the number of meetings held in the health and social care arena, the world for children and their families would be a safe place! None of this is to be cynical about the myriad of successful joint endeavours. However, managers need to recognise that simply meeting as an ACPC or Joint Planning Team does not guarantee good inter-agency working. The key to success is joint agreement to shared objectives that are based on research evidence and a commitment that senior staff will follow through those objectives in their own agencies. The reasons for tensions between agencies are often understood but are not always challenged. The reality is that inter-agency work is complex. Managers need to reflect on their behaviour and perhaps be prepared to give up some of their hallowed ground. Children's needs will only be met when their, and not the organisations', needs are put first.

Summary of key issues

The issue of family support, and in particular the nature of the relationship between child protection and Family Support, is probably the primary policy matter facing child welfare as we approach the twenty first century.

(Frost, in Parton 1997)

Child protection remains central to child welfare but, as Frost indicates and as this chapter has argued, the balance is changing. This chapter has analysed the nature of the family support–child protection debate and its implications for managers. The value of family support services is well-established in the literature, but the imperative of protection must ensure that the child's total needs are not lost.

The dominance of guidance, advice and regulation from all recent governments has been emphasised. Strategic management is faced with macro and micro policy initiatives. The former represents the social policy context – the big picture, a particular feature of the Blair government – and reference has been made to the need to integrate child protection services into that wider picture. Examples include the Anti-Poverty, Community Safety and Partnership agendas that contribute to a safer environment and therefore to child protection. Such major policy thrusts absorb time and energy of managers whose own performance is partly judged on the success of these initiatives. Managers cannot, however, afford to lose sight of the detail and reference has been made to the specific challenges facing child protection and the importance of high quality frontline management to keep this focus.

The new edition of *Working Together to Safeguard Children* and the *Framework for Assessment* have set key objectives for the coming years. The former is unequivocally linked to the latter and sets the initial assessment of children within the context of section 17 of the Children Act 1989, which provides for the assessment and provision of services to children in need and their families. The Government's intention is clear and the spotlight is rightly on outcomes: on promoting access to a range of services for children in need without unnecessarily triggering child protection processes; on work in partnership with families using skilled assessment techniques; and on work across agency boundaries. This agenda poses some challenges for managers in terms of changing organisational cultures. The work of Jones & Ramchandani (1999), albeit concentrating on child sexual abuse, highlights the potential for losing the focus on child protection and for managers and staff there are tensions that need to be openly considered in order to ensure balance is maintained.

Inter-agency issues remain a key area of work. The challenge of working together has been met with varying levels of success. There is potential for conflict between individual organisations as they respond to the imperative for joint work. Maintaining a competitive edge can blur the task of jointly agreeing objectives across boundaries. By creating both a 'league table' mentality (which is very different from good performance management) and the 'joined up working' theme, the Government has added to that tension. The managerial role is to negotiate agreement with colleagues at a strategic level, however, and translate this into action in each agency.

Child protection work is a difficult and complex activity, both for practitioners and managers. Social and health care organisations are large and complex, and keeping a tight focus on child protection means there must be a symbiosis between strategic and operational management. Some of the tensions and difficulties raised by this have been explored but implicit throughout this chapter is that managers need to be proactive. The infrastructure that goes with a safe child protection system requires maintenance. Information technology systems, independent Chairs of child protection conferences, significant event chronologies on files in all agencies, well maintained and updated procedures, and crucially, a training and development programme, are just some key examples. Managers cannot do all these things themselves. They set the context, give permissions, negotiate ownership and evaluate outcomes. There is a fine line, however, between useful performance management and creating a culture amongst staff in which achieving the indicator has become the goal, rather than the provision of services. Child protection requires leadership and the appointment of able key staff to manage the operations.

Conclusion

> A story unfolds in the report of small carelessness, pressures of other work, difficulties of staffing and human procrastinations and failure to co-operate, by which few workers, if they are honest, have not at times been tempted from their standards, but which collectively resulted in individual tragedy and public scandal.
>
> (Jean Heywood (1959) writing about the death of Denis O'Neil)

This chapter has considered the issue of child protection and examined the role of managers in preventing harm to children, and supporting and helping children who have been or are likely to be harmed. Child protection systems are a vital contribution to the fabric of child welfare in a civilised society and the role of strategic management is to shape a system that is workable, respects children and their families, and is robust enough to ensure appropriate intervention.

It is self evident, however, that prevention is better than cure, hence the focus on the links between family support and child protection. The emergence of family support services as a major issue is now well-founded in the research literature and any serious discussion about the management of child protection must now reflect this debate. Placing children centre stage puts that policy into perspective. All agencies involved in child care must continue to develop services that meet the entire range of children's needs and there is now a real opportunity to develop comprehensive services to support children and families. There is some tension, but no contradiction, between support and protection – the role of the manager is to achieve the balance. No mean task – but an exciting one.

Annotated further reading

Publications listed in the references are not repeated here. Recent Department of Health publications listed there are essential reading for managers.

Coady M, Coady C A J 1992 There ought to be a law against it: reflections on child abuse, morality and the law. In: Alston P, Parker S, Seymour J (eds) Children, rights and the law. Oxford University Press, Oxford,
A moral and philosophical discussion about child abuse.
Dent R J 1998 Dangerous care working to protect children. The Bridge Child Care Consultancy, London
An excellent collection; has a review of key research findings.
Department of Health (DOH) 1998 Caring for children away from home: messages from research. John Wiley & Sons, Chichester
These studies deal with culture, safety and management in children's homes.
Dumoi W (ed) 1995 Changing family policies in the member States of the European Union. Commission of The European Communities, Brussels
An international perspective that stimulates lateral thinking about policy.
Hagell P 1999 Dangerous care: reviewing the risks to children from their carers. Policy Studies Institute, London
Discusses risk assessment, dangerousness and a refreshing review of ethical issues in child protection.
Sanders R, Thomas N 1997 Area Child Protection Committees. Ashgate, Aldershot
Surveys the work of ACPCs.

References

Bridge Child Care Consultancy 1995 Paul: death through neglect. Islington ACPC, London
Butler-Sloss Lord Justice E 1988 The report of the inquiry into child abuse in Cleveland 1987. HMSO, London
Davies M 1990 A permanent mark? – management responsibility in child protection. In: NSPCC (ed) Listening to children: the professional response to hearing the abused child. Longman, Harlow
Dent R J 1998 Dangerous care: working to protect children. The Bridge Child Care Consultancy, London
Department of Health (DOH) 1991 Child abuse: a study of inquiry reports 1980–1989. HMSO, London
Department of Health (DOH) 1998a Modernising social services: promoting independence, improving protection, raising standards. The Stationery Office, London
Department of Health (DOH) 1998b Modernising health and social services: national priorities guidance 1999/00–2001/02. The Stationery Office, London
Department of Health (DOH) 1998c Quality Protects Circular. Transforming children's services. Local Authority Circular LAC (98) 28. The Stationery Office, London
Department of Health (DOH) 1998d Families in focus, The Stationery Office, London
Department of Health (DOH) 1999a Working together to safeguard children. A guide to inter-agency working to safeguard and promote the welfare of children. Department of Health, London
Department of Health (DOH) 1999b A new approach to social services performance. Consultation document. The Stationery Office, London

Department of Health (DOH) 1999c Framework for the assessment of children in need and their families. Consultation draft. Department of Health, London

Department of Health (DOH) 1999d The eighth annual report of The Chief Inspector of Social Services. Social Care Group, London

Department of Health Social Care Group 1999 Getting family support right: inspection and delivery of family support services. Department of Health, London

Department of Health and Social Security (DHSS) 1974 Report of the committee of inquiry into the care and supervision provided in relation to Maria Colwell. HMSO, London

Department of Health and Social Security (DHSS) 1982 A study of inquiry reports 1973–1981. HMSO, London

Department of Health and Social Security (DHSS) 1988 Working together. A guide to arrangements for inter-agency cooperation for the protection of children from abuse. HMSO, London

Gibbons J, Conroy S, Bell C 1995 Operating the child protection system: a study of child protection practices in English local authorities. HMSO, London

Flynn N 1997 Public sector management. Prentice Hall/Harvester, London

Hallett C, Birchall E 1992 Coordination and child protection: a review of the literature. HMSO, London

Heywood J 1959 Children in care. Routledge and Kegan Paul, London

Heatherington R, Cooper A, Smith P, Wilford G 1997 Protecting children: messages from Europe. Russell House, Lyme Regis

Home Office 1992 Memorandum of good practice. HMSO, London

Home Office, Department of Health, Department of Education and Science, Welsh Office 1991 Working together under the Children Act 1989. HMSO, London

Hughes J 1998 Making inter-agency work work. In: NOTA News 28. NOTA, Hull

Jones D, Ramchandani P 1999 Child sexual abuse: informing practice from research. Radcliff Medical Press, Abingdon

Kakabadse A, Ladlow R, Vinnicombe S 1988 Working in organisations. Penguin, London

London Borough of Brent 1985 A child in trust: the report of the panel of inquiry into the circumstances surrounding the death of Jasmine Beckford. London Borough of Brent, London

London Borough of Greenwich 1987 A child in mind: protection of children in a responsible society. The report of the commission of enquiry into the circumstances surrounding the death of Kimberley Carlile. London Borough of Greenwich, London

London Borough of Islington 1989 Report into the death of Liam Johnson. London Borough of Islington, London

Parton N 1985 The politics of child abuse. Macmillan, London

Parton N (ed) 1997 Child protection and family support. Tensions, contradictions and possibilities. Routledge & Kegan Paul, London

Parton N, Thorpe D, Wattam C 1997 Child protection. Risk and the moral order. Macmillan, London

Reder P, Duncan S, Gray M 1993 Beyond blame. Routledge, London

Social Services Inspectorate (SSI) 1997 Messages from inspection: child protection inspections 1992–1996. Department of Health, London

Thorpe D 1994 Evaluating child protection. Open University Press, Milton Keynes

Waulby C, Colton M 1999 More children – more problems? Community Care 15–21 July

Warner N 1992 Choosing with care: the report of the committee of inquiry into the selection, development and management of staff in children's homes. HMSO, London

Utting W 1997 People like us. The report of the review of the safeguards for children living away from home. The Stationery Office, London

29 Safeguarding and promoting children's welfare: a question of competence?

Pat Walton

The content, structure and delivery of social work education and training is under review and will be undergoing major change. A key concept within this process is the notion of *competence* and its impact on the world of work in general. This concept, designed originally for use in industrial settings in the USA and subsequently adopted by the UK during the 1980s, has spread gradually to 'the professions' and the development of 'occupational standards' for different professional groups. As the new Training Organisation for the Personal Social Services (TOPSS) informs us, 'National Occupational Standards describe best practice in particular areas of work. These standards bring together the skills, knowledge and values necessary to do the work as statements of competence' (TOPPS 1999).

This chapter draws on the chapter by Jones (1995*a*) in the first edition of the *Handbook* and explores the development of competence and its application to vocational education and training (VET) for professionals in health and social care. These are the people who deliver highly complex services to society's most vulnerable members. The impact of competence-based occupational standards is considered both for practitioners and first-line managers in relation to social work practice.

Social work is becoming increasingly a multi-agency activity. This shift mirrors changes in central government policies, some of which relate primarily to children and families. Key policy issues are considered in the next section which sets the scene for an exploration of the ever more complex nature of social work. Although the chapter's focus is on post-qualifying *social work* education and training, because of certain policy developments, future training within a multi-professional context is also discussed.

Whatever the continuing concerns regarding competence-based assessment and training, the centrality of competence is now well established in the world of work and in VET. However, the concept has not been adopted without controversy. On the one hand, Winter (1992) discusses with enthusiasm a competence-based degree level social work programme developed in partnership between a university and a social services department. He highlights that, among other benefits, competence-based education provides for 'precision and justice in assessment, increased access to educational opportunity and a general "learner centredness" ...' On the other hand, Bates (1995, p. 40) suggests that: 'the rate of development of the competence movement now vastly outstrips our understanding of both its effectiveness and its social significance; more metaphorically, it has become a colossus, skating on very thin ice'.

As Watkins (1999) reminds us, attempts to improve workforce effectiveness using competence-based assessment and training are underway in the USA and Australia as well as in the UK. Additionally, 'the European Union is debating the use of competencies as a means of establishing the mutual recognition of professional qualifications' (Hughes 1994, cited in Watkins 1999, p. 41). All this suggests that competence and its central position in defining occupational standards, assessment and training outcomes is here to stay. It remains to be seen whether such a concept will improve the effectiveness of 'child care' professionals and service delivery to children and families. However, it is possible for those involved in social work education and training, management and direct practice to shape this process. As such, this chapter represents a modest contribution to the debate surrounding competence and child care practice.

Current policies: their impact on 'child care' practice and training

As the twenty-first century begins, major reorganisation of services developed over the past 25 years for children and families is taking place. Since the mid-1970s and the establishment of 'child protection procedures', following the death of Maria Colwell, local authority service provision for children and families has focused increasingly on 'child protection'. As highlighted in this chapter's revised title, a refocusing is underway; coordinated service delivery that assesses and enhances children's development across a broad spectrum is now required of statutory, voluntary and private sector agencies.

The overall aim of current policy development for children and families service provision is to provide a framework for developing preventive rather than reactive services. This aim requires a refocusing of services in order to address children's needs initially at a community-based level of intervention (Hardiker *et al.* 1996).

In May 1998, the Department for Education and Employment (DfEE 1998*a*) published a framework and consultation document, *Meeting the Childcare Challenge*. In its foreword, Tony Blair gave a Government pledge to support families and children as 'the core of our society' and acknowledged that 'they are under pressure' (p. 2). *Meeting the Childcare Challenge* announced the setting up of the National Child Care Strategy and heralded the Government's intention to provide services to meet a wide spectrum of educational, health and direct child care support needs as well as increased welfare benefits and financial help for families on a low income.

One such programme of family support within the 'early years' provision is Sure Start (Glass 1999), which targets families with children under the age of 4. This initiative, set up by the DfEE and the Department of Health (DOH) began in January 1999 with the launch of the first 60 Sure Start programmes. These epitomise current policies designed to promote the refocusing of services, in that service delivery is at a preventive level and encompasses a range of agencies: education, health and social services as well as the voluntary and independent sectors:

It [Sure Start] is part of the Government's policy to prevent social exclusion and aims to improve the life chances of younger children through better access to early education and play, health services for children and parents, family support and advice on nurturing.

(Glass 1999, p. 257)

A significant step in refocusing and improving services for children was the mapping of local authority provision under the *Quality Protects* programme (DOH 1998*a*). One hundred and fifty local authorities submitted to the DOH their Management Action Plans (MAPs) designed to meet eight objectives defined by the DOH for children and families service delivery. These objectives reflected a wider definition of children's needs than that of 'protection' and in order to meet them, it was recognised that agencies would require a workforce whose training would need to reflect this broad spectrum.

Although *Quality Protects* is directed at social services departments, the Government's intention is to establish a strategy for 'connected solutions to joined-up problems' (DOH 1998*b*, p. 12). To further this plan, the Government published a White Paper in November 1998, *Modernising Health and Social Services* which increased the original eight objectives for children's services to 11 (DOH 1998*c*). This paper confirmed the Government's intention to promote closer collaboration between local authority departments, the health service, and the voluntary and independent sectors.

Assessment of children's and families' needs is a key requirement in meeting the *Quality Protects* objectives. In order to help local authorities with this, the Government has produced practice guidelines that reflect the new directions for services for children and families: *Framework for the Assessment of Children in Need and their Families* (DOH 1999*a*) and *Working Together to Safeguard Children: a guide to inter-agency working to safeguard and promote the welfare of children* (DOH *et al.* 1999). These guides are issued initially as consultation drafts.

The Guidance [*Framework for the Assessment of Children in Need*] is a key element of the Department of Health's work to support local authorities in implementing Quality Protects, the Government's £375 m programme for transforming the management and delivery of children's social services … The framework has been developed in parallel with the new Guidance on protecting children from harm (*Working Together to Safeguard Children*).

(DOH 1999*a*, p. i)

Training is being redesigned to provide professionals who can deliver services that reflect these new policies. New social work training will build on current post-qualifying social work programmes established during the 1990s within the 'post-qualifying framework' (Central Council for Education and Training in Social Work (CCETSW) 1992). Importantly, a new post-qualifying child care award (PQCCA) is being developed through eight pilot programmes beginning in January 2000. These will be extended during 2001 with the aim of training social workers to deliver the services to meet the objectives defined by the *Quality Protects* initiative.

These new training programmes will be designed to enable social workers to meet new occupational standards defined by CCETSW in collaboration with social workers' employers and informed by a conceptual framework designed by Jane Aldgate and Richard Coleman, University of Leicester School of Social Work (DOH 1999*b*). Both the conceptual framework and the standards are child-focused and underpinned by a child development perspective, thus reflecting current Government policies for children's services.

In order to ensure that child care social workers will be able to access the new PQCCA, the Department of Health in *Modernising Health and Social Services* (1998*c*) and more recently Local Authority Circular (99)37 (DOH 1999*c*) has announced its intention to ring fence an additional £6 million within local authorities' Training Support Provision (TSP) for the funding of this new training, which will include first-line managers.

The new occupational standards that will underpin the PQCCA have recently been published as an 11th draft by TOPPS (1999). The occupational standards are underpinned by the concept of *competence*. During the past decade, this concept has had a significant impact on social work training as well as on the training of other professionals.

O'Hagan (1996, p. 1) reminds us that the CCETSW's (1989, revised 1991) Paper 30, which established the new Diploma in Social Work, created 'turmoil' with its emphasis on the establishment of partnerships between employers and training institutions and the goal of competence: '... "*competence*" was a major goal: social work training was to be competence-led, competence-dominated, and always competence-seeking'.

Following the new Diploma in Social Work, CCETSW set up in 1992 with the publication of Paper 31 (revised in 1997) the post-qualifying (PQ) framework for social workers' continuing professional development. The PQ framework was underpinned by the same principles and concepts: employer – university partnerships and the demonstration of *competence*. Why the concept of competence has caused so much debate, particularly in the field of higher education, is now considered.

Review of the literature

The complex nature of practice

Jones' chapter in the first edition of the *Handbook* began this section by drawing on the document *The Care of Children: Principles and Practice in Regulations and Guidance* (DOH 1989). In this document the Government offers 26 principles that should underpin child care social work practice. This remains an appropriate place to start as we await the publication of the new requirements for social workers that will underpin their future practice and their new training: the PQCCA.

Requirements of social work practice highlighted by the Government in 1989 were that it should seek:

... to combat racism in all its forms of discrimination against individuals and groups ... Partnership, participation, choice, openness, parental responsibility and [should be aware of] every child's need for both security and family links

(DOH 1989, p. 1)

These principles reflect those of the Children Act 1989, which provides the legal framework for safeguarding and promoting children's welfare. However, research findings from studies published in 1995 (DOH 1995) found that sections of the Act relating to child *protection* (e.g. section 47), rather than those addressing children's broader needs (e.g. section 17), were tending to dominate services. This emphasis by welfare agencies and the ways in which service provision reflected it, was found to be falling short of the principles advocated by central government in their 1989 publication cited above:

The series of child protection research studies (DOH 1995) found that the preoccupation by local authorities on investigation of suspected child abuse had alienated carers and children and had created concerns for social workers. Their efforts to improve children's lives often seemed to cause more distress. These depressing findings were particularly common in relation to children who had been, or were suspected of being, sexually abused (DOH 1995, p. 80). In particular, there were distressing reports from non-abusing or 'safe' carers (usually children's mothers). Once the 'authorities' had decided that children were no longer at risk of sexual abuse, often because their mothers had made difficult changes in their own and their children's lives in order to protect them, any help which had been forthcoming from the 'services' during the child protection investigation ceased.

(Walton 1999*a*, p. 6)

One of the key findings from the DOH (1995) studies was that effective child care practice depends on 'sensitive and informed professional/client relationships [and] on an appropriate balance of power between the key parties ...' (p. 52). The new guidance, *Working Together to Safeguard Children* (DOH *et al.* 1999, pp. 98–99) offers 15 basic principles for working in partnership with children and families. These include (original numbering kept):

4. Be clear with yourself and with family members about your power to intervene, and the purpose of your professional involvement at each stage.
5. Be aware of the effects on family members of the power you have as a professional, and the implications of what you say and do.
14. Take care to distinguish between personal feelings, values, prejudices and beliefs, and professional roles and responsibilities, and ensure that you have good supervision to check that you are doing so.

As discussed later, one of the most swingeing criticisms of competence-based professional practice is its failure to take proper account of issues of power and therefore its potential for misuse in relationships where power is unequal (Dominelli 1996).

Working Together to Safeguard Children (DOH *et al.* 1999) also addresses partnership between professionals and agencies working together to promote children's welfare and to protect them from harm. Multi-professional working is complex, particularly in the field of child protection (Horne 1990, Reder *et al.* 1993*a*, 1993*b*, Hallett & Birchall 1995*a*, 1995*b*, Stevenson 1999, Violence against Children Study Groups 1999). Reder *et al.* (1993*a*, 1993*b*) draw on a systemic conceptual framework in exploring the deaths of children who were the subjects of 35 child abuse inquiries (DOH 1991*a*). A repeated finding from the inquiries was that inter-professional and inter-agency work played a significant part in the failure to protect the children. Their findings concerning inter-professional relationships and communication among professional network members identified four problematic patterns, which they termed 'closed professional system', 'polarisation', 'exaggeration of hierarchy' and 'role confusion' (Reder *et al.* 1993*a*, p. 71):

In a 'closed professional system', one group of workers became united by the dominant view about the case and were less sensitive to conflicting information or observations ... in 'polarisation', schisms developed between groups of workers in which their opinions about the case diverged and they shared less and less information with each other ... in 'exaggeration of hierarchy', workers' presumed status relative to each other was magnified and professionals with lower perceived status deferred to the opinions of others seen as hierarchically superior.

(Reder *et al.* 1993*b*, pp. 92–93)

Good practice depends on appropriate working relationships which support accurate professional judgement based on evidence-based assessment, as part of a process of intervention and evaluation. As Lloyd & Taylor (1995, p. 708) remind us, 'Good practice in social work assessment demands that practitioners be competent, knowledgeable, consistent and accountable, in situations which are frequently chaotic, irrational, hopeless or just plain messy. To do so and remain as human beings relating to other human beings is a complex and risky enterprise'. The new guidance on assessing children's and families' needs produced by the DOH (1999*a*, p. 10) defines ten principles required of practitioners. Assessments should:

- be child-centred
- be rooted in child development
- be ecological in their approach
- ensure equality of opportunity
- require work in partnership with children and families
- build on strengths as well as identify difficulties
- be multi-agency in their approach to assessment and the provision of services
- be a continuing process, not a single event
- be carried out in parallel with other action and providing services
- be grounded in evidence-based knowledge.

This important framework highlights the complexity of making professional judgements in social work which underpin intervention such as removing a child from home, possibly in order to afford protection. As Drury-Hudson (1999, p. 148) points out, 'perhaps no decision in social work poses more awesome responsibilities for the social worker and has more devastating consequences for the child and family ... Research has estimated that 25 per cent of all child fatalities occur in families previously known to, or under the supervision of, social service agencies ...' (Armytage & Reeves 1992, cited in Drury-Hudson 1999). Balancing such knowledge and a fear of media pillorying with an awareness of children's overall developmental needs and findings from research that highlight the poor developmental outcomes for children looked after by local authorities (DOH 1991*b*, Ward 1995), remains a key challenge for front-line child care social workers and their managers.

In addition to the traditional complexity of social work, which involves vulnerable service users and often unpredictable and stressful situations, the shift in our society to a market economy has brought new expectations of social workers. Despite New Labour's emphasis on partnership between informal, voluntary, statutory and private welfare sectors (Page & Silburn 1998), Government administrations during the 1980s and 1990s have continued to apply market forces to the public sector in trying to ensure 'leaner, fitter and more efficient' services (Hodkinson & Issitt 1995, p. 1). To this end, health and social care professionals are being required, increasingly, to act as brokers in the provision of scarce resources (Brown & Bourne 1996). Knowledge and skills to achieve such tasks have to be developed alongside the continuous updating of more familiar knowledge and skills.

These changes in central government ideology and policies and their impact on organisations and professionals contribute to the difficulty in defining new requirements or occupational standards for health and social care professionals.

However, the role of *competence* in defining the requirements of workers during the past decade is now playing a key part in developing new occupational standards across the professions. As the link between professional occupations and training has grown, the concept of competence now informs both.

Defining competence and its influence on education and training

The Health Education Authority (HEA) in their special issue newsletter *The National Occupational Standards for Professional Activity in Health Promotion and Care* (1998, p. 2), inform us that 'Competence is "the ability to do something well or effectively" (*Cobuild Dictionary, Collins*: 1994)'. (Lindsay) Mitchell (Director, Prime Research and Development) suggests that the description of competence falls into three broad patterns:

1. What people bring or what they are like – personal qualities, skills, knowledge, motives and aspirations...
2. What people have to know or be able to do after a period or programme of learning – 'competence-based' programmes...
3. What people have to achieve – the level of expected achievement is set by a process of consensus-forming and negotiation and can focus on minimum standards of safe practice or good practice standards. The principal use of this model is to assess whether individuals meet the standards required for particular areas of work and hence make decisions about education and development needs at an individual or organisational level. (HEA 1998, p. 2).

This description sets the scene for an exploration of competence and its current key position in both the training and assessing of professionals involved in complex practice such as child care work.

Williams & Raggatt (1998) offer an historical and political perspective which sheds some light on the factors surrounding the tenacious hold on the world of work and training in the UK which competence now exerts. They suggest that this is particularly interesting in view of the lack of research into its effectiveness.

Competence-based learning originated in the USA as a response to society's demands for increased competence partly due to '... the feeling that standards of achievement, morality and order were in decline' (Rushton & Martyn 1993, cited in Ashworth & Saxton 1990, p. 4). At the end of the 1970s the youth labour market in Britain had collapsed and new ways of addressing unemployment had to be found. As Williams & Raggatt (1998) remind us, economic recession has an impact on education and generates criticisms of it. Criticisms then directed at education were that it did not provide school-leavers with the knowledge and skills necessary for work.

The Manpower Services Commission (MSC), in seeking a solution to youth unemployment, drew on the American model of behaviourally determined learning and training to establish Youth Training Schemes (YTS) and subsequently Youth Opportunities Programmes (YOPs) in the UK. These provided 162 000 places in 1978–1979, rising to 553 000 in 1981–1982 (Williams & Raggatt 1998). These programmes required the support of work-related and work-based curricula for the young trainees rather than college-based learning ones. 'Thus it is in this context that one can identify an imperative, albeit a somewhat implicit one, to move away from the traditional "input" paradigm towards a model of vocational education and training *in which the outcomes that individuals achieve are given recognition* ...' (Williams & Raggatt 1998, p. 286; my emphasis). Accrediting outcomes was also seen as increasing the credibility of the new scheme and as a way of countering criticisms of it which suggested that it was merely a way of keeping young people off the streets.

The work on developing a curriculum and appropriate accreditation of learning based on outcomes defined by the workplace led to the setting up in 1985 of a new YTS to provide recognised qualifications for all young people in their transition from school to work. It also instituted a Review of Vocational Qualifications in England and Wales (Department of Employment (DE) & Department of Education and Science (DES) 1985), the focus of which was youth training but Williams & Raggatt point out (1998, p. 288) '... the concept of "competence-based" vocational qualifications had become increasingly attractive to policy-makers (see DE & DES 1985, pp. 8–9)'.

Following the publication in 1986 of a White Paper, *Education and Training – Working Together* (DE & DES 1986), the National Council for Vocational Qualifications (NCVQ) was established. Its remit was 'to implement, or secure action to implement, a system of vocational qualifications that will achieve the objectives of comprehensibility, relevance, credibility, accessibility and cost-effectiveness' (cited in Ashworth & Saxton 1990, p. 5).

Jessup (1990), the NCVQ's Scientific Director, outlined the task of the NCVQ. Its function was to put the emphasis on 'outputs', defined as 'standards that need to be achieved at the end of a learning programme', as distinct from 'inputs', which are 'the learning opportunities provided'. 'Standards' specify the level of performance required of a person, and are thus linked to 'statements of competence', which in turn need to incorporate the assessment of 'skills to specified standards; relevant knowledge and understanding; and the ability to use skills and to apply knowledge and understanding to the performance of relevant tasks' (cited in Ashworth & Saxton 1990, p. 5). The NCVQ uses functional analysis to define 'units of competence' and to divide each unit of competence into 'elements of competence'. Employees' abilities to perform to the required standard are assessed against a set of 'performance criteria' which comprises these. Importantly, the required standards were, and still are, *employer-led*:

The system must be planned and led by employers as it is they who are best placed to judge skill needs; it must actively engage individuals of every age, background and occupation, because they have much to gain from appropriate investment in their own training and skills; it must cooperate with the education service.

(DE 1988, p. 38)

NVQs involve ongoing assessment in the workplace and are structured across five levels. Following the implementation of Levels 1, 2 and 3, a Higher-Level Strategy Group was formed in 1991 to extend the NVQ framework to higher-level professional skills and, in 1997, the Qualifications and Curriculum Authority (QCA) was established to develop 'a coherent national framework of qualifications covering "all qualifications at all levels" (QCA press release, June 1998)' (Watkins 1999, p. 42). Levels 4 and 5 approximate to graduate, postgraduate and various professional qualifications such as the accreditation of social workers at PQ level:

Level 4
Competence which involves the application of knowledge in a broad range of complex technical or professional work activities performed in a wide variety of contexts and with a substantial degree of personal responsibility and autonomy. Responsibility for the work of others and allocation of resources is often present.

Level 5
Competence which involves the application of a significant range of fundamental principles and complex techniques across a wide and often unpredictable variety of contexts. Very substantial personal autonomy and often significant responsibility for the work of others and for the allocation of substantial resources feature strongly, as do personal accountabilities for analysis and diagnosis, design, planning, execution and evaluation.

(Watkins 1999, p. 42)

To summarise, the greater control of education by employers and the State afforded by the creation of the NCVQ is reflected in the characteristics of competence-based education and training in Britain:

- Training goals are derived from an analysis of occupational roles, i.e. functional analysis
- These goals are translated into training outputs in the form of performance criteria rather than training 'inputs' such as syllabi
- They offer the opportunity for people to progress at their own speed with readily available performance assessment opportunities rather than coverage of course content, i.e. self-paced learning (Bates 1995, p. 44).

Pillay *et al.* (1998) discuss competence-based education and training in Australia and suggest that there is a lack of evidence that it leads to better outcomes. Citing Mayer (1992) they identify the importance of knowledge and understanding to competent practice: 'competence is underpinned not only by performance but also by knowledge and understanding, and ... competence involves both the ability to perform in a given context and the capacity to transfer knowledge and skills to new tasks and situations'. They highlight the complexity of these abilities and the influence on them of 'many psychosocial factors' (Pillay *et al.* 1998). These complex requirements of professionals are also pinpointed by Hager & Gonczi (1996). This is discussed further in the next section when exploring how professionals apply knowledge and skills in different contexts.

One of the major criticisms of the competence approach is that its focus is on *performance and purpose* rather than *process*. As highlighted earlier (Mitchell 1998, p. 2): 'The principal use of this model is to assess whether individuals meet the standards required for particular areas of work ...' This emphasis is questionable in terms of supporting and developing professional practice. Appropriate knowledge, skills and values and the ability to integrate these determine competent professional practice, rather than the measurement of it against predetermined standards and procedures. For example, candidates at post-qualifying level of the CCETSW PQ framework may be able to work effectively in situations where they carry responsibility for those at serious risk by following procedures alone, but they may have little appreciation of the moral and ethical context of their decision-making. As discussed in the next section, professional practice is unpredictable, requiring practitioners to be able to draw on knowledge, values and skills in different and often complex contexts where interpretation of direct communication, behaviours and interaction within those situations plays a vital role in assessment. It is essential that practitioners learn how to practise as competent professionals under these circumstances. How professionals in the person-centred professions make complex judgements and whether the new competence-based standards will help them to do so is explored further in the next section.

Implications for practice

Competence and practice in the person-centred professions

This section explores some of the concerns highlighted in the literature regarding the application of competence to professional practice and training, together with findings from two studies of post-qualifying programmes involving the compilation of practice portfolios which identify some positive learning outcomes for candidates.

Some of the concerns relating to practice emphasise the detrimental effects on professional judgement and assessments of disaggregating into discrete parts complex tasks and the implications of predetermined occupational standards on service users' rights to be consulted. Issues raised in relation to professional education and training highlight the incompatibility of aims between academic learning and competence-based education and training (CBET) with its emphasis on learning outcomes and occupational performance.

Ethics or 'general principles of what one ought to do' (Robson 1993, p. 30) are integral to professional practice. CCETSW defines the ethical values of social work within the confines of the historical, social and political context of the time. The current definitions were updated in 1995 (CCETSW 1995) and are reflected in the recent DOH (1999*a* guidelines highlighted earlier).

Dominelli (1996) delivers a scathing critique of the NVQ model in which she argues that the competency-based approach is *oppressive* to both service users and workers. She states that the approach individualises and blames workers for structural problems and inadequate resources:

The competency-based approach *presupposes* that:

- what needs to be done in each situation is known and infallible;
- resources are adequate for the tasks at hand; and
- social work relationships operate in a social vacuum (p. 168).

Dominelli (1996) also criticises competency-based practice due to its lack of concern for relationship building and its assumption that there is mutuality between the interests of service providers and service users:

The assessment, planning and intervention stages of social work encompassed by competency based 'case management' systems have become the formal way through which practice skills are defined, elaborated and practised ... it has little scope for involving users in making *real decisions* ... in the market model, the consumer is a passive agent who simply responds to choices which others have laid out. (p. 159)

Also highlighted is the way in which the approach, by attempting to fragment complex professional activity into 'simple' discrete parts, is deprofessionalising social work by the employment of unqualified and low paid workers to perform these seemingly simple tasks.

Issitt & Woodward (1992) also identify a key difficulty in defining competent professional practice using functional analysis:

The essential problem ... is that, at the receiving end, it is the whole interactive performance that is of significance, not bits and pieces assembled or bolted together ... the notion of a 'competent person' ably subtlely and uniquely to care for others in a multitude of situational contexts seems to be lost. (p. 47)

This atomistic reduction of professional activity into separate parts is contrary to holistic professional practice (Jones 1995*b*). Professional practice depends on an ability to synthesise appropriate knowledge, skills and values whilst incorporating contextual feedback. This is the essence of *reflection in and on action*. Schon (1991) likens this ability to that of jazz musicians who are required to integrate into their own playing 'on the spot' feedback from other musicians in order to produce the desired sound.

Hager & Gonczi (1996) highlight professional abilities in critical thinking and problem solving underpinned by an appropriate knowledge base. These factors contribute to practice in a range of different contexts and often unpredictable situations. Several authors (Schon 1991, Clark 1995, Parton 1998) point out that professional reflection underpins the forming of competing hypotheses to decide what the problem is before trying to solve it or test out interventions. 'This ability which Schon (1991: 39–40) describes as 'problem setting' and 'problem solving' is usually carried out in agencies within a context of constraints of various sorts, resources being but one' (Walton 1999*b*). Cognitive skills such as the ability to evaluate, critically analyse, synthesise ideas, innovate and show originality and creativity cannot be developed or assessed solely by using the NVQ model. These abilities, common to the person-centred professions, need to be developed through *reflection on practice* both on training programmes and in the workplace.

Concerns have also been expressed regarding the importance afforded to *underpinning knowledge* within the NVQ model (Ashworth & Saxton 1990, Ashworth 1992). Canning (1999) discusses higher level NVQs and points out that, in part, previous concerns regarding CBET's lack of emphasis on underpinning knowledge are being addressed within revised occupational standards.

> The revised standards have included clearer statements of underpinning knowledge and understanding (DE 1993), offered greater flexibility through devising core and optional modules, and incorporated broader concepts of ethics and values into higher level N/SVQs. They have also attempted to simplify the language used within the standards and to streamline assessment methodologies (Beaumont 1996). However, it is fair to say that the outcome-based competence approach, underpinned by functional analysis, remains the dominant model. The qualifications are driven by criterion-based assessment methodologies and are 'reductionist' and 'technist' in format and style.
>
> (Canning 1999, p. 203)

As Canning informs us, the majority of higher level NVQ programmes now specify a curriculum and related theoretical input. This is the case with the new PQCCA programmes currently being developed. These will be informed by a conceptual framework developed by Leicester University School of Social Work as well as by occupational standards, currently being developed by TOPSS and CCETSW, which incorporate defined competences.

Occupational standards are now being developed across a number of professions (Watkins 1999). He reports on a study of 30 professional institutions including the British Psychological Society, the Law Society and the College of Radiographers and informs us that all professional bodies are trying to find ways of accommodating NVQs:

> However, a typical response is to pilot Level 5 NVQs to ascertain whether they can achieve three essential criteria for professional recognition ... key concerns are:
> - Can aspects of creativity, ethics, etc. be tested meaningfully and incorporated in the qualifications?
> - Can knowledge, understanding and skills be adequately identified?
> - Can assessment be carried out cost effectively and still maintain rigour?
>
> (Watkins 1999, p. 51)

Maynard (1995) offers a critique of competency-based teacher training and highlights the difficulties 'within the competency movement to identify and specify the predicates of transfer ... [there is] some confusion and disagreement between practitioners and experts about core skills and transfer issues in order that courses should have carefully designed elements to develop skills, described in terms of performance, that are transferable' (p. 134).

The new standards for initial teacher training produced by the DfEE (1998*b*) set out the criteria which all courses of initial teacher training must meet. These are designed using a functional analysis methodology as already discussed. However, on page 8 there is a statement which, whilst acknowledging the discrete setting out of each standard, emphasises that 'it is necessary to consider the standards as a whole to appreciate the creativity, commitment, energy and enthusiasm which teaching demands, and the intellectual and managerial skills required of the effective professional'.

Similarly, national occupational standards for health and social care workers have been produced (HEA 1998). The final version of the standards describes 11 key roles and 69 units of competence with each being disaggregated into several elements of competence. 'The elements within each unit include performance criteria by which competent performance will be assessed, the range of contexts in which this work behaviour will take place and the underpinning knowledge, understanding and skills' (Rolls 1998, p. 3). As can be seen, Jessup's (1991) NVQ competence-based approach is reinforced some 8 years later within defined occupational standards for health workers.

Wills (HEA 1998, p. 8) highlights the 'inherent tension between competence-based education and an academic course'. These concern the reconciliation of the aims of academic learning and of training's preoccupation with performance. Academic learning is characterised by 'an interest in the problems of definition and analysis. What underpins the development of the Standards is a wish to specify the necessary learning for performance in a particular role ... The development of broad intellectual abilities of critical thinking, what we regard as academic competence, is not acknowledged'.

Wills also highlights the difference between academic and professional *assessment*. Essentially, students undertaking academic programmes are assessed on their ability to demonstrate not only what they have learned, but also their 'ability to synthesise complex ideas. The Standards judge competence against the performance criteria ...' (Wills 1998, p. 8).

Canning's study of students' experience of higher level NVQ programmes (i.e. at Levels 4 and 5 described earlier) would suggest that the debate about the superficiality of the theoretical basis of competence-based qualifications shows little evidence of change in the way in which knowledge and understanding are identified and assessed (Canning 1999):

The thin specifications of knowledge and understanding in the awards tend to emphasise 'surface level learning' rather than 'deep level learning' (Entwistle 1992) and 'procedural' rather than 'conceptual knowledge' (Billett 1992). If this is the case, the N/SVQ process will tend to value the routine and habitual over the new and innovative. It will also tend *to accredit existing knowledge and practice rather than produce new ways of understanding and behaviour.*

(p. 208; my emphasis)

In Canning's (1999) study students' comments in careers, accountancy and social care professions confirmed the 'primacy' of 'procedural knowledge' in competence-based approaches:

I do not believe evidence of doing and performing tasks is enough to prove competence. I strongly feel that in addition to this it is important to show an understanding of why such tasks are necessary ... For me in care work it is imperative that workers understand why certain tasks are important to perform and why certain attitudes engender certain responses ... (p. 209)

In considering the outcomes of learning, Canning's (1999) study also drew on the process of reviewing professional practice within the context of compiling 'practice' portfolios. This highlighted the limitations of CBET in terms of improving knowledge, understanding and ability. Compiling portfolios was found to have 'very little impact on future performance, as they [N/SVQs] tended simply to accredit current "threshold" competencies ... In other words, the portfolio is confirmation of ... current practice' (Canning 1999, p. 210). One student stated that they had not acquired new skills and knowledge from gaining an NVQ but rather an updating of existing skills.

However, it was highlighted by students that the competence approach does afford greater equal opportunity to further training and to gaining recognised qualifications that are transferable across occupations. Although Canning's study relates to higher level NVQ programmes, rather than post-qualifying programmes, its findings are relevant when considering *competency-based* post-qualifying training such as social work.

More positive outcomes for some candidates from a study by Taylor (1999) regarding a social work practice teacher post-qualifying award were identified. These included new learning concerning time management, the relevance of networking and group learning and the benefits of 'reflecting on one's skills, knowledge and value base ... [and] the attributes to work effectively under considerable pressure' (p. 78).

Similarly, a study (Cayne 1997) relating to the use of portfolios in nurses' professional development found that the reflection on practice which the process generated promoted insight and planning regarding future career directions, i.e. '... portfolio preparation can become a spur to action' (p. 33).

Nevertheless, as Canning (1999) points out, CBET emphasises *assessment* of candidates' existing knowledge and skills, rather than contributing to their ability to internalise new learning in order to improve their future practice. This suggests that there may be a danger that 'we may be simply certificating the 'recycling of inadequacies' in order to meet national education and training targets'. (Canning 1999, p. 211).

Supervisors and mentors hold a key role in guarding against this danger and their responsibilities within the new PQCCA will have a fundamental influence on the level of learning which programmes engender in candidates. Supervisors and mentors already hold an important responsibility for promoting professionals' reflection on their practice because it underpins accurate evaluation and professional judgement. With the development of the PQCCA, this important responsibility will also need to incorporate the support of in-depth learning and the internalisation of new knowledge and understanding which this new training will be designed to generate.

Supervision and mentorship in safeguarding and promoting children's welfare

Good supervision, mentoring and support are essential for health and social care workers. Morrison (Knapman & Morrison 1998) refers to supervision as the hub of two key interlocking systems in health and social care organisations: management and professional practice. Child abuse inquiries have repeatedly identified *supervision*, within the network of services provided by multi-agency professionals, as playing a key role in safeguarding children (DOH 1991a). It is hardly surprising, therefore, that a key task for supervisors is the management of anxiety – their own and that of others. Importantly, these include members of their teams on whose professional judgement, in the first instance, children's lives may depend (Morrison 1999).

Social work supervision, particularly in statutory agencies, usually incorporates both management and mentoring tasks. Power is an important dimension in distinguishing between these two tasks. As highlighted by Gallop (1999), *supervisors* have greater power than those supervised, and accountability is a key concern. Within a mentoring relationship, power is mainly with the person being mentored and the purpose of the relationship is to encourage their professional development. Mutual trust is seen as important in both relationships.

This section considers the impact of the competency approach on supervision, within the context of the rapidly changing expectations of professionals in health and social care services. Importantly, it poses the question of whether the competency approach is likely to alleviate or aggravate the pressures first-line managers face as they juggle the traditionally identified tasks of supervision: to promote and provide competent accountable performance, continuing professional development and personal support of team members (Morrison 1993).

Banks (1995) argues that public sector reforms have led to an emphasis on the managerial aspects of supervision. This is echoed by Sawdon & Sawdon (1995, p. 129): 'Critical enquiries into child protection practice, legislative change, and recurring emphasis on the need for business skills to provide value for money tend to render supervision synonymous with bureaucratic control. Issues of accountability, quality control, and management of resources have inevitably become dominant.' This has raised concerns about the lack of emphasis and time available within supervision for reflection on professional practice. The equally important supervisory tasks of professional development and support to help practitioners make the complex decisions required of them may be given insufficient attention. The new emphasis on assessing competent predetermined *performance*, which characterises the competence approach, could contribute even further to the neglect of these important dimensions of good supervisory practice.

Thompson *et al.* (1996) discuss the findings from a study of 536 field social workers in three local authority social services departments designed to explore the impact on workers' stress levels of organisational cultures. The study revealed that half to three-quarters of the social workers were suffering 'pathological levels of stress' (pp. 658–659). It was also found that supervision and in particular, their *line managers' stress*, had an impact on workers' stress: '... LA1 supervisors are themselves victims of the pervasive "culture of stress" and are too burdened with work to provide the supervision, acknowledgement and support that their stressed social workers need' (Thompson *et al.* 1996, p. 659).

Similarly, in a study by Caughey (1996), 72% of social services employees were found to be displaying signs of 'psychiatric morbidity' (p. 393). This was linked to the impact of several reorganisations resulting in disruption of support systems, increased bureaucracy and anxiety concerning lack of control and meeting performance targets. As discussed earlier, current changes in policy are requiring significant reorganisation of public sector services across the UK.

Morrison (1999) discusses the impact of anxiety on the supervision process. By drawing on Kolb (1988), Jarvis (1995) and Vince & Martin (1993), Morrison analyses the relationship between the organisation, supervision, anxiety and learning: 'Whether anxiety can be harnessed to facilitate practice, or undermines it, depends on the organisational and supervisory context and culture.' As already highlighted the supervisory relationship is of central importance in managing anxiety and 'facilitating practice'. As Jarvis (1995, p. 67) states: 'Learning involves transforming experience into feelings (reflection), knowledge, attitudes, values (conceptualisation), behaviours and skills (active experimentation)' (cited in Morrison 1999, p. 1247). This reflection on practice by workers needs an appropriately supportive context, essentially a relationship characterised by trust and mutual respect where workers can discuss openly attitudes and feelings generated by their practice in order to reach accurate judgements. The impact on this relationship of supervisors also holding responsibilities for assessing workers' performance against predetermined standards needs to be considered.

Morrison (1999) discusses the tensions inherent already in the supervisory task regarding the three areas of responsibility. As already highlighted, given the significant services reorganisation in the public sector, the 'managerial'/accountability function is taking priority. The NVQ model has introduced an emphasis on outcomes and job performance. This brings a danger that assessment and appraisal of practice will squeeze out the other important functions of supervision. As Sawdon & Sawdon (1995) suggest: 'It [assessment] can be seen as a potential driving force, geared to producing measurable outcomes and improved effectiveness through a focus on staff performance ... the pace of appraisal schemes within social services seems likely to quicken' (p. 131).

Kemshall (1993) highlights the potential for misuse of power in the supervisory relationship and how this could be increased with the additional responsibility for assessment by line managers within the PQ framework. Clearly this issue will need to be considered carefully with the advent of the new PQCCA.

The roles of manager, mentor and assessor in the new PQCCA are yet to be clarified by CCETSW. Within the current PQ framework, assessment of candidates' assignments can be carried out outside the management hierarchy. First-line managers of programme candidates are involved in a mentoring role and in the verification of practice evidence. In carrying out this responsibility, they play a key role in supporting team members enrolled on programmes whom they also supervise in the workplace. Gallop (1999) points out that the competence approach can provide a framework within which professional development and performance can be discussed; however, it is important that this is within a 'shared language' (p. 1740). This highlights the importance of supervisors and mentors being involved in post-qualifying training both for themselves and also to facilitate support of team members enrolled on PQCCA programmes. The recent Local Authority Circular (DOH 1999c), which addresses increased staff training provision for local authorities for the PQCCA, also highlights managers' training.

Winter (1992) suggests that: 'NCVQ speak implicitly to us of familiar and acceptable educational themes, such as curriculum relevance, precision and justice in assessment ...' (p. 100). It remains to be seen whether assessment systems within the new PQCCA, which may well involve social workers' immediate line managers, can be 'precise and just' in terms of, for example, uniformity. Given that the DOH intends that all qualified child care social workers should eventually be preparing for, or qualified in, this award (DOH 1999d), the issue of assessment and its possible links to job progression and security becomes even more relevant.

Social work supervisors carry an onerous responsibility for service provision to vulnerable service users. The new PQCCA is likely to have a significant impact on these responsibilities. Adequate training and resourcing seems essential in order to ensure that they are well prepared for these additional challenges.

Summary and conclusion

Bourn (2000) reminds us that the Dearing (1997) report advocates a society committed to life-long learning. Continuing professional development is a key requirement in public service delivery. Services for children and families are being refocused in order to reflect new policy developments. These now require multi-agency services designed to intervene earlier in children's and families' lives. Professional training needs to reflect these new requirements.

As can be seen from this chapter, there remains ongoing concern regarding *competence* and its key position in both practice and training. Some of these concerns relate to its impact on the important task of professional reflection on complex practice. This process is essential in forming professional judgements that underpin assessment, intervention and evaluation. The impact of competence on professional reflection within supervision has also been considered, particularly if supervisors also become assessors within the new PQCCA. These managers will have a key role in ensuring that *competence* supports and enhances learning and professional practice rather than providing a framework for simply ticking discrete competence 'boxes' in order to meet predetermined performance indicators.

The importance of multi-professional and multi-agency training has also been considered as a key factor in the delivery of services which reflect new Government policies for children and families. *Competence* may have a role to play in such training programmes in that some modules, for example the promotion of service users' rights, may be informed by units and elements of competence common to all health and social care professions and underpin their occupational standards.

Research is needed to inform multi-agency post-qualifying training. However, given the important emphasis on professional reflection on practice discussed earlier in this chapter, training that supports multi-professional reflection appears to be important. Issitt (1999) explores the development of anti-oppressive reflective practice in multidisciplinary work. She suggests that 'Professionals with a "duty of partnership" to work together will need to understand methodological approaches and different work rhythms of each other, and recognise and deal with disparities of power. This will require individual and team based reflection in and on action, to understand where each stands, and to identify ways forward for anti-oppressive practice'.

Multi-agency training that emphasises small group reflection on practice may go some way towards guarding against professional competitiveness and the dangerous inter-relationship and inter-communication patterns identified by Reder *et al.* (1993*a*, 1993*b*). It is hoped that this form of training may promote better multi-professional and multi-agency cooperation and collaboration as emphasised by Hallett & Birchall (1995) in their important studies involving health and social care professionals. These are the professionals who hold key responsibilities for safeguarding and promoting children's welfare. Let us hope that the rapidly developing post-qualifying training programmes will offer them help and support in their challenging and responsible work.

Acknowledgements

With thanks to Jocelyn Jones, the author of this chapter in the original text, and to Meg Bond for their comments on earlier drafts of this paper.

References

Armytage P, Reeves C 1992 Practice insights as revealed by child death inquiries in Victoria and overseas. In: Calvert G, Ford A, Parkinson P (eds) The practice of child protection: Australian approaches. Hale & Iremonger, Sydney

Ashworth P, Saxton J 1990 On competence. Journal of Further and Higher Education 14 (2): 3–25

Ashworth P 1992 Being competent and having competencies. Journal of Further and Higher Education 16 (3): 8–17

Banks S 1995 Ethics and values in social work. Macmillan, London

Bates I 1995 The competence movement: conceptualising recent research. Studies in Science Education 25: 39–68

Beaumont G 1996 Review of 100 NVQs and SVQs. Department for Education and Employment, London

Billett S 1992 Towards a theory of workplace learning. Studies in Continuing Education 14 (2): 143–155

Bourn D F 2000 The challenge of delivering a professionally and academically credited post-qualifying social work management programme in supervision and mentorship by distance learning. Journal of Vocational Education and Training (in press)

Brown A, Bourne I 1996 The social work supervisor. Open University Press, Buckingham

Canning R 1999 Discourses on competence: a case study of students' experience of higher level National/Scottish Vocational Qualifications. Journal of Education and Work 12 (2): 201–213

Caughey J 1996 Psychological distress in staff of a social services district office: a pilot study. British Journal of Social Work 26: 389–399

Cayne J V 1997 Portfolios: a developmental influence? In: Abbott P, Sapsford R (eds) Research into practice: a reader. Open University Press, Buckingham

Central Council for Education and Training in Social Work (CCETSW) 1989 (revised 1991) Diploma in social work: requirements and regulations for the Diploma in Social Work. Paper 30. CCETSW, London

Central Council for Education and Training in Social Work (CCETSW) 1992 The requirements for post-qualifying education and training in the personal social services: a framework for continuing professional development. Paper 31. CCETSW, London

Central Council for Education and Training in Social Work (CCETSW) 1995 Rules and requirements for the Diploma in Social Work. Paper 30 revised. CCETSW, London

Central Council for Education and Training in Social Work (CCETSW) 1997 Assuring quality for post-qualifying education and training. CCETSW, London

Clark C 1995 Competence and discipline in professional formation. British Journal of Social Work 25: 563–580

Dearing R 1997 Higher education in the learning society. The National Committee of Inquiry into Higher Education, London

Department for Education and Employment (DfEE) 1998a Meeting the childcare challenge: a framework and consultation document. The Stationery Office, London

Department for Education and Employment (DfEE) 1998b Teaching: high status, high standards: requirements for courses of initial teacher training. Circular 4/98. Department for Education and Employment, London

Department of Employment (DE) 1988 Employment in the 1990s. HMSO, London

Department of Employment (DE) 1993 Knowledge and understanding: its place in relation to NVQs and SVQs. Competence and assessment, briefing series No. 9. Pendragon Press, Cambridge

Department of Employment (DE) & Department of Education and Science (DES) 1985 Education and training for young people. HMSO, London

Department of Employment (DE) & Department of Education and Science (DES) 1986 Working together: education and training. HMSO, London

Department of Health (DOH) 1989 The care of children: principles and practice in regulations and guidance. HMSO, London

Department of Health (DOH) 1991a Child abuse: a study of inquiry reports 1980–1989. HMSO, London

Department of Health (DOH) 1991b Patterns and outcomes in child placement: messages from current research and their implications. HMSO, London

Department of Health (DOH) 1995 Child protection: messages from research. HMSO, London

Department of Health (DOH) 1998a Quality protects: transforming children's services. Local Authority Circular (LAC)(98)28. Department of Health, London

Department of Health (DOH) 1998b Our healthier nation. Cmnd 3852. The Stationery Office, London

Department of Health (DOH) 1998c Modernising health and social services. The Stationery Office, London

Department of Health (DOH) 1999*a* Framework for the assessment of children in need and their families. Consultation draft. Department of Health, London

Department of Health (DOH) 1999*b* Post-qualifying award in child care. Department of Health, London

Department of Health (DOH) 1999*c* Social services training support programme: 1999/2000: additional circular for the new post-qualifying child care award sub-programme. Local Authority Circular (LAC)(99)37. Department of Health, London

Department of Health (DOH) 1999*d* Social services training support programme: 1999/2000: information pack on the new post-qualifying child care award sub-programme. Department of Health, London

Department of Health, Home Office, Department for Education and Employment & The National Assembly for Wales 1999 Working together to safeguard children: a guide to inter-agency working to safeguard and promote the welfare of children. Department of Health, London

Dominelli L 1996 Deprofessionalizing social work: anti-oppressive practice, competencies and postmodernism. British Journal of Social Work 26: 153–175

Drury-Hudson J 1999 Decision-making in child protection: the use of theoretical, empirical and procedural knowledge by novices and experts and implications for fieldwork placement. British Journal of Social Work 29: 147–169

Entwistle N 1992 Teaching and the quality of learning in higher education. In: Entwistle N (ed) Handbook of educational ideas and practices. Routledge, London

Gallop L 1999 The role of the mentor in supporting and facilitating continuing professional development and achievement of competence: study session 20: Certificate in Supervision and Mentorship (Child Care) by Distance Learning. University of Leicester, Leicester

Glass N 1999 Sure Start: the development of an early intervention programme for young children in the United Kingdom. Children and Society 13: 257–364

Hager P, Gonczi A 1996 What is competence? Medical Teacher 18 (1): 15–18

Hallett C, Birchall E 1995*a* Inter-agency coordination. In: Department of Health (ed) Child protection: messages from research. HMSO, London

Hallett C, Birchall E 1995*b* Working together in child protection. In: Department of Health (ed) Child protection: messages from research. HMSO, London

Hardiker P, Exton K, Barker M 1996 A framework for analysing services. Childhood Matters 2 Background Papers. HMSO, London

Health Education Authority (HEA) 1998 The National Occupational Standards for Professional Activity in Health Promotion and Care. PD News (Special Issue). Health Education Authority, London

Hodkinson P, Issitt M 1995 The challenge of competence for the caring professions: an overview. In: Hodkinson P, Issitt M (eds) The challenge of competence: professionalism through vocational education and training. Cassell, London

Horne M 1990 Is it social work? In: Violence Against Children Study Group (eds) Taking child abuse seriously. Routledge, London

Hughes A K 1994 Developing European professions. Bristol University, Bristol

Issitt M 1999 Towards the development of anti-oppressive reflective practice: the challenge for multidisciplinary working. Special Issue: Reflective Practice. Journal of Practice Teaching in Social Work and Health 2(2): 21–36

Issitt M, Woodward M 1992 Competence and contradiction. In: Carter P, Jeffs T, Smith M K (eds) Changing social work and welfare. Open University Press, Buckingham

Jarvis P 1995 Adult and continuing education. Routledge, London

Jessup G 1990 National Vocational Qualifications: implications for further education. In: Bees M, Swords M (eds) National Vocational Qualifications and further education. NCVQ and Kogan Page, London.

Jessup G 1991 Outcomes, NVQs and the emerging model of education and training. Falmer Press, London

Jones J 1995*a* Training for child protection practice: a question of competence? In: Wilson K, James A (eds) The child protection handbook. Ballière Tindall, London

Jones J 1995*b* Professional artistry and child protection: towards a reflective, holistic practice. In: Hodkinson P, Issitt M (eds) The challenge of competence: professionalism through vocational education and training. Cassell, London

Kemshall H 1993 Assessing competence: scientific process or subjective interference? Do we really see it? Social Work Education 12 (1): 36–45

Knapman J, Morrison T 1998 Making the most of supervision in health and social care: a self development manual for supervisees. Pavillion, Brighton

Kolb D 1988 The process of experiential learning. In: Kolb D (ed) Experience as the source of learning and development. Prentice Hall, London

Lloyd M, Taylor C 1995 From Hollis to the Orange Book: developing a holistic model of social work assessment in the 1990s. British Journal of Social Work 25: 691–710

Mayer E (Chair) 1992 Employment-related key competencies: a proposal for consultation. The Mayer Committee, Ministry of Education and Training, Melbourne. Australian Government Publishing Service, Canberra

Maynard C 1995 Competency in practice – Cheshire Certificate in Education: further education. In: Hodkinson P, Issitt M (eds) The challenge of competence: professionalism through vocational education and training. Cassell, London

Mitchell L 1998 Competence and the development of occupational standards: the National Occupational Standards for professional activity in health promotion and care. PD News (Special Issue). Health Education Authority, London

Morrison T 1993 Staff supervision in social care. Longman, Harlow

Morrison T 1999 The supervisory relationship: where macro and micro meet. Study Session 13: Certificate in Supervision and Mentorship (Child Care) by Distance Learning. University of Leicester, Leicester

O'Hagan K 1996 Social work competence: an historical perspective. In: O'Hagan K (ed) Competence in social work practice: a practical guide for professionals. Jessica Kingsley, London.

Page R M, Silburn R 1998 British social welfare in the twentieth century. Macmillan, London

Parton N 1998 Risk, advanced liberalism and child welfare: the need to rediscover uncertainty and ambiguity. British Journal of Social Work 28: 5–27

Pillay H, Brownlee J, McCrindle A 1998 The influence of individuals' beliefs about learning and nature of knowledge on educating a competent workforce. Journal of Education and Work 11 (3): 239–254

Reder P, Duncan S, Gray M. 1993a Beyond blame: child abuse tragedies revisited. Routledge, London

Reder P, Duncan S, Gray M 1993b A new look at child abuse tragedies. Child Abuse Review 2 (2): 89–100

Robson C 1993 Real world research: a resource for social scientists and practitioner-researchers. Blackwell, Oxford

Rolls L 1998 The HEA competences projects and their contribution to the development and piloting of National Occupational Standards for Professional Activity in Health Promotion and Care: The National Occupational Standards for Professional Activity in Health Promotion and Care. PD News (Special Issue). Health Education Authority, London

Rushton A, Martyn H 1993 Learning for advanced practice: a study of away-based training. Paper 31. CCETSW, London

Sawdon C, Sawdon D 1995 The supervision partnership. In: Pritchard J (ed) Good practice in supervision: statutory and voluntary organisations. Jessica Kingsley, London

Schon D A 1991 The reflective practitioner: how professionals think in action. Avebury, Aldershot

Stevenson O 1999 Children in need and abused: inter-professional and inter-agency responses. In: Stevenson O (ed) Child welfare in the UK. Blackwell Science, Oxford

Taylor C 1999 Experiences of a pilot project for the post-qualifying award in social work. Social Work Education 18 (1): 71–82

Thompson N, Stradling S, Murphy M, O'Neill P 1996 Stress and organizational culture. British Journal of Social Work 26: 647–665

Training Organisation for the Personal Social Services (TOPPS) 1999 Draft 11 of The National Occupational Standards for Child Care Post-Qualifying. TOPPS, Leeds

Vince R, Martin L 1993 Inside action learning. Management Education and Development 24 (2): 208–209

Violence Against Children Study Groups (eds) 1999 Children, child abuse and child protection: placing children centrally. John Wiley, Chichester

Walton P 1999a Practitioner research and empowerment. Practice 11 (1): 5–14

Walton P 1999b Using competence as a basis for developing reflective practice: a case study of a post-qualifying framework in child protection. Journal of Practice Teaching (Special Issue: Reflective Practice) 2 (2): 63–76

Ward H (ed) 1995 Looking after children: research into practice. HMSO, London

Watkins J 1999 Educating professionals: the changing role of UK professional associations. Journal of Education and Work 12 (1): 37–56

Williams S, Raggatt P 1998 Contextualising public policy in vocational education and training: the origins of competence-based vocational qualifications policy in the UK. Journal of Education and Work 11 (3): 275–292

Wills J 1998 Using the National Occupational Standards for curriculum planning: The National Occupational Standards for Professional Activity in Health Promotion and Care. PD News (Special Issue). Health Education Authority, London

Winter R 1992 'Quality management' or 'The educative workplace': alternative versions of competence-based education. Journal of Further and Higher Education 16 (3): 100–115

30

Power and partnership: a case study in child protection*

INTRODUC-TION

The complex nature of the responsibilities facing social workers and other professionals working in the field of child protection has been portrayed very clearly in other contributions to this book. While these responsibilities may sometimes weigh on practitioners, our activities are liable to have a much greater and more intrusive impact on the families and children caught up in this work. For this reason, it seemed appropriate to include an account of one family's experience as a 'child protection case'. Where possible, I have tried to link their experience with themes identified by other contributors to the book, but not at the cost of distorting the account.

The account is written from the social worker's perspective; however, the family involved have given their permission for me to write this chapter. The parents also read and approved a draft of it. It is not offered as an example of how child protection work should be carried out in these circumstances. Rather, the process of writing this account has emphasised to me the uniqueness of each family's experience, and the difficulty of making generalised statements about 'good practice'. It is difficult for us to appreciate how our actions and intentions will be interpreted by others, whose previous experiences as children, with parents, social workers and other professionals have been inimical to their welfare.

I have begun with a brief outline of the major events. More detailed information will be shared later in the chapter. All names have been changed, and certain other biographical details have been altered, in an effort to protect the anonymity of the family. It is possible that some readers will think that they recognise the situation as one they were in some way involved with, since across the country there are, no doubt, a number of families with a similar history. Those who do experience this sense of *déjà vu* are asked not to assume that they are right, and in any event to respect the family members' right to confidentiality, and their courage in giving permission for their experience to be shared with the readers of this book.

The Stanley family

Eleanor Stanley was first referred to the local Social Services Department at the end of her first term in Junior School. She was referred because of the Head Teacher's concern that her behaviour indicated that she might be being neglected or abused. She had been stealing food from other pupils, and from the school waste-bins. Her behaviour at other times could be attention seeking and disruptive. The Head Teacher also reported concern about Eleanor's poor physical appearance.

*The author of this chapter was employed in a local authority social services depeartment in the North of England when the work described was carried out. The name of the author has been withheld to protect the identity of the family.

Over the holiday period a social worker tried to investigate these concerns, although without much success. The report was followed by another, some 6 weeks later, from the same source, that Eleanor had been seen at school with a black eye, and said to be looking unhappy. Eight weeks after the initial referral, an initial child protection conference was convened. By this time, Eleanor had been seen by a paediatrician to investigate concerns about her growth, and by a general practitioner (GP) in relation to the black eye. No decision on registration was taken at this initial conference, but when it was reconvened some 4 weeks later, the paediatrician had been able to rule out most possible organic causes for Eleanor's poor growth, and she was registered under the category of emotional abuse. None of her four siblings was registered.

Over the following 9 months, efforts were made to undertake a full assessment of what was going on in Eleanor's family. Many of these efforts met with resistance from the parents. Some medical appointments were missed, and, although the family were referred to a local unit catering for children with mental health needs, which was willing to undertake a full family-centred assessment, the parents did not keep these appointments. However, they did acknowledge that there were grounds for concern about Eleanor's growth, and agreed for her to be admitted to the local hospital children's ward, where her diet could be monitored and the impact on her weight assessed.

Ten months after the initial referral, faced with continuing non-cooperation from the parents, the Local Authority sought and obtained an interim supervision order from the court. This had little effect in overcoming the family's resistance to participating in a full assessment. An interim care order was therefore sought, but was not granted, because at this point the parents agreed, in court, that Eleanor could be accommodated with foster-carers on a voluntary basis for a limited period of time to see how she responded. However, Mr Stanley removed her again on the day she was placed there, and an emergency protection order had to be obtained to retrieve Eleanor. She was then placed with different foster-carers, and an interim care order was granted.

About 2 months after Eleanor was removed from home, Mr Stanley assaulted a member of staff in the Social Services Department; he was charged and remanded in custody, where he remained for several months, before being granted a short period of bail. He subsequently received a prison sentence.

A full care order was granted in respect of Eleanor some 10 months after she was first removed, and almost 22 months after the initial referral. After hearing in court the evidence of the paediatrician that Eleanor's restricted growth could not be the result of any medical condition, Mr and Mrs Stanley changed their position and agreed to take part in a full assessment of the situation. This assessment, which was carried out in the weeks immediately following the making of the care order, resulted in a recommendation that Eleanor could be returned to her parents' care. She was returned home, subject to the Placement with Parents Regulations, some 4 months after the care proceedings were concluded. A period of intensive work with parents and children ensued. A year after the care order was made, a successful application was made to the court for it to be discharged. This account is written several years after the discharge of that order.

Recognition and investigation

Only a fraction of the children who experience maltreatment are referred to the agencies with responsibility for child protection (see Creighton, Chapter 2,

p. 37). The enquiries about Eleanor after the initial referral was made revealed that the concerns had been present since she had started Infants' School. Why had she not been referred earlier?

A failure of inter-agency communication may have played a part. Although Eleanor had been born prematurely, by the time she was 9 months old, her weight and height had reached levels between the 25th and 50th centiles, and her development was considered to be progressing nicely. According to the Health Visitor's notes, this situation had continued until she was 3 years and 6 months, when she had been seen for the last time. When she was weighed and measured by the School Nurse at 5 years and 1 month, her weight had fallen to the 3rd centile, and her height was around the 10th centile. Perhaps these measures should have triggered some concern in their own right, but it appeared that the School Nurse did not know how much better Eleanor had been doing 18 months earlier. This failure to pick up children whose growth is falling away from centile charts was noted by Batchelor (1996). Perhaps the school nurse was also inhibited by the anxiety referred to by Rouse (Chapter 15, p. 309)

In any event, no action was taken at that time. When staff in the infants' school got to know Eleanor, and began to see episodes of her worrying behaviour, they shared those concerns with Mrs Stanley, but did not take the matter any further throughout her career in Infants' School. So, when a referral was made much later, after Eleanor had moved to Junior School, it must have been difficult for Mr and Mrs Stanley to understand why so much concern was generated, when most of the professionals involved, apart from the local authority social workers, had had daily experience of the problem for more than 2 years, without taking any action.

Both parents and professionals alike find it difficult and emotionally taxing to recognise and acknowledge when a child fails to thrive.

(Hanks & Stratton, Chapter 5, p. 102)

In this instance, the parents' bewilderment was probably reinforced by the rapid shift in the attitude of professionals, supporting registration at a child protection conference, after a long period in which the family had not been referred for any help or support. Mr and Mrs Stanley's reaction, which was to retreat into a defensive mode, served to emphasise the growing concerns of the professionals, who were perhaps realising, with the benefit of hindsight, that some action should have been taken earlier. Had the parents shown more willingness to cooperate at this stage, it is possible that the problem would never have escalated as it did. It seems that a key feature of cases filtered out of the child protection system in the course of the investigation is the willingness of parents to cooperate with the professionals (see Wattam, Chapter 11).

However, it could be argued that Eleanor had not shown all the classic symptoms of failure to thrive. Of those listed by Hanks & Stratton (Table 5.1, p. 102), Eleanor did not display the large and swollen stomach, any sign of retarded brain growth, or poor posture. Although her social and behavioural development was immature for her age, other aspects of her development (cognitive and intellectual, in particular) were normal, and even ahead of other children of her age. On the other hand, Eleanor certainly illustrated the observation that children who fail to thrive may show: 'a pattern of unmalleable behaviour, resistance to new routines…' and that their: 'general volatility of mood and behaviour appeared to make them difficult to rear from early life' (Iwaniec *et al.* 1985, p. 251, quoted by Hanks & Stratton, Chapter 5)

The different and conflicting explanations of how Eleanor acquired her black eye made professionals uneasy, but it was never established that this was the result of an assault by a parent: an altercation with her older sister was the most likely alternative explanation.

The schools attended by Eleanor and her sisters served a relatively deprived community, in which many residents were sometimes in conflict with welfare professionals, and where there was a significant problem of drug misuse within young families. The head teachers had good reason to be aware that there may be a conflict between:

... on the one hand, ensuring that the family is experienced by its members as autonomous and the primary sphere for rearing children, while on the other recognising there is a need for intervention in some families where they are seen as failing in their primary task (Parton, Chapter 1)

This case also illustrates Wattam's finding that teachers generally reported their concerns, but in some instances, only after a long interval of consideration (Wattam, Chapter 11). They found the experience difficult, and were reluctant to break their relationship of confidence with the child and family.

Ten months elapsed between the referral and a decision by the Local Authority to institute care proceedings, and a further 3 months passed before Eleanor was removed from home. Undoubtedly this reflects the emphasis in the Children Act 1989 that children are best brought up by their families, and that the provision of services under section 17 to prevent children suffering harm is usually the best policy (Lyon, Chapter 10). In this case, the local authority also found it difficult to establish clearly that Eleanor was suffering 'significant harm', and more particularly, whether the harm was 'attributable to the care being given ... not being what it would be reasonable to expect a parent to give to the child' (Lyon, Chapter 10).

Inter-agency cooperation

All the enquiries into child abuse tragedies have emphasised the risks of failures of communication between the different agencies and professionals involved in working with a child or family where abuse of some kind is suspected. In this situation, 13 agencies or carers, with more than one individual in some instances, quite apart from the parents and child, had to be kept in touch with relevant and significant developments. The task of maintaining effective communication with all these individuals was significant, and from time to time, problems did arise. The parents, foster-carers, and Eleanor sometimes heard information expressed differently by different workers. The need to maintain clear lines of communication became even greater after the assault, because such events arouse strong feelings in colleagues. Sometimes this makes it more difficult to retain an objective perspective.

Assessment

The more complex or severe a child's situation, the more time it may take to understand thoroughly what is happening to the child, the reasons why and the impact on the child; the more it is also likely to involve other agencies in that process.

(Department of Health 1999, p. 14)

The process of assessing Eleanor's needs could be divided into three phases. In the first phase, the focus was predominantly on Eleanor; was she suffering significant harm, and if she was, could this be attributed to a failure of parental care? The key professionals in this phase were the paediatricians who examined Eleanor, and who failed to discover any organic cause for her very poor growth pattern. They also identified that she suffered periodically from a urine infection. Mr and Mrs Stanley confirmed that Eleanor was enuretic most nights, although there had been a period before she was going to school, when she had been dry at night. The urine infection could have contributed to the problem of enuresis, and was probably exacerbated by it, but it was not thought to have had any impact on Eleanor's growth. This combination of factors, together with a bruise observed on Eleanor's thigh, led to suspicions of sexual abuse, even though the parents had offered an innocent explanation of the bruise. A second opinion, obtained from another paediatrician reviewing the medical notes, made explicit the diagnosis of possible sexual abuse.

In this phase, during which Eleanor's weight fluctuated dramatically, the cooperation of her parents with the professionals was, at best, sporadic. Some appointments with doctors were kept; others were not. They agreed to allow Eleanor to be admitted to hospital for observation, and her weight increased by 2 kg in the short period before admission could be arranged. While in hospital, Eleanor's weight increased by a further 2 kg, but in the 3 months after she was discharged back to the care of her family, all this weight increase was lost. After the second paediatric opinion was obtained, and the suggestion of sexual abuse was made explicit, steps were taken to begin care proceedings, and an interim supervision order was obtained. In this period, Eleanor's weight began to increase once more, leading some people to believe that her poor growth was more probably linked to the deliberate withholding of food by her parents; when this regime was relaxed, for whatever reason, her weight would rise.

Parents have a right not to participate in an assessment, although they need to understand the consequences of a refusal.

(Adcock, Chapter 12)

I had no dealings with Mr or Mrs Stanley during this phase of the work, but from my subsequent involvement, I would suggest that they did not understand that the consequence of their refusal to participate in the assessment would be Eleanor's removal from home. It is likely that they did not give professionals the opportunity to explain the consequences of non-participation. What I later realised that they found so difficult to understand was the concept of a direct link between Eleanor's poor growth, which they accepted to be a worry, and her emotional state; and even more difficult to grasp was the possibility that Eleanor's distressed emotional state could be attributed to the state of her relationships with other members of the family. Much later, I wondered to what extent their reluctance to consider this explanation reflected class and cultural differences between the 'respectable' middle-class professional, and the disaffected urban poor. Is it generally more acceptable in middle-class families to link abnormal behaviour from a child to emotional stress, past or present? An alternative explanation, equally plausible, when one learnt more about the parents' own abusive childhood experiences, was that because they had had to suppress the emotional pain they had experienced as children, they were less well equipped to see what their daughter was going through.

Hanks & Stratton (Chapter 5) observe:

... mothers' attributions and belief systems are powerful aspects of a situation when a child is failing to thrive. Understanding how they perceive the causes is crucial to any intervention in this relationship and to aiding the ultimate growth of the child. FTT [failure to thrive] is one situation in which the child's adaptation to mistreatment or mishandling may easily be misconstrued by a parent.

Mr and Mrs Stanley always denied that food had been deliberately withheld from Eleanor, although, much later, they acknowledged that she had sometimes not been given treats offered to her siblings when her behaviour at a mealtime had been particularly objectionable. The idea that Eleanor might have been the victim of sexual abuse was anathema to both parents, and the suggestion undoubtedly reinforced their mistrust of professionals. Clearly, during this phase of assessment, no effective dialogue could be established between the agencies and the parents.

In the second phase, which followed Eleanor's removal from home, difficulties of communication took on a more serious aspect. First, problems were reported at the family centre at which Eleanor had twice-weekly contact with her family: the children were allowed to behave in an unrestrained way by their parents, causing chaos and disorder. Mr Stanley was reported to have obstructed the taxi taking Eleanor back to her foster-home. Lastly, and most seriously, Mr Stanley arrived unannounced at the area office one day, and assaulted a member of the team involved in the work.

Physical assault is not a common experience for social workers, even for those involved in the highly sensitive area of child protection, where an element of intrusion and invasion into private family matters is unavoidable. The impact of such an incident cannot be underestimated: for the victim, whose sense of personal security in their work may be undermined permanently; for the victim's colleagues, whose initial reaction may involve a sense of outrage, but for whom the incident may also be a reminder of their own vulnerability; and for the perpetrator, who is likely to be perceived very differently by professionals as a result of such an incident, and who runs the risk of much more serious punishment than if they had been arrested for a latenight brawl outside a pub.

The incident also raised major questions about how the assessment could be completed. If local authority staff were at risk of assault, it was not reasonable to ask them to continue to work with the family. Eventually, taking into account that Mr Stanley was now remanded in custody, a social work agency from the voluntary sector, not connected with the local authority, agreed to complete the assessment; while a local authority social worker from a different team (myself) was assigned to carry out the essential statutory responsibilities involved in looking after a child subject to care proceedings.

In her foster-home, Eleanor was beginning to thrive. On first arriving, she had been observed to eat voraciously as if she did not know when to stop; she had wet the bed most nights, and had continued to develop urine infections; and her behaviour had been immature and disruptive, particularly in more public social situations. However, within 3 or 4 months, significant positive changes were being reported. She was beginning to gain weight, her enuresis was becoming less regular, and the urine infections were almost eliminated. Her behaviour within the foster-home also began to improve, although this was a slower and more uneven process.

Eleanor had also made various disclosures to the guardian *ad litem*. She had alleged that her mother had sometimes hit her, and that she had been treated unfairly by her, compared with her siblings. However, some of these allegations could not be substantiated. Her behaviour during contact sessions had been difficult, and sometimes almost unmanageable when the whole family had been present. However, after the assault by Mr Stanley and his remand in custody, contact

authority social workers. Work with these parents often revealed that the mistrust had been based either on abuse or neglect at the hands of their own parents, leaving them suspicious and mistrustful of all authority figures. Many of them had also undergone experiences in local authority care that had not enhanced their feelings of security or safety in the care system.

A care order was made by the court, and the care plan was accepted in the knowledge that Mr and Mrs Stanley had shifted their position significantly, and were now offering to engage in a further piece of assessment. This third phase of work was completed within about 8 weeks of the care order being made. An individual agreement was negotiated and adopted by both parents and the local authority, in which the process and outcomes of the assessment were set out. Each of us entered into particular obligations: for example, I agreed to share the notes of each session with each of them, and to correct any factual errors in my records; I also agreed to show a draft of the final report to them, before it was concluded, and to negotiate alterations where appropriate or to indicate those areas in which Mr or Mrs Stanley could not agree with opinions I expressed. I also arranged for a female colleague to undertake the individual sessions with Mrs Stanley, while I met with Mr Stanley in the prison. Perhaps most importantly, our agreement stated explicitly that the purpose of the assessment was to work out the best resolution of the situation for *Eleanor.*

During this phase, my colleague and I had 22 meetings with one or more members of the family. My colleague held several sessions with Mrs Stanley, exploring in some depth her experiences as a child, while I covered similar ground with her husband in the prison. I also spent time with each parent going over their recollections of events and milestones within their own family since they had first begun their relationship. I also made a number of unannounced visits (as part of the agreement we had negotiated) to assess the emotional atmosphere in the home at different times of the day. I also arranged four family events, in which Eleanor was included, where I could observe all the family interacting (except Mr Stanley, of course). These events included a meal at the family centre, a trip to the pantomime, and two family gatherings at the home of Mrs Stanley's mother.

The information emerging from this phase of the assessment amplified rather than contradicted what had been ascertained at earlier stages. However, by getting access to Mr and Mrs Stanley's own recollections of events, it was possible to make more definite links between past events, the meanings attached to those events by the family members, and the situation that had developed. My understanding of the origin of Eleanor's difficulties was greatly enhanced by having this important perspective. I do not know whether Mr or Mrs Stanley agreed entirely with the understanding I built up during this phase of the assessment but sufficient common ground was established to identify appropriate objectives for further work.

The additional information and understanding which emerged, included the following points:

- Mrs Stanley's mother had lost both parents in middle childhood, and had spent the following 12 years in institutional care. This long experience of institutional living, after experiences of major loss, had almost certainly limited her capacity to respond with warmth and in a nurturing way to her own young children.
- Mrs Stanley had never really known her father, but her step-father had been frequently violent towards her mother, and had been punitive and tyrannical towards the children, including Mrs Stanley, in an unpredictable way.

- Mrs Stanley had been small and underweight throughout her childhood and adolescence, possibly herself experiencing undiagnosed failure to thrive.
- Mr Stanley's childhood had also included chronic marital conflict; he recalled one step-father, who had been positive towards and interested in him, until his mother had terminated the relationship when he was about 12 years old.
- Mr Stanley's reaction to this disruption had led his mother to ask the local authority to look after him on the grounds that he was beyond her control.
- Mr Stanley's first offence had involved an assault on a police officer, who had been called to the home to return Mr Stanley to the children's home from which he had run away.
- This, and other subsequent offences, had led Mr Stanley to spend much of his adolescence in institutional care. His sense that his mother had abandoned him became associated with anger towards the local authority social workers who supervised this arrangement.
- When Mr Stanley did return to his family home in his late adolescence, his mother left him to fend for himself, as she moved to another part of the country. Mr Stanley experienced this as a very powerful reminder that other people could not be trusted.
- Mr and Mrs Stanley came together as a couple when both were still young, each with a powerful need for the security of a permanent relationship. With very limited financial and emotional resources, Mrs Stanley was soon faced with the challenge of bringing up two children under a year old, with her husband in prison.
- In spite of these adverse circumstances, both Eleanor and her older sister seemed to thrive until Eleanor reached the age of 3 and a half years.
- When Eleanor was about 18 months old, Mr Stanley suffered a serious road accident, in which he incurred life-threatening injuries. For several weeks, Mrs Stanley was fully involved in nursing him, while relatives looked after the children. Mr Stanley eventually made a good recovery, but was left with other serious after-effects, in the form of chronic headaches and other neurological symptoms.
- One year after the accident, shortly after Mrs Stanley had given birth to Eleanor's next sister, a health visitor had negotiated a place for Eleanor at a local playgroup. According to Mrs Stanley, she had been advised by the playgroup leader to persist in bringing Eleanor, in spite of her strongly expressed protests on being left. Mrs Stanley identified the deterioration in Eleanor's behaviour as beginning at around that time, although she did not make any connection between Eleanor's distress then and her more difficult behaviour later. Mr Stanley, meanwhile, having recovered from his injuries, had resumed a life of crime, and had been given another prison sentence.
- Eleanor's weight declined rapidly over the following 18 months. She had also not only become enuretic, but also liable to wet and soil herself during the day. She went through a phase of smearing her faeces on the bedroom wall. She created tantrums if she was not bought sweets when the family went shopping, and sometimes she stole the sweets. Mrs Stanley found Eleanor's behaviour incomprehensible and acutely embarrassing.
- Even more embarrassing to Mrs Stanley were the later concerns expressed by the infants' school about Eleanor's behaviour there. It seemed that she never reported these concerns to her husband, who claimed to have been unaware of them until the referral was made 2 years later to the Social Services Department.

- An aspect that had not emerged in earlier phases of the assessment was the relationship between Eleanor and her siblings. Eleanor had shared a bedroom with her older sister, Sarah, who had always been close to her mother. As the relationship between Eleanor and her mother had deteriorated, so Sarah had become more negative towards Eleanor, whose bedwetting provided a ready weapon. Eleanor's departure from the family had led to a closer relationship developing between Sarah and her younger sister, Karen. Not only had Eleanor become a scapegoat in the family system, but also, if she was to re-establish herself in the family, significant work would be needed with the sibling group, to prevent the stresses becoming intolerable.

This fuller picture, which emerged during the 8 weeks of intensive assessment, did allow the development of a working hypothesis, which could be shared with Mr and Mrs Stanley as to the origin and history of Eleanor's problem. My colleague and I used the analogy of a wall of invisible bricks being erected between Eleanor and her mother[1] in the period following Mr Stanley's accident, his subsequent imprisonment, the arrival of her younger sister and Eleanor's introduction into playgroup, for which she was emotionally unready. Sarah's more secure attachment to her mother had protected her from some of this stress. Once Eleanor's behaviour had begun to deteriorate, the wall began to get higher. Mrs Stanley lacked the spare emotional resources to reassure her, and had resorted to punishments and the withholding of love. Eleanor's behaviour deteriorated in response to this, and brought shame and embarrassment on Mrs Stanley. It may also have helped to undermine Mrs Stanley's sense of competence as a parent, perhaps more fragile than most, because of her own abusive childhood. Sarah had reinforced the negative dynamic towards Eleanor; we sometimes underestimate the damage to children's self-esteem which can be brought about by siblings in this way. Meanwhile, Mr Stanley, whose relationship with Eleanor had always been close, managed to 'avert his eyes' from what was happening, being either in prison, or engaged in activities that did not involve Eleanor. His view at that time was certainly that child rearing was predominantly a mother's task. The emotional damage inflicted on both parents during their own childhood had made it too painful for them to recognise what was now happening to their own daughter.

Mr and Mrs Stanley were prepared to accept most of this hypothesis, principally because it did not imply that either parent had been deliberately rejecting Eleanor in a calculated fashion. An explanation of this kind also helped to reconcile the apparent conflict between the picture portrayed previously, of a cruel and rejecting mother, with Mrs Stanley's persistent and determined commitment to maintain contact with Eleanor at every opportunity. It was therefore possible to construct a plan of the work needed to bring about Eleanor's return to the family.

Interventions

Efforts to bring about change had been going on in one form or another for some time before the assessment was completed. Eleanor's removal from home had been a crucial intervention, which had had consequences, both negative and positive,

[1] I am indebted to two former colleagues, who developed this analogy for use in direct work involving mothers and children.

for Eleanor, the family and the professionals. The negative consequences have already been spelt out; but some of the positive consequences of this intervention should be mentioned here.

First, the removal of Eleanor to a safe foster-home did give professionals the opportunity to listen to what she was saying. Eleanor described her perspective of her home situation to the guardian *ad litem*, and this indicated the depth of her unhappiness. Perhaps too much attention was paid to establishing whether these disclosures were literally true (some were, others were not), and not enough to the underlying message they conveyed of a child who felt excluded and rejected.

Second, it has to be acknowledged that when Eleanor was removed from home she was quite hard to like. In the foster-home, and at school, she could be attention-seeking, self-centred and aggressive towards younger children. She wet the bed regularly and tried to conceal this. Her table manners were dreadful: she was, by turns, fussy, greedy and thoughtless about the impact of her behaviour on anyone else. She could be dishonest: not only did she sometimes steal things, but she was also able to deny any responsibility for what she had done, even when these actions had been witnessed by others. Fortunately, her very experienced foster-carers were able to bring about a major change in Eleanor's behaviour, using the kind of strategies most parents would want to employ. They were firm about her unacceptable behaviour, while taking every opportunity to convey warmth and positive regard towards Eleanor as a person. They praised and encouraged any positive changes. They did not make the intake of food a source of conflict. They allowed Eleanor to begin to show the more pleasant and likeable aspects of her personality. They also helped to eliminate the enuresis and re-established a normal pattern of growth. These were major achievements, and even though they were not part of a plan, at the time, to enable Eleanor to return home, they would have been necessary tasks if not already completed. The work of the foster-carers demonstrated that there had been a problem, but that it could be addressed with the right approach. It confirmed that Eleanor was not suffering from any underlying physical disorder, and also made her an easier child to like. On the other hand, for Eleanor to make such progress when not in her parents' care could have made her the target for their anger and resentment. Why should Eleanor respond positively to foster-carers when she would not do it for them?

This leads to the third contribution towards positive change. Mrs Stanley may not have been able to restore a good relationship with Eleanor while they were living together, but she strained every sinew, in her own undemonstrative way, to win her back. She swallowed any pride she might have felt, and any anger that Eleanor's changed behaviour might have generated. As she began to see positive changes in Eleanor's behaviour, she began to engage with her more positively in activities, in conversation and, eventually, in setting appropriate boundaries and limits to Eleanor's more disruptive behaviour.

Several bricks in the wall had already been dismantled, therefore, before the third phase of the assessment was begun. Once the recommendation to try to return Eleanor to her family had been agreed in a child care review, it was necessary to plan ways in which what remained of the wall could be dismantled. At the same time, we needed to build in sufficient safeguards to ensure that any relapse in the relationship between Eleanor and other members of her family would be noticed. The areas in which we decided to work, and the work actually undertaken, are summarised here.

- My female colleague agreed to undertake a further series of individual sessions with Mrs Stanley, in which they explored in more depth the impact of her abusive childhood, and endeavoured to connect those experiences with the difficulties she had encountered with Eleanor. This work took place between the time the assessment was concluded and Eleanor's planned return home 3 months later.

- At a less intensive level, I worked with Mr Stanley while he was completing his prison sentence, to identify and develop strategies by which he could support his wife in her efforts to re-establish a positive relationship with Eleanor.

- After Mr Stanley was released, about a month before Eleanor was due to return home, I began to hold regular meetings with Mr and Mrs Stanley together, while the older children were at school, and the two younger children were looked after by a relative. In these sessions, which began on a weekly basis, but reduced to once a fortnight about 3 months after Eleanor's return, we discussed all aspects of the day-to-day parenting tasks: discipline, routines, ways of responding to challenges, how to give each child individual space and attention, and any particular issues involving Eleanor's behaviour. In these sessions, Mr and Mrs Stanley showed a surprisingly creative and imaginative approach. Having a third person there to facilitate open communication between them, and having a set time each week to do this without children to distract them, was all they needed.

- As part of the agreement drawn up prior to Eleanor's return home, Mrs Stanley agreed to ensure that each week she spent some time with Eleanor alone doing something positive with her. Mr Stanley undertook to look after the other children to allow her this space. During our weekly joint sessions, I would try to check up that this part of the agreement was being implemented.

- Before her removal, Eleanor's relationship with her sisters had become very fraught. During contact sessions, a powerful sense of rivalry had also been observed between the three girls, and a lack of skill in peaceful resolution of conflicts. An experienced family centre worker took on the task of working, once a fortnight, with the three girls together, to help them learn skills in cooperative play, and to find ways of enjoying each other's company more. These regular sessions also provided a means of monitoring Eleanor's well-being, independently of me, and of corroborating (or not) what I was hearing from the parents about daily life at home. The dual function of these sessions was made clear to Mr and Mrs Stanley. Our written agreement spelt it out, but also included a commitment that any concerns reported to me by the family centre worker would be discussed with them before any other decisions or actions were taken.

- I also engaged another female colleague (the first having left the organisation) to run fortnightly sessions with me for the whole family; both parents, and all the children. The aim of these sessions was to help the family system re-adjust to Eleanor's return, and also to model some simple techniques of improving communication within the family. We used news-rounds (no interruptions), family games, like charades, which required cooperation between members of different family sub-systems, making things as a family, and other activities of this kind to encourage a sense of the family with Eleanor back in it as a whole and healthy unit. At the end of these sessions, which continued for 6 months, we invited family members to sculpt their image of the family; first, as it had been before Eleanor had left home, and second, as they saw themselves now. Their apparently spontaneous portraits conveyed a much more united family now than 2 years previously.

This was a substantial investment of resources in one family, and it continued at that level for about 6 months after Eleanor's return home. Like most parents, Mr and Mrs Stanley probably tolerated rather than welcomed the high level of intrusion into their private family life; but they never tried to obstruct it, and played a full part in the work, even in the family games, which appeal to most children and embarrass most parents! Whether such a high level of intervention was strictly necessary is doubtful. However, I was aware that a significant risk had been taken in recommending Eleanor's return home at a time when others had felt this was not a safe course of action. A 'belt and braces' strategy, in which several targets were tackled simultaneously by different means, helped to alleviate my own anxiety.

The effects of these interventions are hard to evaluate, but at a more theoretical level another justification for this kind of multi-level approach can be put forward. In Chapter 3, Browne sets out a diagram illustrating the multi-factorial nature of the causality of child abuse and neglect. My understanding of Eleanor's failure to thrive was of a series of factors interacting with each other to create and then maintain the maladaptive interactions between Eleanor and other members of her family. If several factors had been influential, separately and in interaction, then it is reasonable to assume that only a strategy that addressed several of these factors simultaneously would have a positive impact. This is, in my view, an important axiom for those working with chronic complex situations in which a child is suffering significant harm, but where the abuse itself is not so severe or calculated to justify permanent removal of the child. Such situations can be improved, but only (in some cases, at least) with a high investment of resources targeted at several levels, while the changes are being made.

None of these interventions conforms to the models outlined earlier in this book. Instead a series of interventions was developed which tried to meet the specific needs of this family, in venues in which they felt comfortable (their own home, the family centre, or local recreational facilities), and which tried to balance professional expertise with informality and normalisation. The impact of the work done with the three sisters in improving their relationship should not be underestimated, and its importance derives from the greater awareness in child development theory of the role of siblings and peers in the development of a child's sense of identity.

Partnership

Does this account offer any insights into the concept of partnership, and how that might be implemented in analogous situations? Petrie & James refer to the continuum of power relationships, within which the concept of partnership with parents should be placed (Petrie & Corby, Chapter 20). They also quote the view of the Family Rights Group that when agencies take decisions to intervene through court proceedings, partnership may seem a meaningless concept (Petrie & Corby, Chapter 20). In this instance, efforts to establish partnership at any level with the parents were singularly unsuccessful until the local authority had obtained a care order. Once they did have the power to decide Eleanor's future, a kind of partnership could be negotiated, although this would not have lasted long had the assessment concluded that Eleanor should not return to her own family. Nevertheless, after over 2 years of failure, it was eventually possible to build a partnership of sorts, in which the local authority and Mr and Mrs Stanley could agree one joint overall objective, namely that we all wanted the right outcome for Eleanor.

Mr and Mrs Stanley were invited to attend child protection conferences throughout the process, except that Mr Stanley was excluded for a period after he had assaulted a social worker. I do not think that they ever found this a comfortable experience, and indeed, one or both of them often stayed away. It was, nevertheless, important for them to have been invited and to have had access to the minutes of each conference. Mr and Mrs Stanley would certainly endorse Bell's finding that they experienced attendance at some of the conferences 'intensely painful and humiliating' (Bell, Chapter 14).

I found it helpful to draw up written agreements with the parents, at the point of embarking on the third phase of the assessment, when we were proposing to send Eleanor home with a package of support, and again when we were reducing the level of involvement. These agreements, based on a model outlined by Corden (1980), seemed to help to reassure Mr Stanley, since they included specific commitments on our side, as well as requiring similar commitments from him and his wife.

Re-focusing on family support

In the light of the debate that has developed since the publication of *Messages from Research* (DOH 1995) one might reasonably ask what would have happened to this family if the local authority had been trying to refocus its efforts on providing family support at the time. If there had been accessible and non-stigmatising help for parents at the time when Eleanor's behaviour first began to cause concern, would it have been easier for the school nurse or head teacher to make a referral? Would effective help have been offered to Eleanor's mother? Would she have accepted that help? And if not, would a strategy of offering family support, without using the child protection procedures, after Eleanor was eventually referred, have engaged Mr and Mrs Stanley in a more positive and constructive way than we actually managed to do? My answer to the first questions is that a referral would almost certainly have been made. Mrs Stanley might have accepted some help, providing it was offered in an acceptable way. However, similar help might have had to be offered to a substantial number of other parents at the same time, whose children would have been presenting equally worrying behaviour. Most of these would not have gone on to present such worrying symptoms in the longer-term. In other words, several false-positives would have been included in the group considered to need help. This may have been no bad thing, from a social work perspective, but it would have had significant resource implications. It is also appropriate to observe that no additional resources are in place even now, some 6 years later, to provide this earlier support, in that community.

I am much less confident that an offer of family support rather than a series of child protection conferences would have overcome Mr and Mrs Stanley's resistance at the time when Eleanor was eventually referred. It would have been too difficult to engage them successfully in any kind of dialogue at that time, largely because of Mr Stanley's severe mistrust of social workers, and the more acute level of concern.

Evaluating outcome

After 6 months of intensive work together, we reduced our input gradually, so that 1 year after Eleanor's return home, my role was reduced to one of monitoring her welfare. At this point it was agreed that an application could be made to discharge the care order. Mr and Mrs Stanley agreed to take Eleanor back to see the paediatrician 1 year later, and the care order was discharged. Almost 3 years on from Eleanor's return home, and some 6 years after the original referral, she has continued to live at home with her family. No new referrals have been made to the social services department. No support is provided to the family, nor have they requested any. Mr and Mrs Stanley told me that Eleanor has maintained a normal growth rate. Her behaviour is generally typical of a stroppy and lively teenager. Sometimes she has posed more serious challenges to their authority, and at school, but so far Mr and Mrs Stanley have managed to respond appropriately to these issues.

References

Batchelor J A 1996 Has recogniton of failure to thrive changed? Child: Care, Health, and Development 22 (4): 235–240

Corden J 1980 Contracts in social work practice. British Journal of Social Work 10 (2): 143–162

Department of Health (DOH) 1995 Child protection: messages from research. HMSO, London

Department of Health (DOH) 1999 Framework for the assessment of children in need and their families. Consultation draft. The Stationery Office, London

Index

ABC analysis *see* antecedents, behaviour, consequences analysis
abuse *see* child abuse; physical abuse; sexual abuse
Accommodation Syndrome, incest 110
adaptations, behavioural, child abuse 96–7
adolescent abusers, sexual abusers' characteristics 79–81
adoption
   psychology 527–8
   see also out-of-home care
adult survivors, child sexual abuse 498–513
   adult survival strengths 504–5
   boundaries, emotional/physical 502–3
   case study 506–8
   choice 502
   control 502
   false memory 505–6
   framework, therapeutic work 501–4
   power issues 501–2
   seeking help 500–1
   therapeutic contexts 508–10
   trust issues 504
adversarial method, court proceedings 343
African families 141–2
   see also ethnicity issues
Afro-Caribbean families 139–40
   welfare system and 132–5
   see also ethnicity issues
agencies, group work in child protection
alcohol effects
   child abuse 57
   sexual abuse 78
America, historical importance 12, 15, 24
analysing information, case conferences 293–4
antecedents, behaviour, consequences (ABC) analysis, family interactions 445–7
appeals, applications for care/supervision orders 230–1
applications for care/supervision orders 218–31
Area Child Protection Committees, inter-professional cooperation 274, 279–80
art
   childhood memories, reworking of 436–7
   individual work with children 410–11
   see also drawing/writing, children's
Asian families 139–40
   welfare system and 132–5
   see also ethnicity issues
assessing placement needs 516–20
assessing violent families 62–5
assessment 253–71
   carrying out 395–6
   case study 574–81, 579–81
   child and 265–7
   Children Act (1989) 254–5
   completing 269–70

core 261–5
   couple relationship and 267–8
   defined 255–6
   implications for 61–2
   individual adults and 267–8
   initial 261
   manager's perspective 556–7
   nature of 258–9
   parents and 267–9
   parents' rights 575
   partnership with families 256–8
   process 258–9, 260–5
   risk assessments 259–65
   undertaking 260
assessment framework, disability and child abuse 168
attachment relationships, child abuse 97–8
attendance, school 327, 332
attitudes and knowledge, child rearing 62
Audit Commission Report (1994) 21–3

BAPSCAN *see* British Association for the Study and Prevention of Child Abuse and Neglect
BAPT *see* British Association of Play Therapists
battered baby syndrome 12, 15–16
Beck, Frank 177, 178
Beckford inquiry (1985), inter-professional cooperation 276–7
Beckford, Jasmine 17, 311–12, 539
   inter-professional cooperation 275–6
behaviour
   cognitive-behavioural approach, prevention 442–55
   monitoring children's 328, 333–5
behavioural intervention checklist 451
bereavement 477
bias, frequency studies 38–9
blockage, sexual abusiveness factor 81–3
bodily image distortions, sexual abuse 436–7
body language, children's, monitoring and 328, 333–5
boundaries, emotional/physical, adult survivors, child sexual abuse 502–3
bridge placements 518–20
British Association for the Study and Prevention of Child Abuse and Neglect (BAPSCAN), abuse scope 152, 160
British Association of Play Therapists (BAPT) 440
Butler-Sloss L.J.
   applications for care/supervision orders 229
   see also Cleveland inquiry (1988)

CACDP *see* Council for the Advancement of Communication with Deaf People
CAFCASS *see* Children And Family Courts Advisory and Support Service

care
    applications for 218–31
    children in 397
    out-of-home *see* out-of-home care
care system *see* welfare
carers
    skills 530–2
    tasks 530–2
    see also social workers
Carlile, Kimberley 17, 539
case ascertainment, frequency studies 37
case conferences
    children's participation 298–9
    in child protection 288–304
    family participation 296–7
    health visitors 315–16
    information collecting/sharing/analysing
        291–4
    inter-professional cooperation 275
    present situation 289–302
    purpose 290–5
case studies
    adult survivors, child sexual abuse 506–8
    disclosure 506–8
    group work, child protection agencies
        488–91
    power and partnership 571–86
causes, child abuse 53–60
CBT *see* cognitive-behavioural therapy
Central Council for Education And Training in
        Social Work (CCETSW)
    case conferences 298
    Children, Spirituality and Religion 415–16
    Guidance Notes 403, 404
    manager's perspective 554–5
characteristics, abusing families 136–7
Chartered Institute of Public Finance
        Accountancy (CIPFA) 541
child abuse
    behavioural adaptations 96–7
    causes 53–60
    classification 50–3
    consequences 8, 89–113
    defining 7, 50–3, 152
    disability and 147–71
    disappearance 12–19
    discovery 12–19
    effects 8, 89–113
    emergence 13–16
    extent 50–3
    fundamental concepts 94–8
    indicators 89–113, 159–60
    intervention strategies 60–2
    and neglect 457–61
    officially recorded cases, by country 31–3,
        35–6, 39–42
    public awareness levels 29–31
    severity 93–4
    understanding 7–185
Child Assessment Orders 216–17, 245, 312
child care, vs. child protection 7–8
child development, 'spoilt child' 89–94
child-parent attachment quality 64–5
child protection agencies, group work 481–97

child protection plans 211–13
    case conferences 299–300
child protection registers 22, 24–5, 210–11
    case conferences 289–91
    physical maltreatment 98
    placing a child's name on 211–13, 289–91
    rates of registrations 50–3
child protection system, current functioning
        279–81
child protection, vs. child care 7–8
child rearing, knowledge and attitudes 62
child sexual abuse (CSA) *see* sexual abuse
Child Witness Officers (CWOs) 373
ChildLine 176
Children Act (1948) 389
    origins 13–14
Children Act (1989) 19–20, 25, 138, 191–5
    applications for care/supervision orders
        218–31
    assessment 254–9
    child protection plans, written 213
    court structures and proceedings 196
    GALs 355–6
    manager's perspective 555
    out-of-home care 518, 519, 521–2, 531
    partnership 391–2
    prevention 197–204
    processing the investigation 210–11
    Section 37, directions 217
    Section 47, making enquiries under 238–52
    welfare of child 373
Children And Family Courts Advisory and
        Support Service (CAFCASS)
    applications for care/supervision orders 225
    GALs 360
Children and Young Persons Act (1963), origins
        14
Children (Northern Ireland) Order (1995) 191–5
    applications for care/supervision orders
        218–31
    emergency action 214–16
    prevention 197–204
Children (Scotland) Act (1995) 191–5
    emergency action 214–16
    prevention 197–204
Children, Spirituality and Religion 415–16
Children's Rights movement 16–17
children's services, refocusing 21–3
CIPFA *see* Chartered Institute of Public Finance
        Accountancy
civil law
    child protection and 191–237
    see also legal issues
clarification, abuse 473–4
Cleveland inquiry (1988) 17–18, 539
    inter-professional cooperation 277–9
    prevention 202
    recommendations 390–1
cognitive-behavioural approach
    intervention, current policy context 443–5
    prevention 442–55
    theoretical principles 445–9
cognitive-behavioural therapy (CBT) 445
    physical abuse 468–9

Colwell, Maria 16, 17, 137, 390, 538
  inter-professional cooperation 274–5
communication methods
  disabled children 152–8, 160–5
  individual work with children 408–15
communication, opportunities for 405–6
communication stages, investigative interviews
    162–4
comparability, frequency studies 39
competence
  children's welfare 552–70
  defining 558–60
  education and training influence 558–60
  manager's perspective 557–64
competing interests, investigative process 247–8
conferences, decision-making at 396–7
confidentiality
  abused adolescents 434, 435
  individual work with children 407
  investigative process 249
conflicting evidence, evaluating 365
consequences
  child abuse 8, 89–113
  divorce 119–20
  emotional abuse 101–3
  neglect 105–7
  sexual abuse 107–10, 498–9
constructivist approach, family therapy 460
cooperation, inter-professional *see* inter-
    professional cooperation
coordination, inter-agency *see* inter-agency
    coordination
coping mechanisms, sexual abuse 504–5
core assessments 261–5
core group meetings, case conferences 300–1
Council for the Advancement of Communication
    with Deaf People (CACDP) 160
country data, child abuse 31–3, 35–6, 39–42
court craft 342–54
Court of Appeal
  applications for care/supervision orders 220–2
  negligence liability issues 233
court proceedings 342–54
  adversarial method 343
  after giving evidence 353
  after the decision 354
  civil law 195–6
  court hearing 348
  cross-examination 351–3
  directions hearings 347
  examination-in-chief 350–1
  oral evidence 343–4, 348–50
  personal preparations 347–8
  preparing evidence 344–5
  re-examination 353
  research evidence 345–7
  taking instructions 344
  see also criminal justice system
courtroom environment, criminal justice system
    375–6
Crime and Disorder Act (1998) 194
criminal justice system
  child protection and 369–82
  children giving evidence 376–7

courtroom environment 375–6
  implications for practice 372–3
  policy issues analysis 370–2
  welfare of child 373–5
  see also court proceedings
critical incidence model, child abuse causes 56–7
cross-examination, court proceedings 351–3
CSA (child sexual abuse) *see* sexual abuse
cultural perspective, child abuse causes 53–4
culture issues 128–46
  culture, ethnicity and social policy 129–32
  group work, child protection agencies
    485–6
  see also ethnicity issues
current policies, welfare of child 553–5
CWOs *see* Child Witness Officers

Data Protection Act 443
  investigative process 239–40
deaf children 160–5
  see also disability and child abuse; disabled
    children
decision-making
  at conferences 396–7
  investigative process 242–3
  and non-directive play therapy 426–7
denial
  consequences and indicators of child abuse
    91–4
  disabled children and 159
  families 474
disability and child abuse 147–71
  children's ability to tell of abuse 158–60
  communication forms 152–8, 160–5
  Integrated Ecological Model of abuse 147–8,
    168
  investigative interviews 160–5
  missing research 150–1
  myths 149
  negative perception 149
  new developments 166–8
  safety and prevention programmes 153–8
  therapeutic services 165
  useful addresses and information 170–1
disabled children 9
  isolation and risk 158–9
  physical abuse 150
  receptive skills of adults 159
  requirements 169
  sexual abuse 151
  signs and indicators of abuse 159–60
  survival work with 165–6
  trust of adults 159
disclosure 465–6
  case study 506–8
  sexual abuse 470, 504
disinhibition, sexual abusiveness factor 81–3
divorce, consequences 119–20
domestic violence 62–5, 312
drama/role-playing, individual work with
    children 414–15
drawing/writing, children's
  individual work with children 410–11
  monitoring and 329–30, 335–6

early detection 310–12
Ecological Model of abuse, Integrated 147–8,
    168
educating and supporting parents 310
education welfare officers, role 283
effects, child abuse 8, 89–113
emergency action, Children Act (1989) 214–16
Emergency Protection Orders 245
emotional abuse 50–3
    consequences 101–3
    defined 52
    forms 102–3
emotional congruence, sexual abusiveness factor
    81–5
emotional neglect 22
emotional pain, and physical pain 100–1
empathy 406
empowerment 474–5, 481
encapsulation, pain 92
environment, individual work with children
    408–10
environmental perspective, child abuse causes
    53–4
ethnicity issues 128–46, 322
    case conferences 297
    ethnicity of workers 143–4
    group work, child protection agencies 485–6
    out-of-home care 526, 529
    placements 526
    see also culture issues
European Convention on Human Rights
    on prevention 204
    right to a fair trial 371
evaluating outcome, case study 586
evidence-giving, criminal justice system 376–7
examinations, medical 250
exhibitionists 75–6
expert witnesses, court proceedings 345

failure to thrive (FTT) 103–7
    case study 571–86
    intervention 449–50
false memory 505–6
families
    ABC analysis 445–7
    assessing violent 62–5
    assessment 471–2
    assessment and 263
    case conferences participation 296–7
    characteristics of abusing 136–7
    cognitive-behavioural approach 442–55
    conceptual issues 462–5
    disclosure 465–6
    domestic violence 62–5
    new families 467
    planning issues 462–5
    practice issues 465–7
    responsibility, taking 473–4
    treatment aims 471–2
    treatment approaches, sexual abuse 472–8
    working with abusing 456–80
    working with in home 445–7
    see also parents
family group conferences, case conferences 301

family support
    case study 585
    emphasising 11
    meetings, case conferences 301–2
    New Labour 23–4
    re-focusing 585
family therapy 458–67
    constructivist approach 460
    and consultation 462
    indicators 464–5
    motivation issues 463–4
    solution-focused 460
Family Violence Research Program 42–3
fathering, changes in 122–5
female sexual abusers 93
files, access to 443
fixated abusers 78–9
flashbacks
    physical abuse 99–100
    sexual abuse 110
forensic evidence 20
foster homes
    abuse allegations 533
    case study 576–9
    long-term shared care 524–6
    see also out-of-home care
Framework for the Assessment of Children in
    Need and their Families 187–9, 254
    assessment process 258–9, 260–2
    investigative process 241–2
    manager's perspective 549, 554
frequency literature review 29–43
FTT see failure to thrive
fundamental concepts, child abuse 94–8

GALs see guardians ad litem
gender issues
    changing gender relations 118–24
    fathering, changes in 122–5
    female sexual abusers 93
    gender and child abuse 114–27
    gender concept 114–15
    mothering, changes in 120–2, 125
    sexual abusers' characteristics 73–4
generalisability, frequency studies 39
Getting Family Support Right 543
Gillick provision
    applications for care/supervision orders 222–3
    medical examinations 250
Government's Objectives for Children's Services
    179
GPs
    referrals 311–12
    role 281–2
group care placements, long-term 524
group settings, therapeutic contexts 509–10
group work, child protection agencies 481–97
    adolescents 491–2
    adults 492–4
    assessment 484–6
    case study 488–91
    children 487–91
    culture issues 485–6
    ethnicity issues 485–6

functions 481, 482
initial planning 483–4
length/duration 484
methods 487–94
policies 481–3
power issues 482–3
problems 494–5
resources 481–3
running the group 487
selection 484–6
therapeutic methods 489–90
guardians *ad litem* (GALs)
applications for care/supervision orders 221, 224–9
appraisal 358–9
child's best interests 363–5
delay concerns 362–3
financial constraints 361–2
implications for practice 363–6
independence 359–60
research 357–9
resources 360–3
tasks/duties 356–7
work of 355–68
guidance, health visitors 307–8
Guide to Comprehensive Assessment 253
guilt, working with 475

harm
defined 207
see also significant harm
Health Education Authority (HEA) 558
national occupational standards 563
health visitors/visiting
client relationship 308–10
current research summary 308
inter-agency coordination 313–15
policy and guidance 307–8
principles 306–7
public health role 306–7
referrals 310–12
relationships with other disciplines/agencies 313–15
role 282, 305–18
social policing concerns 309
and social workers 313–15
supervision and support 316–17
Henggeler, multi-systemic therapy 469
Henry, Tyra 17, 140
historical overview 7
socio-historical analysis 11–28
House of Lords, applications for care/supervision orders 224–5
Human Rights Act (1998) 192–3
child protection plans, written 213
prevention 203–4

identification process, prevention 205–7
incest 110
sexual abusers' characteristics 74–5
incidence studies 31–3
incidence changes 42–3
Independent Representation of Children in Need (IRCHIN) 359

indicators, child abuse 89–113, 159–60
individual needs, meeting 477–8
individual work with children 403–22
communication methods 408–15
environment 408–10
illustrative case 416–18
professional background 404–8
individually focused models, child abuse causes 54–6
information collecting/sharing/analysing, case conferences 291–4
initial assessment 261
institutional settings, abuse in 9, 172–85
implications for practice 180–1
institutional abuse defined 173, 174
policy issues 177–9
review of literature/research 173–7
Integrated Ecological Model of abuse 147–8, 168
integrated models, child abuse causes 57–60
inter-agency conflict, monitoring and 340
inter-agency coordination 272–87, 313–16, 482
case study 572–4
strategic task 546–8
inter-professional cooperation 272–87, 315–16
current status 281–3
health visitors 313–15
suggestions for improving 283–4
interaction focused models, child abuse causes 56–7
interactions, families, ABC analysis 445–7
interpersonal-interactive perspective, child abuse causes 56
intervention
behavioural intervention checklist 451
case for 43–5
case study 581–4
cognitive-behavioural approach 443–5
effective 444–5
FTT 449–50
issues 383–586
legal basis 11–12
plans 323–4
strategies 60–2
interviews, investigative 249
criminal justice system 378–81
disability and child abuse 160–5
four-phase approach 380–1
investigation process 238–52
prevention 205–7
investigations
carrying out 395–6
case study 572–4
IRCHIN *see* Independent Representation of Children in Need
isolation and risk, disabled children 158–9

joint working
investigative process 240–1
see also inter-agency coordination; inter-professional cooperation
judgements, significant harm 294–5
jurisdiction of the courts 217–18

knowledge and attitudes, child rearing 62
Kolko D J, CBT 468–9

Labour Government 23–4
language, children's, monitoring and 328–9
leading questions, court proceedings 351
learning difficulties, parent training 448–9
legal issues
    applications for care/supervision orders
        218–31
    assessment 254–5
    civil law 191–237
    civil legal framework 197–218
    court structures and proceedings *see* court
        proceedings
    criminal justice system 369–82
    emergency action 214–16
    intervention basis 11–12
    jurisdiction of the courts 217–18
    legalism emphasis 7, 11, 18–19
    legislative changes, recent 19–20
    liability issues, tort of negligence 232–5
    out-of-home care 521–2
    protecting children in care 231–2
    review of literature/research 196–7
liability issues, tort of negligence 232–5
local authority records, monitoring and 338
long-term consequences, sexual abuse 498–9
long-term group care placements 524
long-term shared care 523–6
loss and bereavement 477

Management Action Plans (MAPs), disability
    and child abuse 166–8
manager's perspective
    assessment 545–6
    child protection 538–51
    Children Act (1989) 555
    competence 557–60
    competency-based approach 560–4
    implications for practice 560–4
    literature review 538–43, 555–60
    policy issues 543–8
    research review 538–43
    thresholds 545–6
managing the process, child protection 187–382
mandatory reporting 45
Manpower Services Commission (MSC) 558
MAPs *see* Management Action Plans
marginalisation 8–9
masculine development, psychoanalytic theory
    81–5
maternal issues, changes in mothering 120–2,
    125
meaning of the child, gender issues 117–18
measurement tools, frequency studies 38
medical examinations 250
medicals, monitoring and 330, 336–7
Memorandum of Good Practice
    criminal justice system 377–81
    investigative process 245–7
    manager's perspective 547
    video recordings 20, 138, 160–2, 245–7,
        377–81

memories
    false memory 505–6
    reworking of childhood 436–7
mental illness, child abuse causes 54–5
mentorship, children's welfare 564–6
Messages from Research 21–3, 44, 116
    assessment 253–4
    inter-professional cooperation 281
    manager's perspective 542, 544
    partnership 394–5
    prevention 199–200
methodological factors 34–9
minimisation, working on 474
Modernising Social Services 541, 542, 554–5
monitoring
    body language and 328
    parental involvement and 337–8
    primary school 327–30
    school 324–37
    secondary school 330–7
    teachers and 319–41
    timing of 338–9
monitoring and support, health visitors role
    312–13
monitoring guidelines, professionals' use of 339
monitoring systems, issues arising from 337–40
mood changes, monitoring and 327, 335
mothering, changes in 120–2, 125
motivation issues, family therapy 463–4
MSC *see* Manpower Services Commission
multi-culturalism 131–2, 138
multi-systemic therapy 469
multidisciplinary child protection system 315–16,
    446
multifactor perspective, child abuse causes 57–8
music, individual work with children 411–12
myths 9
    disabled children and abuse 149

National Council for Vocational Qualifications
    (NCVQ) 559–60, 563–4, 566
National Foster Care Association (NFCA),
    sexual abuse risk quantifying 176
National Incidence Studies (NIS-1; NIS-2) 42–3
National Society for the Prevention of Cruelty to
    Children (NSPCC)
    emergency action 214–16
    formation 12–13
    group work 482
    prevention 206–7
NCVQ *see* National Council for Vocational
    Qualifications
neglect
    causes 53–60
    child abuse and 457–61
    consequences 105–7
    defined 51, 106
negligence, liability issues 232–5
New Labour 23–4
New Right, growth 18–19
NFCA *see* National Foster Care Association
NIS-1; NIS-2 *see* National Incidence Studies
non-directive play therapy *see* play therapy, non-
    directive

NSPCC *see* National Society for the Prevention of Cruelty to Children

observation, in school 324–5
occupational standards, national 563
officially recorded cases, child abuse, by country 31–3, 35–6, 39–42
one-to-one settings, therapeutic contexts 508–9
open-ended activities, teachers and 326
oral evidence, court proceedings 343–4, 348–50
out-of-home care 514–37
  abuse allegations 533
  assessing placement needs 516–20
  bridge placements 518–20
  case study 576–9
  Children Act (1989) 518, 519, 521–2, 531
  contact issues 522–3
  duration 521
  ethnicity issues 526, 529
  foster homes, long-term shared care 524–6
  group care placements, long-term 524
  legal status 521–2
  literature on 515–16
  long-term group care placements 524
  long-term shared care 523–6
  permanent placements 527, 529
  placement needs, assessing 516–20
  placement types 518–21
  psychology of adoption 527–8
  with relatives 523–4, 526–7
  residential care placements 525
  respite care 523–4
  shared care 523–6
outcome evaluation, case study 586
outcomes, patterns and 29–49

paediatricians, role 282
paedophilia, defined 72–3
PAIN *see* Parents Against INjustice
pain
  encapsulation 92
  physical and psychological 100–1
parent-child interaction, assessing violent families 63–4
parent training, cognitive-behavioural approach 447–9
parental acceptance-rejection theory 66
parental emotions, assessing violent families 63
parental involvement, monitoring and 337–8
parental perceptions, child behaviour 62–3
parenting style 22, 62–5
parents
  assessment and 267–9
  assessment rights 575
  educating and supporting 310
  partnership with 387–402
  rehabilitation 467
  school settings 327, 332–3
  substitute 532–3
  see also families
Parents Against INjustice (PAIN) 16–17
partners
  partnership 398
  working with 510

partnership
  1970s to 1980s 389–90
  1980s to 1990s 390–1
  assessment 256–8
  case study 584–5
  children in care 397
  current situation 391–2
  decision-making at conferences 396–7
  developing 393–5
  history 388–91
  implications of research for practice 395–6
  investigative process 241
  nature of 387–8
  other professionals 398
  with parents 387–402
  post-war to 1970s 389
  power and partnership case study 571–86
  prior to Children Act (1989) 388–9
  as process 388
  relatives and partners 398
  research findings 392–5
  rights of challenge 398–9
patterns and outcomes 29–49
  implications for practice 43–5
  review of frequency literature 29–43
Patterns and Outcomes in Child Placement 517
PE (physical education), monitoring and 330, 336–7
perceptions of children, 'spoilt child' 89–94
permanent placements 527, 528–30
person-environment interactive perspective, child abuse causes 56–7
physical abuse 50–3, 468–9
  CBT 468–9
  disabled children 150
  flashbacks 99–100
  physical injury, defined 51
  physical maltreatment 98–101
  vs. sexual abuse 321–2
physical consequences, sexual abuse 107
physical education (PE), monitoring and 330, 336–7
'Pindown' practice, institutional abuse 174–6
placements *see* out-of-home care
plans, intervention 323–4
play
  children's, monitoring and 329
  play-related communication 406
  symbolic play 429
play therapy, non-directive 406, 423–41
  abused adolescents 432–9
  broader policy considerations 426–7
  child abuse and 427–31
  development 424
  overview 423–5
  research 425
  statutory considerations 437–9
  statutory settings, within 431–2
  therapist's trustworthiness 435–6
  training programmes 424
  working therapeutically 431–2
police, role 282
policies, child protection agencies 481–3
policies, current, welfare of child 553–5

policy and guidance, health visitors 307–8
policy issues analysis 137–9
    inter-agency coordination 274–9
    investigative process 243–7
policy issues, manager's perspective 543–8
positive feedback, child abuse 58–60
post-traumatic stress, sexual abuse 110
power and partnership, case study 571–86
power issues 474–5
    adult survivors, child sexual abuse 501–2
    empowerment 474–5, 481
    group work, child protection agencies 481,
        482–3
powerlessness, children's 180–1, 474–5, 501–2
PQCCA programmes 566
practice guidances, recent 19–20
predisposing factors, child abuse causes 57–8
preliminary hearings, applications for
        care/supervision orders 225
pressure groups, adult survivors, child sexual
        abuse 509–10
prevalence estimates, abuse 29–43
prevalence studies 34, 35–6
    prevalence changes 42–3
prevention
    civil legal framework 197–204
    cognitive-behavioural approach 442–55
    emphasising 21
    primary 60, 305, 307, 310
    secondary 61, 307, 310–12
    tertiary 61, 307, 312–13
prevention and safety programmes, disabled
        children 153–8
primary prevention 60
    health visitors 305, 307, 310
primary school, monitoring in 327–30
privacy, individual work with children 407
projection of blame 474
Protecting Children 137–8
protecting children, socio-historical analysis
        11–28
psychological abuse see emotional abuse
psychological consequences, sexual abuse
        107–10
psychological pain, and physical pain 100–1
psychological parenting 520
psychology of adoption 527–8
psychopathic perspective, child abuse causes
        54–5
psychosocial perspective, child abuse causes
        57–8
public awareness levels, child abuse 29–31

quality, child-parent attachment 64–5
Quality Protects Programme 195, 547, 554
    disability and child abuse 166–8
    prevention 198, 205
    protecting children in care 232

Race Relations Acts 130–1
racism 128–9, 131, 137, 322
    see also ethnicity issues
rates of registrations, child protection registers
        50–3

receptive skills of adults, disabled children and
        159
recidivism 75–6
recognition, child abuse, case study 572–4
record-keeping
    health visitors 315
    investigation process 250
    local authority records 338
    teachers 325–6
    see also video recordings
Recovery Orders 245
referrals
    case study 572–4
    distribution 243
    health visitors 310–12
    process 247–8
    sources 238–40
registers see child protection registers
regressed abusers 78–9
rehabilitation, parents 467
relationship problems, children's 334–5
relationships
    attachment, child abuse 97–8
    and non-directive play therapy 426
relatives
    partnership 398
    placements with 523–4, 526–7
religion, individual work with children 415–16
reported cases, frequency studies 39–42
reporting, mandatory 45
Reporting Officers (ROs) 355–7
residential care placements 525
resources, child protection agencies 481–3
resources, impact of, prevention 204–5
respite care 523–4
responsibility, taking, families 473–4
rights of challenge, partnership 398–9
risk assessments 259–65
    manager's perspective 540
rivalry, working with 475
role boundaries, families 476–7
role-playing/drama, individual work with
        children 414–15
ROs see Reporting Officers

SACCS see Sexual Abuse: Child Consultancy
        Service
safeguarding children 23–4, 25
Safeguards, Review of 177, 178
safety and prevention programmes, disabled
        children 153–8
safety context, treatment in 466–7
safety of the child, sexual abuse 326
sampling methods, frequency studies 37
school, monitoring in 324–37
schoolteachers see teachers
Scottish Executive Justice Department (SEJD),
        prevention 204
secondary prevention 61
    health visitors 307, 310–12
secondary school, monitoring children in 330–7
secrecy, breaking 504
Section 47, Children Act (1989), making
        enquiries under 238–52

Seebohm Report (1968) 14
SEJD *see* Scottish Executive Justice Department
self-help groups, adult survivors, child sexual
abuse 509–10
self-mutilation 333–4
SENCOs *see* Special Educational Needs
Coordinators
severity, child abuse 93–4
sexual abuse 50–3, 470–1
adult survivors 498–513
bodily image distortions 436–7
characteristics 8
childhood memories, reworking of 436–7
Cleveland inquiry 17–18
consequences 107–10, 498 9
coping mechanisms 504–5
defined 34–7, 52
disabled children 151
disclosure 470, 504
distinctive features 321–2
flashbacks 110
long-term consequences 498–9
and non-directive play therapy 428
vs. physical abuse 321–2
safety of the child 326
sources of help 500–1
survivors, adult 498–513
treatment approaches, family 472–8
Sexual Abuse: Child Consultancy Service
(SACCS) 404
sexual abusers' characteristics 71–88
adolescent abusers 79–81
implications for practice 85–6
methodological issues 72–3
research 73–9
theory of sexual abusiveness 81–5
sexual arousal, sexual abusiveness factor 81–3
sexual feelings/beliefs/activities, work on 476
shared care 523–6
sharing information, case conferences 292–3
sign languages, disabled children 152–8, 160–5
significant harm
acting on suspicions of 216–17
applications for care/supervision orders 220
investigative process 241–2
judgements 294–5
meaning of 207–10
signification regime 539–40
silence, breaking 504
Simon Brown L.J., applications for
care/supervision orders 229
situational stressors, child abuse causes 58–60
social action groups, adult survivors, child sexual
abuse 509–10
social learning perspective, child abuse causes 55
social learning theory 445
social policing concerns, health visitors 309
social policy, culture and ethnicity 129–32
social stress perspective, child abuse causes 53–4
social workers
assessment and 256
case conferences 295–6
and health visitors 313–15
legal mandate 17

and out-of-home care 530–2
role 295–6
stress 565
socio-historical analysis, protecting children
11–28
socio-legal model, child abuse 7, 11, 18–19
sources of help, sexual abuse 500–1
Special Educational Needs Coordinators
(SENCOs), initial contact form 320–1
special victim perspective, child abuse causes 55–6
spirituality, individual work with children
415–16
'spoilt child', perceptions of children 89–94
State, role 18–19
stories/story-telling, individual work with
children 412–14
strategic task, working together 546–8
stress
responses to, assessing violent families 63
social workers 565
substitute parents 532–3
suicide attempts 333–4
supervision and support, health visitors 316–17
supervision, children's welfare 564–6
supervision orders, applications for 218–31
Sure Start programme 23–4, 553
survivors, child sexual abuse *see* adult survivors,
child sexual abuse
suspicions of abuse, teacher's role 323–4
symbolic play 429
symbols communication systems, disabled
children 152–8, 160–5

teachers
confidence 340
enhancing contribution of 319–41
initial contact form 320–1
record-keeping 325–6
role 283, 323–4
technology-aided communication systems,
disabled children 152–8, 160–5
tertiary prevention 61
health visitors 307, 312–13
theory of sexual abusiveness, sexual abusers'
characteristics 81–5
therapeutic groups, adult survivors, child sexual
abuse 509–10
therapeutic services
disabled children 165
individual work with children 405–6
and non-directive play therapy 427
therapy
family therapy 458–67
multi-systemic therapy 469
solution-focused 460
threshold criteria, applications for
care/supervision orders 219–25
time trends, frequency studies 39
TOPPS *see* Training Organisation for the
Personal Social Services
training issues 383–586
NCVQ 559–60
parent training 447–9
TOPPS 552

Training Organisation for the Personal Social Services (TOPSS) 552
transference psychosis, child abuse causes 54–5
trauma, child abuse 94–6
trends
    by country 39–42
    time trends 39
trust issues, adult survivors, child sexual abuse 504
trust of adults
    disabled children 159
    therapist's trustworthiness 435–6

understanding child abuse 7–185
understanding of abuse, child's 503
United Nations Convention on the Rights of the Child 236, 247
    GALs 363–4
unpredictableness, physical maltreatment 101
USA, historical importance 12, 15, 24
Utting Report 177, 178–9, 403

vicious cycle, child abuse 58–60
video recordings 20, 138, 160–2, 245–7, 377–81
violent families, assessing 62–5
vulnerable children
    institutional abuse 180–1
    sexual abusers and 79

Warner Report 177
Waterhouse Report 177
welfare, black minority ethnic groups in 132–5

welfare consensus, collapse 16–19
welfare of child
    criminal justice system 373–5
    current policies 553–5
    focus 538
    gender issues 118–24
    mentorship 564–6
    promoting 552–70
    safeguarding 552–70
    supervision 564–6
welfare reformism, child abuse (re)emergence 13–16
witnesses, court proceedings 342–54
working together, strategic task 546–8
Working Together to Safeguard Children 180, 187–9, 195
    assessment 258–9
    case conferences 288–9
    child protection plans, written 211–13
    initial child protection conference 211
    inter-agency coordination 371–2, 378, 381
    inter-professional cooperation 280
    investigative process 240–1, 243–5
    manager's perspective 546, 549, 554, 556
    prevention 200, 203
    protecting children in care 231
    significant harm, meaning of 209–10

Youth Justice and Criminal Evidence (YJCE) Act (1999) 245–7
    witness special measures 376–7
Youth Opportunities Programmes (YOPs) 5580